Biopharmaceutics and Clinical Pharmacokinetics

Biopharmaceutics and Clinical Pharmacokinetics

MILO GIBALDI, PH.D.

Dean, School of Pharmacy
Associate Vice President,
Health Sciences
University of Washington
Seattle, Washington

FOURTH EDITION

LEA & FEBIGER • Philadelphia • London • 1991

Lea & Febiger
200 Chester Field Parkway
Malvern, Pennsylvania   19355-9725
U.S.A.
(215) 251-2230
1-800-444-1785

Lea & Febiger (UK) Ltd.
145a Croydon Road
Beckenham, Kent BR3 3RB
U.K.

Library of Congress Cataloging-in-Publication Data

Gibaldi, Milo.
    Biopharmaceutics and clinical pharmacokinetics / Milo Gibaldi.—
4th ed.
        p.   cm.
    Includes bibliographical references.
    ISBN 0-8121-1346-2
    1. Biopharmaceutics. 2. Pharmacokinetics. I. Title
    [DNLM: 1. Biopharmaceutics. 2. Pharmacokinetics. QV 38 G437b]
RM301.4.G53   1990
615'.7—dc20
DNLM/DLC
for Library of Congress   90-5614
                                                                      CIP

First Edition, 1971
        Reprinted 1973, 1974, 1975
Second Edition, 1977
        Reprinted 1978, 1979, 1982
Third Edition, 1984
        Reprinted 1988
Fourth Edition, 1991
    First Spanish Edition, 1974
    First Japanese Edition, 1976
    Second Japanese Edition, 1981
    Second Turkish Edition, 1981

The use of portions of the text of USP XX-NF XV is by permission of the USP Convention. The Convention is not responsible for any inaccuracy of quotation or for false or misleading implication that may arise from separation of excerpts from the original context or by obsolescence resulting from publication of a supplement.

Reprints of chapters may be purchased from Lea & Febiger in quantities of 100 or more.

PRINTED IN THE UNITED STATES OF AMERICA

Print no.:   4   3   2   1

To Florence and Ann

Preface

Biopharmaceutics is a major branch of the pharmaceutical sciences; it concerns the relationship between the physical and chemical properties of a drug in a dosage form and the pharmacologic, toxicologic, or clinical response observed after its administration. The study of biopharmaceutics has been extended beyond that of a descriptive discipline by the development of pharmacokinetics, which concerns the study and characterization of the time course of drug absorption, distribution, metabolism, and excretion, as well as the relationship of these processes to the intensity and time course of therapeutic and adverse effects of drugs. Pharmacokinetics involves the application of mathematics and biochemistry in a physiologic and pharmacologic context. The development of clinical pharmacokinetics is the culmination and logical outcome of advances in the areas of pharmacokinetics, clinical pharmacology, toxicology, analytic chemistry, biopharmaceutics, and therapeutics. Simply stated, clinical pharmacokinetics is a health sciences discipline that deals with the application of pharmacokinetics to the safe and effective therapeutic management of the individual patient.

At one time it was common to assume that the response to a drug was simply a function of intrinsic pharmacologic activity, to define potency in terms of a milligram per kilogram dose, and to compare the "potencies" of drugs with similar pharmacologic effects, without a proper frame of reference. Today, it is recognized that dose-response relationships are not the same after oral and parenteral administration of a drug or, in some cases, after different dosage forms of a drug.

It is now evident for most drugs that a more appropriate assessment of potency is realized by considering drug concentration-response rather than dose-response relationships. The concentration of a drug in the plasma depends on the rate and extent of absorption, which in turn is a function of the route of administration, of certain properties of the drug, and of the dosage form. Drug absorption may markedly affect the onset, intensity, and duration of biologic response.

The intrinsic activity of a drug is determined in reference to its biophase or receptor site concentration. For a reversibly acting drug the attainment and maintenance of some minimal concentration in the biophase dictate the onset and duration of biologic response. The maximum level of drug reached at the receptor site determines the intensity of response. To fully appreciate the complexities of a biologic response, one must take into account the distribution and elimination of a drug. The distribution of a drug from the blood to the various tissues and fluids of the body determines what levels are achieved in the biophase. Hence, distribution is an important factor in the onset and intensity of response and may sometimes play a role in the duration of response. Duration of effect, however, is usually related to the elimination rate of the drug from the body. Drug elimination involves renal and biliary excretion as well as biotransformation in the liver and other organs. These processes determine the persistence of drug levels in the biophase.

Clinicians have long appreciated that patient-to-patient variability in response to certain drugs is often great. In the past, these differences were all too frequently ascribed exclusively to individual "sensitivity" or "resistance." We now believe that most of these differences can be explained by intersubject variability in drug absorption, distribution, and elimination. The age, size, and sex of the patient, genetic and disease-related considerations, and concomitant drug therapy can influence these processes. An understanding of the causes of intersubject variability allows the possibility of developing individualized dosing regimens and of improving drug therapy.

Some knowledge of the principles of biopharmaceutics and clinical pharmacokinetics is essential for all health scientists and clinicians concerned with drug therapy. Competence in these principles and the ability to apply this knowledge in the patient setting are imperative for the pharmacist and clinical pharmacologist.

I acknowledge the contributions of scores of scientists and clinicians who are dedicated to the improvement of drug therapy. Without their work, this book could not begin. I am deeply indebted to my staff at the University of Washington for their unflagging support and to my colleagues in Seattle, Washington, Buffalo, New York, and throughout the pharmaceutical industry for the intellectual stimulation they have provided all these many years.

Seattle, Washington MILO GIBALDI

Contents

Introduction to Pharmacokinetics

Advancements in biopharmaceutics have come about largely through the development and application of pharmacokinetics. Pharmacokinetics is the study and characterization of the time course of drug absorption, distribution, metabolism, and excretion, and the relationship of these processes to the intensity and time course of therapeutic and toxicologic effects of drugs. Pharmacokinetics is used in the clinical setting to enhance the safe and effective therapeutic management of the individual patient. This application has been termed *clinical pharmacokinetics*.

DISTRIBUTION AND ELIMINATION

The transfer of a drug from its absorption site to the blood, and the various steps involved in the distribution and elimination of the drug in the body, are shown in schematic form in Figure 1–1. In the blood, the drug distributes rapidly between the plasma and erythrocytes (red blood cells). Rapid distribution of drug also occurs between the plasma proteins (usually albumin but sometimes α_1-acid glycoproteins and occasionally globulin) and plasma water. Since most drugs are relatively small molecules they readily cross the blood capillaries and reach the extracellular fluids of almost every organ in the body. Most drugs are also sufficiently lipid soluble to cross cell membranes and distribute in the intracellular fluids of various tissues. Throughout the body there is a distribution of drug between body water and proteins or other macromolecules that are dispersed in the body fluids or are components of the cells.

The body can be envisioned as a collection of separate compartments, each containing some fraction of the administered dose. The transfer of drug from one compartment to another is associated with a rate constant (k). The magnitude of the rate constant determines how fast the transfer occurs.

The transfer of drug from blood to extravascular fluids (i.e., extracellular and intracellular water) and tissues is called *distribution*. Drug distribution is usually a rapid and reversible process. Fairly quickly after intravenous (iv) injection, drug in the plasma exists in a distribution equilibrium with drug in the erythrocytes, in other body fluids, and in tissues. As a consequence of this dynamic equilibrium, changes in the concentration of drug in the plasma are indicative of changes in drug level in other tissues including sites of pharmacologic effect (bioreceptors).

The transfer of drug from the blood to the urine or other excretory compartments (i.e., bile, saliva, and milk), and the enzymatic or biochemical transformation *(metabolism)* of drug in the tissues or plasma to metabolic products, are usually irreversible processes. The net result of these irreversible steps, depicted in Figure 1–1, is called *drug elimination*. Elimination processes are responsible for the physical or biochemical removal of drug from the body.

The moment a drug reaches the bloodstream, it is subject to both distribution and elimination. The rate constants associated with distribution, however, are usually much larger than those related to drug elimination. Accordingly, drug distribution throughout the body is usually complete while most of the dose is still in the body. In fact, some drugs attain distribution equilibrium before virtually any of the dose is eliminated. In such cases, the body appears to have the characteristics of a single compartment.

This simplification, however, may not be applied to all drugs. For most drugs, concentrations in plasma measured shortly after iv injection reveal a

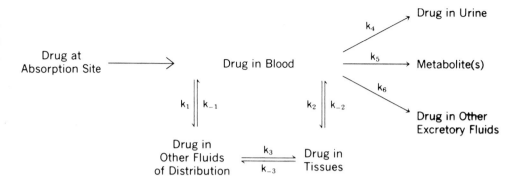

Fig. 1–1. Schematic representation of drug absorption, distribution, and elimination.

distinct distributive phase. This means that a measurable fraction of the dose is eliminated before attainment of distribution equilibrium. These drugs impart the characteristics of a multicompartment system upon the body. No more than two compartments are usually needed to describe the time course of drug in the plasma. These are often called the rapidly equilibrating or central compartment and the slowly equilibrating or peripheral compartment.

PHYSICAL SIGNIFICANCE OF DRUG CONCENTRATION IN PLASMA

Blood samples taken shortly after intravenous administration of equal doses of two drugs may show large differences in drug concentration despite the fact that essentially the same amount of each drug is in the body. This occurs because the degree of distribution and binding is a function of the physical and chemical properties of a drug and may differ considerably from one compound to another.

At distribution equilibrium, drug concentrations in different parts of the body are rarely equal. There may be some sites such as the central nervous system or fat that are poorly accessible to the drug. There may be other tissues that have a great affinity for the drug and bind it avidly. Drug concentrations at these sites may be much less than or much greater than those in the plasma.

Despite these complexities, once a drug attains distribution equilibrium its concentration in the plasma reflects distribution factors and the simple relationship between amount of drug in the body (A) and drug concentration in the plasma (C) shown in Equation 1–1 applies:

$$A = VC \qquad (1-1)$$

The proportionality constant relating amount and concentration is called the apparent volume of distribution (V). In most situations, V is independent of drug concentration. Doubling the amount of drug in the body (e.g., by doubling the iv dose) usually results in a doubling of drug concentration in plasma. This is called *dose proportionality;* it is often used as an indicator of *linear pharmacokinetics.*

The apparent volume of distribution is usually a characteristic of the drug rather than of the biologic system, although certain disease states and other factors may bring about changes in V. The magnitude of V rarely corresponds to plasma volume, extracellular volume, or the volume of total body water; it may vary from a few liters to several hundred liters in a 70-kg man. V is usually not an anatomic volume but is a reflection of drug distribution and a measure of the degree of drug binding.

Acid drugs, such as sulfisoxazole, tolbutamide, or warfarin, are often preferentially bound to plasma proteins rather than extravascular sites. Although these drugs distribute throughout body water, they have small volumes of distribution ranging from about 10 to 15 L in man. A given dose will result in relatively high initial drug concentrations in plasma.

On the other hand, many basic drugs including amphetamine, meperidine, and propranolol are more extensively bound to extravascular sites than to plasma proteins. The apparent volumes of distribution of these drugs are large, ranging from 4 to 8 times the volume of total body water (i.e., 180 to 320 L in a 70-kg man). The frequently small doses and large distribution volumes of these drugs often make their quantitative detection in plasma difficult.

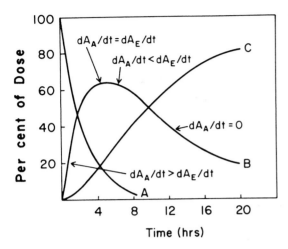

Fig. 1–2. Time course of drug disappearance from the absorption site (curve A) and appearance of eliminated drug in all forms (curve C). The net result is curve B, which depicts the time course of drug in the body.

PHARMACOKINETIC CONSIDERATIONS OF DRUG CONCENTRATIONS IN PLASMA

The plasma contains measurable quantities of many endogenous chemicals. In healthy individuals these biochemicals are present in concentrations that are reasonably constant, and it is appropriate to speak of creatinine or bilirubin levels in the plasma. Drug levels or concentrations in the plasma are rarely level. One usually finds different concentrations of drug in the plasma at different times after administration. These changes reflect the dynamics of drug absorption, distribution, and elimination (Fig. 1–2).

Intravenous Administration

Absorption need not be considered when a drug is given by rapid iv injection. As soon as the drug is administered it undergoes distribution and is subject to one or more elimination pathways. The amount of drug in the body and the drug concentration in plasma decrease continuously after injection. At the same time, there is continuous formation of metabolites and continuous excretion of drug and metabolites. Eliminated products accumulate while drug levels in the body decline.

Most drugs distribute rapidly so that shortly after iv injection, distribution equilibrium is reached. Drug elimination at distribution equilibrium is usually described by *first-order kinetics*. This means that the rate of the process is proportional to the amount or concentration of substrate (drug) in the system. As drug concentration falls, the elimina-

tion rate falls in parallel. The proportionality constant relating rate and amount or concentration is called a rate constant. Accordingly, the elimination rate is written as follows:

$$-\frac{dA}{dt} = \frac{dA_E}{dt} = kA \qquad (1\text{–}2)$$

where A is the amount of drug in the body at time t, A_E is the amount of drug eliminated from the body (i.e., the sum of the amounts of metabolites that have been formed and the amount of drug excreted) at time t, and k is the first-order elimination rate constant.

The elimination rate constant is the sum of individual rate constants associated with the loss of parent drug. For example, the overall elimination rate constant (k) in the model depicted in Figure 1–1 is given by

$$k = k_4 + k_5 + k_6 \qquad (1\text{–}3)$$

Dimensional analysis of Equation 1–2 indicates that the units of k are reciprocal time (i.e., day^{-1}, hr^{-1}, or min^{-1}).

Since there is a relationship between the amount of drug in the body and the drug concentration in the plasma (Eq. 1–1), we may rewrite Equation 1–2 as

$$-\frac{d(VC)}{dt} = -V\frac{dC}{dt} = k(VC)$$

or

$$-\frac{dC}{dt} = kC \qquad (1\text{–}4)$$

Integrating this expression between the limits t = 0 and t = t yields

$$\log C = \log C_o - \frac{kt}{2.303} \qquad (1\text{–}5)$$

Equation 1–5 indicates that a plot of log C versus t will be linear once distribution equilibrium is reached. The term C_o is the intercept on the log concentration axis, on extrapolation of the linear segment to t = 0.

Figure 1–3 shows the average concentration of a semisynthetic penicillin in the plasma as a function of time after an intravenous injection of a 2-g dose. The concentration values are plotted on a log scale; the corresponding times are plotted on a linear scale. The semilogarithmic coordinates make it convenient to plot first-order kinetic data for they

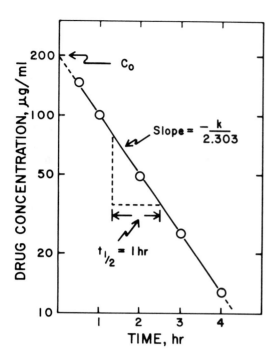

Fig. 1–3. Semilogarithmic plot of penicillin concentrations in plasma after a 2-g intravenous dose. Concentrations decline in a first-order manner with a half-life of 1 hr.

avoid the necessity of converting values of C to log C.

According to Equation 1–5, the linear portion of the semilogarithmic plot of C versus t has a slope corresponding to $-k/2.303$ and an intercept, on the y-axis (i.e., at t = 0), corresponding to C_o. If a drug were to distribute almost immediately after injection, C_o would be a function of the dose and the apparent volume of distribution. Therefore, we would be able to calculate V as follows:

$$V = \frac{iv\ dose}{C_o} \qquad (1\text{–}6)$$

For the data shown in Figure 1–3 we can determine that C_o = 200 mg/ml and that V = 10 L.

This approach, however, is seldom useful; Equation 1–6 usually gives a poor estimate of V, always larger and sometimes substantially larger than the true volume of distribution. Equation 1–6 assumes that drug distribution is immediate, whereas most drugs require a finite time to distribute throughout the body space. Other methods to calculate V will be described subsequently.

Although it is possible to calculate the elimination rate constant from the slope of the line, it is much easier to determine k by making use of the following relationship:

$$k = 0.693/t_{1/2} \qquad (1\text{–}7)$$

where $t_{1/2}$ is the half-life of the drug (i.e., the time required to reduce the concentration by 50%). This parameter is determined directly from the plot (see Fig. 1–3). In a first-order process, the half-life is independent of the dose or initial plasma concentration. One hour is required to observe a 50% decrease of any plasma concentration of the semi-synthetic penicillin, once distribution equilibrium is attained. It follows that the elimination rate constant of this drug is equal to $0.693/t_{1/2}$ or $0.693\ hr^{-1}$. Knowledge of the half-life or elimination rate constant of a drug is useful because it provides a quantitative index of the persistence of drug in the body. For a drug that distributes very rapidly after iv injection and is eliminated by first-order kinetics, one-half the dose will be eliminated in one half-life after administration; three-quarters of the dose will be eliminated after two half-lives. Only after four half-lives will the amount of drug in the body be reduced to less than one-tenth the dose. For this reason, the half-life of a drug can often be related to the duration of clinical effect and the frequency of dosing.

Short-Term Constant Rate Intravenous Infusion

Few drugs should be given as a rapid intravenous injection (bolus) because of the potential toxicity that may result. Many drugs that require intravenous administration, including theophylline, procainamide, gentamicin, and many other antibiotics, are given as short-term constant rate infusions over 5 to 60 min, or longer. The following scheme describes this situation:

Drug in reservoir	$\xrightarrow[\text{rate}]{\text{Constant}}$	Drug in body	$\xrightarrow{k}$	Eliminated drug

The rate of change of the amount of drug in the body (A) during infusion is given by

$$dA/dt = k_o - kA \qquad (1\text{–}8)$$

where k_o is the infusion rate expressed in amount per unit time (e.g., mg/min), kA is the elimination rate, and k is the first-order elimination rate constant. This relationship assumes that the drug reaches distribution equilibrium quickly. Integrating Equation 1–8 from t = 0 to t = t yields

$$A = k_o[1 - \exp(-kt)]/k \qquad (1\text{–}9)$$

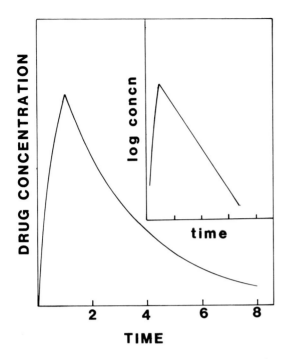

Fig. 1–4. Drug concentration in plasma during and after a 1-hr constant rate intravenous infusion. The inset shows the same data, plotted on semilogarithmic coordinates.

or

$$C = k_o[1 - exp(-kt)]/kV \qquad (1\text{--}10)$$

According to Equation 1–10, drug concentration in plasma increases during infusion. When the entire dose has been infused at time T, drug concentration reaches a maximum given by

$$C_{max} = k_o[1 - exp(-kT)]/kV \qquad (1\text{--}11)$$

and thereafter declines. The declining drug concentration is described by

$$C = C_{max} exp(-kt') \qquad (1\text{--}12)$$

or

$$log\ C = log\ C_{max} - (kt'/2.303) \qquad (1\text{--}13)$$

where $t' = t - T$. Equations 1–12 and 1–13 apply when distribution equilibrium is essentially reached by the end of the infusion. A semilogarithmic plot of C (post-infusion drug concentration in plasma) versus t' yields a straight line, from which the half-life and elimination rate constant can be estimated. The entire drug concentration-time profile during and after a short-term infusion is shown in Figure 1–4.

Equation 1–11 may be arranged to calculate V,

since all other terms are known. This estimate may be less than accurate but it is always better than that provided by Equation 1–6.

The maximum or peak drug concentration in plasma is always lower after intravenous infusion than after bolus injection of the same dose. The more slowly a fixed dose of a drug is infused, the lower the value of C_{max}. Consider a rapidly distributed drug with a half-life of 3 hr. A given dose administered as an iv bolus results in an initial plasma level of 100 units. The same dose, infused over 3 hr ($T = t_{1/2}$) gives a C_{max} value of 50 units ($C_{max}/2$); infused over 6 hr ($T = 2t_{1/2}$), it gives a concentration of 25 units ($C_{max}/4$). Also, since C_{max} is a linear function of k_o, doubling the infusion rate and infusing over the same period of time (i.e., doubling the dose) doubles the maximum concentration.

Extravascular Administration

A more complex drug concentration-time profile is observed after oral, intramuscular, or other extravascular routes of administration because absorption from these sites is not instantaneous, nor does it occur at a constant rate. As shown in Figure 1–2, the rate of change of the amount of drug in the body (dA/dt) is a function of both the absorption rate (dA_A/dt) and the elimination rate (dA_E/dt); that is,

$$\frac{dA}{dt} = \frac{dA_A}{dt} - \frac{dA_E}{dt} \qquad (1\text{--}14)$$

or

$$\frac{dC}{dt} = \frac{1}{V}\left[\frac{dA_A}{dt} - \frac{dA_E}{dt}\right] \qquad (1\text{--}15)$$

where V is the apparent volume of distribution. When the absorption rate is greater than the elimination rate (i.e., $dA_A/dt > dA_E/dt$), the amount of drug in the body and the drug concentration in the plasma increase with time. Conversely, when the amount of drug remaining at the absorption site is sufficiently small so that the elimination rate exceeds the absorption rate (i.e., $dA_E/dt > dA_A/dt$), the amount of drug in the body and the drug concentration in the plasma decrease with time. The maximum or peak concentration after drug administration occurs at the moment the absorption rate equals the elimination rate (i.e., $dA_A/dt = dA_E/dt$). The faster a drug is absorbed, the higher is the maximum concentration in plasma after a given dose, and the shorter is the time after administration when the peak is observed.

First Order In—First Order Out

Many drugs appear to be absorbed in a first-order fashion and the following scheme often applies:

$$\text{Drug at} \xrightarrow{k_a} \text{Drug in} \xrightarrow{k} \text{Eliminated}$$
$$\text{absorption site} \qquad \text{body} \qquad \text{drug}$$

Under these conditions

$$dA/dt = k_a A_A - kA \qquad (1\text{-}16)$$

where k_a is the apparent first-order absorption rate constant, k is the first-order elimination rate constant, A is the amount of drug in the body, and A_A is the amount of drug at the absorption site. Integrating Equation 1–16 from $t = 0$ to $t = t$ and converting amounts to concentrations results in the complicated equation shown below:

$$C = k_a FD[\exp(-kt)$$
$$- \exp(-k_a t)]/V(k_a - k) \qquad (1\text{-}17)$$

where F is the fraction of the administered dose (D) that is absorbed and reaches the bloodstream, V is the apparent volume of distribution, and C is the drug concentration in plasma any time after administration. Equation 1–17 is often used to describe drug concentrations in plasma after extravascular administration.

The absorption rate constant of a drug is frequently larger than its elimination rate constant. In this case, at some time after administration, the absorption rate term in Equation 1–15 approaches zero, indicating that there is no more drug available for absorption, and Equation 1–17 simplifies to

$$C = k_a FD[\exp(-kt)]/V(k_a - k) \qquad (1\text{-}18)$$

or

$$C = C_o{}^* \exp(-kt) \qquad (1\text{-}19)$$

and

$$\log C = \log C_o{}^* - \frac{kt}{2.303} \qquad (1\text{-}20)$$

Equation 1–18 assumes that distribution equilibrium is essentially reached by the end of the absorption phase.

When absorption is complete, the rate of change of the amount of drug in the body equals the elim-

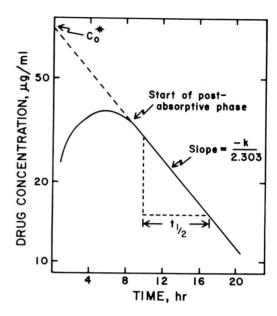

Fig. 1–5. Typical semilogarithmic plot of drug concentration in plasma following oral or intramuscular administration of a slowly absorbed form of the drug.

ination rate, and Equation 1–15 reduces to Equation 1–4. The portion of a drug concentration in the plasma versus time curve, commencing at the time absorption has ceased, is called the postabsorptive phase. During this phase, the decline in drug concentration with time follows first-order-kinetics. A semilogarithmic plot of drug concentration in the plasma versus time after oral or other extravascular routes of administration usually shows a linear portion that corresponds to the postabsorptive phase. A typical plot is shown in Figure 1–5; the slope of the line is equal to $-k/2.303$.

The intercept of the extrapolated line ($C_o{}^*$) is a complex function of absorption and elimination rate constants, as well as the dose or amount absorbed and the apparent volume of distribution. It is incorrect to assume that the intercept approximates the ratio of dose to volume of distribution unless the drug is very rapidly and completely absorbed, and displays one-compartment characteristics (i.e., distributes immediately). This rarely occurs.

Occasionally, the absorption of a drug is slower than its elimination, a situation that may be found with drugs that are rapidly metabolized or excreted and with drugs that are slowly absorbed because of poor solubility or administration in a slowly releasing dosage form. When this occurs, a semilogarithmic plot of drug concentration versus time (see Fig. 1–5) after oral administration cannot be used to estimate k or half-life because the slope is related to the absorption rate constant rather than the elimination rate constant. The drug must be administered in a more rapidly absorbed form or given intravenously.

Patient-To-Patient Variability

The time course of drug in the plasma after administration of a fixed dose may show considerable intersubject variability. The variability after intravenous administration is due to differences between patients in distribution and elimination of the drug. These differences may be related to disease or concomitant drug therapy or they may be genetic in origin. Variability is greater after intramuscular administration because, in addition to differences in distribution and elimination, absorption may be variable. Differences in absorption rate after intramuscular injection have been related to the site of injection and the drug formulation. Still greater variability may be found after oral administration. The absorption rate of a drug from the gastrointestinal tract varies with the rate of gastric emptying, the time of administration with respect to meals, the physical and chemical characteristics of the drug, and the dosage form, among other factors. Similarly, the amount of an oral dose of a drug that is absorbed depends on biologic, drug, and dosage form considerations. Many commonly used drugs are less than completely available to the bloodstream after oral administration because of incomplete absorption or presystemic metabolism.

Absorption Rate and Drug Effects

The influence of absorption on the drug concentration-time profile is shown in Figure 1–6. Administration of an equal dose in three different dosage forms results in different time courses of drug in the plasma. The faster the drug is absorbed, the greater is the peak concentration and the shorter is the time required after administration to achieve peak drug levels.

Many drugs have no demonstrable pharmacologic effect or do not elicit a desired degree of pharmacologic response unless a minimum concentration is reached at the site of action. Since a distribution equilibrium exists between blood and tissues, there must be a minimum therapeutic drug concentration in the plasma that corresponds to, though may not equal, the minimum effective con-

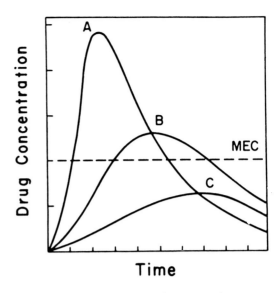

Fig. 1–6. The effects of absorption rate on drug concentration-time profile. The same amount of drug was given orally with each dosage form. The drug is absorbed most rapidly from dosage form A. Drug absorption after administration of dosage form C is slow and possibly incomplete. The dotted line represents the minimum effective concentration (MEC) required to elicit a pharmacologic effect.

centration (MEC) at the site of pharmacologic effect. Thus, the absorption rate of a drug after a single dose may affect the clinical response. For example, it is evident from Figure 1–6 that the more rapid the absorption rate, the faster is the onset of response. The drug is absorbed so slowly from dosage form C that the minimum effective level is never attained. No effect is observed after a single dose, but effects may be seen after multiple doses.

The intensity of many pharmacologic effects is a function of the drug concentration in the plasma. The data in Figure 1–6 suggest that administration of dosage form A may evoke a more intense pharmacologic response than that observed after administration of dosage form B since A produces a higher concentration of drug. When dosage form C is considered, it is clear that an active drug may be made to appear inactive by administering it in a form that results in slow or incomplete absorption.

BIOAVAILABILITY

The bioavailability of a drug is defined as its rate and extent of absorption. Rapid and complete absorption is usually desirable for drugs used on an acute or "as needed" basis for pain, allergic response, insomnia, or other conditions. As suggested in Figure 1–6, the more rapid the absorption, the shorter is the onset and the greater is the intensity of pharmacologic response. The efficacy of a single dose of a drug is a function of both the rate and extent of absorption. In such cases, there is no assurance of the bioequivalence of two dosage forms of the same drug simply because the amount of drug absorbed from each is equivalent; the absorption rate of drug from each drug product must also be comparable. Rapid absorption may also reduce the frequency and severity of gastrointestinal distress observed after oral administration of certain drugs, including aspirin and tetracycline, by reducing the contact time in the gastrointestinal tract.

Usually, a useful estimate of the relative absorption rate of a drug from different drug products or under different conditions (e.g., with food or without food) can be made by comparing the magnitude and time of occurrence of peak drug concentrations in the plasma after a single dose.

Estimating the Extent of Absorption

The extent of absorption or relative extent of absorption of a drug from a product can be estimated by comparing the total area under the drug concentration in plasma versus time curve (AUC), or the total amount of unchanged drug excreted in the urine after administration of the product to that found after administration of a standard. The standard may be an intravenous injection, an orally administered aqueous or water-miscible solution of the drug, or even another drug product accepted as a standard. When an iv dose is used as the standard and the test product is given orally (or via some other extravascular route), we determine absolute bioavailability. If, following equal doses of the test product and the iv standard, the AUC values are the same, we conclude that the drug in the test product is completely absorbed and not subject to presystemic metabolism.

Frequently, however, the standard is an oral solution or an established product. If, following equal doses of the test product and standard, the AUC values are the same, we conclude that the test product is 100% bioavailable, *relative* to the standard; we need use the word relative because we do not know *a priori* that the standard is completely absorbed or completely available. When two products produce the same peak concentration of drug in

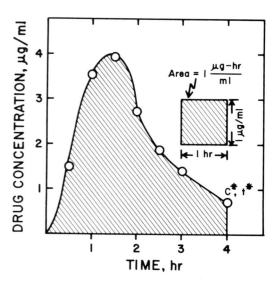

Fig. 1–7. Typical rectilinear plot of drug concentration in the plasma following an oral dose. The area under the concentration-time plot from t = 0 to t = 4 hrs is denoted by shading.

plasma and the same AUC, the products are *bio-equivalent*.

The area under a drug concentration in the plasma versus time curve has the units of concentration-time (e.g., $\mu g - hr/ml$), and can be estimated by several methods. One method is to use a planimeter, an instrument for mechanically measuring the area of plane figures. Another procedure, known as the "cut and weigh method," is to cut out the area under the entire curve on rectilinear graph paper and to weigh it on an analytical balance. The weight thus obtained is converted to the proper units by dividing it by the weight of a unit area of the same paper (Fig. 1–7). The most common method of estimating area under curves is by means of the trapezoidal rule, which is described in Appendix I.

Sometimes, single dose bioavailability studies are not carried out long enough to allow drug concentrations to fall to negligible levels. We cannot determine directly the total AUC, only the partial AUC. In this case, a widely used method is to determine the AUC from t = 0 to the last sampling time (t*), by means of the trapezoidal rule, and to estimate the missing area by means of the equation

$$\text{Area from t* to } \infty = C^*/k \qquad (1\text{–}21)$$

where C^* is the drug concentration at t = t*, and k is the apparent first-order elimination rate constant. This area must be added to the area calculated from time zero to t* to obtain the total area under the curve.

The total area under the drug level-time curve for drugs eliminated by first-order kinetics is given by

$$\text{AUC} = \frac{\text{Amount of drug reaching the bloodstream}}{k \cdot V} \qquad (1\text{--}22)$$

It follows that the bioavailability (F) of a drug from a drug product may be determined from the expression

$$F = \frac{(\text{AUC})_{\text{Drug product}}}{(\text{AUC})_{\text{Standard}}} \qquad (1\text{--}23)$$

when equal doses are administered. If different doses of the product and standard are given, the area estimates should be scaled appropriately to permit comparison under conditions of equivalent doses, assuming AUC is proportional to dose.

The amount of drug excreted unchanged in the urine (A_u) after administration is given by

$$A_u = F \cdot \text{Dose} \cdot (k_u/k) \qquad (1\text{--}24)$$

where k_u is the urinary excretion rate constant and k is the overall elimination rate constant. It follows that the fraction of the dose absorbed from a drug product relative to that absorbed from a standard may be calculated from the expression

$$F = \frac{(A_u)_{\text{Drug product}}}{(A_u)_{\text{Standard}}} \qquad (1\text{--}25)$$

The usefulness of Equation 1–25 depends on how much of the drug is eliminated by urinary excretion, the sensitivity of the assay for drug in urine, and the variability in urinary output of the drug. Many drugs are extensively metabolized and little, if any, appears unchanged in the urine. In such cases, bioavailability is estimated from plasma concentration data.

CONTINUOUS DRUG ADMINISTRATION

Most drugs are administered in a constant dose given at regular intervals for prolonged periods of time. For some of these drugs a therapeutic plasma concentration range has been identified. By prescribing a drug in an appropriate dosing regimen, the physician hopes to elicit a prompt and adequate clinical response. This is often predicated upon the prompt attainment of adequate drug concentration in the plasma.

Constant Rate Infusion

It is convenient to consider first the simpler case of continuous administration of a drug by intravenous infusion; this method of drug administration results in a plasma concentration-time profile that is similar in many ways to that found on intermittent repetitive dosing. Figure 1–8 illustrates the time course of drug concentration in plasma during and after infusion at a constant rate. At the outset, drug concentration increases gradually but at a diminishing rate. If infusion is continued, drug concentration eventually reaches a plateau or steady state. A steady state is reached because the amount of drug in the body reaches a level where the elimination rate, given by kA, is equal to the infusion rate (k_o). Whenever input rate equals output rate, $dA/dt = 0$, $dC/dt = 0$, and steady state exists.

By considering Equation 1–10, which describes drug concentration in plasma during constant rate infusion, at times that are sufficiently large so that $\exp(-kt)$ approaches zero, drug concentration at steady state (C_{ss}) is given by

$$C_{ss} = k_o/kV \qquad (1\text{--}26)$$

Since attainment of steady state often represents the stabilization of a patient on a given course of therapy, it is of interest to know how long it takes to reach steady state. For drugs with pharmacokinetic characteristics that can be described by a one-compartment model (i.e., drugs that distribute rapidly) we have a relatively simple relationship between attainment of steady state and the half-life of the drug. One half the steady-state concentration is reached within a period of time equal to the half-life of the drug. Following a period of infusion equal to four times the half-life, the plasma concentration is within 10% of the eventual steady-state concentration.

If the time to reach steady-state represents an unacceptable delay, one may wish to use an iv bolus loading dose or a series of iv bolus minidoses before starting the infusion. The loading dose is estimated from the ratio of infusion rate (k_o) to elimination rate constant (k). This approach works well for most drugs given intravenously.

If one knows the drug level (C_{ss}) needed to produce a satisfactory response, Equation 1–26 can be used to calculate the infusion rate (k_o) needed to reach the desired level. Under these conditions, $k_o = C_{ss} \cdot k \cdot V$ and loading dose $= C_{ss} \cdot V$.

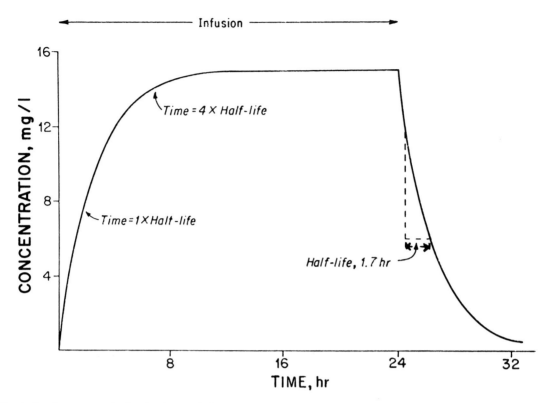

Fig. 1–8. Drug concentration in plasma during and after prolonged constant rate intravenous infusion. (From Gibaldi, M., and Levy, G.: Pharmacokinetics in clinical practice. II. Applications. JAMA, 235:1987, 1976. Copyright 1976, American Medical Association.)

Repetitive Dosing

Turning now to the more common case of repetitive oral administration of the same dose of a drug at regular intervals (Fig. 1–9), we find that although drug accumulates in much the same way as during constant infusion, drug concentrations in plasma during a dosing interval first increase and then decrease as a result of absorption, distribution, and elimination. The magnitude of the concentration difference in a dosing interval depends on the rates of absorption and distribution and on the half-life of the drug; this concentration difference increases with increasing absorption rate and decreasing half-life. Drugs with long half-lives or slow absorption show rather constant blood levels at steady state.

Drug concentration at any time during a dosing interval at steady state can usually be described by the following equation:

$$C_{ss} = \frac{k_a FD}{V(k_a - k)} \left[\frac{\exp(-kt)}{1 - \exp(-k\tau)} - \frac{\exp(-k_a t)}{1 - \exp(-k_a \tau)} \right] \quad (1\text{–}27)$$

where τ is the dosing interval. Equation 1–27 is too complicated to be of routine use; however, if we could estimate the maximum and minimum drug concentrations, we would be able to characterize steady state. Solving Equation 1–27 for the maximum drug concentration at steady state yields an equally complex equation. Better results are obtained when we solve for the minimum concentration at steady state, particularly if we assume that a dose is always given in the postabsorptive phase of the previous dose. Under these conditions,

$$(C_{min})_{ss} = \frac{k_a FD \exp(-k\tau)}{V(k_a - k)[1 - \exp(-k\tau)]} \quad (1\text{–}28)$$

Since the minimum drug concentration after the first dose of a repetitive dosing regimen is given by

$$C_{min} = k_a FD \exp(-k\tau)/V(k_a - k) \quad (1\text{–}29)$$

we can write a relatively simple expression for the degree of drug accumulation during multiple dosing by comparing the minimum drug concentration

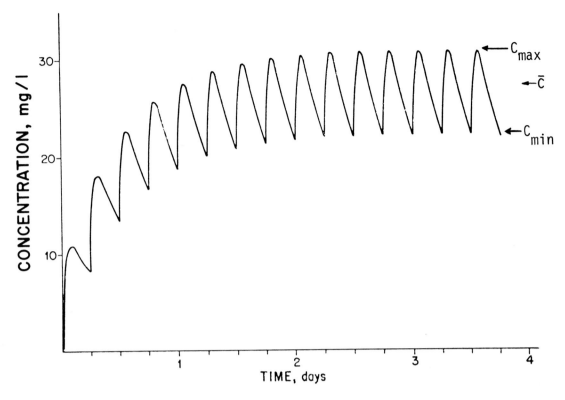

Fig. 1–9. Drug concentration in plasma during repetitive oral administration of 250 mg every 6 hr. The maximum (C_{max}), minimum (C_{min}), and average ($\overline{C}$) drug concentrations at steady state are noted. (From Gibaldi, M., and Levy, G.: Pharmacokinetics in clinical practice. II. Applications. JAMA, 235:1987, 1976. Copyright 1976, American Medical Association.)

at steady state to that after the first dose. Dividing Equation 1–28 by Equation 1–29 yields

$$\text{Accumulation} = (C_{min})_{ss}/C_{min}$$
$$= 1/[1 - \exp(k\tau)] \quad (1\text{–}30)$$

Therefore, by merely knowing the elimination rate constant (k) or half-life of a drug we can predict the degree of accumulation for a given dosing regimen. If a drug is given every half-life ($\tau = t_{1/2}$) the accumulation at steady state will be about 2-fold relative to the first dose.

Some drugs, including the penicillins and cephalosporins, are given less frequently than once every half-life. These drugs have half-lives in the order of 1 hr, but are usually given every 6 to 8 hr. Virtually no accumulation is observed on repeated administration. Many drugs, such as diazepam, amiodarone, phenobarbital, and digoxin, are given more frequently than once every half-life. For these drugs the half-life is greater than one day but they are given either several times a day or once a day. Drug accumulation may be substantial.

When appropriate, it has become increasingly common to administer a drug once every half-life. The current use of theophylline, procainamide, phenytoin, and tricyclic antidepressants reflects this trend.

Average Drug Concentration at Steady State

An alternative and simpler way of describing steady state is to consider the average drug concentration ($\overline{C}_{ss}$), which is analogous to the steady-state concentration during continuous infusion. If drug concentration during each dosing interval is viewed in terms of an average concentration, we can express the intermittently administered dose in terms of an average dosing rate. For example, 100 mg given every 4 hr can be viewed as a 25 mg/hr average dosing rate. When based on these considerations, Equation 1–26 for a constant rate intravenous infusion can be applied to the intermittent oral administration of a drug with one additional provision; allowance must be made for the possibility that absorption of the drug is less than complete. Then,

$$\overline{C}_{ss} = F(\text{average dosing rate})/Vk \quad (1\text{--}31)$$

where F is the fraction of the administered dose that actually reaches the bloodstream. The properties and usefulness of $\overline{C}_{ss}$ are discussed in greater detail in Chapter 2.

Loading Dose

Whether a drug is given by continuous intravenous infusion or by repetitive oral administration, it usually requires about 4 times the half-life of the drug to reach an average concentration within 10% of the steady-state concentration. In some instances, this may represent too long a period to wait for optimum drug effects, and an initial loading dose is used.

Assuming that it is clinically acceptable to do this in a single dose, one can estimate a loading dose based on the usual maintenance dose and elimination rate constant of the drug as follows:

$$\text{Loading dose} = \frac{\text{Maintenance dose}}{1 - \exp(-k\tau)} \quad (1\text{--}32)$$

This loading dose will provide a drug concentration τ hr after administration that is equal to the minimum drug concentration at steady state following repetitive administration of the maintenance dose. If a drug is administered every half-life, the appropriate loading dose is 2 times the maintenance dose. Therapy with tetracycline ($t_{1/2}$ = 8 hr) is often initiated with a 500-mg loading dose followed by 250 mg every 8 hr.

The difference between loading dose and maintenance dose depends on the dosing interval and the half-life of the drug. Digoxin, which has a half-life of about 44 hr but is administered once a day, is typically given as a loading dose of 1.0 to 1.5 mg followed by daily doses of 0.125 to 0.5 mg; the ratio of loading dose to maintenance dose is about 3 or 4. The half-life of digitoxin is about 6 days; typically digitoxin therapy is initiated with a loading dose of up to 1.6 mg followed by daily doses of 0.1 to 0.2 mg; the ratio of loading dose to maintenance dose is usually about 10. The smaller the ratio of dosing interval to half-life, the larger is the ratio of loading dose to maintenance dose.

Loading of drugs may be hazardous, particularly for those drugs which distribute slowly or to which patients become accustomed only gradually. Caution should be applied at all times. With digoxin or digitoxin therapy, loading (or digitalization) is almost always carried out with 3 or 4 divided doses over the first 1 or 2 days of therapy.

Treatment of epileptic patients with phenytoin is often initiated with a regular maintenance dose, divided or single, of 300 to 400 mg daily. When phenytoin therapy is begun in this manner, steady-state plasma phenytoin levels are achieved after 7 to 10 days. Some clinicians believe, however, that in the patient with frequent seizures a delay in reaching the therapeutic steady-state phenytoin plasma level may be detrimental because attacks may occur before the drug develops its full anticonvulsant effect. Several clinical investigators have suggested initial loading of selected patients with phenytoin.[1,2] In one study,[2] 61 patients received a 1-g loading dose of phenytoin followed by a constant daily maintenance dose of 300 to 400 mg. Seizure control was obtained promptly in all patients who responded to the drug. Patients tolerated the loading doses well, and therapeutic phenytoin levels were achieved rapidly. Studies in children have confirmed the efficacy but have raised questions regarding the safety of this approach.[3]

It is well recognized that more than a week of treatment with a given maintenance dose of guanethidine may be required to produce the maximum antihypertensive effect of this dose. This results from the fact that elimination of the drug from the body is slow (average half-life about 5 days). A regimen has been devised for achieving the pharmacologic effects of guanethidine relatively rapidly, using the concept of loading and maintenance doses based on the kinetics of guanethidine elimination.[4] This regimen was tested in 6 hypertensive patients. Reduction of blood pressure was achieved with individualized divided loading doses of 150 to 525 mg guanethidine administered over a period of 1 to 3 days. Maintenance doses ranging from 20 to 65 mg per day were calculated from the loading dose by assuming a daily loss of about one seventh of the body stores of drug. Satisfactory control of blood pressure was maintained following the guanethidine load, without side effects.

Dosing Interval

The frequency of dosing is often based on tradition and usage (e.g., the t.i.d. or q.i.d. regimen). From a pharmacokinetic point of view, however, a rational dosing interval for most drugs approximates the biologic half-life. Thus, it has been found that the traditional 3-times-a-day dose of phenytoin, a drug with an average half-life of about one day, is unnecessary in many patients and that the total daily dose can often be administered once a day.[5]

Similar conclusions have been reached with respect to dosing of griseofulvin. Comparable steady-state plasma levels of griseofulvin are achieved whether the drug is given in doses of 125 mg 4 times a day or in a single daily dose of 500 mg.[6] Apparently, treatment with griseofulvin can be simplified to once-a-day administration with no loss of efficacy or safety.

Many neuroleptics and tricyclic antidepressants have rather long biologic half-lives. Almost from the beginning of psychopharmacotherapy, certain clinicians have recognized that the traditional t.i.d. or q.i.d. division of drug administration is not as necessary as generally believed and that single daily doses are sufficient for many patients, particularly those on maintenance therapy.[7]

For the past 15 years, the most commonly used dosage of allopurinol has been 100 mg 3 times a day. Although the half-life of allopurinol is only about 1 hr, the half-life of its active metabolite, oxypurinol, is much longer, about 30 hr. In recognition of this, it has been suggested that allopurinol be administered as a single daily dose. When 300 mg of allopurinol given in a single daily dose was compared with 100 mg given 3 times a day, it was found to be equally effective in reducing and controlling uric acid levels and equally well tolerated.[8,9] A more recent study confirmed these results and found that 27 of 33 patients preferred the once-a-day regimen to the divided-dose regimen because it was easier to remember or easier to take and more convenient.[10]

Less frequent dosing may not be feasible with some rapidly absorbed drugs that produce high peak concentrations in the plasma, resulting in adverse effects. This problem may be overcome by using slow-release dosage forms. Thus, slow-release forms may be rational even for some drugs with long biologic half-lives. Presumably, once-a-day dosing of griseofulvin and certain phenytoin products is well tolerated because these drugs are absorbed rather slowly. High doses of most neuroleptics and tricyclic antidepressants tend to sedate and, for most patients, late evening administration of the total dose is preferable. This may offer the additional advantage of avoiding the need for a hypnotic drug.

REFERENCES

1. Kutt, H., et al.: Diphenylhydantoin metabolism, blood levels, and toxicity. Arch. Neurol., *11*:642, 1964.
2. Wilder, B.J., Serrano, E.E., and Ramsay, R.E.: Plasma diphenylhydantoin levels after loading and maintenance doses. Clin. Pharmacol. Ther., *14*:797, 1973.
3. Wilson, J.T., Höjer, B., and Rane, A.: Loading and conventional dose therapy with phenytoin in children: Kinetic profile of parent drug and main metabolite in plasma. Clin. Pharmacol. Ther., *20*:48, 1976.
4. Shand, D.G., et al.: A loading-maintenance regimen for more rapid initiation of the effect of guanethidine. Clin. Pharmacol. Ther., *18*:139, 1975.
5. Buchanan, R.A., et al.: The metabolism of diphenylhydantoin (dilantin) following once-daily administration. Neurology, *22*:1809, 1972.
6. Platt, D.S.: Plasma concentrations of griseofulvin in human volunteers. Br. J. Dermatol., *83*:382, 1970.
7. Ayd, F.D.: Once-a-day neuroleptic and tricyclic antidepressant therapy. Int. Drug Ther. Newsletter, *7*:33, 1972.
8. Brewis, I., Ellis, R.M., and Scott, S.T.: Single daily dose of allopurinol. Ann. Rheum. Dis., *341*:256, 1975.
9. Rodman, G.P., et al.: Allopurinol and gouty hyperuricemia. Efficacy of a single daily dose. JAMA, *231*:1143, 1975.
10. Currie, W.J.C., Turner, P., and Young, J.H.: Evaluation of once a day allopurinol administration in man. Br. J. Clin. Pharmacol., *5*:90, 1978.

2

Compartmental and
Noncompartmental Pharmacokinetics

The basic principles outlined in Chapter 1 are useful for many drugs but they do not apply to all drugs. When a drug distributes relatively slowly, the relationships that have been described do not strictly apply; rigorous pharmacokinetic analysis is much more complicated. The purpose of this chapter is to describe the difficulties encountered with drugs that impart multicompartmental characteristics to the body, and to introduce methods that permit noncompartmental pharmacokinetic analysis of drugs, irrespective of their distribution characteristics.

MULTICOMPARTMENTAL CHARACTERISTICS

On intravenous bolus administration, many drugs distribute sufficiently slowly so that a significant fraction of the dose is eliminated before distribution equilibrium is achieved. When this occurs, a semilogarithmic plot of drug concentration in plasma versus time looks like the curve shown in Figure 2–1. The data cannot be described by a single exponential expression (i.e., a single compartment). At the outset drug concentrations decline rapidly; ultimately, a linear relationship between log concentration and time is observed. The entire curve can usually be described by a mathematical expression that contains either two or three exponential terms [e.g., $C = A \exp(-\alpha t) + B \exp(-\beta t)$].

The mathematical models that apply to this situation are shown in Figure 2–2. In the simpler of the two models (the two-compartment model), the drug is assumed to distribute instantaneously into a space called the central compartment; the appar-

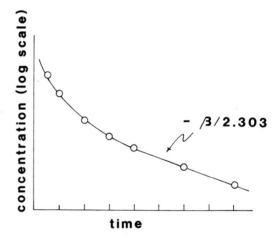

Fig. 2–1. Semilogarithmic plot of plasma concentration versus time after intravenous bolus administration of a drug with multicompartment pharmacokinetic characteristics. The slope of the terminal linear segment of the curve is indicated.

ent volume of this space is usually larger than blood volume. The drug is simultaneously but more slowly distributed into a second space (the peripheral or tissue compartment) and eliminated. The three-compartment model assumes that there are two distinct spaces to which the drug distributes from the central compartment at measurably different rates. In either model, after administration, the apparent volume of the drug increases and the rate constant associated with the rate of decline of drug concentrations in plasma decreases until distribution equilibrium is achieved.

The kinetics of the situation might be better understood by considering the mathematical relationships that apply. For the two-compartment model,

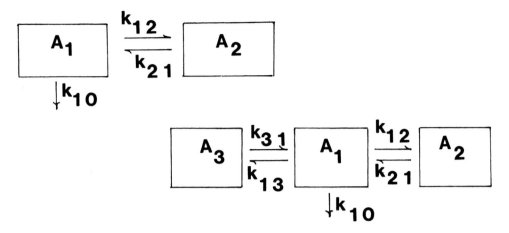

Fig. 2–2. Examples of a two- and three-compartment pharmacokinetic model. A_1 denotes the central compartment in each model and A_2 and A_3 are peripheral compartments. Immediately after an iv bolus injection, the central compartment contains an amount of drug equal to the dose. The general case for extravascular administration assumes that drug is transferred from the absorption site to the central compartment.

$$\begin{array}{c}\text{Rate of loss of drug} \\ \text{from central compartment}\end{array} = \begin{array}{c}\text{Rate of} \\ \text{distribution}\end{array} + \begin{array}{c}\text{Rate of} \\ \text{elimination}\end{array} - \begin{array}{c}\text{Rate of} \\ \text{redistribution}\end{array} \qquad (2\text{–}1)$$

where

$$\begin{array}{c}\text{Rate of loss of drug} \\ \text{from central compartment}\end{array} = -dA_1/dt \qquad (2\text{–}2)$$

$$\text{Rate of distribution} = k_{12}A_1 \qquad (2\text{–}3)$$

$$\text{Rate of elimination} = k_{10}A_1 \qquad (2\text{–}4)$$

$$\text{Rate of redistribution} = \qquad (2\text{–}5)$$

where A_1 and A_2 represent the amounts of drug in the central and peripheral compartments, respectively (see Fig. 2–2).

Immediately after administration, $-dA_1/dt$ is at a maximum equal to the product of $(k_{12} + k_{10})$ and dose; since there is no drug in the tissue compartment, there is no redistribution. As drug levels (A_1) in the central compartment decline because of distribution and elimination, there is a corresponding fall in $-dA_1/dt$, but as drug levels build up in the tissue compartment and the rate of redistribution becomes significant, there is a braking effect on the rate of decline of A_1.

At distribution equilibrium a fixed relationship exists between A_1 and A_2 such that

$$A_2 = \mathbb{Z}A_1 \qquad (2\text{–}6)$$

where $\mathbb{Z}$ is a complex constant incorporating both distribution and elimination parameters. Under these conditions

$$-dA_1/dt = k_{12}A_1 + k_{10}A_1 - k_{21}\mathbb{Z}A_1 \qquad (2\text{–}7)$$

or

$$-dA_1/dt = (k_{12} + k_{10} - k_{21}\mathbb{Z})A_1 \qquad (2\text{–}8)$$

Expressing Equation 2–8 in terms of drug concentrations rather than amounts yields

$$-dC/dt = (k_{12} + k_{10} \\ - k_{21}\mathbb{Z})C = \beta C \qquad (2\text{–}9)$$

where $\beta = k_{12} + k_{10} - k_{21}\mathbb{Z}$. Equation 2–9 is a typical first-order rate expression. Thus, irrespective of the complexity of the model, drug concentrations in the plasma decline in a first-order manner once distribution equilibrium is achieved. The rate constant describing this first-order portion of the curve is usually termed β.

Data Analysis at Distribution Equilibrium

Integration of Equation 2–9 indicates that the log-linear region of the curve shown in Figure 2–1 will have a slope equal to $(-\beta/2.303)$. Therefore, for drugs that require multicompartmental description, a terminal half-life may be defined as

$$t_{1/2} = 0.693/\beta \qquad (2\text{--}10)$$

It is important to remember that this half-life reflects the persistence of only a fraction of the dose; the balance of the dose is eliminated more rapidly. It is also important to note that, irrespective of the model, the half-life of a drug always reflects both distribution and elimination. This is evident when Equation 2–9 is considered.

The mathematical relationships that apply when distribution equilibrium is reached also make it possible to calculate an apparent volume of distribution. This apparent volume, usually termed V_β, is given by

$$V_\beta = \frac{\text{iv dose}}{(\text{AUC})\beta} \qquad (2\text{--}11)$$

where AUC denotes the total area under the drug concentration-time profile and β is the terminal first-order elimination rate constant. V_β is a proportionality constant relating the amount of drug in the body to drug concentration in the plasma during the terminal (log-linear) phase of drug elimination (i.e., at distribution equilibrium).

An analogous expression that can be applied to drugs that distribute rapidly is

$$V = \frac{\text{iv dose}}{(\text{AUC})k} \qquad (2\text{--}12)$$

where k is the first-order elimination rate constant.

Equations 2–11 and 2–12 can usually be applied to data obtained after intramuscular administration of a drug; in this case, the term ''iv dose'' is replaced by ''im dose.'' These equations should not ordinarily be applied to data obtained after oral administration. If they are, the term ''iv dose'' must be replaced by ''amount absorbed'' or, more precisely, by ''amount of drug actually reaching the bloodstream.''

Equation 2–12 is a mathematically rigorous and widely applied equation for the estimation of apparent volume of drugs that distribute rapidly once they reach the bloodstream. Equation 2–11 is a useful approximation of the volume of distribution of most drugs that require a multicompartmental

description. However, V_β has several inherent problems not the least of which is that it reflects elimination as well as distribution. In all cases, V_β will overestimate the volume of distribution of a drug; in most cases, the overestimate is small and of little consequence, but it can be unacceptably large for drugs with pronounced multicompartmental characteristics. The dependence of V_β on drug elimination also means that changes in drug elimination may cause a change in V_β even though the perturbation has no effect on distribution per se.[1]

Sometimes it is also useful to calculate the apparent volume of the central compartment (V_1). This is usually done by curve-fitting the concentration-time data after iv bolus injection, by means of a computer-based nonlinear regression program, to an equation of the form

$$C = A\exp(-\alpha t) + B\exp(-\beta t) \qquad (2\text{--}13)$$

where $\alpha > \beta$. The iv dose divided by the sum of the coefficients is equal to the volume of the central compartment, i.e.

$$V_1 = \text{iv dose}/(A+B) \qquad (2\text{--}14)$$

V_1 is always smaller than the total volume of distribution (V). For this reason, high drug concentrations (i.e. dose/V_1) may occur immediately after a rapid iv injection. These levels fall quickly but could be dangerous. Good sense dictates that iv injections be given relatively slowly.

In the previous chapter, it was noted that the peak concentration of a drug is always smaller after iv infusion than after iv bolus. The difference in concentration for drugs that distribute immediately is a function of the infusion time and half-life of the drug. Strictly speaking, a drug must be infused over at least one half-life to see a 50% change in peak concentration. In practice, much shorter infusion times are almost always helpful because most drugs display a distributive phase and multicompartment characteristics on iv administration.

The initial rapid fall in drug levels after iv bolus injection, the distribution-elimination phase, is sometimes characterized by a half-life, the so-called alpha half-life (i.e., $0.693/\alpha$). The alpha half-life is usually much smaller than the beta half-life (i.e., $0.693/\beta$). Under these conditions, the difference in peak concentration after an iv bolus and an iv infusion is a function of the alpha half-life.

Consider a drug that shows two-compartment

characteristics after iv administration. Assume that the iv dose is 1 g, V_1 = 10 L, α half-life = 15 min, and β half-life = 6 hr. After an iv bolus, the initial drug concentration is 100 mg/L. In contrast, the peak concentration of the drug is only about 25 mg/L when it is infused over 30 minutes.

Other Problems with Multicompartmental Analysis

The number of exponentials and, therefore, the number of compartments required to describe the decline of drug concentration after intravenous bolus injection is not well defined, but depends on both the frequency and timing of blood samples. More frequent sampling right after administration tends to yield data that must be described by equations containing more exponential terms than would be required by less frequent sampling. Thus, the compartmental model required to describe the pharmacokinetics of a drug depends, in part, on the experimental design. In turn, estimates of half-life are dependent on the model selected.

Various statistical considerations are useful in minimizing the problems associated with model selection, but they do not overcome them. Studies with a single drug in a group of patients may result in some patients requiring a two-compartment model to describe the pharmacokinetics of the drug, whereas others require a three-compartment model. We frequently find that drugs requiring multicompartmental analysis after intravenous administration can be described by a one-compartment model after oral administration. Since pharmacokinetic analysis based on compartmental models can lead to unreconcilable difficulties, more and more investigators and clinicians who use pharmacokinetics are turning to noncompartmental approaches that can be applied to all drugs.

NONCOMPARTMENTAL METHODS

Noncompartmental methods for calculating absorption, distribution, and elimination parameters are based on the theory of statistical moments.[2,3] The zero moment of a drug concentration in plasma versus time curve is the total area under the curve from time zero to infinity (AUC), which has been described in Chapter 1. Estimates of AUC are not only useful for calculating bioavailability, but can also be used for calculating drug clearance, which is equal to the ratio of the intravenous dose to AUC.

The first moment of a plasma concentration-time profile is the total area under the curve resulting

Table 2–1. Drug Concentration and Drug Concentration-Time Data, During and After a 1-hr Constant Rate Intravenous Infusion

Time (hr)	Concentration (μg/ml)	Concentration-Time (μg/ml)(hr)
0.5	3.2	1.6
1.0	5.9	5.9
2.0	4.2	8.4
3.0	3.0	9.0
4.0	2.1	8.4
5.0	1.5	7.5
6.0	1.1	6.6
8.0	0.5	4.0

from a plot of the product of drug concentration and time versus time. Table 2–1 shows concentration data obtained after constant rate intravenous infusion of a drug. Also listed are the values of C · t. These values are plotted versus time in Figure 2–3. The area under the C · t versus t plot from t = 0 to the last sampling time, t*, can be calculated by means of the trapezoidal rule (see Appendix I). Provided that blood samples have been collected for a sufficiently long period of time so that the last sample may be considered in the postabsorptive and, where applicable, postdistributive

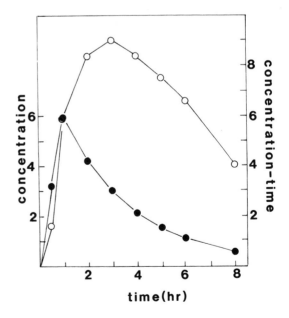

Fig. 2–3. Plots of drug concentration (μg/ml) (●) and drug concentration-time (μg-hr/ml) (○) versus time, during and after a 1-hr constant rate intravenous infusion. The area under the drug concentration versus time plot to infinity is AUC; the area under the drug concentration-time versus time plot to infinity is AUMC.

phase of the curve, the area from t* to ∞ may be estimated from the following equation:[4]

$$\int_{t^*}^{\infty} t \cdot C = \frac{t^* \, C^*}{\beta} + \frac{C^*}{\beta^2} \qquad (2\text{--}15)$$

where the integral term on the left-hand side of the equation is the partial area under the curve, C^* is drug concentration at the last sampling time, t^*, and β is the terminal first-order elimination rate constant. This area is then added to the area from $t = 0$ to $t = t^*$, determined by the trapezoidal rule, to estimate the total area. The total area under the $C \cdot t$ versus t plot is termed the AUMC or area under the first moment curve.

The ratio of AUMC to AUC for any drug is a measure of its mean residence time (MRT).[5,6] MRT calculated after intravenous administration is the statistical moment analogy to drug half-life; it provides a quantitative estimate of the persistence of a drug in the body. Like half-life, MRT is a function of both distribution and elimination.

Comparison of MRT values after intravenous bolus administration with the MRT after some other route of administration provides information regarding the mean absorption time.[7] Similar comparisons can be made between two dosage forms given orally to obtain relative absorption data.

One of the most useful properties of statistical moments is that they permit the estimation of a volume of distribution that is independent of drug elimination.[4,6] Using these methods, the volume of distribution of a drug is given by the product of the intravenous bolus dose and the ratio of AUMC to AUC squared.

Drug Clearance

Clearance is a function of both the intrinsic ability of certain organs, such as the kidneys and liver, to excrete or metabolize a drug and the blood flow rate to these organs. This concept is best illustrated by considering elimination in a single organ as depicted schematically in Figure 2–4. Under these conditions, the venous concentration of drug (C_V) will always be less than the arterial concentration (C_A) because some of the drug is eliminated or extracted during the passage of the blood through the organ. The rate at which drug enters the organ is equal to the product of blood flow (Q) and arterial concentration. The rate at which drug leaves the organ is equal to the product of blood flow and venous concentration. The difference between the

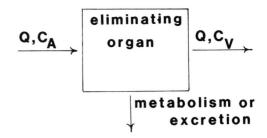

Fig. 2–4. Schematic representation of drug elimination by a single organ. Blood flows through the organ at a rate equal to Q. Drug concentration entering the organ is C_A; drug concentration leaving the organ is C_V; C_V is less than C_A.

input rate and the output rate is the rate of elimination of drug by the organ;

$$\text{Elimination rate} = Q(C_A - C_V) \qquad (2\text{--}16)$$

The ratio of the elimination rate to the drug input rate (QC_A) is termed the extraction ratio (ER) and is given by

$$ER = (C_A - C_V)/C_A \qquad (2\text{--}17)$$

The extraction ratio of a drug ranges from 0 to 1 depending on how well the organ eliminates or extracts the drug from the blood flowing through it. If the organ does not eliminate the drug, then $C_V = C_A$ and $ER = 0$; if the organ avidly extracts the drug so that $C_V \cong 0$, then $ER = 1$.

By definition, the organ clearance (Cl) of a drug represents the volume of blood cleared per unit time. It may be viewed as a proportionality constant relating the elimination rate of a drug to the drug concentration in the blood, as expressed in the following equation:

$$Cl = \text{Elimination rate}/C_A \qquad (2\text{--}18)$$

It follows from Equation 2–16 that

$$Cl = Q(C_A - C_V)/C_A \qquad (2\text{--}19)$$

or, according to Equation 2–17

$$Cl = Q(ER) \qquad (2\text{--}20)$$

Thus, clearance is equal to the product of blood flow and extraction ratio. Since elimination rate is expressed in units of amount per unit time, and concentration is expressed in units of amount per unit volume, it follows that clearance has units of volume per unit time (e.g., ml/min or L/hr), the same as flow rate. If drug elimination is a first-order process, then clearance is independent of drug concentration.

These equations, which have been developed for a single organ, can be extended to the elimination of a drug from the body. The total body clearance of a drug from the blood is equal to the ratio of the overall elimination rate of the drug to the drug concentration in blood, where the overall elimination rate is the sum of the elimination processes occurring in all organs.

By means of integral calculus, it can be shown that the ratio of the overall elimination rate of a drug to its concentration in the blood is equal to the ratio of the amount of drug ultimately eliminated to the total area under the drug concentration-time curve. Since, after intravenous administration, the amount eliminated is equal to the dose, clearance can be expressed as

$$Cl = dose/(AUC) \qquad (2-21)$$

Equation 2–21 provides the basis for the routine estimation of the total body clearance of a drug after a single dose. To estimate clearance, drug is ordinarily given intravenously, but Equation 2–21 usually applies as well to intramuscular administration. Clearance cannot be estimated after oral administration unless it can be assumed that the total dose reaches the bloodstream. Application of Equation 2–21 to data obtained after oral administration when bioavailability is incomplete results in an overestimate of clearance.

Clearance can also be estimated at steady state after prolonged constant rate intravenous infusion. Under these conditions

$$Cl = k_o/C_{ss} \qquad (2-22)$$

where k_o is the infusion rate and C_{ss} is the drug concentration at steady state.

It is sometimes useful to keep in mind that clearance can also be expressed as the product of V_β and β. For drugs that distribute rapidly and can be described by a single compartment, $Cl = Vk$.

Apparent Volume of Distribution

The most useful volume term in pharmacokinetics is the apparent volume of distribution at steady state or V_{ss}. It represents the proportionality constant relating the amount of drug in the body at steady state after prolonged constant rate intravenous infusion or repetitive administration to the drug concentration or average drug concentration at that time. V_{ss} is independent of drug elimination and reflects solely the anatomic space occupied by

a drug and the relative degree of drug binding in the blood and extravascular space.

Estimation of V_{ss} does not require data obtained at steady state; this distribution parameter can be calculated after a single dose of a drug by means of the following equation:[4,6]

$$V_{ss} = iv\ dose(AUMC)/(AUC)^2 \qquad (2-23)$$

where AUMC is the total area under the first moment curve.

Although Equation 2–23 applies only to intravenous bolus administration, the relationship can be modified easily to accommodate the different ways drugs are administered. If a drug is given by a short-term constant rate intravenous infusion,[8] then

$$V_{ss} = \frac{infused\ dose(AUMC)}{(AUC)^2} - \frac{infused\ dose(T)}{2(AUC)} \qquad (2-24)$$

where T is the duration of infusion. Since the infused dose is equal to k_oT, we can also express Equation 2–24 as

$$V_{ss} = \frac{k_oT(AUMC)}{(AUC)^2} - \frac{k_oT^2}{2(AUC)} \qquad (2-25)$$

Relationship of Half-Life, Clearance, and Volume of Distribution

Earlier, we noted that clearance is equal to the product of V_β and β. This relationship does not imply, however, that clearance is dependent on volume of distribution and half-life. Both clearance and distribution volume are independent parameters, although both may be affected by a change in plasma protein binding. Half-life is a dependent parameter. For a multicompartment model, $t_{1/2} = 0.693\ V_\beta/Cl$.

This relationship shows that the larger is the distribution volume, the longer is the half-life. Independently, the larger is the clearance of a drug, the smaller is the half-life. An increase in half-life should not be interpreted as a decrease in drug elimination; it may merely reflect an increase in distribution volume. Changes in elimination are represented by changes in clearance.

Mean Residence Time

The mean residence time (MRT) of a drug after administration of a single dose is given by

$$MRT = (AUMC)/(AUC) \qquad (2-26)$$

The MRT of a drug after intravenous bolus administration provides a useful estimate of the persistence time in the body and in this sense is related to half-life. When applied to drugs that distribute rapidly it can be shown that

$$MRT_{iv} = 1/k \qquad (2\text{--}27)$$

where k is the first-order elimination rate constant. The half-life of a drug is equal to 0.693/k. Half-life tells us the time required to eliminate 50% of the dose; MRT_{iv} tells us the time required to eliminate 63.2% of the dose.

The MRT of a drug that distributes slowly and requires multicompartment characterization is a complex function of the model rate constants for distribution and elimination. However, in noncompartmental terms, the following relationship is useful:

$$MRT_{iv} = 1/\bar{k} \qquad (2\text{--}28)$$

where $\bar{k}$ is a rate constant equal to the ratio of clearance to V_{ss}. For drugs with multicompartment characteristics, $\bar{k} > \beta$. For drugs that distribute almost immediately, $\bar{k} = k$. In many cases, the ratio of 0.693 to $\bar{k}$ serves as the effective half-life of a drug.

Irrespective of the distribution characteristics of a drug, MRT represents the time required for 63.2% of an intravenous bolus dose to be eliminated. As such, it may be possible to determine MRT from urinary excretion data alone by determining the time required to excrete 63.2% of that amount which is ultimately excreted as unchanged drug.

Mean residence time is a function of how we give the drug. The MRT values for noninstantaneous administrations will always be greater than the MRT following intravenous bolus administration. However, the MRT_{iv} can be estimated following other modes of drug administration. For example, following a constant rate intravenous infusion

$$MRT_{iv} = MRT_{inf} - (T/2) \qquad (2\text{--}29)$$

where T is the duration of the infusion. MRT_{inf} is calculated according to Equation 2–26.

DRUG ABSORPTION

Noncompartmental methods for estimating the extent of absorption of a drug after oral or other extravascular routes of administration have been described in Chapter 1. Essentially, these methods require a comparison of areas under the curve. The fraction of an oral dose that actually reaches the bloodstream can be estimated from the ratio of AUC after oral administration to AUC after intravenous administration of equivalent doses of the drug. The extent of absorption of drug in a test dosage form relative to its absorption from a standard dosage form, such as an aqueous solution, can be estimated from the ratio of AUC after the test dose to AUC after the standard.

Noncompartmental methods for estimating the rate of absorption of a drug after extravascular administration are based on differences in MRT after different modes of administration. In general,[7]

$$MAT = MRT_{ni} - MRT_{iv} \qquad (2\text{--}30)$$

where MAT is the mean absorption time, MRT_{ni} is the mean residence time after administration of the drug in a noninstantaneous manner, such as orally, intramuscularly, or by iv infusion and MRT_{iv} is the mean residence time after intravenous bolus administration.

When absorption is a first-order process

$$MAT = (1/k_a) \qquad (2\text{--}31)$$

where k_a is the first-order absorption rate constant. Under these conditions, $k_a = 1/MAT$, and the absorption half-life is given by 0.693 (MAT). When absorption or input is a zero-order process

$$MAT = (T/2) \qquad (2\text{--}32)$$

where T is the time over which absorption or input takes place.

Moment analysis and the concept of MRT may also be useful for comparing the absorption characteristics of a drug from different formulations. This application is considered in Chapter 8.

A limitation of moment theory is seen when the difference between MRT_{ni} and MRT_{iv} is small. In this case, it may be difficult to estimate MAT with adequate accuracy.

A useful application of moment theory, to evaluate the pharmacokinetics of furosemide after iv and oral administration, has been reported.[9] The mean MRT after an iv dose of the loop diuretic to eight healthy subjects was less than 1 hr, suggesting an effective half-life of about 40 min. Absorption after oral administration, however, was slow and incomplete. Bioavailability was only about half the dose. The difference in MRT after oral and iv administration (MAT) was 84 min. The mean absorption time for furosemide was significantly larger than the MRT_{iv}, suggesting absorption rate-limited elimination of the drug.

Predicting Steady-State Concentrations

When a drug is given continuously or intermittently for a sufficient period of time it accumulates and eventually reaches a steady state with respect to drug concentration in the blood (see Figs. 1–8 and 1–9). Drug concentration at steady state is solely a function of the effective rate of dosing and the total body clearance of the drug in the patient, both of which are noncompartmental parameters.

The steady-state concentration (C_{ss}) following constant rate intravenous infusion may be determined by rearranging Equation 2–22 which yields

$$C_{ss} = k_o/Cl \qquad (2\text{--}33)$$

where k_o is the infusion rate and Cl is the clearance of the drug.

A similar equation can be written to describe the average drug concentration at steady state ($\overline{C}$) following repetitive intermittent administration of a fixed dose (D) given at fixed intervals (τ) (see Fig. 1–9). Under these conditions,

$$\overline{C} = F(DR)/Cl \qquad (2\text{--}34)$$

where F is the fraction of the administered dose that actually reaches the bloodstream and DR is the average dosing rate; if a drug is given in a dose of 400 mg every 8 hr, then DR = 50 mg/hr.

If a drug is given at irregular intervals during the day (e.g., 3 times a day or after meals and at bedtime rather than every 8 hr or every 6 hr), one can use Equation 2–34 to calculate the average drug concentration over the day by setting DR equal to (total daily dose)/24 hr.

A still simpler method for estimating average drug concentration at steady state than that suggested by Equation 2–34 is also available. As may be seen in Figure 1–9, $\overline{C}$ is a concentration intermediate between the maximum and minimum drug concentrations at steady state. Specifically,

$$\overline{C} = AUC_{ss}/\tau \qquad (2\text{--}35)$$

where AUC_{ss} is the area under the curve from t = 0 to t = τ during a dosing interval at steady state. In other words, $\overline{C}$ is the height of a rectangle of width τ that has an area ($\overline{C} \times \tau$) equal to the area under the curve during a dosing interval at steady state. Steady-state bioavailability studies comparing AUC_{ss} for test product and reference standard are widely used for evaluating sustained-release

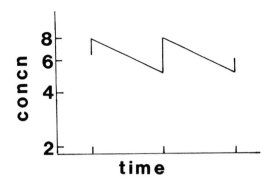

Fig. 2–5. Steady-state concentrations after repetitive administration of a rapidly distributing drug with a 12-hr half-life given every 8 hr. The ratio of C_{max} to C_{min} is 1.6.

dosage forms. By definition, AUC_{ss} is equal to AUC, the total area under the curve from t = 0 to t = ∞ after a single dose. Under these conditions

$$\overline{C} = AUC/\tau \qquad (2\text{--}36)$$

By merely knowing the AUC of a drug after a single dose administered in the same way that will be used for repetitive dosing, we can predict the average drug concentration at steady state.

Although $\overline{C}$ is a useful parameter and easy to calculate, we must remember that it tells us nothing about the time course of drug concentrations during a dosing interval. This limitation is of little consequence for drugs with long half-lives that distribute rapidly and are dosed relatively frequently (i.e., $\tau < t_{1/2}$). In this case, the steady-state ratio of C_{max} to C_{min} will be less than 2 and the drug concentration profile at steady state will be relatively flat (Fig. 2–5). On the other hand, large fluctuations may be seen with drugs having relatively short half-lives that are given less frequently than every half-life (Fig. 2–6) and with drugs that distribute slowly and display multicompartment characteristics (Fig. 2–7). In these cases, the steady-state ratio of C_{max} to C_{min} will exceed 2. For certain drugs, the attainment of an acceptable value of $\overline{C}$, well within the therapeutic concentration range, may belie the fact that C_{max} is too high and adverse effects may result or that C_{min} is too low and for some time during the dosing interval the patient may not be receiving the optimal benefit of the drug. Noncompartmental methods are generally not useful for describing the time course of drug in the blood. It is probably best to handle such considerations with the concept of half-life and the application of compartmental analysis. Questions

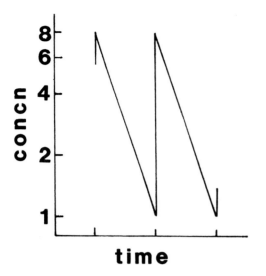

Fig. 2–6. Steady-state concentrations after repetitive administration of a rapidly distributing drug with a 2-hr half-life given every 6 hr. The ratio of C_{max} to C_{min} is 8.

regarding drug accumulation and loading dose may also be better answered by applying compartment theory, as described in Chapter 1. A noncompartmental alternative based on the principle of superposition is described in Appendix II.

Predicting the Time to Steady State

The time required to reach steady state on continuous constant rate intravenous infusion of a drug that distributes rapidly is a function of the half-life of the drug. After a period of infusion equal to 4 half-lives, the drug concentration in blood or plasma will be within 90% of the steady-state concentration; after a period equal to 7 half-lives, drug concentration is within 99% of the steady-state level. The same drug given as repetitive intravenous boluses of fixed doses at fixed intervals will

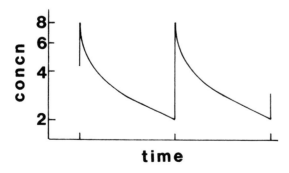

Fig. 2–7. Steady-state concentrations after repetitive administration of a slowly distributing drug with a 12-hr half-life given every 12 hr. The ratio of C_{max} to C_{min} is 4.

show similar characteristics; after a period of dosing equal to 4 half-lives, the average drug concentration will be within 90% of the average steady-state concentration.

In practice, the time after the start of dosing to attain a certain fraction (e.g., 90%) of the steady-state concentration is not only a function of half-life, but also of the way we give the drug and of the distribution characteristics of the drug. Repetitive extravascular or noninstantaneous administration of a drug requires a longer period to attain steady state than we would predict from its half-life. On the other hand, repetitive administration of a drug that distributes slowly and shows multicompartment characteristics requires a shorter period to reach steady state in the plasma than we would predict from its terminal half-life. Exact equations to solve for the time after starting dosing at which a certain percentage of steady state is reached for different drugs under different conditions of use are both complex and difficult to solve.

Moment analysis provides a unique solution to this problem. Chiou has shown that by means of AUC analysis one can calculate the time to steady state for any drug after a single dose given in the same way that will be used for repetitive dosing.[10] In essence, the time required after giving the dose for the partial area under the curve (AUC_0^t) to be equal to a certain fraction of the total area under the curve (AUC) is the same as the time required to reach the same fraction of steady state on repetitive dosing of the drug.[11] This idea is expressed in the following equation:

$$f_{ss} = AUC_0^t/AUC \qquad (2\text{--}37)$$

where f_{ss} is the fraction of the steady-state concentration reached at time t on repetitive dosing and the area terms refer to a single dose.

When using Equation 2–37, one does not explicitly solve for time. Rather, one selects a time after giving the dose and carries out an area analysis to calculate f_{ss}. The time required to reach a desired f_{ss} (e.g., 90%) is estimated by trial and error. Usually two trials followed by interpolation should be sufficient to provide a useful estimate of the required time.

Parameters Based on Free Drug Concentration

The noncompartmental methods described in this chapter are based on total drug concentrations in blood or plasma. Most drugs are bound to some extent to plasma proteins and formed elements in the blood. Therefore, we can speak of a free drug concentration and a total drug concentration (free plus bound) in blood or plasma.

The usual analytic methods determine total drug concentration in plasma (C). Total drug concentration in blood (C_b) can be estimated by the following equation:

$$C_b = C_{rbc} \cdot HCT + C(1 - HCT) \quad (2–38)$$

where C_{rbc} is drug concentration in the red blood cell and HCT is hematocrit.

The ratio of free (C_f) to total drug concentration in blood or plasma is termed the free fraction (f). Free fraction is usually determined in plasma (f_p) by means of equilibrium dialysis or ultrafiltration. Free fraction in blood is calculated by the following equation:

$$f_b = f_p C / C_b \quad (2–39)$$

The plasma or blood binding of most drugs given in usual doses is independent of drug concentration. Therefore, by determining total drug concentration and by determining free fraction at a given concentration, we can calculate free drug concentration.

In theory, free rather than total drug concentration in blood or plasma is more closely related to pharmacologic effects. There is some experimental and clinical data to support this idea. In the absence of inter- or intrasubject differences in binding, a given total drug concentration always reflects the same free drug concentration. However, some patients bind a drug much more or much less effectively than average because of disease-related factors. During a course of therapy, there may be a change in binding because of concomitant drug therapy. Therefore, an undesirably low or high total drug concentration may not reflect a corresponding low or high free drug concentration.

Total drug concentration at steady state is a function of clearance (see Eq. 2–34). The clearance of drugs with a low hepatic or renal extraction ratio depends on binding as well as the efficiency of the eliminating organs. The clearance of total drug may increase or decrease simply because of a change in binding. In this case, there will be a change in the steady-state concentration of total drug but not of free drug. Since free drug concentration at steady state is unchanged, an unusually high or low total drug concentration may not require a change in dosing rate.

Under these conditions, it may be desirable to determine the clearance of free drug (Cl_f) as well as the clearance of total drug. Free drug clearance from plasma is given by the following equation:

$$Cl_f = Cl / f_p \quad (2–40)$$

CONCLUSIONS

The noncompartmental methods described in this chapter permit a comprehensive pharmacokinetic analysis without resort to curve-fitting, computers, or tedious mathematical equations. Although these methods cannot be applied to all pharmacokinetic problems, they are useful for most problems and are particularly useful for the clinical application of pharmacokinetics. In the following pages, you will find many of these relationships used to answer important clinical questions.

REFERENCES

1. Jusko, W.J., and Gibaldi, M.: Effects of change in elimination on various parameters of the two-compartment model. J. Pharm. Sci., 61:1270, 1972.
2. Yamaoka, K., Nakagawa, T., and Uno, T.: Statistical moments in pharmacokinetics. J. Pharmacokinet. Biopharm., 6:547, 1978.
3. Cutler, D.J.: Theory of the mean absorption time, an adjunct to conventional bioavailability studies. J. Pharm. Pharmacol., 30:476, 1978.
4. Benet, L.Z., and Galeazzi, R.L.: Noncompartmental determination of the steady-state volume of distribution. J. Pharm. Sci., 68:1071, 1979.
5. Perl, W., and Samuel, P.: Input-output analysis for total input rate and total traced mass of body cholesterol in man. Circ. Res., 25:191, 1969.
6. Oppenheimer, J.H., Schwartz, H.L., and Surks, M.I.: Determination of common parameters of iodothyronine metabolism and distribution in man: noncompartmental analysis. J. Clin. Endocrinol. Metab., 41:319, 1975.
7. Riegelman, S., and Collier, P.: The application of statistical moment theory to the evaluation of in vivo dissolution time and absorption time. J. Pharmacokinet. Biopharm., 8:509, 1980.
8. Lee, C.S., Brater, D.C., Gambertoglio, J.G., and Benet, L.Z.: Disposition kinetics of ethambutol in man, J. Pharmacokinet. Biopharm., 8:335, 1980.
9. Hammarlund, M.M., Paalzow, L.K., and Odlind, B.: Pharmacokinetics of furosemide in man after intravenous and oral administration. Application of moment analysis. Eur. J. Clin. Pharmacol., 26:197, 1984.
10. Chiou, W.L.: Rapid compartment- and model-independent estimation of times required to attain various fractions of steady-state plasma level during multiple dosing of drugs obeying superposition principle and having various absorption or infusion kinetics. J. Pharm. Sci., 68:1546, 1979.
11. Perrier, D., and Gibaldi, M.: General derivation of the equation for the time to reach a certain fraction of steady-state. J. Pharm. Sci., 71:474, 1982.

3

Gastrointestinal Absorption—
Biologic Considerations

Drugs are most commonly given orally and the gastrointestinal tract plays a major role in determining the rate and extent of drug absorption. In this chapter, the more important biologic factors that influence drug absorption are considered.

MEMBRANE PHYSIOLOGY

The gastrointestinal barrier that separates the lumen of the stomach and intestines from the systemic circulation and the sites of drug action is a complex structure composed of lipids, proteins, lipoproteins, and polysaccharides. The barrier has the characteristics of a semipermeable membrane, permitting the rapid passage of some chemicals while retarding or preventing the passage of others. Amino acids, sugars, fatty acids, and other nutrients required for life readily cross the barrier in the healthy individual. At the same time the barrier can be highly restrictive. For example, there is virtually no leakage of plasma protein into the gastrointestinal tract in the healthy mammalian adult. Certain toxins, which would produce lethal effects if present in the circulation in minute quantities, are harmless if ingested because of their inability to traverse the barrier. Most drugs used in clinical practice are administered orally and must cross this barrier before reaching the systemic circulation. Thus, the characteristics of the gastrointestinal barrier are of considerable importance in biopharmaceutics.

Lipid-soluble molecules as well as small, hydrophilic molecules and ions are readily absorbed from the gastrointestinal tract in an apparently passive manner. Certain larger polar molecules with molecular weights up to several hundred are also absorbed but in a manner suggesting the active participation of components of the membrane. Accordingly, the biologic membrane may be viewed as a dynamic lipoid sieve, a semipermeable lipoid membrane containing numerous aqueous pores or channels, too small to be seen, and a host of carrier molecules that shuttle back and forth across the membranes like ferries.

Lipid-soluble molecules penetrate the barrier directly through the fat-like portion of the lipoprotein membrane. The aqueous pores render the epithelial membranes freely permeable to water, to monovalent ions, and to hydrophilic solutes of small molecular size such as urea. By introducing aqueous solutions of molecules of graduated size into the human intestine, and by determining the facility of absorption, it has been estimated that the hypothetical pores in the proximal intestine (jejunum) have an average radius of 7.5 A (7.5×10^{-7} mm) and those in the distal intestine (ileum), one of about 3.5 A.[1] The molecular size of most drug molecules suggests that pore transport is of minor importance in drug absorption.

The digestive end products of dietary carbohydrates and proteins are hexose and amino acid molecules that are water soluble but usually too large to flow easily through the system of pores. The carriers in the membrane transport these water-soluble substances through the lipid, perhaps by interacting with the solute to render it temporarily fat soluble.

Membrane transport of drugs and other chemicals directly through the lipid or aqueous channels is called *passive diffusion*. Carrier-mediated transfer of polar molecules is called *facilitated diffusion* or, in some cases, *active transport*.

Passive Diffusion

The transfer of most drugs across biologic membranes occurs by passive diffusion from a region of higher concentration to one of lower concentration. Passive transport is described by Fick's first law which states that the rate of diffusion across a membrane (dC/dt) is proportional to the difference in drug concentration on each side of the membrane (ΔC); that is,

$$-dC/dt = k\ \Delta C = k(C_1 - C_2) \quad (3-1)$$

where C_1 and C_2 denote the drug concentrations on each side of the membrane and k is a proportionality constant. By convention, we assume that $C_1 > C_2$ and that there is net transport of drug from region 1 to region 2. The proportionality constant incorporates the diffusion coefficient of the drug, the thickness and area of the biologic membrane, and the permeability of the membrane to the specific drug.

The gastrointestinal absorption of a drug from an aqueous solution requires diffusion in the lumen to the gut wall and penetration of the epithelial barriers to the capillaries of the systemic circulation. Upon emerging in the blood, the drug distributes rapidly into an apparent volume that is usually considerably larger than blood volume. Thus, during absorption, drug concentration in the blood will be much lower than at the absorption site. In essence, the general circulation functions like a sink for the drug in the gastrointestinal tract, and a large concentration gradient is maintained throughout the absorption phase; that is, $C_1 \gg C_2$. Consequently, the concentration gradient (ΔC) is nearly equal to C_1, and Equation 3–1 may be rewritten as

$$-dC/dt \cong k\ C_1 \quad (3-2)$$

which is the familiar form of a first-order rate equation.

The gastrointestinal absorption of most drugs from solution may be described by first-order kinetics; the rate of absorption is proportional to drug concentration over a wide concentration range indicating passive absorption. For example, the absorption rate of hydrocortisone from the human small intestine is proportional to the concentration of the drug over a 2000-fold concentration range (from 0.05 to 100 mg/L).[2] The passive absorption process is driven solely by the effective concentration gradient that exists across the gastrointestinal barrier.

Carrier-Mediated Transport

Although most drugs are absorbed from the gastrointestinal tract by passive diffusion, certain compounds of therapeutic interest and many substances of nutritional concern are absorbed by an apparently *carrier-mediated* transport mechanism.

Active absorption takes place when the intestine transports a substance *uphill* against a concentration gradient. This phenomenon is easily demonstrated by placing identical solutions of glucose on either side of an excised segment of intestine. After a while, if the segment is kept viable, the concentration of glucose is found to be decreased on the mucosal (lumen) side, whereas its concentration on the serosal side has increased over the initial level. The epithelial cells have apparently pumped glucose uphill. *Facilitated diffusion* takes place when the intestine transports certain solutes *downhill* but at rates much greater than would be anticipated based on the polarity of the solute and its molecular size.

Active or facilitated absorption is usually explained by assuming that carriers in the lipoprotein membranes of the intestinal epithelial cells are responsible for shuttling these solutes in a mucosal-to-serosal direction. The major substances that are believed to be actively transported are sodium, other ions such as calcium and iron, glucose, galactose, amino acids, bile salts, and vitamin B_{12}. A larger number of substances, including other vitamins, such as riboflavin and thiamine, and certain drugs, are believed to be absorbed by facilitated diffusion.

The number of apparent carriers in the intestinal membranes is limited. Therefore, the rate of carrier-mediated transport must be described by the following equation:

$$\text{Absorption rate} = \frac{V_{max}C}{K_M + C} \quad (3-3)$$

where C is the solute concentration at the absorption site and V_{max} and K_M are constants. At low solute concentrations, such that $K_M \gg C$,

$$\text{Absorption rate} = \frac{V_{max}}{K_M}C = k\ C \quad (3-4)$$

and apparent first-order kinetics are observed. Under these conditions there are a sufficient number of carriers so that a constant proportion of solute molecules presented to the epithelial surface is transported. As the solute concentration increases

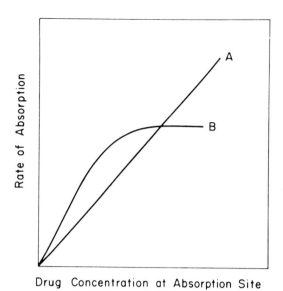

Drug Concentration at Absorption Site

Fig. 3–1. Relationship between absorption rate and drug concentration for a passive process (curve A) and a carrier-mediated process (curve B).

the number of unoccupied carriers is reduced and the proportion of solute molecules that actually gets across the membrane declines until a maximum absolute number is reached. When $C >> K_M$, then

$$\text{Absorption rate} = V_{max} \qquad (3\text{–}5)$$

Further increases in solute concentration are not associated with any increase in the rate of absorption.

Absorption rate-concentration relationships for carrier-mediated and passive diffusion processes are shown in Figure 3–1. The plot describing the passive process is linear over the entire concentration range (see Eq. 3–2). The absorption rate of a substance that is transported by active absorption or facilitated diffusion shows linear dependence on concentration only at low concentrations (see Eq. 3–4). As the concentration increases the rate of ascent of the curve decreases, and eventually the absorption rate becomes invariant with concentration (see Eq. 3–5). The plateau region of the curve reflects saturation of the carrier mechanism. This type of rate process is termed a *capacity-limited process.*

There appear to be several carrier-mediated transport systems in the small intestine. Each is characterized by both structural and site specificity. For example, amino acids and monosaccharides such as glucose and galactose are absorbed in a specialized fashion but by different carrier systems.

The amino acid system is specific and strongly favors the transport of the L-stereoisomeric form as opposed to the D-form of amino acids. The hexose system requires the particular molecular configuration of glucose; a wide variety of other 6-carbon sugars are unacceptable to the carrier. Independent carrier-mediated processes have been identified for the absorption of bile salts and pyrimidines.

Competition between two similar substances for the same transfer mechanism and inhibition of absorption of one or both compounds are other characteristics of carrier-mediated transport. Inhibition of absorption may also be observed with agents, such as sodium fluoride, cyanide, or dinitrophenol, that interfere with cell metabolism.

If the structure of a drug is sufficiently similar to that of a substance absorbed by carrier-mediated transport, there is the likelihood that the drug may also be absorbed in this manner. Methyldopa and levodopa are both absorbed by active transport via an amino acid transport mechanism. Penicillamine, an amino acid analog used in the treatment of Wilson's disease and lead poisoning, is actively transported across the rat intestine.[3] Uphill transport is found with the L-isomer but not with the D-form. Active transport of penicillamine is decreased in the presence of cyanide and certain L-amino acids. Serine and threonine derivatives of nitrogen mustard, which have been investigated for antitumor activity, are also absorbed by a carrier-mediated process.[4] Another antitumor agent, 5-fluorouracil, is actively transported across the small intestine by the pyrimidine transport system.[5]

Some substances may be absorbed by simultaneous carrier-mediated and passive transport processes. Certain pyrimidines such as uracil and thymine are a case in point.[6] The contribution of each process to the total absorption rate varies with concentration. The contribution of the carrier-mediated process to the overall absorption rate decreases with concentration and at sufficiently high concentrations is negligible.

The capacity-limited characteristics of carrier-mediated processes suggest that the bioavailability of a drug absorbed in this manner should decrease with increasing dose. Figure 3–2 shows that the relative availability of riboflavin in man decreases with increasing amounts of administered vitamin.[7] Above a certain dose, the *amount* of riboflavin absorbed remains constant regardless of the size of the dose. Similar findings are reported for thiamine

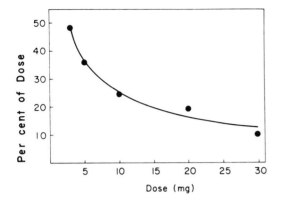

Fig. 3–2. Relative bioavailability of riboflavin (expressed as percent of dose) as a function of oral dose administered to fasting subjects. (Data from Levy, G., and Jusko, W.J.[7])

and ascorbic acid.[8,9] The use of large single oral doses of these vitamins is irrational. If relatively large daily doses are required, one should use divided doses.

GASTROINTESTINAL PHYSIOLOGY

The major components of the gastrointestinal tract are the stomach, small intestine, and large intestine or colon (Fig. 3–3). The small intestine includes the duodenum, jejunum, and ileum. The major segments of the gastrointestinal tract differ from one another both anatomically and morphologically, as well as with respect to secretions and pH.

The stomach is a pouch-like structure lined with a relatively smooth epithelial surface. Extensive absorption of weakly acidic or nonionized drugs and certain weakly basic drugs can be demonstrated

in the stomach under experimental conditions. Ethanol is rapidly and completely absorbed from the ligated stomach pouch of the dog. Similar findings with sulfaethidole and barbital have been reported in surgically altered rats.[10] However, under normal conditions, when gastric emptying is not impeded, the stomach's role in drug absorption is modest. The absorption of aspirin and ethanol from the human stomach after oral administration of aqueous solutions to healthy subjects has been estimated to be about 10% and 30% of the dose, respectively.[11,12] In each case, the balance of the dose is absorbed from the small intestine.

The small intestine is the most important site for drug absorption in the gastrointestinal tract. The epithelial surface area through which absorption can take place in the small intestine is extraordinarily large because of the presence of villi and microvilli, finger-like projections arising from and forming folds in the intestinal mucosa. The irregularities in the mucosal surface caused by the microvilli, villi, and submucosal folds increase the area available for absorption by more than 30 times that which would be present if the small intestine were a smooth tube.[13] Based on studies in the rat, one can estimate that the effective surface area of the small intestine is about 10 times that of the stomach.[10] Other studies conclude that surface area decreases sharply from proximal to distal small intestine. The surface area in man has been estimated to range from 80 cm²/cm serosal length just beyond the duodenojejunal flexure to about 20 cm²/cm serosal length just before the ileocecal valve.[14] There is also a progressive decrease in the average

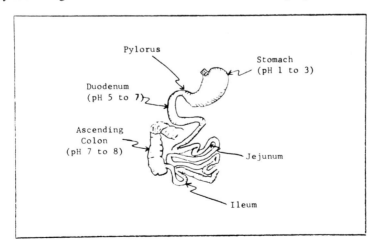

Fig. 3–3. Representation of the human gastrointestinal tract.

size of aqueous pores from proximal to distal small intestine and colon.[1,15]

The small intestine is also the most important region of the gastrointestinal tract with respect to carrier-mediated transport. The proximal small intestine is the major area for absorption of dietary constituents including monosaccharides, amino acids, vitamins, and minerals. However, both vitamin B_{12} and bile salts appear to have specific absorption sites in the ileum.[16]

The large intestine, like the stomach, has a considerably less irregular mucosa than that of the small intestine. This segment serves as a reserve area for the absorption of drugs that have escaped absorption proximally because of their physiochemical properties or their dosage form (e.g., enteric-coated tablets and sustained-release products). The large intestine is not an ideal absorption site, however, and incomplete absorption may result if a large fraction of the dose of a drug reaches the colon. On the other hand, the large intestine may play an important role in the efficacy of orally administered drugs, such as sulfasalazine, that require metabolism (reduction) by intestinal bacteria in the ileum and colon for bioactivation.

Gastrointestinal Blood Flow

The blood perfusing the gastrointestinal tract plays an important role in drug absorption by continuously maintaining the concentration gradient across the epithelial membrane. The dependence of intestinal absorption on blood flow rate changes from blood flow-independent to blood flow-limited as the absorbability of the substance increases.[17] Polar molecules that are slowly absorbed show no dependence on blood flow; the absorption of lipid soluble molecules and molecules that are small enough to easily penetrate the aqueous pores is rapid and highly dependent on the rate of blood flow. The absorption rate of most drugs probably shows an intermediate dependence on blood flow rate; relatively large decreases from normal mesenteric blood flow rate are required to produce an important change in absorption rate. In general, the rate of drug absorption is unaffected by normal variability in mesenteric blood flow. Ordinarily, changes in mesenteric blood flow that result from disease or drug effects must be substantial and sustained to significantly influence drug absorption.

The entire blood supply draining most of the gastrointestinal tract returns to the systemic circulation by way of the liver. Therefore, the entire dose of a drug that is given orally and completely absorbed is exposed to the liver before reaching the bloodstream. Since the liver is the most important organ in the body for drug metabolism and metabolizes some drugs rapidly, there is the possibility that a large fraction of the dose will never reach the systemic circulation because of hepatic metabolism during absorption. This phenomenon is known as the hepatic first-pass effect and is responsible for the less-than-complete bioavailability of many drugs given orally. Metabolism of a drug during absorption by enzymes found in the gut wall may also reduce bioavailability. A more detailed discussion of these aspects of drug metabolism is presented in Chapter 8.

Gastrointestinal pH

There may be as much as a 10 million-fold difference in hydrogen ion concentration between the stomach and the colon. An exceedingly abrupt, 10 thousand-fold difference in hydrogen ion concentration exists between the stomach and the duodenum. The pH at the absorption site is an important factor in drug absorption because many drugs are either weak organic acids or bases. In solution, organic electrolytes exist in a nonionized (usually lipid-soluble) and an ionized (usually poorly lipid-soluble) form. The fraction of each species depends on the pH of the solution. Since the gastrointestinal barrier (as well as many other barriers and membranes in the body) is much more permeable to uncharged, lipid-soluble solutes, a drug may be well absorbed from one segment of the gastrointestinal tract, where a favorable pH exists, but poorly absorbed from another segment, where a less favorable pH is found. The absorption of weakly basic drugs such as antihistamines and antidepressants is favored in the small intestine where such drugs exist largely in a nonionized form. On the other hand, the acidic gastric fluids tend to retard the absorption of weak bases but promote the absorption of weakly acidic drugs such as sulfonamides and nonsteroidal anti-inflammatories. Changes in the pH of the fluids in a given segment of tract may improve or impede the absorption of a drug.

The pH of gastric fluid varies considerably. Gastric secretions have a pH of less than 1, but the pH of gastric contents is usually between 1 and 3 because of dilution and diet. The pH of the stomach contents is distinctly but briefly elevated after a meal; pH values of 5 are not unusual. Fasting tends to decrease the pH of gastric fluids. Disease may also influence the pH of the stomach. The average gastric pH is significantly lower in patients with a duodenal ulcer than in healthy individuals. Fats and fatty acids in the diet have been found to inhibit gastric secretions. A major clinical effect of antispasmodic drugs, such as atropine and propantheline, and H_2-blockers, such as cimetidine and ranitidine, is a reduction in gastric acid. Some anticholinergic activity, including suppression of gastric secretions, is commonly found with many other drugs. Antacid products are widely used for the purpose of neutralizing gastric acidity and elevating the pH of gastric contents. Disease or drug-related changes in gastric pH may influence the dissolution, stability, and/or absorption of certain drugs.

GASTRIC EMPTYING AND GASTROINTESTINAL MOTILITY

In theory, weakly acidic drugs should be better absorbed from the stomach than from the intestine, because a larger fraction of the dose is in a non-ionized, lipid-soluble form. However, the limited residence of the drug in the stomach and the relatively small surface area of the stomach more than balance the influence of pH in determining the optimal site of absorption. Thus, factors that promote gastric emptying tend to increase the absorption rate of all drugs. The converse is also true. Slow gastric emptying can delay the onset of effect of drugs such as analgesics or sedatives in situations requiring prompt clinical response. Prompt gastric emptying is important for drugs that are unstable in stomach fluids because of low pH or enzyme activity. For example, the extent of degradation of penicillin G after oral administration depends on its residence time in the stomach and on the pH of the stomach fluids.

Gastric emptying often appears to be an exponential process. Standard low bulk meals and liquids are transferred from the stomach to the duodenum in an apparent first-order fashion, with a half-life of 20 to 60 min in the healthy adult. However, many factors can influence the rate of this process. Gastric emptying is retarded by fats and fatty acids in the diet, high concentrations of electrolytes or hydrogen ion, high viscosity or bulk, mental depression, lying on the left side, diseases such as gastroenteritis, pyloric stenosis, gastric ulcer, gastroesophageal reflux, Crohn's disease, celiac disease, and hypothyroidism, and during the luteal phase of the menstrual cycle. Many drugs including atropine and propantheline, narcotic analgesics, amitriptyline, imipramine, desipramine, chlorpromazine, and aluminum hydroxide can also retard gastric emptying. Propantheline has been found to double the mean gastric half-emptying time of a test meal in man.[18] After placebo the mean half-emptying time was 68 min and after 30 mg of propantheline bromide it was 135 min. Gastric emptying is promoted by fasting or hunger, alkaline buffer solutions, anxiety, lying on the right side, diseases such as hyperthyroidism, and drugs such as metoclopramide, a dopaminergic blocker, widely used for nausea and vomiting associated with cancer chemotherapy.

Gastric emptying of liquids is much faster than that of food or solid dosage forms. It has been found in normal subjects that complete gastric emptying of enteric-coated barium granules, administered in a standard breakfast, requires about 4 to 8 hr.[19] When considering the emptying of a single object from the stomach, such as an enteric-coated tablet, terms such as half-life are meaningless. Emptying of a single unit is a random process. Intact tablets have been observed in the stomach as long as 6 hr after ingestion of an enteric-coated product with a meal.[20]

Gastric emptying is one of the more important factors contributing to the unusually large inter-subject variability in the absorption of drugs from enteric-coated tablets. As a means of reducing this variability, it has been suggested that enteric-coated medication be administered in the form of small, individually coated granules that would empty gradually but continuously into the duodenum.[21]

Differences in gastric emptying among patients also contribute to the variability in absorption rate of drugs from conventional dosage forms. For example, after administration of 1.5 g (3 tablets) acetaminophen to 14 convalescent hospital patients, the maximum concentration in the plasma ranged from 7.4 to 37.0 μg/ml, and the time required to reach the maximum concentration ranged from 30 to 180 min.[22] Both these indices of absorption rate were linearly related to the gastric emptying half-life found in each patient (Fig. 3–4). Despite the marked variability in absorption rate, little difference in the extent of absorption of acetaminophen was found among patients. A similar correlation between absorption rate and gastric emptying has been observed in man with cimetidine.[23]

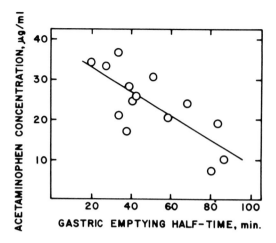

Fig. 3–4. Relationship between peak concentration of acetaminophen in plasma and gastric emptying half-time after a single oral dose. Rapid gastric emptying results in high peak levels. (Data from Heading, R.C., et al.[22])

Posture, which affects gastric emptying, also affects the absorption of acetaminophen.[24] Acetaminophen absorption was markedly delayed in all subjects lying on the left side compared to that observed when the same subjects were ambulatory (Fig. 3–5). This effect must be taken into account in drug absorption studies conducted in hospitalized patients.

Tablets and capsules are commonly swallowed with little or no water and many patients in bed swallow them lying down. Under these conditions, a solid dosage form may lodge in the esophagus

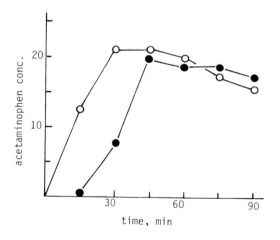

Fig. 3–5. Mean acetaminophen concentrations in plasma (μg/ml) after a single oral dose to ambulatory (○) and supine (●) subjects. The supine position results in delayed gastric emptying and absorption of acetaminophen. (Data from Nimmo, W.S., and Prescott, L.F.[24])

and stay there until it disintegrates. This may cause damage to the esophageal mucosa, leading to ulceration and later to stricture or perforation.

Esophageal ulceration has been described for many drugs including aspirin and other nonsteroidal anti-inflammatory drugs (NSAIDs), slow-release KCl, tetracycline, doxycycline, clindamycin, quinidine, and iron salts. One case report[25] cites a patient with mild asthma who on one occasion, after forgetting to take the evening dose of slow-release theophylline, swallowed his medication without water when he went to bed. The tablets seemed to lodge in his esophagus; he ignored this sensation, swallowed several times, and went to sleep. On awakening, the patient experienced severe, sharp retrosternal pain; this persisted for 2 weeks. A large local esophageal erosion was identified on esophagoscopy and the patient was treated with hourly antacids; symptoms resolved within one week.

Slow esophageal transit also delays drug absorption. Twenty patients awaiting cardiac catheterization swallowed a single tablet containing acetaminophen and barium sulfate. The first 11 subjects swallowed the tablet with up to 15 ml water while supine; the tablet's progress down the esophagus was followed by fluoroscopy. In 10 of these subjects, transit of the tablet was delayed in the esophagus. The 9 subjects who followed, swallowed the tablet while standing; in all cases, it entered the stomach immediately.[26]

The mean peak plasma concentration of acetaminophen in the patients who experienced no esophageal delay was 8.8 μg/ml and the median time to peak was 35 min, whereas mean peak concentration was 5.9 μg/ml and median time to peak was 105 min in those where tablet transit was delayed in the esophagus. When there is delayed esophageal transit, absorption in the first 60 min is much less than when normal transit occurs.

Patients should be advised that tablets and capsules must be taken with several swallows (at least 2 ounces) of water or other beverages, while standing or sitting upright. This is particularly important for drugs that may damage the esophageal mucosa or that need to be absorbed rapidly to induce sleep or relieve pain.

On the basis of aspirin absorption studies, it has been suggested that migraine causes a significant delay in gastric emptying.[27] Thirty minutes after 900 mg of effervescent aspirin the mean plasma salicylate concentration in 35 patients during a migraine attack was 5 mg/100 ml, compared with a value of about 7 mg/100 ml in 14 control patients. Impairment of absorption correlated with the severity of the headache and the gastrointestinal symptoms at the time of treatment. There is the possibility that severe pain in general may retard gastric emptying.

The effect of acute migraine attack on the absorption of tolfenamic acid, an NSAID, was studied in 7 female patients.[28] Migraine attacks delayed absorption. At 2 hr after oral administration mean drug concentration in plasma was about 4 μg/ml in the absence of an attack but only 1.8 μg/ml during an attack; mean peak concentrations were found at 2 hr and 4 hr, respectively. These findings are probably the result of the delay in gastric emptying that accompanies a migraine attack. Rectal metoclopramide accelerates gastric emptying and absorption of oral tolfenamic acid; the combination may be useful for the treatment of migraine in certain patients.

Not only is gastric emptying an important determinant of the overall absorption rate, in some cases it may be rate limiting. In other words, the apparent absorption rate constant of a drug determined from pharmacokinetic studies may actually equal the first-order rate constant for gastric emptying. This hypothesis was recently tested and confirmed by simultaneously measuring gastric emptying and the rate of appearance in blood of acetaminophen after oral administration to healthy subjects.[29] The emptying pattern and the plasma acetaminophen concentration-time profile were closely related. For example, when the start of gastric emptying was delayed, there was a corresponding lag period during which the plasma concentration did not rise or rose slightly. On the other hand, the most rapid increases in plasma acetaminophen concentrations were found when a substantial proportion of the dose emptied in an initial squirt. In those cases where gastric emptying could be described as a simple monoexponential process, there was agreement between the apparent absorption rate constant (determined from the blood data) and the gastric emptying rate constant (Fig. 3–6). These findings confirm that gastric emptying, rather than transmucosal transfer from the lumen of the small intestine, is the rate-limiting step in the absorption of acetaminophen given orally in solution. In all cases, the calculated rate constant for transfer of drug from the small intestine to the bloodstream was greater than the rate constant for

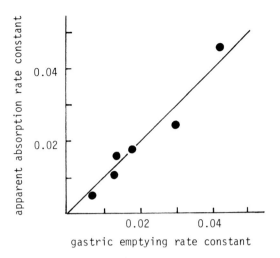

Fig. 3–6. Relationship between the apparent absorption rate constant (min^{-1}) and the gastric emptying rate constant (min^{-1}) after a single oral dose of acetaminophen in healthy subjects who emptied the drug from their stomachs in a monoexponential manner. The line of identity is shown. Under certain conditions, the absorption rate of a drug is rate-limited by gastric emptying. (Data from Clements, J.A., et al.[29])

gastric emptying. Once the drug reached the small intestine, absorption was rapid (mean absorption half-life of about 7 min).

There are many examples of the influence of drugs that affect gastric emptying on the absorption rate of other drugs administered concomitantly (Fig. 3–7). Propantheline has been found to reduce the absorption rate of riboflavin, sulfamethoxazole, ethanol, and acetaminophen.[30–33] Intramuscular administration of meperidine or heroin produces a profound delay in the gastric emptying and absorption of acetaminophen.[34] On the other hand, metoclopramide increases the absorption rate of ethanol,[32] acetaminophen,[33] tetracycline,[35] and pivampicillin.[36] In most of these cases, there is little effect on the extent or completeness of absorption.

The motility of the small intestine as indicated by small bowel transit time also plays a role in drug absorption. The mean transit time of unabsorbed food residues or insoluble granules through the human small intestine is estimated to be about 4 hr.[37]

Intestinal transit of pharmaceutical dosage forms—solutions, small pellets, and several unit forms such as nondisintegrating capsules and tablets—ranged from 3 to 4 hr, independent of the dosage form and whether the subjects were fed or fasted.[38] The gastrointestinal transit (i.e., the time

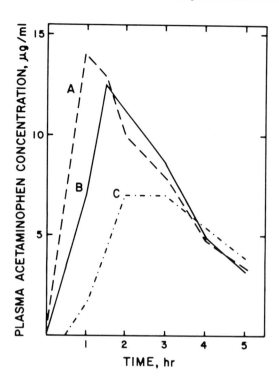

Fig. 3–7. The effects of metoclopramide (A) and propantheline (C) on acetaminophen concentrations in plasma (μg/ml) after a single oral dose of acetaminophen. The middle plot (B) shows the drug level-time curve in control subjects. Metoclopramide promotes absorption and propantheline retards absorption by affecting gastric emptying. (Data from Nimmo, J., et al.[33])

to reach the cecum after oral administration) of a constant release-rate tablet was 7.6 hr, on the average, in 4 subjects. Stomach emptying averaged 3.1 hr. Therefore, intestinal transit time was 4.5 hr.[39] The rather short residence in the small intestine has implications for the design of prolonged-release dosage forms. A product designed to release drug over a 6-hr period may demonstrate poor bioavailability if it is rapidly emptied from the stomach and the drug is poorly absorbed in the large bowel.

Propantheline and similar drugs increase small bowel transit time, whereas metoclopramide accelerates transit through the small intestine. The extent of absorption of drugs that are incompletely absorbed may be dependent on intestinal motility. Clinical studies show that propantheline increases the absorption of riboflavin by more than twofold in healthy subjects,[30] enhances the absorption of hydrochlorothiazide by about one third[40] and nitrofurantoin by about 50%,[41] and markedly increases the steady-state serum concentration of digoxin in patients on maintenance digoxin therapy.[42] In an-

other group of patients, the concomitant administration of metoclopramide reduced the steady-state serum concentration of digoxin.[42] The effects of propantheline and metoclopramide on digoxin levels in serum are the result of changes in the extent of absorption of digoxin.

Drug absorption studies based on recovery of unchanged drug in the urine after a single oral dose indicate that the bioavailability of chlorothiazide is only about 20% after a 500 mg dose, but increases to 50% when the dose is reduced to 50 mg. These nonlinear characteristics suggest the possibility of saturable or site-specific gastrointestinal absorption, sensitive to changes in gastric emptying and intestinal transit.

To test this hypothesis, the bioavailability of chlorothiazide 500 mg was studied in fasted subjects on three different occasions, the drug given alone, given with propantheline 30 mg, or given with metoclopramide 20 mg.[43] Urinary recovery of unchanged drug was 23% of the dose when chlorothiazide was given alone, increased to 55% when propantheline was co-administered, and decreased to 13% when given with metoclopramide. The bioavailability of chlorothiazide doubled when stomach emptying rate and intestinal transit were decreased by propantheline and was cut in half when emptying and transit were accelerated by metoclopramide.

Other factors that influence motility also influence the bioavailability of certain drugs. For example, riboflavin is well absorbed in children with hypothyroidism but poorly absorbed in children with hyperthyroidism, compared with gastrointestinal absorption in healthy children.[44] Treatment of the thyroid disorder results in normalization of riboflavin absorption. These findings are consistent with the known effects of thyroid disease on intestinal transit. Accelerated intestinal transit induced by a laxative (bisacodyl) markedly decreased the azo reduction of sulfasalazine to 5-amino-salicylic acid (5-ASA) and sulfapyridine in the large bowel.[45] Urinary recovery of 5-ASA after a single dose was reduced to one-third control levels. Since 5-ASA appears to be the active component of sulfasalazine, the efficacy of sulfasalazine in the treatment of colitis may be reduced in patients with profuse diarrhea.

EFFECTS OF FOOD ON DRUG ABSORPTION

In general, gastrointestinal absorption is favored by an empty stomach, but the interaction between food and drugs during regular treatment with oral medication is almost inevitable. Furthermore, one should not give all drugs on an empty stomach; some are irritating and should be administered with or after a meal.

There is considerable evidence that food sometimes has a marked but unpredictable effect on the rate and extent of drug absorption. Food tends to decrease the rate of stomach emptying, due to feedback mechanisms from receptors in the proximal small intestine, and often delays the rate of drug absorption. Food tends to increase gastric pH, which may increase or decrease the dissolution or chemical degradation of some drugs. Food appears to interact directly with certain drugs either to enhance or to reduce the extent of absorption. Food stimulates gastrointestinal secretions, which may facilitate the dissolution of poorly water soluble drugs. Food also stimulates hepatic blood flow, which may have implications for the bioavailability of drugs subject to first-pass hepatic metabolism.

The potential for food-drug interactions is sufficiently great that the US Food and Drug Administration now requires studies as to the effects of food on drug absorption as part of the biopharmaceutic characterization of almost every new drug intended for oral administration. This requirement is also being applied to new dosage forms of established drugs.

Welling,[46] a leading authority in this particular area of drug interactions, has reviewed the literature on the effects of food on drug absorption. In general, the absorption of drugs taken 30 min or more before a meal is not affected by food. This guideline, however, does not apply to drugs given in slowly dissolving or prolonged-release dosage forms. The potential for interaction is greatest when drugs are given with a meal or within 30 min after a meal. Food appears to have little effect on drug absorption when the drug is given 2 hr or more after a meal. In his review, Welling[46] places drug-food interactions into one of four categories: interactions resulting in unaffected, delayed, reduced, and increased drug absorption.

In most of the cases reported to date, food appears to have either little effect on drug absorption or, at worst, it decreases the rate but not the extent of drug absorption. Examples include digoxin, acetaminophen, pentobarbital sodium, various sulfonamides, and cephalexin.[47–52]

The most dramatic delays in drug absorption have been observed with enteric-coated tablets, which pass intact from the stomach to the small intestine and do not release drug until reaching the intestine. Less important effects are observed with well-dispersed dosage forms (e.g., solutions, suspensions, and rapidly disintegrating tablets and capsules), particularly when the drugs in question are water soluble. It follows that the effect of food on drug absorption may depend on the dosage form used. For example, food delays the absorption of enteric-coated aspirin tablets and digoxin tablets but has no effect on the absorption of enteric-coated aspirin granules and digoxin elixir.

Recent studies have shown that food has little effect on the absorption of enalapril,[53] an angiotensin-converting enzyme (ACE) inhibitor, and isosorbide mononitrate.[54] Enalapril is a prodrug, activated by deesterification to enalaprilat, the diacid form of the drug. The time course of serum concentrations and urinary excretion of enalaprilat after a single 40-mg oral dose of enalapril is virtually identical whether the drug is given to healthy subjects after fasting or after a standardized heavy breakfast. The oral administration of isosorbide mononitrate after a light breakfast results in a slight delay in achieving peak concentrations in plasma and a slight decrease in those concentrations, consistent with the slowing of gastric emptying, but causes no important changes in the area under the drug-concentration time curve. Similar findings have been reported for isosorbide dinitrate.[55]

The lack of effect of food on the absorption of enalapril is in contrast to the substantial effect of food on the absorption of captopril, a related drug. Singhvi et al.[56] have shown that oral administration of [^{14}C]captopril after breakfast decreases the recovery of total radioactivity in the urine from 76% (fasted state) to 49% of the administered dose. Comparing the effect of food on the absorption of enalapril and captopril, Swanson et al.[53] suggested that "oral absorption of enalapril may . . . be more complete than captopril because the sulfhydryl group of [captopril] binds to other thiol groups in food." The absorption of penicillamine, another sulfhydryl-containing drug, is reduced by about 50% when given after a meal compared with the results observed in fasting subjects.[57]

Most of the penicillins and tetracyclines, certain erythromycin preparations, lincomycin, and rifampin fall into the category of significantly reduced absorption after a meal.[58–67] Absorption of almost all tetracyclines is also markedly reduced when these drugs are taken with milk or milk products, presumably because of an interaction with calcium resulting in a poorly soluble complex.[66] The influence of food on the absorption of antimicrobial agents is the subject of a comprehensive review.[67]

The absorption of other drugs may also be seriously impaired when given with food. For example, administration of the anticholinergic drug propantheline immediately after a meal virtually abolished its effects on salivation, suggesting a substantial decrease in absorption. In contrast, hyoscyamine suppressed salivation to the same extent whether given after a meal or to fasted subjects.[68]

Another example is hydralazine. Shepherd et al.[69] studied the effect of food on hydralazine levels and hemodynamic response in 6 patients with essential hypertension. A single oral dose of hydralazine (1 mg/kg) was given in solution after fasting and after a standardized breakfast.

Hydralazine blood levels were reduced almost 50% when the drug was given after a meal compared with the fasting state. The higher blood levels of hydralazine observed in fasted subjects produced a greater change in mean arterial pressure (MAP). Overall, a statistically significant linear correlation was observed between the percent decrease in MAP and the log of peak hydralazine concentration in blood. The authors concluded that the reduction of vasodepressor response when hydralazine is taken after breakfast suggests that patients with hypertension should take the drug at a fixed time in relation to meals.

Food dramatically affects the absorption of nifedipine.[70] After a single 10-mg dose, peak concentration was 136 ng/ml when the subjects were fasted, but only 43 ng/ml after a meal. Time to peak concentration shifted from about 1 hr to 3.5 hr. The mean AUC for nifedipine over the first 6 hr was reduced by nearly 50% when the calcium channel blocker was given after breakfast. The high C_{max} value observed in fasted subjects was associated with a large drop in blood pressure and tachycardia. Although the effects of nifedipine were less intense when taken with a meal, they remained clinically significant. Taking nifedipine after food may reduce vasodilator side effects while retaining therapeutic efficacy.

Tolbutamide taken 30 min before a meal lowers blood glucose in patients with diabetes more effectively than when it is taken with a meal.[71] This finding is clinically relevant and probably reflects both better absorption when taken in the fasted state and higher blood levels of tolbutamide at peak glu-

Table 3–1. Effect of Dose on the Absorption of Riboflavin in Fasting and Nonfasting Healthy Subjects*

Dose (mg)	Percent absorbed	
	Fasting	Nonfasting
5	48	62
10	30	63
15	16	61

*Data from Levy, G., and Jusko, W.J.[7]

cose load when it is taken 30 min before rather than with a meal.

Increased absorption of drugs after a meal is usually rationalized in terms of the following mechanisms: (a) delayed gastric emptying causing more drug to dissolve before reaching the small intestine or a longer residence time at specific absorption sites in the small intestine; (b) increased gastrointestinal secretions (e.g., bile) improving drug solubility; (c) direct interaction and solubilization of drug by food (e.g., high-fat meals); (d) food-related increases in hepatic blood flow causing a decrease in first-pass metabolism. According to Welling,[46] "the increased absorption of riboflavin and also chlorothiazide in nonfasting subjects is probably related to nonsaturation of active absorption processes or to slow passage of drug past a gastrointestinal 'absorption window'."

The absorption of riboflavin is much greater when it is taken after a standard breakfast.[7] The data in Table 3–1 suggest that the effect of the meal increases with increasing dose of the vitamin. The substantial increase in the bioavailability of griseofulvin when given with a high-fat meal may be related to solubilization of the water-insoluble drug by lipid components of the meal and by stimulated bile secretions.[72,73]

A 20% increase in the urinary excretion of hydrochlorothiazide was found after oral administration of the drug with food compared to that observed in fasted subjects.[74] The bioavailability of chlorothiazide is doubled when taken immediately following a meal compared to that found in fasting subjects.[75] Studies in children suggest that administration of erythromycin ethylsuccinate after a meal results in a substantial improvement in bioavailability.[76]

Colburn et al.[77] recently reported that food increases the bioavailability of isotretinoin (*cis*-retinoic acid), a retinoid with low aqueous solubility indicated for the treatment of severe recalcitrant

Table 3–2. Effect of Food on the Bioavailability of Nitrofurantoin, as Determined from Urinary Excretion*

Dosage form	Percent excreted	
	Fasting	Nonfasting
Capsule (macrocrystalline)	22	40
Tablet (microcrystalline)	36	44

*Data from Bates, T.R., Sequeira, J.A., and Tembo, A.V.[79]

cystic acne. The standard dosage form of isotretinoin is a soft gelatin capsule containing the drug dispersed in lipid; bioavailability of the drug in fasted subjects is 50% or less. Increases in the bioavailability of isotretinoin of 50 to 100% were observed when the retinoid was given with a meal or 1 hr after the meal compared with the results observed in fasted subjects. The authors suggest the "stimulation of bile flow due to meal anticipation and ingestion could have enhanced the solubilization [and bioavailability] of isotretinoin."

Still greater effects of food have been reported with etretinate, another retinoid used in the treatment of psoriasis.[78] A high fat meal or two glasses of milk increased the peak concentration following a single dose of etretinate 100 mg by more than threefold and the total AUC by 3- to 4-fold.

Administration of nitrofurantoin in commercial capsules containing macrocrystalline drug or tablets containing microcrystalline drug after a standard breakfast results in more complete absorption of the antibacterial agent compared to that obtained after administration to fasting subjects.[79] The effect of food, however, is much more pronounced with the macrocrystalline form of the drug (Table 3–2). In fact, although there are substantial differences in bioavailability between the two products in fasted subjects, no significant differences were observed when the products were compared in nonfasted individuals. These findings are important because both products are recommended to be taken with food to improve gastrointestinal tolerance. The common practice of using only fasted subjects in bioavailability studies would appear to be inappropriate for drugs that are normally administered with meals.

Food increases the bioavailability of hydrochlorothiazide (HCT) and triamterene (T) from an incompletely absorbed combination product, but has no effect on the absorption of these diuretics from a well-absorbed product.[80] Studies in fasted subjects indicated that 30 to 45% of administered

HCT and less than 25% of administered T was absorbed after product I, compared with 55 to 60% absorption for each drug after product II. Following administration of I with a high fat meal, the absorption of both drugs increased; the percentage of the dose of HCT and T absorbed from product I was directly related to the fat content of the meal. Food did not affect the absorption of either drug in product II.

In another study, lithium sulfate was given as a single dose in slow-release tablets to 30 healthy subjects, fasting and after a standard meal.[81] Postprandial administration produced practically no adverse effects, whereas lithium on an empty stomach caused diarrhea in about 20% of the subjects. Absorption was estimated by determining the amount of lithium excreted in the urine in a group of 10 subjects. The drug was well absorbed when given after food, but when given on an empty stomach the absorption was lower in most subjects, apparently owing to more rapid gastrointestinal passage in connection with diarrhea. The investigators propose that slow-release lithium preferably be administered after meals.

Clinical investigations convincingly demonstrate that the bioavailability of certain drugs subject to first-pass hepatic metabolism during absorption is increased after a meal. For example, administration of hydralazine following a meal results in a two- to threefold increase in bioavailability.[82]

Food has also been found to substantially increase the serum levels of propranolol and metoprolol after a single dose;[83] the propranolol data are described in Figure 3–8. Other studies have shown that the increase in propanolol bioavailability is related to the protein content of the meal.[84]

The influence of a high-protein meal on the kinetics of simultaneous iv (unlabeled) and oral (deuterated) doses of propranolol was studied in 6 healthy subjects.[85] The clearance of propranolol, as determined from the iv dose, was nearly rate-limited by hepatic blood flow. The high-protein meal increased systemic clearance from about 1.0 L/min to 1.4 L/min; bioavailability [(oral AUC × 100)/iv AUC] increased from 27% (fasting) to 45.5% (after meal).

These findings are probably the result of the well-known effect of food on splanchnic blood flow. Meals, particularly meals high in protein content, increase splanchnic blood flow transiently but substantially over fasting values. Olanoff and his colleagues,[85] found that hepatic blood flow, estimated by indocyanine green (ICG) clearance, in-

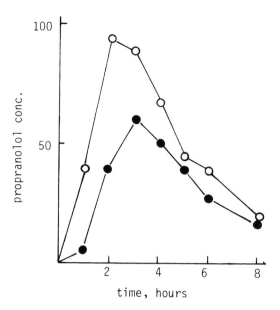

Fig. 3–8. Propranolol concentrations (ng/ml) in serum after a single oral dose to fasted (●) and fed (○) subjects. Oral administration of propranolol after a meal results in higher serum levels. (Data from Melander, A., et al.[83])

creased by 34% 60 min after the meal, from 1.7 L/min to 2.3 L/min. In theory, a transient increase in hepatic blood flow rate during absorption would allow a larger fraction of the oral dose to evade first-pass metabolism and result in an increased bioavailability.[86]

MALABSORPTION

Malabsorption may be defined as any disorder with impaired absorption of fat, carbohydrate, protein, vitamins, electrolytes, minerals, or water. Drug-induced malabsorption has been observed after administration of neomycin, phenytoin, aminosalicylate, and certain antineoplastic agents such as methotrexate.[87] 5-Fluorouracil (5-FU) damages the gastrointestinal epithelium and impairs the function of the mucosa to serve as a barrier to large polar molecules. The absorption of polyvinylpyrolidone (PVP) and tobramycin, both of which are ordinarily rather poorly absorbed, is substantially enhanced in patients receiving a course of 5-FU therapy.[88] Patients with intestinal malabsorption invariably lose weight. The most important clinical phenomena are usually those of lipid deprivation, including signs of fat-soluble vitamin (i.e., vitamins A, D, E, and K) deficiencies.

Chronic alcoholism may also lead to a leaky gut.[89] Intestinal permeability was investigated with a labeled marker in alcoholic patients and found to be significantly higher than in control subjects, even after up to 4 days of abstinence from alcohol. In several cases, increased permeability was evident up to 2 weeks after cessation of drinking. The investigators suggest that increased intestinal permeability could result in the absorption of toxic, ordinarily non-absorbable compounds (MW <5000), which might accelerate the extraintestinal tissue damage common in alcoholics.

Studies concerned with drug absorption in patients with malabsorption have been limited, and the results of such studies generally have not been remarkable. For example, the absorption of isoniazid, chloramphenicol, salicylate, and cycloserine in 10 patients with demonstrable villous atrophy, 8 of whom absorbed xylose to a limited extent, was similar to that measured in 10 healthy control subjects matched for age and sex.[90] The investigators suggest that the intestinal absorption of drugs by passive diffusion may remain largely unaltered in states in which histologic and/or abnormal results from nutrient absorption tests indicate intestinal injury.

Although some studies have shown that the absorption of digoxin is reduced in malabsorptive states,[91] others have found digoxin absorption to be normal in such patients.[92] Reduced bioavailability of digoxin in patients with malabsorption syndrome may be the result of delayed or impaired dissolution rather than a defect in the intrinsic absorption of the drug. For example, one case report showed that a patient with a radiation-induced malabsorption syndrome absorbed digoxin poorly from a tablet preparation but that substitution of digoxin elixir overcame the bioavailability problem.[93] Other investigators[94] have shown that high-dose chemotherapy [carmustine (BCNU) or cyclophosphamide] and radiation therapy decreased the absorption of digoxin by about 50%, when the drug was given in the form of a tablet. A much smaller effect, a reduction of only 15%, was noted when the drug was given as a solution inside a capsule. Chemotherapy- and radiation-induced malabsorption of digoxin can be influenced by the pharmaceutical formulation.

The difficulty of maintaining a therapeutic phenytoin concentration in a patient who developed seizures while undergoing treatment for a malignant tumor with cisplatinum, vinblastine, and bleomycin was documented by Sylvester et al.[95] Low serum levels and poor control were observed during chemotherapy despite relatively high oral doses of phenytoin. The investigators related these findings to changes in the intestinal mucosa induced by the cytotoxic drugs, resulting in impaired absorption of phenytoin. Based on serum levels and urinary excretion data, the authors calculated that the patient absorbed only about 20% of the administered dose of phenytoin; bioavailability of phenytoin in healthy volunteers is greater than 80%.

An investigation of propranolol found that bioavailability on oral administration was similar in normal subjects and patients with untreated celiac disease.[96] Direct perfusion of the proximal jejunum, however, indicated that propranolol absorption is reduced about 70% in celiac patients compared to normal subjects. The results suggest that, ordinarily, propranolol is absorbed in the duodenum; morphologic changes in the intestine distal to the optimum absorption site have no effect on propranolol bioavailability. On the other hand, the absorption of propranolol from prolonged-release products may be impaired in patients with active celiac disease.

Concern that serum levels of cyclosporine may be inadequate in some patients prompted Atkinson et al.[97] to determine cyclosporine concentrations during oral and iv therapy in 56 patients receiving bone marrow transplants for treatment of hematologic malignancy or severe aplastic anemia. Patients with no clinical intestinal dysfunction (no vomiting or diarrhea) consistently demonstrated high serum levels after an oral dose. In contrast, patients with intestinal disease (e.g., chemoradiation enteritis, graft-versus-host disease of the intestine, or *Candida* enteritis) showed poor absorption of oral cyclosporine. Intestinal disease had no effect on serum levels of cyclosporine after iv infusions. The authors concluded that the iv infusion of cyclosporine is reliable and is the indicated route when malabsorption or intolerance of the oral preparation occurs.

Surgical resection of the small bowel can result in impaired absorption of digoxin as well as other drugs. Reduced bioavailability of digoxin was found in 5 of 9 patients who had undergone jejunal bypass surgery.[92] A strong correlation was noted between the length of jejunum remaining in continuity and the area under the digoxin concentration in serum versus time curve. The bioavailability of hydrochlorothiazide is reduced by 50% in patients who had undergone intestinal shunt operations for obesity.[98] Epileptic patients with an ileojejunal by-pass receiving phenytoin are likely to require much higher oral doses to achieve adequate blood levels of the drug because absorption is only about 30% of normal.[99] In some cases, bioavailability in intestinal bypass patients may be improved by giving a more rapidly absorbed form of the drug.

REFERENCES

1. Fordtran, J.S., et al.: Permeability characteristics of the human small intestine. J. Clin. Invest., *44*:1935, 1965.
2. Schedl, H.P.: Absorption of steroid hormones from the human small intestine. J. Clin. Endocrinol. Metab., *25*:1309, 1965.
3. Wass, M., and Evered, D.F.: Transport of penicillamine across mucosa of the rat small intestine in vitro. Biochem. Pharmacol., *19*:1287, 1970.
4. Evered, D.F., and Randall, H.G.: Absorption of amino acid derivatives of nitrogen mustard from rat intestine in vitro. Biochem. Pharmacol., *11*:372, 1962.
5. Schanker, L.S., and Jeffrey, J.J.: Active transport of foreign pyrimidines across the intestinal epithelium. Nature, *190*:727, 1961.
6. Schanker, L.S., and Tocco, D.J.: Active transport of some pyrimidines across the rat intestinal epithelium. J. Pharmacol. Exp. Ther., *128*:115, 1960.
7. Levy, G., and Jusko, W.J.: Factors affecting the absorption of riboflavin in man. J. Pharm. Sci., *55*:285, 1966.
8. Thomson, A.D., and Leevy, C.M.: Observations on the mechanism of thiamine hydrochloride absorption in man. Clin. Sci., *43*:153, 1972.
9. Mayersohn, M.: Ascorbic acid absorption in man-pharmacokinetic implications. Eur. J. Pharmacol., *19*:140, 1972.
10. Crouthamel, W.G., et al.: Drug absorption. IV. Influence of absorption kinetics of weakly acidic drugs. J. Pharm. Sci., *60*:1160, 1971.
11. Cooke, A.R., and Hunt, J.N.: Absorption of acetylsalicylic acid from unbuffered and buffered gastric contents. Am. J. Dig. Dis., *15*:95, 1970.
12. Cooke, A.R., and Birchall, A.: Absorption of ethanol from the stomach. Gastroenterology, *57*:269, 1969.
13. Granger, B., and Baker, R.F.: Electron microscope investigation of the striated border of intestinal epithelium. Anat. Rec., *107*:423, 1950.
14. Wilson, J.P.: Surface area of the small intestine in man. Gut, *8*:618, 1967.
15. Chadwick, V.S., Phillips, S.F., and Hofmann, A.F.: Measurement of intestinal permeability using low molecular weight polyethylene glycols (PEG 400). II. Application to normal and abnormal permeability states in man and animals. Gastroenterology, *73*:247, 1977.
16. Booth, C.C.: Sites of absorption in the small intestine. Fed. Proc., *26*:1563, 1967.
17. Winne, D.: Influence of blood flow on intestinal absorption of xenobiotics. Pharmacology, *21*:1, 1980.
18. Hurwitz, A., Robinson, R.G., and Herrin, W.F.: Prolongation of gastric emptying by oral propantheline. Clin. Pharmacol. Ther., *22*:206, 1977.
19. Horton, R.E., Ross, F.G.M., and Darling, G.H.: Determination of the emptying time of the stomach by use of enteric-coated barium granules. Br. Med. J., *1*:1537, 1965.
20. Blythe, R.H., Grass, G.M., and MacDonnell, D.R.: Formulation and evaluation of enteric-coated aspirin tablets. Am. J. Pharm., *131*:206, 1959.
21. Wagner, J.G., Veldkamp, W., and Long, S.: Enteric coatings. IV. In vivo testing of granules and tablets coated with styrene-maleic acid copolymer. J. Pharm. Sci., *49*:128, 1960.

22. Heading, R.C., et al.: The dependence of paracetamol absorption on the rate of gastric emptying. Br. J. Pharmacol., 47:415, 1973.
23. Logan, R.F.A., et al.: Effect of cimetidine on serum gastrin and gastric emptying in man. Digestion, 18:220, 1978.
24. Nimmo, W.S., and Prescott, L.F.: The influence of posture on paracetamol absorption. Br. J. Clin. Pharmacol., 5:348, 1978.
25. Enzenauer, R.W., Bass, J.W., and McDonnell, J.T.: Esophageal ulceration associated with oral theophylline. N. Engl. J. Med., 310:261, 1984.
26. Channer, K.S., and Roberts, C.J.C.: Effect of delayed esophageal transit on acetaminophen absorption. Clin. Pharmacol. Ther., 37:72, 1985.
27. Volans, G.N.: Absorption of effervescent aspirin during migraine. Br. Med. J., 4:265, 1974.
28. Tokola, R.A., and Neuvoncn, P.J.: Effects of migraine attack and metoclopramide on the absorption of tolfenamic acid. Br. J. Clin. Pharmacol., 17:67, 1984.
29. Clements, J.A., et al.: Kinetics of acetaminophen absorption and gastric emptying in man. Clin. Pharmacol. Ther., 24:420, 1978.
30. Levy, G., Gibaldi, M., and Procknal, J.A.: Effect of an anticholinergic agent on riboflavin absorption in man. J. Pharm. Sci., 61:798, 1972.
31. Antonioli, J.A., et al.: Effect of gastrectomy and of an anticholinergic drug on the gastrointestinal absorption of sulfonamide in man. Int. J. Clin. Pharmacol., 5:212, 1971.
32. Gibbons, D.O., and Lant, A.F.: Effects of intravenous and oral propantheline and metoclopramide on ethanol absorption. Clin. Pharmacol. Ther., 17:578, 1975.
33. Nimmo, J., et al.: Pharmacological modification of gastric emptying: Effects of propantheline and metoclopramide on paracetamol absorption. Br. Med. J., 1:587, 1973.
34. Nimmo, W.S., et al.: Inhibition of gastric emptying and drug absorption by narcotic analgesics. Br. J. Clin. Pharmacol., 2:509, 1975.
35. Nimmo, J.: The influence of metoclopramide on drug absorption. Postgrad. Med. J., 49(Suppl.):25, 28, 1973.
36. Gothoni, G., et al.: Absorption of antibiotics: Influence of metoclopramide and atropine on serum levels of pivampicillin and tetracycline. Ann. Clin. Res., 4:228, 1972.
37. Eve, I.S.: A review of the physiology of the gastrointestinal tract in relation to radiation doses of radioactive materials. Health Phys., 12:131, 1966.
38. Davis, S.S., Hardy, J.G., and Fara, J.W.: Transit of pharmaceutical dosage forms through the small intestine. Gut, 27:886, 1986.
39. Wilson, C.G., and Hardy, J.G.: Gastrointestinal transit of an osmotic tablet drug delivery system. J. Pharm. Pharmacol., 37:573, 1985.
40. Beermann, B., and Groschinsky-Grind, M.: Enhancement of the gastrointestinal absorption of hydrochlorothiazide by propantheline. Eur. J. Clin. Pharmacol., 13:385, 1978.
41. Jaffe, J.M.: Effect of propantheline on nitrofurantoin absorption. J. Pharm. Sci., 64:1729, 1975.
42. Manninen, V., et al.: Altered absorption of digoxin in patients given propantheline and metoclopramide. Lancet, 1:398, 1973.
43. Osman, M., and Welling, P.G.: Influence of propantheline and metoclopramide on the bioavailability of chlorothiazide. Curr. Ther. Res., 34:404, 1983.
44. Levy, G., MacGillivray, M.H., and Procknal, J.A.: Riboflavin absorption in children with thyroid disorders. Pediatrics, 50:896, 1972.
45. VanHees, P.A.M., et al.: Influence of intestinal transit time on azo-reduction of salicyazosulphapyridine. Gut, 20:300, 1979.
46. Welling, P.G.: Interactions affecting drug absorption. Clin. Pharmacokin., 9:404, 1984.
47. White, R.J., et al.: Plasma concentrations of digoxin after oral administration in the fasting and postprandial state. Br. Med. J., 1:380, 1971.
48. Jaffe, J.M., Colaizzi, J.L., and Barry, H.: Effects of dietary components on gastrointestinal absorption of acetaminophen tablets in man. J. Pharm. Sci., 60:1646, 1971.
49. Smith, R.B., et al.: Pharmacokinetics of pentobarbital after intravenous and oral administration. J. Pharmacokinet. Biopharm., 1:5, 1973.
50. MacDonald, H., et al.: Effect of food on absorption of sulfonamides in man. Chemotherapy, 12:282, 1967.
51. Harvengt, C., et al.: Cephradine absorption and excretion in fasting and nonfasting volunteers. J. Clin. Pharmacol., 13:36, 1973.
52. Welling, P.G.: Influence of food and diet on gastrointestinal drug absorption: a review. J. Pharmacokinet. Biopharm., 5:291, 1977.
53. Swanson, B.N., and Vlassess, P.H.: Influence of food on the bioavailability of enalapril. J. Pharm. Sci., 73:1655, 1984.
54. Laufen, H., and Leitold, M.: The effect of food on the oral absorption of isosorbide-5-mononitrate. Br. J. Clin. Pharmacol., 18:967, 1984.
55. Taylor, T., et al.: Isosorbide dinitrate pharmacokinetics. Arzneim. Forsch., 32:1329, 1982.
56. Singhvi, S.M., et al.: Effect of food on the bioavailability of captopril in healthy subjects. J. Clin. Pharmacol., 22:135, 1982.
57. Osman, M.A., et al.: Reduction in oral penicillamine absorption by food, antacid, and ferrous sulfate. Clin. Pharmacol. Ther., 33:465, 1983.
58. Kirby, W.M.M., Roberts, C.E., and Bardick, R.E.: Comparison of two new tetracyclines with tetracycline and demethylchlortetracycline. Antimicrob. Agents Chemother., 1961, p. 286.
59. Klein, J.O., and Finland, M.L.: The new penicillins. N. Engl. J. Med., 269:1019, 1963.
60. Welling, P.G., et al.: Bioavailability of ampicillin and amoxicillin in fasted and nonfasted subjects. J. Pharm. Sci., 66:549, 1977.
61. Kaplan, K., Chew, W.H., and Weinstein, L.: Microbiological, pharmacological and clinical studies of lincomycin. Am. J. Med. Sci., 250:137, 1965.
62. Siegler, D.I., et al.: Effect of meals on rifampicin absorption. Lancet, 2:197, 1974.
63. Welling, P.G., et al.: Bioavailability of tetracycline and doxycycline in fasted and nonfasted subjects. Antimicrob. Agents Chemother., 11:462, 1977.
64. Welling, P.G., et al.: Bioavailability of erythromycin stearate: Influence of food and fluid volume. J. Pharm. Sci., 67:764, 1978.
65. Rutland, J., Berend, N., and Marlin, G.E.: The influence of food on the bioavailability of new formulations of erythromycin stearate and base. Br. J. Clin. Pharmacol., 8:343, 1979.
66. Rosenblatt, J.E., et al.: Comparison of in vitro activity and clinical pharmacology of doxycycline and other tetracyclines. Antimicrob. Agents Chemother., 1966, p. 134.
67. Welling, P.G.: The influence of food on the absorption of antimicrobial agents. J. Antimicrob. Chemother., 9:7, 1982.
68. Ekenved, G., et al.: Influence of food on the effect of propantheline and l-hyoscyamine on salivation. Scand. J. Gastroenterol., 12:963, 1977.
69. Shepard, A.M.M., Irvine, N.A., and Ludden, T.M.: Effect of food on blood hydralazine levels. Clin. Pharmacol. Ther., 36:14, 1984.

70. Hirasawa, K., et al.: Effect of food ingestion on nifedipine absorption and haemodynamic response. Eur. J. Clin. Pharmacol., 28:105, 1985.

71. Samanta, A., et al.: Improved effect of tolbutamide when given before food in patients on long-term therapy. Br. J. Clin. Pharmacol., 18:647, 1984.

72. Crounse, R.G.: Human pharmacology of griseofulvin: the effect of fat intake on gastrointestinal absorption. J. Invest. Dermatol., 37:529, 1961.

73. Kabasakalain, P., et al.: Parameters affecting absorption of griseofulvin in a human subject using urinary metabolite excretion data. J. Pharm. Sci., 59:595, 1970.

74. Beermann, B., and Groschinsky-Grind, M.: Gastrointestinal absorption of hydrochlorothiazide enhanced by concomitant intake of food. Eur. J. Clin. Pharmacol., 13:125, 1978.

75. Welling, P.G., and Barbhaiya, R.H.: Influence of food and fluid volume on chlorothiazide bioavailability: comparison of plasma and urinary excretion methods. J. Pharm. Sci., 71:32, 1982.

76. Coyne, T.C., et al.: Bioavailability of erythromycin ethylsuccinate in pediatric patients. J. Clin. Pharmacol., 18:194, 1978.

77. Colburn, W.A., et al.: Food increases the bioavailability of isotretinoin. J. Clin. Pharmacol., 23:534, 1983.

78. Colburn, W.A., et al.: Effect of meals on the kinetics of etretinate. J. Clin. Pharmacol., 25:583, 1985.

79. Bates, T.R., Sequeira, J.A., and Tembo, A.V.: Effect of food on nitrofurantoin absorption. Clin. Pharmacol. Ther., 16:63, 1974.

80. Williams, R.L., et al.: Effects of formulation and food on the absorption of hydrochlorothiazide and triamterene or amiloride from combination diuretic products. Pharm. Res., 4:348, 1987.

81. Jeppson, J., and Sjogren, J.: The influence of food on side effects and absorption of lithium. Acta Psychiatr. Scand., 51:258, 1975.

82. Melander, A., et al.: Enhancement of hydralazine bioavailability by food. Clin. Pharmacol. Ther., 22:104, 1977.

83. Melander, A., et al.: Enhancement of the bioavailability of propranolol and metoprolol by food. Clin. Pharmacol. Ther., 22:108, 1977.

84. Walle, T., et al.: Food-induced increase in propranolol bioavailability—Relationship to protein and effects on metabolites. Clin. Pharmacol. Ther., 30:790, 1981.

85. Olanoff, L.S., et al.: Food effects on propranolol systemic and oral clearance: support for a blood flow hypothesis. Clin. Pharmacol. Ther., 40:408, 1986.

86. McLean, A.J., et al.: Food, splanchnic blood flow, and bioavailability of drugs subject to first-pass metabolism. Clin. Pharmacol. Ther., 24:5, 1978.

87. Rahman, F., and Cain, G.D.: Current concepts in therapy: Drug-induced malabsorption—A review. South. Med. J., 66:724, 1973.

88. Siber, G.R., Mayer, R.J., and Levin, M.J.: Increased gastrointestinal absorption of large molecules in patients after 5-fluorouracil therapy for metastatic colon carcinoma. Cancer Res., 40:3430, 1980.

89. Bjarnason, I., Ward, K., and Peters, T.J.: The leaky gut of alcoholism: possible route of entry for toxic compounds. Lancet, 1:179, 1984.

90. Mattila, J.J., Jussila, J., and Takki, S.: Drug absorption in patients with intestinal villous atrophy. Arzneimittelforsch., 23:583, 1973.

91. Hall, W.H., and Doherty, J.E.: Tritiated digoxin. XXII. Absorption and excretion in malabsorption syndromes. Am. J. Med., 56:437, 1974.

92. Gerson, C.D., Lowe, E.H., and Lindenbaum, J.: Bioavailability of digoxin tablets in patients with gastrointestinal dysfunction. Am. J. Med., 69:43, 1980.

93. Jusko, W.J., et al.: Digoxin absorption from tablets and elixir. The effect of radiation-induced malabsorption. JAMA, 230:1554, 1974.

94. Bjornsson, T.D., et al.: Effects of high-dose cancer chemotherapy on the absorption of digoxin in two different formulations. Clin. Pharmacol. Ther., 39:25, 1986.

95. Sylvester, R.K., et al.: Impaired phenytoin bioavailability secondary to cis-platinum, vinblastine, and bleomycin. Ther. Drug Monitor, 6:302, 1984.

96. Sandle, G.I., et al.: Propranolol absorption in untreated coeliac disease. Clin. Sci., 63:81, 1982.

97. Atkinson, K., et al.: Detrimental effect of intestinal disease on absorption of orally administered cyclosporine. Transplant Proc., 15:2446, 1983.

98. Backman, L., et al.: Malabsorption of hydrochlorothiazide following intestinal shunt surgery. Clin. Pharmacokinet., 4:63, 1979.

99. Kennedy, M.C.V., and Wade, D.N.: Phenytoin absorption in patients with ileojejunal bypass. Br. J. Clin. Pharmacol., 7:515, 1979.

4

Gastrointestinal Absorption— Physicochemical Considerations

Drug absorption is influenced by many physiologic factors, but it also depends on the solubility, particle size, chemical form, and other physicochemical characteristics of the drug itself. Clinically significant differences in the absorption of closely related drugs such as lincomycin and clindamycin, ampicillin and pivampicillin, or secobarbital and sodium secobarbital are the result of differences in physicochemical properties.

ABSORPTION OF DRUGS FROM SOLUTION

The dissociation constant and lipid solubility of a drug, as well as the pH at the absorption site, dictate the absorption characteristics of a drug from solution. The interrelationship among these parameters is known as the pH-partition theory of drug absorption. This theory has been advanced by extensive investigations in laboratory animals[1-5] and in man,[6] and provides a basic framework for the understanding of drug absorption from the gastrointestinal tract and drug transport across biologic barriers in the body.

The pH-partition theory of drug absorption is based on the assumption that the gastrointestinal tract is a simple lipid barrier to the transport of drugs and chemicals. Accordingly, the nonionized form of an acid or basic drug, if sufficiently lipid soluble, is absorbed but the ionized form is not. The larger the fraction of drug in the nonionized form at a specific absorption site, the faster is the absorption. Acid and neutral drugs may be absorbed from the stomach but basic drugs are not. The rate of absorption is related to the oil-water partition coefficient of a drug; the more lipophilic the compound, the faster is its absorption.

Drug pKa and Gastrointestinal pH

The fraction of drug in solution that exists in the nonionized form is a function of both the dissociation constant of the drug and the pH of the solution. The dissociation constant is often expressed for both acids and bases as a pKa (the negative logarithm of the acidic dissociation constant). The pKa values of several drugs and the relative acid or base strengths of these compounds are shown in Figure 4–1. The relationship between pH and pKa, and the extent of ionization is given by the Henderson-Hasselbalch equation:

for an acid

$$pKa - pH = \log (fu/fi)$$

and for a base

$$pKa - pH = \log (fi/fu)$$

where fu and fi are the fractions of the drug present in the un-ionized and ionized forms, respectively.

Most acid drugs are predominantly un-ionized at the low pH of gastric fluids and may be absorbed from the stomach as well as from the intestines. The pH range found in the gastrointestinal tract from the stomach to the colon is about 1 to 8. Very weak acids (pKa > 8) such as phenytoin, theophylline, or glutethimide are essentially un-ionized throughout the gastrointestinal tract. The ionization of weak acids with pKa values ranging from about 2.5 to 7.5 is sensitive to changes in pH. More than 99% of the weak acid aspirin (pKa = 3.5) exist as un-ionized drug in gastric fluids at pH 1. On the other hand, only about 0.1% of aspirin is un-ionized at pH 6.5 in the fluids of the small intestine. Despite this seemingly unfavorable ratio of non-

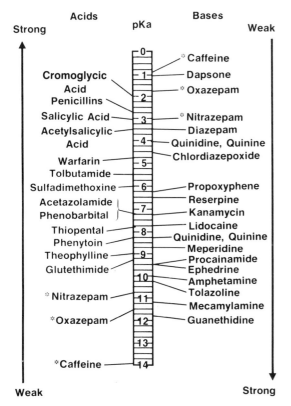

Fig. 4–1. The pKa values of certain acidic and basic drugs. Those drugs denoted with an asterisk* are ampho-teric. (From Rowland, M., and Tozer, T.N.[7])

ionized to ionized drug, aspirin and most weak acids are well absorbed in the small intestine. A large surface area and a relatively long residence time in the small intestine are contributing factors. These factors minimize the need for a large fraction of the drug to be in an un-ionized form in the small intestine. Strong acids (e.g., cromolyn) are ionized throughout the gastrointestinal tract and are poorly absorbed.

Table 4–1. Comparison of Gastric Absorption at pH 1 and pH 8 in the Rat*

	pKa	% Absorbed at pH 1	% Absorbed at pH 8
Acids			
5-Sulfosalicylic	<2.0	0	0
5-Nitrosalicylic	2.3	52	16
Salicylic	3.0	61	13
Thiopental	7.6	46	34
Bases			
Aniline	4.6	6	56
p-Toluidine	5.3	0	47
Quinine	8.4	0	18
Dextromethorphan	9.2	0	16

*Data from Schanker, L.S., et al.[2]

Table 4–2. Comparison of Intestinal Absorption in the Rat at Several pH Values*

		% Absorbed at			
	pKa	pH 4	pH 5	pH 7	pH 8
Acids					
5-Nitrosalicylic	2.3	40	27	0	0
Salicylic	3.0	64	35	30	10
Acetylsalicylic	3.5	41	27	—	—
Benzoic	4.2	62	36	35	5
Bases					
Aniline	4.6	40	48	58	61
Amidopyrine	5.0	21	35	48	52
p-Toluidine	5.3	30	42	65	64
Quinine	8.4	9	11	41	54

*Data from Schanker, L.S., et al.[3]

Most weak bases are poorly absorbed, if at all, in the stomach since they are largely ionized at low pH. Codeine, a weak base with a pKa of about 8 will have only 1 of every million molecules in the nonionized form in gastric fluid at pH 1. The pH range of the intestines from the duodenum to the colon is about 5 to 8. Weakly basic drugs (pKa < 5), such as dapsone, diazepam, or chlordiazepoxide, are essentially un-ionized throughout the intestines. Strong bases, those with pKa values of 5 to 11, show pH-dependent absorption. Stronger bases, such as mecamylamine or guanethidine, are ionized throughout the gastrointestinal tract and tend to be poorly absorbed.

Convincing evidence of the importance of dissociation in drug absorption is found in the results of studies in which the pH at the absorption site is changed. According to the Henderson-Hasselbalch equations, an increase in the pH of the stomach should retard the absorption of weak acids but promote the absorption of weak bases; this is evident in Table 4–1. A clinical study has found similar results in healthy subjects. The gastric absorption of aspirin is considerably reduced when the drug is given in a buffered solution (gastric pH about 5) compared to the results following administration of aspirin in an unbuffered solution (gastric pH about 2). The data in Table 4–2 permit a comparison of the intestinal absorption of several drugs from buffered solutions ranging from pH 4 to pH 8. These results are consistent with pH-partition theory.

Lipid Solubility

Certain drugs may be poorly absorbed after oral administration even though they are largely un-ionized in the small intestine; low lipid solubility

Table 4–3. Comparison of Barbiturate Absorption in Rat Colon and Partition Coefficient (Chloroform/Water) of Undissociated Drug*

Barbiturate	Partition coefficient	% Absorbed
Barbital	0.7	12
Aprobarbital	4.9	17
Phenobarbital	4.8	20
Allylbarbituric acid	10.5	23
Butethal	11.7	24
Cyclobarbital	13.9	24
Pentobarbital	28.0	30
Secobarbital	50.7	40
Hexethal	>100	44

*Data from Schanker, L.S.[5]

of the uncharged molecule may be the reason. A guide to the lipophilic nature of a drug is its partition coefficient between a fat-like solvent, such as chloroform or butanol, and water or an aqueous buffer. The effect of lipid solubility on the absorption of a series of barbituric acid derivatives is shown in Table 4–3. Each compound has about the same pKa. In this case, an almost perfect rank correlation exists between partition coefficient and extent of absorption.

The critical role of lipid solubility in drug absorption is a guiding principle in drug development. Polar molecules such as gentamicin, ceftriaxone, heparin, and streptokinase are poorly absorbed after oral administration and must be given by injection. Lipid soluble drugs with favorable partition coefficients are usually well absorbed after oral administration. The selection of a more lipid soluble compound from a series of research compounds often results in improved pharmacologic activity.

Occasionally, the structure of an existing drug can be modified to develop a similar compound with improved absorption. The development of clindamycin, which differs from lincomycin by the single substitution of a chloride for a hydroxyl group, is an example. Even slight molecular modification, however, runs the risk of also changing the efficacy and safety profile of the drug. For this reason, medicinal chemists prefer the development of lipid soluble prodrugs of a drug with poor oral absorption characteristics.

A prodrug is a chemical modification, frequently an ester, of an existing drug that reverts back to the parent compound because of metabolism or chemical reaction in the body. An ideal prodrug is not found in the systemic circulation and has no

intrinsic biologic activity. Prodrugs are developed to overcome one or more undesirable characteristics of the parent drug, i.e., bitter taste, poor solubility, pain on injection, poor distribution, or poor absorption.

Prodrugs designed to improve permeability and oral absorption are more lipid soluble than the parent drug and should be rapidly converted to the parent compound during absorption, in the gut wall or the liver. Pivampicillin, the pivaloyloxymethyl ester of ampicillin, is more lipid soluble and efficiently absorbed than the parent compound.[8] The ester appears to undergo rapid and essentially complete hydrolysis to ampicillin during absorption.

Another prodrug of ampicillin, bacampicillin, a semisynthetic carbonate ester of ampicillin, has also been introduced in the United States. It is rapidly and completely absorbed after oral administration, and completely hydrolyzed to ampicillin; no bacampicillin is detected in blood or tissues. Peak blood levels of ampicillin after oral administration of the prodrug are reached more quickly and are twice those found after an equivalent oral dose of the parent drug.[9] The poor oral absorption of carbenicillin has also been overcome to some degree by synthesizing a lipid-soluble indanyl ester that, once absorbed, is said to be rapidly hydrolyzed to the parent drug.[10]

Cefuroxime axetil is an oral form of the second-generation parenteral cephalosporin cefuroxime. The oral absorption of cefuroxime is negligible. The axetil form of the drug, an acetoxyethyl ester of cefuroxime, has increased lipid solubility, better gastrointestinal absorption, and sufficient oral bioavailability to be clinically useful. Bioavailability has varied from 35 to 50%. After absorption, it is hydrolyzed to cefuroxime.

Factors affecting the absorption of lipid-soluble prodrugs have been studied by Sommers, et al.,[11] who specifically examined the effect of food and of an increased gastric pH on the bioavailability of bacampicillin and cefuroxime axetil. In one study, healthy subjects received each of the prodrugs alone and after treatment with ranitidine and sodium bicarbonate to elevate gastric pH.

Reduced gastric acidity dramatically decreased the bioavailability of bacampicillin (as ampicillin) and cefuroxime axetil (as cefuroxime). The area under the curve (AUC) for serum levels of cefuroxime decreased from 36 (control) to 13 mg-hr/L (after ranitidine and bicarbonate administration) and urinary recovery decreased from 40 to 12% of the dose. The authors indicated that the most likely explanation of the results with bacampicillin is that the ester becomes partially hydrolyzed before absorption when the gastric acidity is reduced by pretreatment with an H_2-receptor blocker and antacid. In the case of cefuroxime axetil, the authors suggest that optimum absorption of the prodrug requires a sufficiently low pH level in the stomach to allow the drug to dissolve in gastric juice.

Food also decreased the bioavailability of bacampicillin. In contrast, the gastrointestinal absorption of cefuroxime axetil was enhanced when the prodrug was taken after breakfast. The investigators suggested that the findings with cefuroxime axetil may be rationalized in terms of delayed gastric emptying and gastrointestinal transit allowing more complete dissolution or prolonged residence at optimal absorption sites in the small intestine.

The oral absorption of terbutaline may be improved considerably by administering it in the form of the dibutyrl ester.[12] Levodopa can be used to deliver dopamine in the treatment of heart failure.[13] We are familiar with the use of levodopa in Parkinson's disease, where levodopa crosses the blood-brain barrier and delivers dopamine to the central nervous system. A large amount of dopamine is also formed outside the CNS. Levels are sufficiently high and sustained to produce improvements in cardiac function in patients with severe heart failure.

Enalaprilat is a potent angiotensin-converting enzyme (ACE) inhibitor, effective in the treatment of hypertension, but its use is restricted to iv administration. It is a diacid, fully ionized in the small intestine and poorly absorbed. Enalapril, its inactive prodrug, has one carboxyl group esterified and is well-absorbed after oral administration and converted in the liver to enalaprilat.

DEVIATIONS FROM THE pH-PARTITION THEORY

The pH-partition theory provides a basic framework for understanding drug absorption, but it is an oversimplification of a more complex process. For example, theory indicates that the relationship between pH and permeation or absorption rate is described by an S-shaped curve corresponding to the dissociation curve of the drug (see Fig. 4–2). For a simple acid or base, the inflection point of the pH-absorption curve should occur at a pH equal to the pKa of the drug. This is rarely observed experimentally. In general, pH-absorption curves are less steep than expected and are shifted to

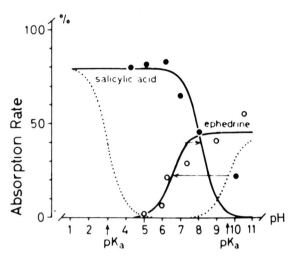

Fig. 4–2. Relationship between absorption rates of salicylic acid and ephedrine and bulk phase pH in the rat small intestine in vivo. Dashed lines indicate curves predicted by the pH-partition theory in the absence of an unstirred layer. (From Winne, D.[17])

higher pH values for acids and to lower pH values for bases. The pH-absorption curves for salicylic acid (a weak acid with a pKa of about 3) and for ephedrine (a weak base with a pKa of about 9.5) have inflection points at about pH 8 and pH 6.5, respectively.[17] Theory predicts little absorption of salicylic acid at pH 8 because at this pH the drug would be almost completely ionized; in fact, the absorption rate of salicylate across the small intestine at pH 8 is about 50% of the maximum absorption rate.

Many investigators have attempted to rationalize the experimental deviations from the unmodified pH-partition theory and there is no lack of suggestions. Several of the more interesting factors that may contribute to the deviations are absorption of the ionized form of the drug, the presence of an unstirred diffusion layer adjacent to the cell membrane, and a difference between lumenal pH and the pH at the surface of the cell membrane.

Absorption of the Ionized Form of a Drug

Certain quaternary ammonium drugs elicit systemic pharmacologic effects after oral administration, suggesting that the restriction to ionized forms of a drug by the gastrointestinal barrier may not be absolute. Several in situ and in vivo studies support this idea. It is conceded today that absorption of organic anions and cations does take place in the small intestine but at a much slower rate than the corresponding un-ionized form of the drug. Crout-hamel et al.[14] have estimated that the permeability ratio of un-ionized to ionized drug across the rat small intestine is about 3 for barbital and about 5.5 for sulfaethidole, but these estimates may be low because they do not take into account the presence of a stagnant aqueous diffusion layer or a difference between lumenal and microclimate pH. Hogerle and Winne,[15] using a more comprehensive absorption model, suggest a ratio of about 190 for benzoic acid. The absorption of ionized forms of a drug would cause the pH-absorption curve to shift to the right for a weak acid and to the left for a weak base; the extent of the shift depends on the relative permeability of the ionized form of the drug.

Mucosal Unstirred Layer

The aqueous stagnant layer is now a well-recognized component of the gastrointestinal barrier to drug absorption (see Fig. 4–3). It is found at the villous surface of the mucosa. The thickness of the layer in the small intestine has been estimated at several hundred micrometers. The unstirred layer is particularly important for drugs that penetrate the barrier rapidly; its role in absorption also varies directly with the effective molecular weight of the drug. The unstirred layer is the rate-limiting barrier for the intestinal absorption of lipids from micellar solutions.[17]

The thickness of the unstirred layer can be reduced by, in effect, stirring the drug solution in the intestinal lumen. The absorption rate of butanol, antipyrine, salicylic acid, and urea from rat jejunal loops perfused in vivo is increased significantly if the intraluminal solution is mixed more efficiently by the simultaneous perfusion of air.[18] The increased absorption rate is mainly the result of reducing the effective thickness of the unstirred layer.

The net effect of the unstirred layer on the pH-absorption profile of a weak electrolyte is a reduction in absorption rate, particularly and perhaps exclusively with respect to the un-ionized form of the drug, and a shift in the inflection point of the curve to the right for acids and to the left for bases.[14,19,20]

A similar unstirred layer over the gastric mucosa, estimated to be 800 to 1000 μm thick, may protect the stomach against injury from certain drugs and chemicals. Duane et al.[21] have specifically considered the role of the unstirred layer in protecting the gastric mucosa from bile salt arising from reflux of duodenal contents into the stomach. Some believe that this reflux is a factor in certain forms of gastritis.

Damage to the gastric mucosa by bile salts results from dissolution of mucosal membrane lipids by lumenal micelles. This damage is associated with increased back-diffusion of hydrogen ions. Duane et al. propose that "the presence of an unstirred water layer on the surface of the gastric mucosa could protect against bile salt injury either by creating a concentration gradient of bile salt from lumen to mucosal surface or by slowing diffusion of lipid-laden mixed micelles away from the mucosal surface."

To support this hypothesis, Duane et al. measured the back-diffusion of hydrogen ions across the rat gastric mucosa before and after exposure to a bile salt solution that was either unmixed or mixed by continuous withdrawal and injection. Continuous mixing of gastric contents decreased the thickness of the unstirred water layer by 45%, from 880 to 448 μm. Mixing also increased back-diffusion of hydrogen ions by about 60% and nearly doubled the efflux of mucosal phospholipid and cholesterol in the bile salt solution. These findings provide

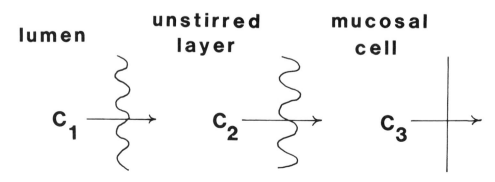

Fig. 4–3. Schematic representation of barriers to gastrointestinal absorption.

evidence that the unstirred water layer helps protect the gastric mucosa from bile-salt injury.

Drug-related gastric injury probably involves mechanisms different from those associated with bile-salt damage. Nevertheless, there is merit in considering the role of the unstirred layer in local adverse effects of drugs. One could imagine that a steep concentration gradient across an unstirred layer could lower drug concentration at the mucosal surface and reduce toxicity.

Microclimate pH

Another factor that can contribute to the deviation of pH-absorption curves from those predicted by the unmodified pH-partition theory is a difference between the lumenal pH and the microclimate or virtual pH at the cell membrane. The microclimate-pH hypothesis is supported by the fact that H^+ ions are secreted into the intestinal lumen.

Hogerle and Winne[15] attempted to characterize the microclimate directly by measuring the pH at the surface of the jejunal mucosa in vivo. The pH of the lumenal solutions was varied over a pH range of 4 to 10.8. In all cases, after lowering the pH electrode down to the tips of the villi, the pH shifted towards neutral. At a lumenal pH of 7, the microclimate pH was 6.4. Microclimate pH varied relatively little with changes in lumenal pH, ranging from about 5.7 to 7.4 over the entire lumenal pH range. The authors proposed the following relationship between microclimate pH and lumenal pH:

$$MpH = A + B (LpH - 7)$$
$$+ C (LpH - 7)^3, \quad (4\text{--}1)$$

where MpH is the microclimate pH, LpH is the lumenal pH, $A = 6.36$, $B = 12.2 \times 10^{-2}$, and $C = 10.3 \times 10^{-3}$. The authors also proposed that a microclimate pH must be invoked to adequately explain the pH-absorption profile for benzoic acid in the rat jejunum.

A Unifying Hypothesis

Hogerle and Winne[15] have developed a model for intestinal absorption that accounts for the factors discussed above. According to this model, the absorption rate of a drug may be described by the following equation:

$$absorption\ rate = (C \times A)/[(T/D)$$
$$+ 1/Pu(fu + fi \times Pi/Pu)] \quad (4\text{--}2)$$

where C is drug concentration in the lumen, A is the absorptive surface area, T is the thickness of the unstirred layer, D is the diffusion coefficient of the drug, *fu* and *fi* are the fractions of the un-ionized and ionized forms of the drug, and *Pu* and *Pi* are the permeability coefficients for the un-ionized and ionized forms of the drug.

The extent of dissociation is a function of the pKa of the drug and microclimate pH; *fu* and *fi* are calculated from the Henderson-Hasselbalch equation. For a weak acid,

$$pKa - MpH = log\ (fu/fi) \quad (4\text{--}3)$$

and for a weak base,

$$pKa - MpH = log\ (fi/fu) \quad (4\text{--}4)$$

The microclimate pH (MpH) is a function of lumenal pH (LpH), according to Equation 4–1.

Equation 4–2 has been used to describe the pH-absorption rate profiles for benzoic acid and aminopyrine under stirred and unstirred conditions.[15] The extension of the pH-partition theory to incorporate the effects of the unstirred layer and microclimate pH provides a far more satisfactory rationalization of the experimental data.

ABSORPTION OF DRUGS FROM SOLID DOSAGE FORMS AND SUSPENSIONS

When a drug is given orally in the form of a tablet, capsule, or suspension, the rate of absorption is often controlled by how fast the drug dissolves in the fluids at the absorption site. In other words, dissolution rate is often the *rate-limiting* (slowest) step in the sequence,

Solid drug $\xrightarrow{\text{Dissolution}}$

Drug in solution at absorption site $\xrightarrow{\text{Absorption}}$ Drug in systemic circulation

When dissolution is the controlling step in the overall process, absorption is said to be *dissolution rate limited*. An example of dissolution rate-limited absorption is shown in Figure 4–4, which depicts the absorption of aspirin in man from solution and from two different types of tablets.[22] Absorption from solution proceeds more rapidly than from tablets. Whenever a drug is more rapidly absorbed from solution than from a solid dosage form, it is likely that absorption is rate-limited by dissolution.

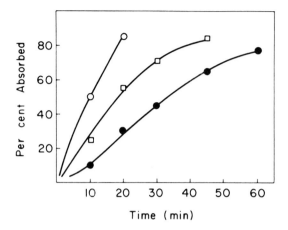

Fig. 4–4. Absorption of aspirin after oral administration of a 650-mg dose in solution (○), in buffered tablets (□), or in regular tablets (●). (Data from Levy, G., Leonards, J.R., and Procknal, J.A.[22])

A general relationship describing the dissolution process was first observed by Noyes and Whitney.[23] The Noyes-Whitney equation states that:

$$dC/dt = kS \, (C_s - C) \qquad (4\text{–}5)$$

where dC/dt is the dissolution rate, k is a constant, S is the surface area of the dissolving solid, C_s is the solubility of the drug or chemical in the solvent, and C is the concentration of the material in the solvent at time t. The constant k has been shown to be equal to D/h, where D is the diffusion coefficient of the dissolving material, and h is the thickness of the *diffusion layer*. The diffusion layer, like the unstirred water layer in the intestine, is a thin, stationary film of solution adjacent to the surface of the solid. The layer is saturated with drug; drug concentration in the layer is equal to C_s. The term $(C_s - C)$ in Equation 4–5 represents the concentration gradient between the diffusion layer and the bulk solution. If absorption is dissolution rate-limited, C is negligible compared to C_s. Under these conditions, Equation 4–5 may be written as:

$$dC/dt = DSC_s/h \qquad (4\text{–}6)$$

Equation 4–6 describes a diffusion-controlled dissolution process.

It is envisioned that when the solid is introduced to the dissolution medium, the drug rapidly saturates the diffusion layer. Drug molecules diffuse from the saturated layer to the bulk (the slow step in the dissolution process) but are immediately replaced in the diffusion layer from the solid surface.

Equation 4–6 is an oversimplified representation

of the dynamics of dissolution; nevertheless, it is qualitatively useful and permits a consideration of the effects of certain important factors on dissolution rate. The solubility (C_s) of many drugs increases with increasing temperature. Therefore, dissolution is temperature-dependent. The diffusion coefficient (D) is inversely related to viscosity; dissolution rate decreases as the viscosity of the solvent increases. The degree of agitation or stirring of the solvent can affect the thickness of the diffusion layer (h). The greater the agitation, the thinner is the layer and the more rapid is the dissolution. Changes in the characteristics of the solvent, such as pH, that affect the solubility of the drug affect the dissolution rate accordingly. Similarly, the use of different salts, or other chemical or physical forms of a drug, which have a solubility or effective solubility different from that of the parent drug, usually affect dissolution rate. Increasing the surface area (S) of drug exposed to the dissolution medium, by reducing the particle size or by attaining more effective wetting of the solid by the solvent, usually increases the dissolution rate. In the discussion that follows, some of the more important factors affecting dissolution are considered in greater detail.

Dissolution and pH

The solubility of a weak acid or base can change considerably as a function of pH. Therefore, differences in dissolution rate are expected in different regions of the gastrointestinal tract.

The total solubility (C_s) of a weak acid is given by:

$$C_s = [HA] + [A^-] \qquad (4\text{–}7)$$

where [HA] is the intrinsic solubility of the nonionized acid (denoted as C_o) and $[A^-]$ is the concentration of its anion, which is infinitely soluble. The concentration of the anion can be expressed in terms of the dissociation constant, Ka, and C_o; that is,

$$C_s = C_o + \frac{KaC_o}{[H^+]} \qquad (4\text{–}8)$$

In a similar manner, the solubility of a weak base is given by:

$$C_s = C_o + \frac{C_o[H^+]}{Ka} \qquad (4\text{–}9)$$

By substituting Equations 4–8 and 4–9 into

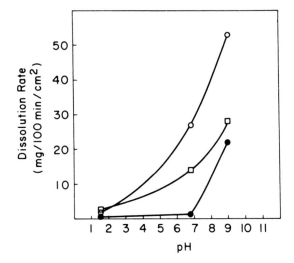

Fig. 4–5. pH-Dependent dissolution of salicylic acid (○), benzoic acid (□), and phenobarbital (●).

Equation 4–6 (the modified Noyes-Whitney relationship), the following dissolution rate equations are obtained:

for a weak acid

$$\frac{dC}{dt} = K' \left[C_o + \frac{Ka\, C_o}{[H^+]} \right] \quad (4\text{–}10)$$

or

$$\frac{dC}{dt} = K' C_o \left[1 + \frac{Ka}{[H^+]} \right] \quad (4\text{–}11)$$

and for a weak base

$$\frac{dC}{dt} = K' C_o \left[1 + \frac{[H^+]}{Ka} \right] \quad (4\text{–}12)$$

where K' is equal to DS/h.

Equations 4–11 and 4–12 indicate that the dissolution rate of weak acids increases with increasing pH (i.e., decreasing $[H^+]$), whereas the dissolution rate of weak bases decreases with increasing pH. The dissolution rate of weak bases is at a maximum in gastric fluids but that of weak acids is at a minimum. The dissolution rate of a weak acid increases as the undissolved drug particles are transported to the more alkaline regions of the gastrointestinal tract. Dissolution rates of some weak acids as a function of pH are shown in Figure 4–5.

It is important for poorly soluble weakly basic drugs to dissolve rapidly in the stomach, since the dissolution rate of undissolved drug in the small intestine may be too low to permit complete absorption. Ketoconazole, a systemic antifungal agent, is a weak base that requires acidity for dissolution and absorption. Patients also being treated with antacids, anticholinergics, or H_2-blockers, which reduce gastric acidity, should take these drugs at least two hours after ketoconazole. This also applies to diazepam and dipyridamole. We are usually less concerned with prompt dissolution of weakly acid drugs in gastric fluids because both dissolution and absorption proceed efficiently in the small intestine.

The relatively poor dissolution of weak acids at the pH of gastric fluids diminishes further the importance of the stomach as a drug absorption site. Although gastric absorption of weak acids may occur from solutions, it is unlikely that much drug dissolves and is absorbed during the limited residence of a solid dosage form in the stomach. Dissolution and gastrointestinal absorption studies with a series of sulfonamides (weak acids) suggest that the importance of gastric absorption is a function of drug solubility at gastric pH.[24] The investigators proposed that the critical value of solubility that distinguishes acid drugs according to their absorption site, stomach or intestine, is about 3 mg/ml in 0.1 N HCl, when 1 g of the drug is given orally to fasted subjects. If the solubility of the drug is less than 3 mg/ml, virtually no absorption occurs in the stomach.

Changes in gastric pH alter the solubility of certain drugs and may affect dissolution and absorption rate. Patients with achlorhydria have a distinctly higher gastric pH and absorb aspirin (pKa = 3.5) more rapidly than healthy subjects.[25] No differences between normal subjects and patients with achlorhydria were found with respect to the absorption rate of acetaminophen, a much weaker acid (pKa = 9.5), whose solubility would be unaffected by changes in gastric pH.

Defective absorption of calcium has been thought to exist in patients with achlorhydria. This has been documented with calcium carbonate.[26] Based on serum and urine levels of calcium, only about 25% of the dose of calcium carbonate was absorbed in patients with achlorhydria compared with that observed in healthy subjects. Curiously, calcium absorption after calcium citrate was twice as effective in patients with achlorhydria than in normal subjects. Both calcium carbonate and citrate were equally well absorbed in normal subjects.

Malabsorption of calcium due to achlorhydria may affect a large population because acid output decreases considerably after the age of 60 years, and calcium carbonate is the most widely used supplement and prophylactic for osteoporosis. Fortunately, the absorption defect is largely overcome when calcium carbonate is given with breakfast.

Differences in gastric and intestinal pH between man and dog have raised questions as to the suitability of a canine model for studying bioavailability. One study found that fasting gastric pH in the dog was significantly higher than in humans (1.8 versus 1.1), and that fasting intestinal pH in dogs was consistently higher than in humans (7.3 versus 6.0).[27]

The pH profiles suggest that absorption of certain drugs would vary between dog and man as a result of pH differences. For example, chlorothiazide (a weak acid, pKa = 6.7) is more efficiently absorbed in the dog than in human subjects. The lower bioavailability in humans may be due to their lower intestinal pH, leading to incomplete dissolution at pH values below the pKa.

Another area of concern in using dogs as an absorption model is the release of drug from enteric-coated products. The polymers used for enteric coating have highly pH-dependent dissolution profiles. An increase in pH of 1 or 2 units could change rapid dissolution to virtually no dissolution. Controlled-release dosage forms sometimes exhibit pH-dependent release profiles, so their performance may also change under different conditions of GI pH.

Diffusion Layer pH

The relationships that have been described between dissolution rate and hydrogen ion concentration (Eqs. 4–11 and 4–12) are approximations because they do not fully account for the influence of the unstirred diffusion layer. These equations tend to overpredict the dissolution rate of weak acids in the small intestine and the dissolution rate of weak bases in the stomach. Strictly speaking, the hydrogen ion concentration of the bulk, $[H^+]$, is not equal to the hydrogen ion concentration of the diffusion layer, $[H^+]_d$. In general:

$$[H^+]_d > [H^+], \text{ for weak acids}$$

and

$$[H^+]_d < [H^+], \text{ for weak bases}$$

The hydrogen ion concentration of the diffusion layer at a given bulk pH may be approximated by determining the pH of an appropriate aqueous buffer solution saturated with the drug. A saturated solution of a weak acid, like that found in the diffusion layer, tends to depress the neutral pH of the intestinal fluids, whereas a saturated solution of a weak base tends to elevate the low pH of gastric fluid.

These differences are probably of limited importance for the absorption of weakly acidic or basic drugs administered as such, but they are important when drugs are given in the form of salts.

Salts

The dissolution rate of a particular salt is usually different from that of the parent compound. Sodium or potassium salts of weak acids dissolve more rapidly than the free acids, regardless of the pH of the dissolution medium.[28] The same is true of the HCl or other strong acid salts of weak bases. Comparative dissolution rates of some weak acids and their sodium salts as a function of pH are shown in Table 4–4.

The effect of salt formation on dissolution rate cannot be explained in terms of solubility and bulk pH, but requires a consideration of the pH of the diffusion layer. At a fixed pH, a drug will have a fixed solubility, irrespective of whether the free acid (or base) or its salt is dissolving. Thus, classical solution theory (see Eqs. 4–8 and 4–9) does not predict the rapid dissolution of salt forms of a drug. In this case, the concept of a diffusion layer becomes helpful.

The pH of the diffusion layer at any given bulk pH is always greater for the sodium or potassium salt of a weak acid than for the corresponding free acid. On the other hand, the pH of the diffusion layer of an HCl or other strong acid salt of a weak base is always smaller than the diffusion layer pH of the corresponding free base. It has been noted that the pH of the diffusion layer may be approximated by determining the pH of an appropriate aqueous buffer saturated with either the drug or its salt. A solution of 0.1 N HCl saturated with sodium salicylate will have a higher pH than the same solution saturated with salicylic acid. It follows that the *effective* solubility and, therefore, the dissolution rate of a soluble salt is always greater than its corresponding free acid or base.

Many examples of the effects of soluble salts on drug absorption can be found. Some studies also report significant differences in clinical response.

Table 4–4. Dissolution Rate of Weak Acids and Their Sodium Salts*

| Compound | pKa | Dissolution rate (mg/100 min/cm²) | | |
		0.1 N HCl pH 1.5	0.1 M Phosphate pH 6.8	0.1 M Borate pH 9.0
Benzoic acid	4.2	2.1	14	28
Sodium salt		980	1770	1600
Phenobarbital	7.4	0.24	1.2	22
Sodium salt		~200	820	1430
Salicylic acid	3.0	1.7	27	53
Sodium salt		1870	2500	2420
Sulfathiazole	7.3	<0.1	~0.5	8.5
Sodium salt		550	810	1300

*Data from Nelson, E.[28]

Marked differences have been observed in the rate and extent of absorption of novobiocin, a weak acid, when administered as such or in the form of a salt.[29] The bioavailability of the drug after oral administration of the sodium salt was twice that of the calcium salt and 50 times that of the free acid.

The potassium salt of penicillin V yields higher peak concentrations of antibiotic in plasma than does the free acid. Oral administration of the calcium salt yields peak plasma levels intermediary to those of the sodium salt and free acid. Differences in absorption rates are consistent with differences in the dissolution rates of the three forms of the drug.[30]

An example of the difference in pharmacologic response that may result from administering two different chemical forms of the same drug is found in studies with tolbutamide and its sodium salt.[31] The dissolution rate of tolbutamide sodium in 0.1 N HCl is about 5000 times greater than that of the free acid. At pH 7.2 the dissolution rate of the sodium salt is about 275 times greater than that of tolbutamide. Oral administration of the sodium salt results in a rapid and pronounced reduction in blood glucose to about 65 to 70% of control levels. The response is comparable to that observed after intravenous administration. The more slowly dissolving free acid produces a gradual decrease in blood sugar to about 80% of control levels, which is observed about 5 hr after administration. It has been suggested that the sodium salt of tolbutamide would produce an undesirable degree of hypoglycemia and that the free acid is the more useful form of the drug for treatment of diabetes.

Barbiturates are often available in the form of sodium salts to achieve a rapid onset of sedation. The findings of several studies support this practice. For example, the average sleep induction times in dogs after oral administration of equivalent doses of secobarbital or secobarbital sodium were 23 min and 8 min, respectively. The sodium salt not only produced a more rapid onset of sleep but its effects were also more predictable. The range of induction times in 6 dogs given the sodium salt was 7.5 to 8.5 min, whereas the range in dogs given secobarbital was 12 to 45 min. Peak drug concentrations in the blood were found within 10 min following administration of secobarbital sodium but not until about 80 min after administration of the free acid.[32]

In a double-blind study of 41 healthy subjects, the sodium salts of phenobarbital and secobarbital were found to produce more rapid and more profound impairment of performance on a variety of tests than the corresponding acid forms.[33] The basis for the observed differences between acids and salts in speed of action is presumably more rapid absorption of the salt form from the gastrointestinal tract. Comparison of heptabarbital and heptabarbital sodium in healthy subjects indicates more rapid absorption after giving the salt form of the drug.[34]

The nonsteroidal anti-inflammatory drug naproxen was originally marketed as the free acid for the treatment of rheumatoid- and osteoarthritis. New indications of the drug for the treatment of mild to moderate pain, including dysmenorrhea, prompted the development of naproxen sodium. The sodium salt is absorbed faster and is more effective in postpartum pain than the free acid.[35]

Certain salts have a lower solubility and dissolution rate than the parent drug, e.g., the aluminum salts of weak acids, and the pamoate salts of weak bases. In these particular examples, insoluble films of either aluminum hydroxide or pamoic acid appear to form over the dissolving solids when the salts are exposed to an alkaline or acidic environment, respectively. These insoluble films further reduce the rate of dissolution.

Use of the relatively insoluble aluminum salt of aspirin has been considered for chewable tablets to minimize the taste of the drug, but aluminum aspirin is more slowly absorbed and less available than aspirin after oral administration.[36]

In general, poorly soluble salts delay the onset of drug effect. Studies with a series of salts of benzphetamine and etryptamine have shown that the median lethal time of death (LT_{50}) of mice following a lethal dose and the median lethal dose (LD_{50}) are inversely related to the dissolution rates of the salts at pH 7.2.[37] The experimental data suggest that salt formation is a potentially useful means of obtaining slow absorption and prolonged effects of certain drugs. The pamoate salt of imipramine has been marketed as a slow-release form of the drug.

Sometimes, problems with chemical stability preclude the use of salts of a drug in a dosage form. Aspirin, for example, is much more prone to hydrolysis in the form of sodium acetylsalicylate than as the free acid. One way to overcome this problem is to form the salt in situ, during dissolution in the gastrointestinal tract. If a mixture of a weakly acidic drug and a nontoxic basic salt is administered, faster dissolution and absorption may be obtained than if the drug were administered alone. When the mixture reaches the gastric fluids, the diffusion layer becomes saturated with both the drug and the basic salt. Accordingly, the pH of the diffusion layer is greater than that for the drug alone. Thus, the solubility of the drug in the diffusion layer and its dissolution rate is increased.

The effects of in situ salt formation on dissolution rate have been demonstrated with benzoic acid.[38] The addition of trisodium phosphate to benzoic acid increases the dissolution rate at pH 1 about 75 times that observed with benzoic acid alone. The principle of in situ salt formation is the basis for the enhanced dissolution and absorption of aspirin from buffered tablets (i.e., tablets of aspirin mixed with small amounts of alkaline materials).[39] Since occult gastrointestinal blood loss produced by therapeutic doses of aspirin is a local effect of the drug,[40] blood losses from aspirin can be reduced by administering the drug in buffered, rapidly dissolving tablets.[41]

Soluble Prodrugs

Most efforts with prodrugs have been directed at improving lipid solubility to increase permeability and absorption after oral administration. The development of a prodrug may also offer an alternative for drugs that show incomplete absorption because of limited water solubility. The minor tranquilizer clorazepate is a prodrug of nordiazepam, an active metabolite of the widely used benzodiazepine diazepam, and is marketed as a dipotassium salt that is freely soluble in water, in contrast to the poorly soluble nordiazepam. Clorazepate, like most prodrugs, has little intrinsic biologic activity, but must be converted to nordiazepam. The prodrug is unstable at low pH; gastric fluid is the principal site of conversion.

A prodrug of the poorly soluble anticonvulsant phenytoin has been described.[42] The sulfate salt of this compound is 9,000 to 15,000 times more soluble in water than phenytoin. The prodrug is unstable at neutral pH and degrades with a half-life of about 7 min.

A general strategy for using soluble prodrugs to improve the gastrointestinal absorption of water-insoluble compounds has been reported.[43] The prodrug is designed to be a substrate for enzymes in the surface coat of the brush border region of the microvillous membrane. Consequently, the properties of the compound are changed from polar to nonpolar, just before reaching the membrane.

The incomplete absorption of acyclovir, an antiherpes drug, when given orally to patients infected with herpesvirus has prompted efforts to develop a water-soluble prodrug that would be better absorbed from the GI tract and then converted to acyclovir. One such compound, desciclovir, lacks the 6-hydroxy group and is also called 6-deoxyacyclovir. Although desciclovir lacks appreciable activity against herpes simplex type 1 virus in vitro, it is readily oxidized in vivo to acyclovir by xanthine oxidase and is far better absorbed than acyclovir after oral administration.

Studies in rats indicate that only about 15% of an orally administered dose of acyclovir is excreted in the urine. When the same rats were given equivalent doses of desciclovir, they excreted 66% of the dose as acyclovir. The urinary excretion of acyclovir in two human volunteers following a 200-mg oral dose of the prodrug was 65% and 68%, respectively. In comparison, about 12% of the dose is recovered in the urine after oral administration of acyclovir and about 70% after intravenous administration of acyclovir.[44] The area under the acyclovir concentration in plasma-versus-time curve in these two individuals was five to six times greater after oral desciclovir than after oral acyclovir.

Petty et al.[45] gave desciclovir 250 mg orally 3 times daily for 10 days to healthy human subjects. Absorption was at least 75% of the dose and almost two-thirds of the administered dose was recovered in the urine as acyclovir. The levels of acyclovir in plasma were of the same magnitude as those found in subjects given intravenous acyclovir 2.5 mg/kg, and about 10 times higher than levels attained after administration of oral acyclovir 200 mg every 4 hr. The peak ratio of acyclovir to desciclovir in plasma was about 4:1. The mean half-life of desciclovir was 0.85 hr., compared with 2.6 hr. for acyclovir, suggesting rapid conversion of desciclovir to acyclovir.

Surface Area and Particle Size

A drug dissolves more rapidly when its surface area is increased. This is usually accomplished by reducing the particle size of the drug. Many poorly soluble, slowly dissolving drugs are marketed in micronized or microcrystalline form. Particle size reduction usually results in more rapid and complete absorption.

The problems associated with low water solubility were not fully appreciated when certain drugs were first introduced. For example, since the original marketing of spironolactone, the therapeutic dose has been reduced twentyfold (from 500 to 25 mg) by reformulation, including micronization of the drug. A similar situation has occurred with griseofulvin. The currently marketed formulation, containing micronized griseofulvin, requires a daily dose of 0.5 g, which is one half that needed when the drug was originally marketed.

Particle size may also be an important factor in the bioavailability of digoxin.[46] A digoxin powder, widely used in the United Kingdom for tablet manufacture, was found to have a mean particle size diameter of 20 to 30 μm. This material was slowly and incompletely absorbed, compared with a solution of digoxin. Reduction in digoxin particle size by ball milling to a mean diameter of 3.7 μm led to an increase in the rate and extent of absorption of the drug.

Another study examined the influence of both particle size and gastrointestinal motility on the absorption of digoxin.[47] In this study, healthy subjects received 0.5 mg digoxin as standard tablets, or tablets containing micronized digoxin or large particle size digoxin. Tablets were given 30 min after 15 mg propantheline (which increases residence time in the small intestine), 10 mg metoclopramide (which decreases residence time in the small intestine), or placebo, and following an overnight fast. The extent of absorption was estimated by determining the cumulative urinary excretion of digoxin over 4 days. Assigning a value of 100% for the bioavailability of digoxin in subjects who took the micronized tablet, Johnson and associates calculated that the relative bioavailability of digoxin taken with placebo was 94% after the standard tablets, but only 43% after the large particle size tablets.[47] Propantheline improved the absorption of digoxin from these large particle size tablets by an average of about 15%, whereas metoclopramide further reduced bioavailability from 43% to 31%. Neither propantheline nor metoclopramide had an effect on the absorption of digoxin after standard or micronized tablets. A general principle derived from these studies is that the bioavailability of slowly dissolving drugs may be sensitive to normal variation and other changes in gastrointestinal motility.

The gastrointestinal absorption of medroxyprogesterone acetate from tablets containing 10 mg of either micronized or nonmicronized drug was compared in a crossover fashion in healthy subjects.[48] The micronized material had 99.9% of the particles smaller than 10 μm. The specific surface areas of micronized and nonmicronized medroxyprogesterone acetate were 7.4 M^2/g and 1.2 M^2/g, respectively. Micronization led to a twofold increase in the extent of absorption of the steroid.

In a clinical study of pyrvinium pamoate in the treatment of patients infested with pinworms, the cure rate for the suspension form of the drug was significantly higher than the cure rate for the existing tablet form (100% versus 61%). In further studies, the efficacy of a new tablet formulation, with particles less than 10 μm in diameter, in contrast to the 50 to 90 μm particles in the original tablet, was compared with that of the suspension. Cure rates with both the new tablet and suspension were similar and exceeded 90%.[49]

The bioavailability of benoxaprofen, an anti-inflammatory agent withdrawn from the market because of serious side effects, was determined in healthy subjects after oral administration of two capsule formulations containing 200 mg of drug in

Table 4–5. Maximum Plasma Phenacetin Concentrations and Urinary Recovery of Phenacetin Metabolites Following Oral Administration of Different Suspensions Each Containing 1.5 g Phenacetin to 6 Healthy Subjects*

Preparation	Average maximum plasma phenacetin concentration (µg/ml)	Urinary recovery†
Fine suspension with polysorbate 80	13.5	75
Fine suspension	9.6	51
Medium suspension	3.3	57
Coarse suspension	1.4	48

*Data from Prescott, L.F., Steel, R.F., and Ferrier, W.R.[51]
†Amount recovered in 24 hr, expressed as percent of dose.

the form of either small crystals (mean = 18.5 µm) or large crystals (mean = 610 µm).[50] The percent absorbed relative to an aqueous solution was found to be 94 to 98% for the small crystals and 39 to 43% for the large crystals. A higher dose of the large crystal formulation resulted in still lower bioavailability; an 800 mg dose was only 22% bioavailable.

The effective surface area of hydrophobic drug particles may be increased by the addition of a wetting agent to the formulation. In one investigation, 6 volunteers received 1.5 g of phenacetin as a fine suspension (particle size less than 75 µm) with and without polysorbate 80 (a wetting agent), as a medium suspension (particle size 150 to 180 µm), and as a coarse suspension (particle size greater than 250 µm).[51] Drug absorption was assessed by determining phenacetin concentrations in the plasma and urinary excretion of drug metabolites. The maximum phenacetin concentrations in the plasma and the urinary recovery of phenacetin metabolites, after administration of the different forms of the drug, are presented in Table 4–5. The importance of particle size in phenacetin absorption is evident. Polysorbate 80 significantly enhances the rate and extent of absorption of phenacetin, probably by increasing the wetting and solvent penetration of the particles and by minimizing aggregation of the suspended particles. Physiologic surface active agents, like bile salts and lysolecithin, probably facilitate the dissolution and absorption of poorly water-soluble drugs in the small intestine.[52]

Effective absorption of cyclosporine appears to require the presence of bile in the small intestine. Absorption studies shortly after liver transplanta-

tion with bile drained through a T-tube found that the AUC over a dosing interval was only 5.2 ng-hr/ml; blood levels peaked at about 250 ng/ml. Some time later, when bile was returned to the small intestine, AUC was 15.8 ng-hr/ml and peak concentrations exceeded 1500 ng/ml.[53] Bile may increase the solubility of cyclosporine by means of micellar solubilization.

There are instances in which particle size reduction fails to increase the absorption rate of a drug. One reason may be that dissolution is not the rate-limiting step in the absorption process. Weak bases dissolve readily in the acidic gastric fluid; gastric emptying, rather than dissolution, is the slow step in the absorption of these drugs.

Micronization sometimes increases the tendency of a drug powder to aggregate, which may lead to a decrease in effective surface area. This problem may be overcome by adding a wetting agent or other excipients to the formulation.

Another approach to deaglomeration is to intimately mix the hydrophobic drug with an excess of a hydrophillic carrier. This is sometimes called an ordered mixture because we strive to have the fine drug particles distributed fairly evenly on course carrier particles. Micronized griseofulvin mixed with sodium chloride crystals dissolves much more rapidly than micronized griseofulvin alone.[54] Extremely rapid dissolution has also been observed when micronized griseofulvin was mixed with lactose.[55] Under these conditions, drug appears to be delivered as free, well-dispersed primary particles after rapid dissolution of the carrier. Mixing griseofulvin with a hydrophobic carrier (paraffin) results in poorer dissolution than with griseofulvin alone.

The advantages to be derived from the use of micronized particles may be reduced or even eliminated by compaction of the particles during tablet compression. For example, the effect of particle size reduction on the absorption of griseofulvin is much greater when the micronized drug is given in a suspension rather than as a tablet.[56]

Certain drugs such as penicillin G and erythromycin are unstable in gastric fluids. Chemical degradation is minimized if the drug does not dissolve readily in the stomach. Particle size reduction and the attendant increase in dissolution rate may result in more extensive degradation of the drug. It has been shown that the addition of a wetting agent to a formulation of erythromycin propionate results in considerably lower drug levels in the blood, apparently owing to increased dissolution and degradation of the antibiotic in gastric fluids.[57]

Crystal Form

Many drugs can exist in more than one crystalline form, a property known as *polymorphism*. The drug molecules exhibit different space-lattice arrangements in the crystal from one polymorph to another. Although the drug is chemically indistinguishable in each form, polymorphs may differ substantially with respect to physical properties such as density, melting point, solubility, and dissolution rate. At any one temperature and pressure only one crystal form will be stable. Any other polymorph found under these conditions is metastable and will eventually convert to the stable form, but the conversion may be slow. The metastable polymorph is a higher energy form of the drug and usually has a lower melting point, greater solubility, and greater dissolution rate than the stable crystal form. Accordingly, the absorption rate and clinical efficacy of a drug may depend on which crystal form is administered.

Some drugs also occur in an amorphous form showing little crystallinity. The energy required for a drug molecule to transfer from the lattice of a crystalline solid to a solvated state is much greater than that required from an amorphous solid. For this reason, the amorphous form of a drug is always more soluble than the corresponding crystalline forms.

Two polymorphs of novobiocin have been identified, one of which is crystalline and the other amorphous. The amorphous material is at least 10 times more soluble than the crystalline form. Studies in dogs fail to detect any absorption of novobiocin after oral administration of the crystalline solid, whereas the amorphous form is rapidly absorbed.[58]

Chloramphenicol palmitate exists in four polymorphs: three crystalline forms (A, B, and C) and an amorphous one. Aqueous suspensions of polymorphs A and B yielded average peak chloramphenicol concentrations in blood of 3 and 22 μg/ml, respectively, on oral administration. Similar differences were noted with respect to the extent of absorption of the two polymorphs.[59]

Studies with sulfameter have indicated the occurrence of six polymorphs. Crystalline form II is about twice as soluble as crystalline form III. Studies in normal human subjects show that the rate and extent of absorption of the sulfonamide are

about 40% greater after administration of form II than after administration of form III.[60]

MacGregor et al.[61] prepared and evaluated tablets of amorphous chlorthalidone stabilized by the addition of polyvinylpyrollidone (PVP). Studies in the dog indicated that these experimental tablets were bioequivalent in both rate and extent of absorption to an oral solution of the thiazide-related diuretic, and more rapidly and efficiently absorbed than the standard commercial tablet. These differences were also seen in bioavailability studies with normal healthy subjects.[62] The tablet with amorphous chlorthalidone appeared to deliver all the drug, whereas the commercial tablet delivered 80% of the drug.

Vardan et al.[63] compared the efficacy of a 15-mg tablet containing amorphous chlorthalidone with that of a 25-mg commercial tablet in a double-blind placebo-controlled trial in patients with mild hypertension. At the end of 12 weeks, a decrease in standing diastolic blood pressure from baseline of at least 5 mm Hg was seen in 61% of the patients on the 15-mg experimental tablet, 72% of the patients on the 25-mg commercial tablet, and 31% of the patients on placebo. Both active drug groups were significantly different from the placebo group but not from each other.

Fewer adverse events were reported in the placebo and 15-mg groups than in the 25-mg group. The decline in potassium was significantly greater in the 25-mg group than in the 15-mg group. At 12 weeks there were four patients with potassium levels below 3 meq/L in the 25-mg group but none in the 15-mg group. The results demonstrate that 15-mg chlorthalidone administered in a superbioavailable dosage form was as effective as the 25-mg commercial tablet in lowering systolic blood pressure; this was accomplished with a reduced incidence of hypokalemia.

Many drugs can associate with solvents to produce crystalline forms called *solvates*. When the solvent is water, the crystal is termed a *hydrate*. Consistent with theory, the anhydrous forms of caffeine, theophylline, and glutethimide dissolve more rapidly in water than do the hydrous forms of these drugs.[64] The anhydrous form of ampicillin is about 25% more soluble than is the trihydrate. A similar difference has been found with respect to the extent of absorption of ampicillin from the two forms of the drug in man.[65]

Several reports suggest that solvate forms of a drug with organic solvents may dissolve faster than the nonsolvated form. This has been observed with the n-pentanol and ethyl acetate solvates of fludro-cortisone, and with the n-pentanol solvate of suc-cinylsulfathiazole.[66] Studies in man indicate that the rate and extent of absorption of griseofulvin were significantly increased after administration of the chloroform solvate compared to that observed after administration of the nonsolvated form of the drug. These findings are consistent with the greater solubility and dissolution rate of the solvate in sim-ulated intestinal fluid.[67]

DRUG STABILITY AND HYDROLYSIS IN THE GASTROINTESTINAL TRACT

Acid and enzymatic hydrolysis of drugs in the gastrointestinal tract is sometimes the reason for poor bioavailability. The hydrolysis and inactiva-tion of penicillin G in the stomach is one example. The half-life of degradation of penicillin G is less than 1 min at pH 1 and about 9 min at pH 2. The stability of methicillin is equally poor. Other pen-icillins, notably ampicillin, are considerably more resistant to acid hydrolysis. The degradation rate of penicillin G decreases sharply with increasing pH; the drug is essentially stable in the small in-testine. Chemical inactivation in the stomach is responsible in part for the relatively low bioavail-ability of penicillin G and methicillin.

The absorption of digoxin is less than complete after oral administration, even when the drug is given in solution. Studies indicate that hydrolysis of digoxin in gastric fluid to digoxigenin and its mono- and bis-digitoxosides contributes to the bio-availability problem.[68–70] Hydrolysis of digoxin at 37°C and pH 3 is minimal after 90 min of incu-bation but increases with increasing acidity; more than 70% is hydrolyzed at pH 1.2 after 30 min and more than 96% after 90 min incubation.[68] Extensive intragastric hydrolysis and reduced bioavailability of digoxin may occur in man under conditions of maximum acid output.

When a drug is unstable in gastric fluids, rapid dissolution may reduce bioavailability. Investiga-tions with a series of erythromycin esters, unstable in the stomach, have shown that bioavailability is inversely proportional to dissolution rate in simu-lated gastric fluid (pH 1). The propionyl ester is absorbed to the greatest extent but dissolves most slowly at pH 1. With such drugs it is desirable to have minimal dissolution in the stomach and rapid dissolution in the small intestine.[71]

Certain prodrugs must be hydrolyzed to the par-ent drug in gastrointestinal fluids to produce clin-ical effects. Clorazepate is rapidly converted to the anxiolytic nordiazepam at low pH. The only site for effective conversion is gastric fluid. Failure to achieve complete conversion results in absorption of the prodrug itself which has little, if any, tran-quilizer activity. Some reports have suggested that the absorption of clorazepate could be adversely affected by giving the drug with antacids, which elevate gastric pH and reduce the rate of conversion to nordiazepam.[72,73] Clinical studies with single oral doses of clorazepate and single or multiple doses of a commercial aluminum-magnesium ant-acid indicate that although antacids reduce the rate of appearance of nordiazepam in plasma, they have no effect on the extent of conversion of clorazepate to nordiazepam.[74]

Chloramphenicol is sometimes given as the pal-mitate or stearate ester, particularly in pediatric practice. The low water solubility of the esters min-imizes the objectionable taste of the drug and fa-cilitates its use in oral suspensions. However, the esters are poorly absorbed; adequate drug absorp-tion requires conversion of the prodrug to chloram-phenicol in the small intestine.[75] Clinical studies in children with serious bacterial infections, who were given the palmitate ester, suggest that conversion is about 70% complete, on the average, and results in satisfactory serum levels of chloramphenicol.[76]

Failure to effectively convert a prodrug to parent drug in the gastrointestinal fluids, gut wall, or liver during absorption results in the prodrug reaching the systemic circulation in relatively large amounts. Chemical or enzymatic conversion of the prodrug to parent drug in blood or tissues may be limited and the prodrug may be metabolized or excreted unchanged. Since the prodrug ordinarily has little or no clinical activity, the net result of these events may be inadequate bioavailability with respect to active drug.

This problem is evident with prodrugs of eryth-romycin. Erythromycin base is unstable in gastric fluid, which leads to poor bioavailability when the drug is given as such. Various esters of erythro-mycin have been investigated to find compounds with a low dissolution rate in gastric fluid and high acid stability and lipid solubility. Two prodrugs with these characteristics, the lauryl sulfate salt of the propionate ester of erythromycin (erythromycin estolate) and the ethylsuccinate ester of erythro-mycin, are marketed in the United States. How-ever, both prodrugs are absorbed directly into the bloodstream; conversion to erythromycin in the blood and tissues is incomplete. High blood levels of total drug, particularly after the estolate, are misleading because the esters have little antibacterial activity. Certain microbiologic assays for estimating antibacterial activity are misleading, because the assay procedure permits in vitro conversion of the ester to erythromycin during incubation. Despite the incomplete conversion to erythromycin, these prodrugs are clinically effective.

A second important problem that may be encountered when prodrugs reach the systemic circulation in relatively large amounts is the appearance of toxicity distinct from that observed with the parent drug. In general, the safety record of the erythromycins has been good; the only major adverse effect of erythromycin therapy is hepatotoxicity, more frequently associated with the estolate and ethylsuccinate forms of the drug.[77]

Alternatives to ester prodrugs of erythromycin include erythromycin stearate, a salt form of the drug, and enteric-coated products of erythromycin base. The stearate is more resistant to acid degradation than the free base. Prolonged retention in the stomach however may result in breakdown of the drug. Food reduces the bioavailability of erythromycin stearate by more than 50%; when used in this form, the drug should be given 1 hr before or 2 hr after meals to obtain maximum bioavailability. Enteric-coated products of erythromycin base do not dissolve in the stomach but allow rapid absorption of the drug in the small intestine. Administration of these products with meals has no effect on bioavailability.

PHYSICAL-CHEMICAL MODELS OF DRUG ABSORPTION

Clinical effectiveness after oral administration is a decided advantage in the development of new drugs. Principal reasons for inadequate bioavailability are low aqueous solubility, poor lipid solubility, drug degradation in the gut lumen, or presystemic metabolism, and dosage form characteristics that limit the dissolution or release rate of the drug. Dissolution rate considerations are important for poorly water soluble drugs, whereas intestinal wall permeability may be rate controlling for polar drugs. Dosage form characteristics may be important for drugs with low aqueous solubility and for delayed-release and prolonged-release preparations.

The earliest quantitative studies on gastrointes-

tinal (GI) absorption focused on permeability and demonstrated that when drugs were administered in aqueous solution, absorption potential was a function of the pH of GI fluids as well as the pK and partition coefficient of the drug. These principles remain conceptually useful but cannot be applied directly because most drugs are given in solid dosage forms, and dissolution and aqueous solubility play an important role in determining absorption. More recent efforts at predicting drug absorption have attempted to relate in vitro dissolution with in vivo absorption characteristics, assuming that dissolution in the GI fluids is the rate-limiting step in drug absorption. These approaches permit differentiation of dosage forms from which a given drug is absorbed at different rates but are less useful for predicting the extent of absorption of a drug. Dressman et al.[78] have developed an equation for calculating absorption potential that for the first time takes both intestinal permeability and drug solubility into account. The strength of their method of prediction lies in its simplicity; the paradigm is based entirely on easily obtained physical-chemical data.

The investigators assumed that the absorption potential of a drug is a function of the membrane-water partition coefficient, which can be correlated to the octanol/water partition coefficient, P; the intrinsic solubility (i.e., the water solubility of the nonionized species at 37°), S; the dose, D; the fraction in nonionized form at pH 6.5, f; and the volume of the lumenal contents, V. Absorption potential, AP, is defined as follows:

$$AP = \log (PfSV/D) \qquad (4\text{--}13)$$

Several drugs covering a wide range of absorption characteristics were selected to evaluate the ability of the estimated absorption potential to predict bioavailability. The drugs varied widely in their physical-chemical characteristics. Partition coefficients covered the range from 0.018 (acyclovir) to 295 (phenytoin). Acyclovir was also the most soluble (1.3 mg/ml), whereas griseofulvin and phenytoin were the least soluble (< 0.02 mg/ml). Griseofulvin, prednisolone, and digoxin are nonionizable; pKa values for acyclovir, chlorothiazide, hydrochlorothiazide, and phenytoin range from 6.7 to 9.5. The lumenal volume was set at 250 ml for all compounds.

The correlation between absorption potential and fraction of the dose absorbed was excellent and indicates for the compounds chosen that absorption potential is a good predictor of bioavailability. Negative AP values (acyclovir and hydrochlorothiazide) suggest poor drug absorption; values of 1.0 or above (phenytoin, prednisolone, and digoxin in solution) suggest nearly complete absorption. Compounds with intermediate AP values (micronized griseofulvin and hydrochlorothiazide) show intermediate bioavailability.

Predictions of percent absorption, however, will not correlate with the bioavailability of compounds subject to substantial first-pass metabolism in the intestinal epithelium or liver or degradation in the gut lumen. Under these conditions, the absorption potential may be considerably greater than systemic availability. For example, propranolol is completely absorbed, but bioavailability is less than 30% after a single oral dose.

Absorption potential as described by Dressman et al.[78] is likely to be a useful tool in drug development so long as it is understood that the parameter is exclusively concerned with the physical-chemical characteristics of the drug and that it cannot be used as the sole indicator of bioavailability. Furthermore, the dissolution rate of a drug but not its solubility is affected by characteristics of the dosage form such as particle size; this distinction may be a significant factor in determining the fraction absorbed when drug solubility is in the μg/ml range. Dressman et al. note that for these cases, the absorption potential is an indicator of how well the drug might be absorbed provided dissolution rate limitations are circumvented by micronizing the drug (griseofulvin), using a solid solution formulation, or giving a solution of the drug in a soft gelatin capsule (digoxin).

More recently, Dressman and Fleisher[79] have investigated the role of dissolution in the absorption of very poorly soluble drugs. They simulated absorption profiles based on a theoretical mixing tank model that takes into account dissolution, absorption, and residence time in the small intestine (assumed to be the site of absorption).

Griseofulvin (G) and digoxin (D) were chosen as examples of drugs that exhibit dissolution rate controlled absorption. Both compounds have low aqueous solubilities (G = 15 μg/ml, D = 25 μg/ml) and high partition coefficients (G = 151, D = 56).

Despite the similar physical-chemical characteristics of griseofulvin and digoxin, estimates of their absorption potential (G = 0.36, D = 3.1) indicate that digoxin is potentially completely absorbed,

whereas griseofulvin is not. This difference is consistent with the results of bioavailability studies in human subjects and is probably related to the markedly different doses of these drugs (G = 500 mg, D = 0.25 mg). There is a 3000-fold difference between griseofulvin and digoxin in terms of the ratio of dose to solubility.

The simulations predict that about 40% of a 500-mg dose of micronized griseofulvin (particles 4 μm in diameter) will be absorbed over a 5-hr period, whereas about 20% of the same dose of "regular" griseofulvin (30 μm mean diameter) will be absorbed over the same period. These estimates are in good agreement with values in the literature from studies in human subjects. The results indicate that even with small particles, the absorption of griseofulvin does not approach 100%. "This suggests that the dose-to-solubility ratio as well as the dissolution rate is a significant limitation to griseofulvin absorption."[79]

The model also predicts that the absorption of micronized griseofulvin is dose-dependent. The fraction absorbed increases from about 40 to 80% as the dose is decreased from 500 to 100 mg. This finding implies that small doses of micronized griseofulvin given more frequently may result in higher drug levels in blood and greater effectiveness.

In summary, the model adequately simulates the gastrointestinal absorption of griseofulvin over a wide range of particle sizes and other conditions. The results indicate that the large dose-to-solubility ratio for this drug restricts the fraction absorbed, even when dissolution rate effects are minimized by administering very fine particles of the drug. "At usual doses of griseofulvin, reducing the particle size below the compendial requirement for the micronized form is not predicted to result in significantly better bioavailability."[79]

Simulations of digoxin absorption present a different picture, principally because of the much smaller doses that are required. As with griseofulvin, the absorption of digoxin is strongly dependent on particle size, but the model predicts that a particle diameter of 5 μm or less will result in complete absorption.

Mean residence time in the small intestine also has a substantial effect on digoxin absorption. With the usual range of residence times (100 to 250 min), the percentage absorbed can vary from 60 to 90%. These predictions are consistent with the effects of metoclopramide and propantheline, drugs that modify gastric emptying and intestinal transit, on the bioavailability of digoxin from certain preparations.

The theoretical considerations proposed by Dressman et al.[78,79] are a substantial contribution to our understanding of drug absorption from the gastrointestinal tract. It appears that quantitative estimates of drug absorption may be made, based solely on certain physical-chemical properties of the drug and several assumptions as to the characteristics of the gut. These advances, however, do not minimize the need for continued improvements in our ability to predict drug absorption after oral administration of solid dosage forms, particularly controlled-release forms.

COMPLEXATION

Complexation of a drug in gastrointestinal fluids may alter the rate and, in some cases, the extent of absorption. The complexing agent may be a substance normal to the gastrointestinal tract, a dietary component, or a component of the dosage form. Intestinal mucus, which contains the polysaccharide mucin, can avidly bind streptomycin and dihydrostreptomycin.[63] This binding may contribute to the poor absorption of these antibiotics. Bile salts in the small intestine interact with certain drugs, including tubocurarine, neomycin, and kanamycin, to form insoluble, nonabsorbable complexes.[81,82]

Tetracyclines form insoluble complexes with calcium. Absorption of these antibiotics is substantially reduced if they are taken with milk, certain foods, or other sources of calcium such as antacids. Similar effects are observed with aluminum antacids. Incorporation of dicalcium phosphate as a filler in a tetracycline dosage form substantially reduces the bioavailability of the drug.

Complexation probably occurs often in pharmaceutical dosage forms. Complex formation between drugs and gums, cellulose derivatives, polyols, or surfactants is common. Such complexes have a much higher molecular weight and are usually considerably more polar than the drug itself. The physicochemical properties of these complexes suggest poor absorption characteristics. Fortunately, most complexes are freely soluble in the fluids of the gastrointestinal tract and dissociate rapidly. Therefore, little or no effect on absorption is noted. There are, however, some exceptions. Amphetamine interacts with carboxymethylcellulose to form a poorly soluble complex that leads to reduced absorption of the drug.[83] Phenobarbital

forms an insoluble complex with polyethylene glycol 4000. The dissolution and absorption rates of phenobarbital from tablets containing this polyol are markedly reduced.[84]

Drug complexes usually differ appreciably from the free drug with respect to water solubility and lipid-water partition coefficient. Many investigators have pursued the possibility that certain polar drugs, which are poorly absorbed, may be made more permeable by forming lipid-soluble complexes. For example, certain dialkylamides can enhance the intestinal absorption of prednisone in the rat. These amides presumably form well-absorbed lipid-soluble complexes with the steroid.[85] The usefulness of this approach to increasing the absorption of certain drugs may be seriously limited by the residence time of the complexing agent in the gastrointestinal tract. If the complexing agent is more rapidly absorbed than the complex, the concentration of complex at the absorption site decreases rapidly and enhanced absorption of the drug may be short-lived.

Perhaps a more rewarding application of complex formation is the administration of water-soluble complexes of drugs that are incompletely absorbed because of poor water solubility. For example, inclusion complex formation of a drug with cyclodextrin is known to increase solubility and dissolution rate.[86]

Hydroquinone forms a water-soluble, rapidly dissolving complex with digoxin.[87] The complex is quickly and completely dissociated when dissolved. An oral tablet formulation containing the complex resulted in significantly faster absorption of digoxin than did a standard tablet of digoxin, but only small differences were found with respect to the extent of absorption.[88] Relative to an intravenous injection of digoxin, the bioavailability of the complex was 70% whereas that of the standard tablet was 65%. In the same subjects, the bioavailability of digoxin from an elixir was about 80%.

ADSORPTION

Certain insoluble substances may adsorb coadministered drugs. This often leads to poor absorption. Studies of the effects of attapulgite or charcoal on promazine absorption in man are illustrative. Attapulgite is used as an active component in antidiarrheal mixtures. Charcoal has been used for various gastrointestinal disorders and is considered to be an efficient antidote in drug intoxication.

Promazine was administered to healthy subjects as a solution in water or as a mixture containing either charcoal or attapulgite. About 80% of the drug was adsorbed initially in the attapulgite preparation and about 50% in the charcoal preparation. Attapulgite decreased the rate but not the extent of absorption of promazine. Charcoal significantly reduced both the rate and extent of drug absorption. In vitro studies indicated that the promazine-charcoal adsorbate had little tendency to dissociate. Apparently, only the fraction of the dose that is initially unadsorbed in the mixture is available for absorption. On the other hand, dissociation of drug from the promazine-attapulgite adsorbate is rapid. Therefore, the extent of adsorption in a dosage form may not be related directly to the effect on absorption. The ease with which the adsorbate dissociates may be the more important factor.[89]

In another investigation, serum concentrations and urinary excretion of lincomycin were determined under the following conditions: (1) 0.5 g in a capsule taken orally with 3 fl oz of water; (2) 3 fl oz of a commercial kaolin-pectin mixture taken 2 hr *before* the capsule; (3) 3 fl oz of the antidiarrheal mixture taken 2 hr *after* the capsule; and (4) 3 fl oz of the mixture taken *with* the capsule. The relative bioavailabilities were 1.00, 0.71, 0.69, and 0.20 for conditions (1), (2), (3), and (4), respectively.[90] Parallel in vitro studies showed that the mixture strongly binds lincomycin. The effect of the antidiarrheal mixture on lincomycin absorption is reduced by administering the drug and the mixture several hours apart.

Cholestyramine and colestipol are insoluble anionic exchange resins used to lower serum cholesterol levels in patients with hypercholesterolemia. These agents bind cholesterol metabolites and bile salts in the intestinal lumen and prevent enterohepatic cycling. They also bind and reduce the absorption of many drugs.

Clinical studies show that fecal radioactivity after oral administration of thyroxine I-131 is markedly increased in patients receiving cholestyramine. Absorption, as determined by whole-body retention and cumulative urinary radioactivity, is correspondingly reduced. If a 4- to 5-hr period exists between the ingestion of cholestyramine and the ingestion of thyroxine, the absorption of the hormone approaches normal in most subjects. Hypothyroid patients receiving thyroxine and cholestyramine, at the same time, should be examined periodically for evidence of lack of efficacy. Ad-

justments in thyroxine dose and in the time interval between the two drugs should be made, if appropriate.[91]

Single-dose studies in adult subjects have shown that cholestyramine significantly reduces the absorption of the anticoagulants warfarin[92] and phenprocoumon.[93] Cholestyramine also affects the bioavailability of digoxin.

Brown et al.[94] studied the effect of continuous treatment with cholestyramine on steady-state levels of digoxin resulting from either two 0.25-mg digoxin tablets or two 0.2-mg digoxin capsules (containing a solution of the drug) once a day for 2 weeks. Bioavailability was determined from the steady-state 24-hr area under the serum concentration-time curve (AUC, ng $\times$ hr/ml).

The AUC values for tablets alone and with the resin were 32.8 and 22.4, a decrease of about 32%. For the capsules alone and with cholestyramine, AUC values were 31.7 and 24.7, a decrease of about 22%. The results show that the 0.2-mg capsule of digoxin is bioequivalent to the 0.25-mg tablet with respect to AUC. The results also suggest that cholestyramine may have a greater effect on the more slowly dissolving tablets than on the capsules of digoxin.

Unlike cholestyramine, colestipol had no apparent effect on phenprocoumon absorption.[95] On the other hand, colestipol has been found to decrease chlorothiazide absorption by 50% even when the drug was taken 1 hr after the resin.[96] Doses of cholestyramine (8 g) and colestipol (10 g), equieffective in lipid lowering, produce similar reductions in the bioavailability of propranolol when given with the drug.[97] Additional examples of drug-drug interactions affecting absorption are described in Chapter 14.

REFERENCES

1. Shore, P.A., Brodie, B.B., and Hogben, C.A.M.: Gastric secretion of drugs—a pH partition hypothesis. J. Pharmacol. Exp. Ther., *119*:361, 1957.
2. Schanker, L.S., et al.: Absorption of drugs from the stomach. I. The rat. J. Pharmacol. Exp. Ther., *120*:528, 1957.
3. Schanker, L.S., et al.: Absorption of drugs from the rat small intestine. J. Pharmacol. Exp. Ther., *123*:81, 1958.
4. Hogben, C.A.M., et al.: On the mechanism of intestinal absorption of drugs. J. Pharmacol. Exp., Ther., *125*:275, 1959.
5. Schanker, L.S.: On the mechanism of absorption from the gastrointestinal tract. J. Med. Pharm. Chem., *2*:343, 1960.
6. Hogben, C.A.M., et al.: Absorption of drugs from the stomach. II. The human. J. Pharmacol. Exp. Ther., *120*:540, 1957.
7. Rowland, M., and Tozer, T.N.: Clinical Pharmacokinetics: Concepts and Applications. 2nd Ed. Philadelphia, Lea & Febiger, 1989.

8. Foltz, E.L., et al.: Clinical pharmacology of pivampicillin. Antimicrob. Agents Chemother., 1970. p. 442.

9. Anon.: Bacampacillin hydrochloride (Spectrobid). Med. Lett., *23*:49, 1981.

10. Knirsch, A.K., Hobbs, D.C., and Korst, J.J.: Pharmacokinetics, toleration, and safety of indanyl carbenicillin in man. J. Infect. Dis., *127*:S105, 1973.

11. Sommers, DeK., et al.: Influence of food and reduced gastric acidity on the bioavailability of bacampicillin and cefuroxime axetil. Br. J. Clin. Pharmacol., *18*:535, 1984.

12. Hornblad, Y., et al.: The metabolism and clinical activity of terbutaline and its prodrug ibuterol. Eur. J. Clin. Pharmacol., *10*:9, 1976.

13. Rajfer, S.I., et al.: Beneficial hemodynamic effects of oral levodopa in heart failure. Relation to the generation of dopamine. N. Engl. J. Med., *310*:1357, 1984.

14. Crouthamel, W.G., et al.: Drug absorption. IV. Influence of pH on absorption kinetics of weakly acidic drugs. J. Pharm. Sci., *60*:1160, 1971.

15. Hogerle, M.L., Winne, D.: Drug absorption by the rat jejunum perfused *in situ*. Dissociation from the pH-partition theory and role of microclimate-pH and unstirred layer. Naunyn Schmiedebergs Arch. Pharmacol., *322*:249, 1978.

16. Wilson, F.A., Sallee, V.L., and Dietschy, J.M.: Unstirred water layers in intestine: rate determinant of fatty acid absorption from micellar solutions. Science, *174*:1031, 1971.

17. Winne, D.: The influence of unstirred layers on intestinal absorption. *In* Intestinal Permeation, Workshop Conference Hoechst. Vol. 4. Edited by M. Kramer and F. Lauterbach. Amsterdam-Oxford: Excerpta Medica International Congress Series No. 391, 1977, pp. 58–64.

18. Winne, D.: Dependence of intestinal absorption *in vivo* on the unstirred layer. Naunyn Schmiedebergs Arch. Pharmacol., *304*:175, 1978.

19. Suzuki, A., Higuchi, W.I., and Ho, N.F.H.: Theoretical model studies of drug absorption and transport in the gastrointestinal tract. I. J. Pharm. Sci., *59*:644, 1970.

20. Suzuki, A., Higuchi, W.I., and Ho, N.F.H.: Theoretical model studies of drug absorption and transport in the gastrointestinal tract. II. J. Pharm. Sci., *59*:651, 1970.

21. Duane, W.C., et al.: Role of the unstirred layer in protecting the murine gastric mucosa from bile salt. Gastroenterol., *91*:913, 1986.

22. Levy, G., Leonards, J.R., and Procknal. J.A.: Development of *in vitro* dissolution tests which correlate quantitatively with dissolution-rate limited absorption. J. Pharm. Sci., *54*:1719, 1965.

23. Noyes, A.A., and Whitney, W.R.: The rate of solution of solid substances in their own solutions. J. Am. Chem. Soc., *19*:930, 1897.

24. Ogata, H., et al.: Studies on dissolution tests of solid dosage forms. IV. Relation of absorption sites of sulfonamides administered orally in solid dosage form to their solubilities and dissolution rates. Chem. Pharm. Bull., *27*:1281, 1979.

25. Pottage, A., Nimmo, J., and Prescott, L.F.: The absorption of aspirin and paracetamol in patients with achlorhydria. J. Pharm. Pharmacol., *26*:144, 1974.

26. Recker, R.R.: Calcium absorption and achlorhydria. N. Engl. J. Med., *313*:70, 1985.

27. Lui, C.Y., et al.: Comparison of gastrointestinal pH in dogs and humans: implications on the use of the beagle dog as a model for oral absorption in humans. J. Pharm. Sci., *75*:271, 1986.

28. Nelson, E.: Comparative dissolution rates of weak acids and their sodium salts. J. Am. Pharm. Assoc. (Sci. Ed.), *47*:297, 1958.

29. Furez, S.: Blood levels following oral administration of different preparations of novobiocin. Antibiot. Chemother., *8*:448, 1958.

30. Juncher, H., and Raaschou, F.: Solubility of oral preparations of penicillin V. Antibiot. Med., *4*:497, 1957.

31. Nelson, E., et al.: Influence of absorption rate of tolbu-

tamide on rate of decline of blood sugar levels in normal humans. J. Pharm. Sci., *51*:509, 1962.

32. Anderson, K.W.: Oral absorption of quinalbarbitone and its sodium salt. Arch. Int. Pharmacodyn. Ther., *147*:171, 1964.

33. Epstein, L.C., and Lasagna, L.: A comparison of the effects of orally administered barbiturate salts and barbiturate acids on human psychomotor performance. J. Pharmacol. Exp. Ther., *164*:433, 1968.

34. Breimer, D.D., and deBoer, A.G.: Pharmacokinetics and relative bioavailability of heptabarbital and heptabarbital sodium after oral administration to man. Eur. J. Clin. Pharmacol., *9*:169, 1975.

35. Sevelius, H., et al.: Bioavailability of naproxen sodium and its relationship to clinical analgesic effects. Br. J. Clin. Pharmacol., *10*:259, 1980.

36. Levy, G., and Sahli, B.A.: Comparison of the gastrointestinal absorption of aluminum acetylsalicylate and acetylsalicylic acid in man. J. Pharm. Sci., *51*:58, 1962.

37. Morozowich, W., et al.: Relationship between in vitro dissolution rates, solubilities, and LT_{50}'s in mice of some salts of benzphetamine and etryptamine. J. Pharm. Sci., *51*:993, 1962.

38. Nelson, E.: Dissolution rate of mixtures of weak acids and tribasic sodium phosphate. J. Am. Pharm. Assoc. (Sci. Ed.), *47*:300, 1958.

39. Levy, G., and Hayes, B.A.: Physico-chemical basis of the buffered acetylsalicylic acid controversy. N. Engl. J. Med., *262*:1053, 1960.

40. Leonards, J.R., and Levy, G.: Aspirin-induced occult gastrointestinal blood loss: Local versus systemic effects. J. Pharm. Sci., *59*:1511, 1970.

41. Leonards, J.R., and Levy, G.: Effect of pharmaceutical formulation on gastrointestinal bleeding from aspirin tablets. Arch. Intern. Med., *129*:457, 1972.

42. Anon.: Prodrugs: safer and more effective. Chem. Eng. News, Sept. 23, 1974, pp. 26–27.

43. Amidon, G.L., Leesman, G.D., and Elliott, R.L.: Improving intestinal absorption of water-insoluble compounds: a membrane metabolism strategy. J. Pharm. Sci., *69*:1363, 1980.

44. Krenitsky, T.A., et al.: 6-Deoxyacyclovir: a xanthine oxidase-activated prodrug of acyclovir. Proc. Natl. Acad. Sci., *81*:3209, 1984.

45. Petty, B.G., et al.: Pharmacokinetics and tolerance of desciclovir, a prodrug of acyclovir, in healthy human volunteers. Antimicrob. Agents Chemother., *31*:1317, 1987.

46. Shaw, T.R.D., and Carless, J.E.: The effect of particle size on the absorption of digoxin. Eur. J. Clin. Pharmacol., *7*:269, 1974.

47. Johnson, B.F., O'Grady, J., and Bye, C.: The influence of digoxin particle size on absorption of digoxin and the effect of propantheline and metoclopramide. Br. J. Clin. Pharmacol., *5*:465, 1978.

48. Smith, D.L., Pulliam, A.L., and Forist, A.A.: Comparative absorption of micronized and nonmicronized medroxyprogesterone acetate. J. Pharm. Sci., *55*:398, 1966.

49. Buchanan, R.A., et al.: Pyrvinium pamoate. Clin. Pharmacol. Ther., *16*:716, 1974.

50. Wolen, R.L., et al.: The effect of crystal size on the bioavailability of benoxaprofen: studies utilizing deuterium labeled drug. Biomed. Mass Spectrom., *6*:173, 1979.

51. Prescott, L.F., Steel, R.F., and Ferrier, W.R.: The effects of particle size on the absorption of phenacetin in man. A correlation between plasma concentration of phenacetin and effects on the central nervous system. Clin. Pharmacol. Ther., *11*:496, 1970.

52. Miyazaki, S., et al.: Interaction of drugs with bile components. II. Effect of bile on the absorption of indomethacin and phenylbutazone in rats. Chem. Pharm. Bull., *28*:323, 1980.

53. Mehta, M.U., et al.: Effect of bile on cyclosporin absorp-

tion in liver transplant patients. Br. J.Clin. Pharmacol., 25:579, 1988.

54. Nystrom, C., Westerberg, M.: The use of ordered mixtures for improving the dissolution rate of low solubility compounds. J. Pharm. Pharmacol., 38:161, 1985.

55. Westerberg, M., Jonsson, B., Nystrom, C.: Physicochemical aspects of drug release. IV. The effect of carrier particle properties on the dissolution rate from ordered mixtures. Int. J. Pharmac., 28:23, 1986.

56. Levy, G.: Effect of particle size on dissolution and gastrointestinal absorption rates of pharmaceuticals. Am. J. Pharm., 135:78, 1963.

57. Stephens, V.C., Conine, J.W., and Murphy, H.W.: Esters of erythromycin. IV. Alkyl sulfate salts. J. Am. Pharm. Assoc. (Sci. Ed.), 48:620, 1959.

58. Mullins, J.D., and Macek, T.J.: Some pharmaceutical properties of novobiocin. J. Am. Pharm. Assoc. (Sci. Ed.), 49:245, 1960.

59. Aguiar, A.J., et al.: Effect of polymorphism on the absorption of chloramphenicol from chloramphenicol palmitate. J. Pharm. Sci., 56:847, 1967.

60. Khalil, S.A., et al.: GI absorption of two crystal forms of sulfameter in man. J. Pharm. Sci., 61:1615, 1972.

61. MacGregor, T.R., et al.: Chlorthalidone pharmacodynamics in beagle dogs. J. Pharm. Sci., 74:851, 1985.

62. Farina, P.R., et al.: Relative bioavailability of chlorthalidone in humans after single oral doses. J. Pharm. Sci., 74:995, 1985.

63. Vardan, et al.: Efficacy and reduced metabolic side effects of a 15-mg chlorthalidone formulation in the treatment of mild hypertension. JAMA, 258:484, 1987.

64. Shefter, E., and Higuchi, T.: The influence of hydrate and solvate formation on rates of solution and solubility of drugs. J. Pharm. Sci., 52:781, 1963.

65. Poole, J.W., et al.: Physicochemical factors influencing the absorption of the anhydrous and trihydrate forms of ampicillin. Curr. Ther. Res., 10:292, 1968.

66. Ballard, B.E., and Biles, J.A.: Effect of crystallizing solvent on absorption rates of steroid implants. Steroids, 4:273, 1964.

67. Bates, T.R., et al.: Comparative bioavailability of anhydrous griseofulvin and its chloroform solvate. Res. Commun. Chem. Pathol. Pharmacol., 11:233, 1975.

68. Gault, M.H., et al.: Hydrolysis of digoxin by acid. J. Pharm. Pharmacol., 29:27, 1977.

69. Gault, M.H., et al.: Influence of gastric pH on digoxin biotransformation. I. Intragastric hydrolysis. Clin. Pharmacol. Ther., 27:16, 1980.

70. Gault, M.H., et al.: Influence of gastric pH on digoxin biotransformation. II. Extractable urinary metabolites. Clin. Pharmacol. Ther., 29:181, 1981.

71. Nelson, E.: Physicochemical factors influencing absorption of erythromycin and its esters. Chem. Pharm. Bull., 11:1099, 1962.

72. Abruzzo, C.W., et al.: Differential pulse polarographic assay procedure and in vivo biopharmaceutic properties of dipotassium clorazepate. J. Pharmacokin. Biopharm., 4:29, 1976.

73. Shader, R.I., and Greenblatt, D.J.: Clinical implications of benzodiazepine pharmacokinetics. Am. J. Psychiatry, 134:652, 1977.

74. Chun, A.H.C., et al.: Effect of antacids on absorption of clorazepate. Clin. Pharmacol. Ther., 22:329, 1977.

75. Glazko, A.J., Dill, W.A., and Wolf, L.M.: Further observations on metabolic fate of chloramphenicol. Fed. Proc., 9:48, 1950.

76. Pickering, L.K., et al.: Clinical pharmacology of two chloramphenicol preparations in children: sodium succinate (iv) and palmitate (oral) esters. J. Pediatr., 96:757, 1980.

77. Fraser, D.G.: Selection of an oral erythromycin product. Am. J. Hosp. Pharm., 37:1199, 1980.

78. Dressman, J.B., Amidon, G.L., Fleisher, D.: Absorption potential: estimating the fraction absorbed for orally administered compounds. J. Pharm. Sci., 74:588, 1985.

79. Dressman, J.B., Fleisher, D.: Mixing tank model for predicting dissolution rate control of oral absorption. J. Pharm. Sci., 75:109, 1986.

80. Nelson, E.: Unpublished data.

81. Mahfouz, M.: Fate of tubocurarine in the body. Br. J. Pharmacol., 4:295, 1949.

82. Faloon, W.W., et al.: Effect of neomycin and kanamycin on intestinal absorption. Ann. N.Y. Acad. Sci., 132:879, 1966.

83. Wagner, J.G.: Biopharmaceutics: Absorption aspects. J. Pharm. Sci., 50:359, 1961.

84. Singh, P., et al.: Effect of inert tablet ingredients on drug absorption. I. Effect of PEG 4000 on intestinal absorption of four barbiturates. J. Pharm. Sci., 55:63, 1966.

85. Hayton, W.L., Guttman, D.E., and Levy, G.: Enhancement of steroid absorption by dialkylamides. J. Pharm. Sci., 59:575, 1970.

86. Tokumura, T., et al.: Enhancement of bioavailability of cinnarizine from its beta-cyclodextrin complex on oral administration with DL-phenylalanine as a competing agent. J. Pharm. Sci., 74:498, 1985.

87. Higuchi, T., and Ikeda, M.: Rapidly dissolving forms of digoxin: Hydroquinone complex. J. Pharm. Sci., 63:809, 1974.

88. Bochner, F., et al.: Bioavailability of digoxin-hydroquinone complex: a new oral digoxin formulation. J. Pharm. Sci., 66:644, 1977.

89. Sorby, D.L.: Effect of adsorbents on drug absorption. I. Modification of promazine absorption by activated attapulgite and activated charcoal. J. Pharm. Sci., 54:677, 1965.

90. Wagner, J.G.: Design and data analysis of biopharmaceutical studies in man. Paper presented to the American Pharmaceutical Association National Meeting, Dallas, Texas, 1966.

91. Northcutt, R.C., et al.: The influence of cholestyramine on thyroxine absorption. JAMA, 208:1857, 1969.

92. Robinson, D.S., Benjamin, D.M., and McCormack, J.J.: Interaction of warfarin and nonsystemic gastrointestinal drugs. Clin. Pharmacol. Ther., 12:491, 1971.

93. Hahn, K.J., et al.: Effect of cholestyramine on the gastrointestinal absorption of phenprocoumon and acetylsalicylic acid in man. Eur. J. Clin. Pharmacol., 4:142, 1972.

94. Brown, D.D., et al.: A steady-state evaluation of the effects of propantheline bromide and cholestyramine on the bioavailability of digoxin when administered as tablets or capsules. J. Clin. Pharmacol., 25:360, 1985.

95. Harvengt, C., and Desager, J.P.: Effect of colestipol, a new bile acid sequestrant, on the absorption of phenprocoumon in man. Eur. J. Clin. Pharmacol., 6:19, 1973.

96. Kauffman, R.E., and Azarnoff, D.L.: Effect of colestipol on gastrointestinal absorption of chlorothiazide in man. Clin. Pharmacol. Ther., 14:886, 1973.

97. Hibbard, D.M., Peters, J.R., Hunninghake, D.B.: Effects of cholestyramine and colestipol on the plasma concentrations of propranolol. Br. J. Clin. Pharmacol., 18:337, 1984.

5

Gastrointestinal Absorption— Role of the Dosage Form

Most of the drugs used today are potent and, increasingly, specific. However, finding a chemical that selectively binds to an enzyme in the myocardium or inhibits the synthesis of a key element in blood clotting does not constitute drug discovery. Among the requirements for a drug, we must be able to administer it to the whole animal and it must find its way to the site of action. In this sense, the modern dosage form is a *drug delivery system;* its selection may be as important to the clinical outcome of a given course of therapy as is the selection of the drug. With virtually any drug, one can routinely produce a 2- to 5-fold difference in the rate or extent of gastrointestinal absorption, depending on the dosage form or its formulation.[1] In some cases, even greater differences may be observed. A difference of more than 60-fold has been found in the absorption rate of spironolactone from the worst formulation to the best formulation.[2-4] The peak concentration of spironolactone metabolites in the plasma after a single dose of the drug in different dosage forms ranged from 0.06 to 3.75 µg/L per mg of administered drug.

From first principles, one would expect the bioavailability of a drug to decrease in the following order: solution > suspension > capsule > tablet > coated tablet. Although this ranking is not universal, it provides a useful guideline. The results of bioavailability studies with pentobarbital in man are summarized in Figure 5–1. The absorption rate of pentobarbital after administration in various oral dosage forms decreased in the following order: aqueous solution > aqueous suspension of the free acid ≈ capsule of the sodium salt > tablet of the free acid.[5] These findings demonstrate how the dosage form can influence drug absorption.

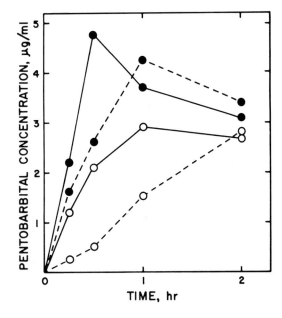

Fig. 5–1. Pentobarbital concentrations in plasma after a single 200-mg dose in various oral dosage forms. ●—aqueous solution, ●– – – aqueous suspension, ○— capsule (sodium salt), ○– – – tablet (acid). (Data from Sjögren, J., Sölvell, L., and Karlsson, I.[5])

This chapter deals with the biopharmaceutic characteristics of dosage forms. The first section is an overview of the potential effects on absorption that may be observed with conventional oral dosage forms, including solutions, suspensions, capsules, tablets, and coated tablets. Special enteral dosage forms, like buccal or sublingual tablets and rectal preparations, are discussed in Chapter 6; prolonged-release medication is considered in Chapter 7. The second section deals with the correlation of drug absorption in man with in vitro parameters such as the disintegration time of the dosage form or the dissolution rate of the drug from the dosage form.

DOSAGE FORMS

Solutions

The solution dosage form is widely used for cough and cold preparations and for many other drugs, particularly in pediatric and geriatric patients. With rare exception, drugs are absorbed more rapidly when given as a solution than in any other oral dosage form. The rate-limiting step in the absorption of a drug from a solution dosage form is likely to be gastric emptying, particularly when the drug is given after a meal.

When an acidic drug is given in solution in the form of a salt, there is the possibility of precipitation in gastric fluid. Experience suggests that these precipitates are usually finely subdivided and easily redissolved. However, with highly water-insoluble drugs, like phenytoin or warfarin, this may not be the case; one may find that the absorption rate or extent of absorption from a well-formulated suspension of the free acid is greater than from a solution of the sodium salt.

Many drugs, unless converted to a water-soluble salt, are poorly soluble. Solutions of these drugs can be prepared by adding cosolvents, such as alcohol, propylene glycol, polyethylene glycol 400, agents that form water-soluble complexes with the drug, or surfactants in sufficient quantity to exceed the critical micelle concentration and to effect solubilization. After administration of such water-miscible preparations, dilution with gastrointestinal fluids may result in precipitation of the drug. Again experience suggests that in most cases rapid redissolution takes place. Reversible interactions that occur between the drug and solubilizing agent or other component of the formulation are unlikely to affect drug absorption if the interaction product is water-soluble.

Serajuddin et al.[6] studied the physical properties and bioavailability of a poorly water-soluble drug dissolved in polyethylene glycol (PEG) 400 or polysorbate 80. On dilution of the water-miscible solutions with simulated gastric fluid, the drug immediately formed saturated solutions and the excess drug separated as finely divided emulsified oily globules with a high surface area. The average globule size of the oily form was 1.6 μm or less,

as compared with a particle size of 5 to 10 μm for the solid drug.

Absorption studies in the rat using labeled drug resulted in 54% of the radioactivity excreted in the urine when the PEG solution was given and 41% when the polysorbate 80 solution was used, but only 19% of the radioactivity was found in the urine when an aqueous suspension of the drug was administered. The large surface area of drug separating from water-miscible solvents on dilution with water facilitates its dissolution and absorption.

Certain materials such as sorbitol or hydrophilic polymers are sometimes added to a solution dosage form, to improve pourability and palatability by increasing the viscosity of the preparation. The higher the viscosity of the formulation, the slower are gastric emptying and absorption. Such effects, however, are unlikely to be clinically important.

There has been some interest in giving drugs dissolved in oil. Rapid and complete absorption may be observed in some instances, particularly if the oil is administered in emulsified form. Early clinical studies with indoxole, a poorly water-soluble, investigational, nonsteroidal anti-inflammatory agent, suggested incomplete absorption of the drug from a suspension or capsule dosage form. Administration of indoxole dissolved in the oil phase of Lipomul-Oral, a commercially available oil-in-water emulsion, resulted in a threefold improvement in the extent of absorption compared to that observed after administration of an aqueous suspension and a ninefold improvement compared to a hard gelatin capsule.[7]

Serajuddin et al.[6] found that a solution of a poorly water-soluble drug in peanut oil gave nearly 75% greater bioavailability than an aqueous suspension of the drug when both dosage forms were studied in the rat. Bioavailability from the water-immiscible peanut oil solution, however, was not as great as that found when the drug was dissolved in PEG 400 or polysorbate 80 to form water-miscible solutions.

Certain nontoxic but unpalatable solvents may be used for solubilizing drugs if the solution can be encapsulated. This approach can, in some cases, dramatically improve the absorption of water-insoluble drugs. For example, the bioavailability of indoxole after administration of a soft elastic capsule containing the drug dissolved in polysorbate 80 was comparable to that found after administration of the drug dissolved in the oil phase of an oil-in-water emulsion.[7]

Suspensions

As a drug delivery system, the well-formulated aqueous suspension is second in efficiency only to the solution dosage form. Usually, the absorption rate of a drug from a suspension is dissolution-rate limited; however, drug dissolution from a suspension is often rapid because a large surface area is presented to the fluids at the absorption site. Drug contained in a capsule or tablet may never achieve the state of dispersion in the gastrointestinal tract that is attained with a finely subdivided, well-formulated suspension.

Several studies have demonstrated the superior bioavailability characteristics of suspensions compared to those of solid dosage forms. For example, the blood levels of trimethoprim and sulfamethoxazole were compared in 24 healthy subjects following oral administration of 3 forms (tablet, capsule, and suspension) of the antibacterial combination. The absorption rate of each drug was significantly greater with the suspension than with the tablet or capsule.[8] There were no significant differences between the preparations in the extent of absorption of either drug. Similar results have been found with pentobarbital[5] and penicillin V.[9]

Among the more important factors to consider in formulating suspension dosage forms for maximum bioavailability are particle size, inclusion of wetting agents, formation of insoluble complexes, crystal form, and viscosity. Figure 5–2 compares the serum levels of phenytoin after a single 600-mg dose in the form of an aqueous suspension containing either micronized (Formulation G) or conventional (Formulation F) drug. Based on the total area under the drug concentration in serum versus time curve (AUC), almost twice as much phenytoin is absorbed after the micronized suspension.[10]

The higher the viscosity of a suspension, the slower is the dissolution rate of the drug. The inclusion of methylcellulose in an aqueous suspension of nitrofurantoin has been found to impair its rate and extent of absorption.[11]

Merely shaking some drug powder in an aqueous solution of a gum such as acacia neither constitutes a well-formulated suspension nor guarantees good absorption. This extemporaneous approach to formulation is sometimes used in screening drugs for biologic activity and in the safety assessment of promising compounds in laboratory animals. More sophisticated methods than these are called for to

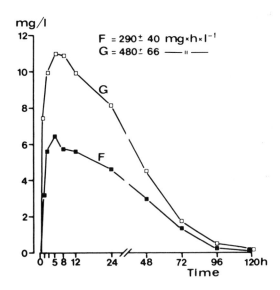

Fig. 5–2. Phenytoin concentrations (mg/L) in serum after a 600-mg oral dose in aqueous suspensions containing either micronized (G) or conventional (F) drug. The area under the serum level-time curve is noted for each formulation. (From Neuvonen, P.J., Pentikäinen, P.J., and Elfving, S.M.[10])

avoid costly mistakes regarding a drug's safety or efficacy.

Bioavailability studies with drugs suspended in oil-in-water emulsions have yielded some promising results. One study compared the absorption of micronized griseofulvin after its administration to healthy subjects in a corn oil-in-water emulsion (in which the drug was suspended), an aqueous suspension, and two different commercial tablets.[12] Based on cumulative urinary excretion of griseofulvin metabolites, the extent of absorption of the drug after administration of the emulsion was about twice that observed after administration of the aqueous suspension or tablets. A mechanism based on the ability of fatty acids, liberated during the digestion of corn oil, to inhibit gastrointestinal motility (which would increase the residence time of the drug in the small intestine) and to stimulate gallbladder evacuation and, thereby, elevate the concentrations of surface-active bile constituents in the intestine (which would promote dissolution of the drug) may explain the results.

Capsules

The capsule dosage form has the potential to be an efficient drug delivery system. The hard gelatin shell encapsulating the formulation should disrupt quickly, and expose the contents to the gastrointestinal fluids. However, this will not be the case if the formulation or the method of manufacture imparts a hydrophobic nature to the shell.

Drug particles in a capsule are not subjected to high compression forces that tend to compact the powder and to reduce the effective surface area. On disruption of the shell, the encapsulated powder mass should disperse rapidly to expose a large surface area to the gastrointestinal fluids. However, with some formulations the rate of dispersion has been found to be unacceptably slow. Thus, although one might expect better bioavailability characteristics of a drug from a capsule than from a compressed tablet, this is not always so. For example, tablets and capsules of a combination product containing triamterene and hydrochlorothiazide were compared in single-dose studies in normal subjects using cumulative urinary excretion of apparent drug as an index of the extent of absorption.[13] The capsule was a simple formulation containing the drugs, lactose, and a small amount of magnesium stearate. The tablet was a more complex formulation that included a large amount of glycine, used as a water-soluble diluent. The excretion of hydrochlorothiazide after the tablet was twice as much as that found after the capsule. A 3-fold difference in the cumulative excretion of triamterene was observed. The tablets also consistently produced an earlier and a greater peak increase in sodium excretion.

It is usually necessary to have a suitable diluent in a capsule dosage form, particularly when the drug is hydrophobic. Figure 5–3 shows the change in dissolution rate that can be effected by the incorporation of hydrophilic diluents.[14] The diluent serves to disperse the drug particles, minimize aggregation, and maximize the effective surface area and dissolution rate. The incorporation of a wetting agent in the formulation may also be advantageous.

Other attempts to modify the wetting characteristics of poorly water-soluble drugs have included treating the drug with a solution of a hydrophilic polymer such as methylcellulose. Phenytoin was found to dissolve and be absorbed considerably faster from capsules containing drug treated with methylcellulose compared to capsules containing untreated drug.[15]

Many pharmacologic and toxicologic studies with investigational drugs in dogs and monkeys use hand-packed, hard gelatin capsules of the drug alone as the delivery system. This practice may

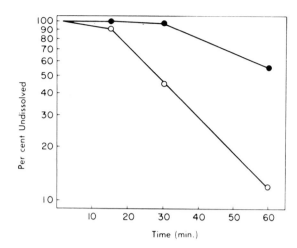

Fig. 5–3. Dissolution from hard gelatin capsules containing drug alone (●) or drug plus diluents (○). The diluents serve to disperse the drug and enhance wetting and dissolution. (Data from Paikoff, M., and Drumm, G.[14])

lead to erratic and incomplete drug absorption, and should be strongly discouraged.

The diluents of a capsule dosage form should have little tendency to adsorb or otherwise interact with the drug. The use of dicalcium phosphate as a diluent in tetracycline capsules has been found to significantly impair absorption, presumably because a poorly soluble calcium-tetracycline complex is formed in the powder mass or during dissolution.[16]

Factors that influence drug absorption from capsule dosage forms include particle size and crystal form of the drug, and selection of diluents and fillers.

Attempts to improve the oral absorption of digoxin has led to renewed interest in the use of soft elastic capsules as a solid oral dosage form. The soft elastic capsule has a gelatin shell somewhat thicker than that of hard gelatin capsules, but the shell is plasticized by the addition of glycerin, sorbitol, or a similar material. Unlike the hard gelatin capsule, the soft elastic capsule may contain nonaqueous solutions of a drug, or drugs that are liquids (e.g., the antitussive drug, benzonatate) or semisolids (e.g., certain vitamins).

A formulation consisting of digoxin dissolved in a mixture of polyethylene glycol, ethanol, and propylene glycol, prepared as a liquid concentrate in soft elastic capsules, has been developed and found to have good bioavailability characteristics. The encapsulated liquid concentrate of digoxin is consistently better absorbed than the standard commercial tablet of the drug.[17-22]

A soft elastic capsule containing 0.4 mg of digoxin is about equivalent to a tablet containing 0.5 mg of the drug. In one study, mean absorption was 75% of the dose from the tablet and 97% from the capsule.[18] Surprisingly, some studies[18,21] but not all[22] suggest that the bioavailability of digoxin from the soft elastic capsule is greater than from an aqueous solution of the drug. The superior bioavailability of the encapsulated liquid concentrate over an aqueous solution may result from less chemical breakdown in the stomach when the capsule is given. Whatever the mechanism, we can conclude that the absorption of digoxin from soft elastic capsules is clearly better than from conventional tablets and at least comparable to an aqueous solution of the drug.

Tablets

Compressed tablets are the most widely used dosage form. They are usually produced by either wet granulation or direct compression. Wet granulation consists of mixing the drug with other powdered materials and wetting the mixture with an aqueous solution of a suitable binder such as gelatin or starch. The damp mass is forced through a 6- or 8-mesh screen and dried to produce cohesive granules. These granules usually flow easily through the tablet press and are easily compressed.

Increasing attention is being given to manufacturing tablets by direct compression. As its name implies, direct compression consists of compressing tablets directly from powdered material without modifying the physical characteristics of the material itself. For tablets in which the drug constitutes a major portion of the total tablet weight, the drug itself must have the physical attributes (crystallinity and cohesiveness) needed for the formulation to be compressed directly. Direct compression can almost always be used for tablets containing 25% or less of the total weight as drug, by formulating with suitable diluents which act as a carrier or vehicle for the drug. These diluents include processed forms of common tablet materials such as dicalcium phosphate dihydrate, tricalcium phosphate, calcium sulfate, anhydrous lactose, and mannitol, as well as spray-dried lactose, pregelatinized starch, compressible sugar, and microcrystalline cellulose.

Most bioavailability problems with compressed tablets are related to the large reduction in effective surface area that results from the tablet manufacturing process, as well as to the difficulty in regenerating well-dispersed primary drug particles in the gastrointestinal tract. After ingestion, the tablet first breaks down to granules and then to primary drug particles. Granules resulting from directly compressed tablets may be softer and more easily wetted than those produced by tablets prepared with the wet-granulation process, but it is difficult to generalize. The disintegration and dissolution processes that take place in the gastrointestinal fluids after oral administration of a tablet are presented in schematic form in Figure 5–4.

The effective surface area of drug in an intact tablet is so limited that k_1, the dissolution rate constant, is usually negligible, except for drugs that

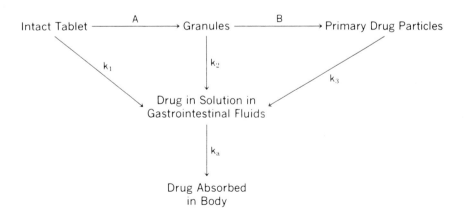

Fig. 5–4. Schematic representation of disintegration (A, B) and dissolution (k_1, k_2, k_3) processes that precede drug absorption after administration of a tablet dosage form. The term k_a is a first-order rate constant characterizing drug absorption from solution in the fluids of the gastrointestinal tract.

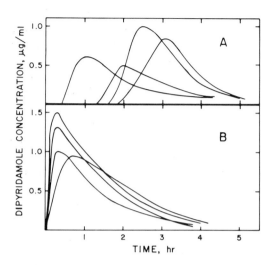

Fig. 5–5. Dipyridamole concentrations in serum of individual subjects after a 25-mg oral dose as intact tablets (A) or crushed tablets (B). When the tablets are chewed before swallowing, the peak concentration tends to be higher and the peak time tends to be earlier. (Data from Mellinger, T.J., and Bohorfoush, J.G.[23])

are extremely water-soluble. Tablet disintegration (step A) greatly increases the effective surface area of the drug. A further increase in surface area is attained upon granule disintegration; accordingly, $k_3 >> k_2 >> k_1$. The dissolution rate from the granules may be likened to that observed with a coarse, aggregated drug suspension, whereas the dissolution rate from the primary particles is probably comparable to that observed with a fine, well-dispersed drug suspension. Poorly water-soluble drugs are likely to dissolve mainly after granule disintegration.

Tablet disintegration and granule disintegration are important steps in the absorption process. A tablet that fails to disintegrate or disintegrates slowly may result in incomplete absorption or an undue delay in the onset of clinical response. The importance of disintegration in drug absorption is evident from the results of clinical studies with dipyridamole.[23] Curves of serum concentrations of dipyridamole versus time after administration are shown in Figure 5–5. When the tablets were taken intact, the appearance of drug in blood was delayed and variable. When the tablets were chewed before swallowing, the drug appeared in the blood within 5 or 6 min. In every patient, the peak drug concentration was higher after the crushed tablet than after swallowing the intact tablet. Similar results have been observed with thioridazine tablets.[24]

Studies in the United Kingdom have shown that when commercial digoxin tablets, from which the drug is incompletely absorbed, are crushed and given in a capsule, much higher digoxin levels are obtained.[25]

Tablet disintegration, although important, is unlikely to be the rate-limiting step in the absorption of drugs administered as conventional tablets. In most instances, granule disintegration and drug dissolution occur at a slower rate than tablet disintegration.

Many factors related to the formulation or production of tablets may affect drug dissolution and absorption. Most formulations require the incorporation of hydrophobic lubricants, such as magnesium stearate, to produce an acceptable tablet. In general, the larger the quantity of lubricant in a formulation, the slower is the dissolution rate.[26]

Even seemingly modest changes in formulation may lead to significant effects on dissolution and availability. A classic example has been reported with tolbutamide.[27] Two formulations of the drug were compared in healthy subjects with respect to bioavailability (serum tolbutamide levels) and therapeutic efficacy (hypoglycemic response). One tablet was the commercial product and the other was identical in all respects except for a halving of the amount of a disintegrant. Both tablets met United States Pharmacopeia (USP) specifications. Both tablets disintegrated in vitro within 10 min.

Despite the similar specifications, the experimental formulation was inferior to the commercial product. The area under the average serum tolbutamide curve over an 8-hr observation period was more than 3 times greater with the commercial product than with the experimental formulation. The average cumulative reduction of serum glucose over the 8-hr period after administration of the commercial tablet was twice that after administration of the experimental tablet (Fig. 5–6).

Compression force may also be an important factor in drug bioavailability from compressed tablets. The in vitro disintegration time of tablets has been shown to be directly proportional to compression force and tablet hardness.[28] High compression forces may also increase the strength of the internal structure of the granules and retard dissolution of drug from the granules and disintegration of the granules.

The effect of particle size reduction on dissolution and absorption may be reduced by compression.[29] Studies in man showed that a 3.8-fold

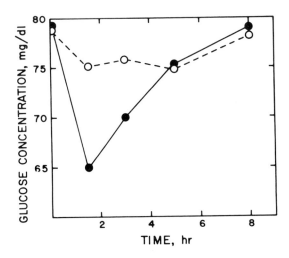

Fig. 5–6. Serum glucose levels after 0.5-g tolbutamide in a commercial tablet (●) or an experimental tablet containing less disintegrating agent (○). (Data from Varley, A.B.[27])

increase in the specific surface area of griseofulvin led to a 2.3-fold increase in blood concentration after administration of a suspension, but only a 1.5-fold increase after administration of a tablet.

A novel approach to enhance the availability of poorly water-soluble drugs from tablets has been used in a marketed griseofulvin product.[30] A molecular dispersion of the drug in polyethylene glycol 6000, a water-soluble, waxy polymer that congeals at about 60°C, is prepared and suitably modified for incorporation into a tablet dosage form. The absorption of griseofulvin from this product appears to be complete and about twice that observed from commercial tablets containing micronized drug.

Coated Tablets

Tablet coatings are used to mask unpleasant tastes and odors, to protect an ingredient from decomposition during storage, or simply to improve the appearance of a tablet. The most common coated medications are sugar-coated and film-coated tablets. Not only do these dosage forms present all the potential problems discussed earlier with respect to compressed tablets, but they also impose an additional barrier between the gastrointestinal fluid and the drug. The coating must dissolve or disrupt before tablet disintegration and drug dissolution can occur. The disintegration of certain coated tablets appears to be the rate-limiting

process in drug absorption, since correlations have been found between bioavailability and in vitro disintegration time.

The venerable sugar-coated tablet is still used today. The sugar coating formulation is complex; the coating process is time consuming and requires skill. The first step of the process is the application of a nonaqueous, sealing solution to protect the tablet and its ingredients from the aqueous solutions used in subsequent steps. A special grade shellac dissolved in alcohol is commonly used to seal tablets. Other materials that have been used include fatty glycerides, beeswax, and silicone resins. The other steps of the coating process add bulk and modify the shape of the tablets. Other ingredients of the coating formulation may include talc, acacia, flour, starch, and calcium carbonate, in addition to sucrose.

The application of the sealing coat and the development of a relatively dense crystalline barrier around the tablet retard the release of drug in the gastrointestinal tract. In general, we must assume that a sugar coating may affect the bioavailability of a drug. This dosage form should not be used when a prompt clinical response is desired.

The basic disadvantages of sugar coating have stimulated a search for alternatives. These alternatives include the film-coated tablet and the press-coated tablet. Film-coated tablets are compressed tablets that are coated with a thin layer or film of a material that is usually water soluble or dispersible. A number of polymeric substances with film-forming properties may be used including hydroxypropyl methylcellulose and carboxymethylcellulose. Aqueous vehicles are preferred but a nonaqueous vehicle may be used when moisture is detrimental to the product being coated. A mixture of cellulose acetate phthalate and polyethylene glycol can be applied from aqueous or nonaqueous solvents. Care should be taken when selecting coating materials. Methylcellulose, for example, has been reported to retard drug dissolution.[31]

The film coat masks objectionable tastes and protects, to some degree, tablet ingredients from moisture during storage. The film coat should disrupt quickly in the fluids of the gastrointestinal tract, independent of pH. A well-formulated product should show little difference in bioavailability compared with that of an uncoated tablet.

Press-coated or dry-coated tablets are prepared by feeding previously compressed tablets into a special tableting machine and compressing another granulation layer around the preformed tablet. Press-coated tablets appear to retain all the attributes of compressed tablets but provide the advantages of sugar-coated tablets. Ideally, there should be little difference in disintegration time between press-coated and uncoated tablets.

Enteric-Coated Tablets

An enteric coat is usually a special film coat designed to resist gastric fluids and to disrupt or dissolve in the small intestine. The enteric coat is used to protect a drug from degrading in the stomach (e.g., erythromycin), or to minimize gastric distress caused by some drugs (e.g., aspirin). Enteric-coated tablets must empty from the stomach before drug absorption can begin. The rate of appearance of drug in the blood after giving an enteric-coated tablet is, therefore, a function of gastric emptying. Differences in gastric emptying from one patient to another or in the same patient from one administration to another contribute to the large variability in drug absorption commonly found with this dosage form.

The time course of an enteric coated aspirin tablet from the stomach to the small intestine was monitored in dogs using radiotelemetry.[32] A 500-mg enteric coated tablet was attached to a Heidelberg capsule calibrated to pH 1 and pH 7. Gastric pH was about 1.5. As the tablet was emptied into the small intestine, the monitored pH rose to about 7. This time interval was termed the gastric emptying time. The pH in the small intestine remained relatively constant until the enteric coating dissolved and aspirin was released. At this time, the monitored pH dropped to about 3.8, close to the pK_a of aspirin. This time interval was defined as the coating dissolution time.

As a result of carrying out four replicates in each of 4 dogs both inter- and intrasubject variability could be evaluated. In 1 dog the gastric emptying time ranged from 7 to 40 min and in another from 8 to 115 min. Mean gastric emptying times varied from 24 to 63 min. Coating dissolution time seemed to be less variable. In 1 dog the dissolution times ranged from 23 to 49 min and in another from 26 to 77 min. Mean coating dissolution times varied from 34 to 57 min. The variable onset of aspirin appearance in the plasma is the result of variance in both gastric emptying time and coating dissolution time, with the variance in gastric emptying time being significantly larger.

The modern approach to enteric-coating makes use of polymers like cellulose acetate phthalate that are "insoluble" at pH 1 to 3 but "soluble" at pH 5 to 7. These materials are polymeric acids with ionizable carboxyl groups. The apparent pKa of these polymers is important. If the pKa is too low, appreciable ionization takes place at low pH, and the coating will dissolve in the stomach. A high pKa may prevent release of drug in the small intestine. In practice, polymers with pKa values ranging from 4 to 7 have been found useful.

In one investigation, a series of half-esters of the copolymer poly (vinyl methyl ether-maleic anhydride) was prepared. The in vitro dissolution pH (i.e., the pH of complete solubility) of films of these polymers varied from 4.25, for the ethyl derivative, to 6.25, for the cyclopentyl half-ester. The bioavailability of aspirin was studied in normal subjects following administration of tablets coated with these copolymers. An inverse correlation was observed between absorption rate and the in vitro dissolution pH. Twelve hr after administration of tablets coated with the ethyl half-ester, 87% of the dose was recovered in the urine, compared to a urinary recovery of 53% after administration of tablets coated with the cyclopentyl half-ester.[33]

The thickness of the coating may also affect bioavailability. Studies with quinine tablets coated with cellulose acetate phthalate show a decrease in both rate and extent of absorption with increasing thickness of the coating.[34] A particular problem with shellac as an enteric coating is that the water solubility of the film decreases with age; an enteric-coated tablet with acceptable bioavailability characteristics at the time of manufacture may perform poorly some time later.

A considerable delay may be observed between the administration of an enteric-coated tablet and the appearance of drug in the bloodstream. This is evident from bioavailability studies with prednisolone and aspirin. Enteric-coated prednisolone has been available for many years because some believe that chronic steroid therapy predisposes to gastric ulceration. Studies comparing blood levels after a single dose of prednisolone in the form of ordinary or enteric-coated tablets show that although the extent of absorption (AUC) and maximum blood levels are comparable, there is, on the average, a 3-hr difference in the time required to attain the peak concentration of the drug (Table 5–1).[35]

Aspirin has maintained an important place in the treatment of rheumatic diseases despite the intro-

Table 5–1. Peak Concentration of Prednisolone in Plasma, Time to Peak, and Total Area Under the Plasma Level-Time Curve (AUC) After an Oral Dose*

Formulation	Peak concentration	AUC	Time (min)
Tablet	1383	347	84
Enteric-coated tablet	1267	311	260
Significance	NS	NS	p <0.001

*Data from Lee, D.A.H., et al.[35]

duction of many other nonsteroidal anti-inflammatory drugs (NSAIDs). However, gastric intolerance and injury are commonly observed with the high doses required for optimal effects. One of the traditional methods of overcoming the gastric side effects of aspirin has been to formulate the drug as an enteric-coated tablet. A well-formulated enteric-coated tablet of aspirin has been compared with uncoated tablets with respect to time of appearance of salicylate in the plasma after a single dose.[36] The results in a representative subject are shown in Figure 5–7. Salicylate was detected in the plasma of all 18 subjects within 1 hr after giving the uncoated tablet but not until 3 hr, on the average, after the enteric-coated tablet. Two subjects showed no salicylate in the plasma for 8 hr after the coated tablets.

Fenoprofen is another NSAID available as an enteric coated tablet. The effects of plain and enteric coated fenoprofen calcium on gastrointestinal microbleeding were studied in healthy male subjects.[37] A one-week baseline (placebo) period preceded two weeks of fenoprofen therapy (enteric coated or plain tablets, 600 mg 4 times a day). Fecal blood loss was estimated by a ^{51}Cr-tagged erythrocyte assay and was averaged over days 4 to 7 (baseline) and days 18 to 21 (active treatment). At the end of the active drug period, mean daily fecal blood loss was lower with enteric coated fenoprofen than with plain tablets, 1.1 ml/day *versus* 1.7 ml/day. Gastric and duodenal mucosal damage, however, as evaluated by endoscopy, was similar for both dosage forms.

The delay in drug absorption typically found after administration of enteric-coated tablets could be the result of prolonged gastric emptying or, alternatively, slow dissolution of the coating after the tablet reaches the small intestine. In most cases, slow gastric emptying appears to be the principal reason for the delay because coadministration of metoclopramide, a drug that accelerates gastric emptying, can dramatically decrease the lag time.[36,38]

Since gastric emptying of the enteric-coated dosage unit plays an important role in the onset of drug absorption, it is to be expected that administration of this dosage form after a meal will further delay absorption. Paull and associates report that giving an enteric-coated aspirin tablet immediately after a heavy breakfast markedly delays the appearance of salicylate in saliva, compared to that observed after giving the tablet 2 hr after a light breakfast.[38]

The Heidelberg capsule, a radiotelemetric indicator of gastrointestinal pH, has also been used in human subjects to evaluate the relationship between gastric residence time (GRT) and variability in aspirin absorption from enteric coated tablets.[39] In a crossover study, subjects received enteric coated aspirin together with the Heidelberg capsule while fasting or with food (breakfast, followed 4 hr later by lunch).

The mean time to peak salicylate concentration was 8.3 hr when the subjects were fasted and 13.8 hr when fed. This shift was related to gastric emptying. Mean GRT was markedly delayed by food,

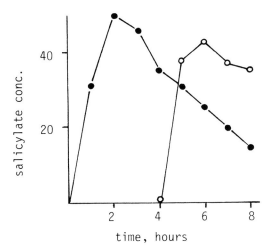

Fig. 5–7. Salicylate concentrations in plasma (μg/ml) after a 650-mg dose of aspirin in conventional tablets (●) or enteric-coated tablets (○). (Data from Day, R.D., et al.[36])

going from about 1 hr to about 6 hr. Time to appearance of salicylate in plasma (lag time) was also delayed when enteric coated aspirin was given with food, from about 3 to 9 hr. There was an excellent correlation (r = 0.94) between the lag time for appearance of salicylate in plasma and GRT.

The effect of food on the absorption of quinidine from an enteric-coated tablet has also been studied.[40] In fasting subjects, the delay in the start of absorption after a single dose ranged from 2 to 8 hr (mean = 4.8 hr); in nonfasting subjects the delay ranged from 3 to 10 hr (mean = 6.1 hr). Whether or not the dosage form was given with food, intersubject variability in the length of the delay before the onset of absorption was substantial; in some subjects the delay was longer than the usual dosing interval for the drug. Other studies with this enteric-coated quinidine product suggested that absorption began later and was slower at night, consistent with the fact that gastric emptying is slower when the patient is in the prone position.[40]

The enteric-coated tablet dosage form has been the object of well-deserved criticism in recent years. Many reports of clinical failure because of erratic and incomplete absorption can be found in the literature. Far fewer problems are found with newer products, but variability remains a substantial concern. One approach that appears to minimize variability is the use of individually enteric-coated granules.[41] These granules may be compressed into rapidly disintegrating tablets or administered in capsules. After disintegration of the dosage form in the stomach, gradual but continual emptying of the granules into the intestine is anticipated.

A theoretical analysis of blood level profiles resulting from enteric-coated granules has been published.[42] It concludes that:

an enteric-coated tablet may take from approximately 0.5 to more than 8 hr. to pass from the stomach to the duodenum. On the other hand, enteric-coated pellets are subjected to dispersion in the stomach and they pass through the pyloric sphincter after a mean residence time in the stomach that would not be different from that exhibited by a suspension dosage form.

Investigators in Sweden have compared the absorption of aspirin from two different enteric-coated dosage forms, tablets and granules, in healthy subjects under fasting and nonfasting conditions.[43] Under fasting conditions, the absorption of aspirin from both preparations was complete. When the dosage forms were taken after a meal,

the enteric-coated tablets gave much lower concentrations of salicylate in plasma than under fasting conditions, and absorption was incomplete in some subjects. Neither the rate nor extent of aspirin absorption from the enteric-coated granules was affected by food.

Drug absorption from enteric-coated granules appears to be more consistent than from enteric-coated tablets. Do the granules protect the GI mucosa as well as the tablets? A placebo-controlled study has been reported comparing the effects of aspirin formulated as enteric-coated granules or as buffered tablets on gastric mucosa, as determined by endoscopic examination 2 hours after a single 975-mg dose in fasted subjects.[44] A grading scale of 0 (no damage) to 4 (severe damage) was used.

The granules produced a much lower severity and incidence of gastric lesions than the buffered aspirin formulation. The mean severity score was 0.4 for the granules and 3.0 for the buffered tablet. All subjects receiving the buffered tablet showed one or more sites of submucosal hemorrhage or erosion, compared with 36% of those given the enteric-coated granules. None of the lesions produced by the granules or the placebo was considered clinically significant, whereas nearly two-thirds of the subjects given buffered aspirin had clinically important stomach damage.

Although incomplete and variable absorption has been the most common problem found with enteric-coated tablets, a far more serious problem brought national attention to this dosage form. This problem was the life-threatening toxicity associated with enteric-coated potassium chloride tablets. Enteric-coated KCl was developed to minimize gastric irritation and to enhance palatability and compliance. However, from 1964 to 1974 numerous cases of small bowel ulceration associated with the administration of enteric-coated potassium chloride, alone or in combination with thiazide diuretics, were reported.[45] This serious adverse effect was not found with liquid or effervescent tablet forms of potassium chloride.

The cause of the problem can be found in the crystalline nature and compression characteristics of KCl itself. Tablets of this salt are easily made but do not disintegrate easily. When the enteric-coated tablet empties from the stomach and the film coating dissolves, what remains is a poorly disintegrating tablet of almost pure potassium chloride resting on the mucosa of the small intestine. The limited surface area of the intact tablet results in slow dissolution and prolonged and corrosive contact. Of the dozens of enteric-coated KCl products that were on the market in the United States, none remains. Today, the need for a solid dosage form of potassium chloride is met by slow-release tablets in which the KCl is embedded in a wax matrix and by tablets or capsules containing small microencapsulated particles of KCl. These preparations are marked improvements over enteric-coated tablets.

Sulfasalazine is used in the treatment of ulcerative colitis. It is poorly absorbed in the small intestine, allowing essentially all of an oral dose to reach the large intestine where bacteria split the diazo bond, forming sulfapyridine and 5-aminosalicylic acid (5-ASA).

There is controversy as to which drug(s) is the active species. Sulfapyridine appears to contribute little or nothing to the effectiveness of sulfasalazine and may be responsible for most of its side effects. Many believe that 5-ASA is the active drug and that sulfasalazine is simply a prodrug for delivery of 5-ASA to the colon. Supporting this idea is the observation that topical (rectal) administration of 5-ASA is in fact effective in ulcerative colitis restricted to the distal large intestine.

There is interest in the development of an oral preparation that retains the activity of 5-ASA, while eliminating sulfapyridine as a source of unwanted effects. One product contains 5-ASA particles coated with an acrylic resin that disintegrates at pH 7 or above. These pH conditions ordinarily occur only in the distal ileum and colon.

Riley et al.[46] studied the ileostomy excretion of this dosage form in human subjects who previously had undergone a colectomy. Following a single dose given after an overnight fast, 5-ASA first appeared in the effluent between 4 and 6 hours in 6 subjects and between 6 and 8 hours in the other two. Within 12 hr of taking the tablet, an average of 88% (range 69 to 114%) of the 400-mg dose was recovered in the effluent as unchanged 5-ASA, indicating that little absorption of resin-coated 5-ASA takes place in the small intestine.

An in vitro dissolution study[46] indicated that at pH values above 7.0, dissolution of the protective coat was rapid. Between pH 6.0 and 7.0, dissolution was considerably delayed. At pH 2.0 and 4.0, the coat remained intact for more than three days.

The results of open-label studies have suggested that the preparation of coated 5-ASA is tolerated well by patients who previously had adverse re-

actions to sulfasalazine.[47] Other investigators found that administration of 4.8 g per day of coated 5-ASA to patients with mildly or moderately active ulcerative colitis resulted in a complete response in 24% of the patients and a partial response in 50%. This dose is equivalent in terms of 5-ASA content to a 12 g dose of sulfasalazine, "a dosage that could not be tolerated by most patients."[48]

The use of acid-resistant coatings to deliver drugs to the colon has also been applied to cholestyramine.[49] Ileal resection causes malabsorption of bile acid; the increased load of bile acids in the colon induces increased secretion of salt and water and leads to diarrhea. A double blind crossover trial was carried out with placebo and cholestyramine coated with cellulose acetate phthalate. During treatment with cholestyramine, the daily fecal output and the number of defecations each week decreased, and patient acceptance of the preparation was high.

A somewhat different approach to drug delivery has been proposed for peptides.[50] The oral administration of peptide drugs is precluded because they are digested in the stomach and small intestine. As a new approach to oral delivery, vasopressin and insulin were coated with polymers cross-linked with azoaromatic groups to protect them from digestion. When the azopolymer-coated drug reached the large intestine, the indigenous microflora reduced the azo bonds, broke the cross-links, and degraded the polymer film, thereby releasing the drug into the lumen of the colon for local action or for absorption. The feasibility of delivering insulin to lower blood glucose was demonstrated in rats made diabetic with streptozotocin.

IN VITRO CORRELATES OF DRUG ABSORPTION

The advantages to be gained in developing in vitro tests that are predictive of drug absorption in man are considerable and have stimulated an overwhelming number of investigations by pharmaceutical scientists throughout the world. These efforts have focused largely on disintegration and dissolution tests.

Disintegration Tests

The first official method for tablet disintegration was described in a Swiss pharmacopeia in 1934. The United States Pharmacopeia (U.S.P.) has recognized one test or another for tablet disintegration since 1950. The latest revision of the U.S.P.

(U.S.P. XXI) published in 1985 also includes a disintegration test for hard gelatin capsules.

The following is taken directly from U.S.P. XXI.

⟨701⟩ DISINTEGRATION

This test is provided to determine compliance with the limits on *Disintegration* stated in the individual monographs except for soft gelatin capsules and where the label states that the tablets or capsules are intended for use as troches, or are to be chewed, or are designed to liberate the drug content gradually over a period of time or to release the drug over two or more separate periods with a distinct time interval between such release periods. Determine the type of units under test from the labeling and from observation, and apply the appropriate procedure to 6 or more dosage units.

For the purposes of this test, disintegration does not imply complete solution of the unit or even of its active constituent. Complete disintegration is defined as that stage in which any residue of the unit, except fragments of insoluble coating or capsule shell, remaining on the screen of the test apparatus is a soft mass having no palpably firm core.

Apparatus

The apparatus[1] consists of a basket-rack assembly, a 1000-mL, low-form beaker for the immersion fluid, a thermostatic arrangement for heating the fluid between 35° and 39°, and a device for raising and lowering the basket in the immersion fluid at a constant frequency rate between 29 and 32 cycles per minute through a distance of not less than 5.3 cm and not more than 5.7 cm. The volume of the fluid in the vessel is such that at the highest point of the upward stroke the wire mesh remains at least 2.5 cm below the surface of the fluid and descends to not less than 2.5 cm from the bottom of the vessel on the downward stroke. The time required for the upward stroke is equal to the time required for the downward stroke, and the change in stroke direction is a smooth transition, rather than an abrupt reversal of motion. The basket-rack assembly moves vertically along its axis. There is no appreciable horizontal motion or movement of the axis from the vertical.

Basket-rack Assembly—The basket-rack assembly consists of six open-ended glass tubes, each 7.75 ± 0.25 cm long and having an inside diameter of approximately 21.5 mm and a wall approximately 2 mm thick; the tubes are held in a vertical position by two plastic plates, each about 9 cm in diameter and 6 mm in thickness, with six holes, each about 24 mm in diameter, equidistant from the center of the plate and equally spaced from one another. Attached to the under surface of the lower plate is 10-mesh No. 23 (0.025-inch) W. and M. gauge woven stainless-steel wire cloth having a plain square weave. The parts of the apparatus are assembled and rigidly held

by means of three bolts passing through the two plastic plates. A suitable means is provided to suspend the basket-rack assembly from the raising and lowering device using a point on its axis.

The design of the basket-rack assembly may be varied somewhat provided the specifications for the glass tubes and the screen mesh size are maintained.

Disks[2]—Each tube is provided with a slotted and perforated cylindrical disk 9.5 ± 0.15 mm thick and 20.7 ± 0.15 mm in diameter. The disk is made of a suitable, transparent plastic material having a specific gravity of between 1.18 and 1.20. Five 2-mm holes extend between the ends of the cylinder, one of the holes being through the cylinder axis and the others parallel with it equally spaced on a 6-mm radius from it. Equally spaced on the sides of the cylinder are four notches that form V-shaped planes that are perpendicular to the ends of the cylinder. The dimensions of each notch are such that the openings on the bottom of the cylinder are 1.60 mm square and those on the top are 9.5 mm wide and 2.55 mm deep. All surfaces of the disk are smooth.

Procedure

Uncoated Tablets—Place 1 tablet in each of the six tubes of the basket, add a disk to each tube, and operate the apparatus, using water maintained at $37 \pm 2°$ as the immersion fluid unless another fluid is specified in the individual monograph. At the end of the time limit specified in the monograph, lift the basket from the fluid, and observe the tablets: all of the tablets have disintegrated completely. If 1 or 2 tablets fail to disintegrate completely, repeat the test on 12 additional tablets: not less than 16 of the total of 18 tablets tested disintegrate completely.

Plain Coated Tablets—Place 1 tablet in each of the six tubes of the basket and, if the tablet has a soluble external coating, immerse the basket in water at room temperature for 5 minutes. Then add a disk to each tube, and operate the apparatus, using simulated gastric fluid TS maintained at $37 \pm 2°$ as the immersion fluid. After 30 minutes of operation in simulated gastric fluid TS, lift the basket from the fluid, and observe the tablets. If the tablets have not disintegrated completely, substitute simulated intestinal fluid TS maintained at $37 \pm 2°$ as the immersion fluid, and continue the test for a total period of time, including previous exposure to water and simulated gastric fluid TS, equal to the time limit specified in the individual monograph plus 30 minutes, lift the basket from the fluid, and observe the tablets: all of the tablets have disintegrated completely. If 1 or 2 tablets fail to disintegrate completely, repeat the test on 12 additional tablets: not less than 16 of the total of 18 tablets tested disintegrate completely.

Enteric-coated Tablets—Place 1 tablet in each of the six tubes of the basket and, if the tablet has a soluble external coating, immerse the basket in water at room temperature for 5 minutes. Then operate the apparatus, without adding the disks, using simulated gastric fluid

---

[1]A suitable apparatus, meeting these specifications, is available from laboratory supply houses, from Van-Kel Industries, Inc., P.O. Box 311, Chatham, N.J. 07928, or from Hanson Research Corp., P.O. Box 35, Northridge, Calif. 91324.

[2]Disks meeting these specifications are obtainable from Van-Kel Industries, Inc.

TS maintained at $37 \pm 2°$ as the immersion fluid. After 1 hour of operation in simulated gastric fluid TS, lift the basket from the fluid, and observe the tablets: the tablets show no evidence of disintegration, cracking, or softening. Then add a disk to each tube, and operate the apparatus, using simulated intestinal fluid TS maintained at $37 \pm 2°$ as the immersion fluid, for a period of time equal to 2 hours plus the time limit specified in the individual monograph, or, where only an enteric-coated tablet is recognized, for only the time limit specified in the monograph. Lift the basket from the fluid, and observe the tablets: all of the tablets disintegrate completely. If 1 or 2 tablets fail to disintegrate completely, repeat the test on 12 additional tablets: not less than 16 of the total of 18 tablets tested disintegrate completely.

Buccal Tablets—Apply the test for *Uncoated Tablets,* but omit the use of the disks. After 4 hours, lift the basket from the fluid, and observe the tablets: all of the tablets have disintegrated. If 1 or 2 tablets fail to disintegrate completely, repeat the test on 12 additional tablets: not less than 16 of the total of 18 tablets tested disintegrate completely.

Sublingual Tablets—Apply the test for *Uncoated Tablets,* but omit the use of the disks. Observe the tablets within the time limit specified in the individual monograph: all of the tablets have disintegrated. If 1 or 2 tablets fail to disintegrate completely, repeat the test on 12 additional tablets: not less than 16 of the total of 18 tablets tested disintegrate completely.

Hard Gelatin Capsules—Apply the test for *Uncoated Tablets,* but omit the use of disks. In place of disks attach a removable 10-mesh wire cloth,[3] as described under *Basket-rack Assembly,* to the surface of the upper plate of the basket-rack assembly. Observe the capsules within the time limit specified in the individual monograph: all of the capsules have disintegrated except for fragments from the capsule shell. If 1 or 2 capsules fail to disintegrate completely, repeat the test on 12 additional capsules: not less than 16 of the total of 18 capsules tested disintegrate completely.

The testing fluid for uncoated tablets and hard gelatin capsules is usually water at 37°C, but in some cases (e.g., alumina and magnesia tablets, benzthiazide tablets) the monograph directs that simulated gastric fluid be used. Tests for enteric-coated tablets call for initial immersion for a specific period of time in simulated gastric fluid, followed by immersion in simulated intestinal fluid. Maximum disintegration times are included in some of the individual tablet monographs but in many cases, a dissolution test has replaced the disintegration test. For most uncoated tablets and capsules, the specified disintegration time is 30 min or less. Exceptions include erythromycin tablets (60 min) and griseofulvin tablets (60 min). For coated tablets, up to 2 hr may be permitted. These specifications are based largely on the disintegration properties of commonly available products of the drug, rather than on bioavailability considerations.

One should expect the disintegration of a tablet in the gastrointestinal tract to take longer than that observed in the U.S.P. apparatus. The disintegration test subjects the tablet to a great deal of abrasion and turbulence, which facilitate disintegration. This is not encountered in the gastrointestinal tract. Since it is unlikely that disintegration would be the rate limiting step in the absorption of drugs from tablets, it is not surprising that the results of in vitro disintegration tests have been found to be of limited value in predicting drug absorption.

Successful correlations between parameters of drug absorption and disintegration times have been reviewed by Wagner.[51] The few quantitative correlations that have been reported involve only sugar-coated or enteric-coated tablets. Results with uncoated tablets have been disappointing. For example, studies with different commercial aspirin tablets showed that their disintegration times had no relation to the rate of absorption of aspirin in human subjects.[52]

There are also reports indicating that although certain enteric-coated products conform to compendial standards for disintegration, they may in fact be poorly absorbed. Bioavailability studies with a marketed enteric-coated aspirin tablet showed incomplete absorption, ranging from 0 to 25% of the dose in 3 of 4 subjects. The fourth subject absorbed the entire dose. Tablet disintegration times, determined by the U.S.P. XVI procedure for enteric-coated tablets, which represents the disintegration time in simulated intestinal fluid after 1-hr exposure to simulated gastric fluid, ranged from 18 to 25 min, well within the 125-min requirement extant at the time.[53] Still another example is a brand of enteric-coated tablets of aminosalicylic acid that met all U.S.P. specifications, including disintegration, but failed to yield detectable blood levels of the drug in 8 normal adults.[54]

The test for tablet disintegration is useful for quality control purposes in manufacturing; however, it is generally recognized that the in vitro disintegration test is a poor index of bioavailability. Conformance of a tablet or capsule product to compendial standards for disintegration does not guarantee adequate drug absorption. On the other hand, failure to conform to a standard for disintegration

---

[3]A suitable wire cloth cover is available as Van-Kel Industries Part TT-1030.

time surely signals a potential bioavailability problem.

Dissolution Tests

The documented inability of disintegration tests to provide an index of bioavailability intensified interest in the development of dissolution tests that might better serve as predictors of drug absorption. The results of these efforts have been more encouraging. From first principles, one would expect a closer relationship between drug absorption and dissolution rather than disintegration, particularly for poorly water-soluble drugs.

The United States Pharmacopeia has played an important role in the development of dissolution standards. For many tablets recognized in U.S.P. XXI, the monographs direct compliance with specifications for dissolution rather than disintegration. Although these specifications are primarily for the purpose of quality control, they represent a first step in the assurance of bioavailability.

The following is taken from U.S.P. XXI as amended in its fifth Supplement.

⟨711⟩ DISSOLUTION

This test is provided to determine compliance with the dissolution requirements where stated in the individual monograph for a tablet or capsule dosage form, except where the label states that the tablets are to be chewed. Requirements for *Dissolution* do not apply to liquid-filled soft gelatin capsules. Where the label states that an article is enteric-coated, and a dissolution or disintegration test that does not specifically state that it applied to enteric-coated articles is included in the individual monograph, the test for *Delayed-release Articles* under *Drug Release* ⟨724⟩ is applied unless otherwise specified in the individual monograph. Of the types of apparatus described herein, use the one specified in the individual monograph.

Apparatus 1—The assembly consists of the following: a covered vessel made of glass or other inert, transparent material[1]; a motor; a metallic drive shaft; and a cylindrical basket. The vessel is partially immersed in a suitable water bath of any convenient size that permits holding the temperature inside the vessel at $37 \pm 0.5°$ during the test and keeping the bath fluid in constant, smooth motion. No part of the assembly, including the environment in which the assembly is placed, contributes significant motion, agitation, or vibration beyond that due to the smoothly rotating stirring element. Apparatus that permits observation of the specimen and stirring element during the test is preferable. The vessel is cylindrical, with a hemispherical bottom. It is 160 mm to 175 mm high, its inside diameter is 98 mm to 106 mm,

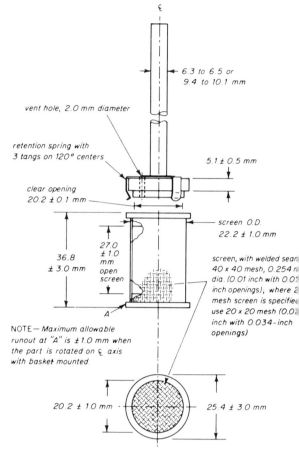

Fig. 1. Basket Stirring Element.

and its nominal capacity is 1000 mL. Its sides are flanged at the top. A fitted cover may be used to retard evaporation.[2] The shaft is positioned so that its axis is not more than 2 mm at any point from the vertical axis of the vessel and rotates smoothly and without significant wobble. A speed-regulating device is used that allows the shaft rotation speed to be selected and maintained at the rate specified in the individual monograph, within $\pm 4\%$.

Shaft and basket components of the stirring element are fabricated of stainless steel, type 316 or equivalent, to the specifications shown in Figure 1. Unless otherwise specified in the individual monograph, use 40-mesh cloth. A basket having a gold coating 0.0001 inch (2.5 μm) thick may be used. The dosage unit is placed in a dry basket at the beginning of each test. The distance between the inside bottom of the vessel and the basket is maintained at 25 ± 2 mm during the test.

Apparatus 2—Use the assembly from *Apparatus 1*, except that a paddle formed from a blade and a shaft is used as the stirring element. The shaft is positioned so

---

[1]The materials should not sorb, react, or interfere with the specimen being tested.

[2]If a cover is used, it provides sufficient openings to allow ready insertion of the thermometer and withdrawal of specimens.

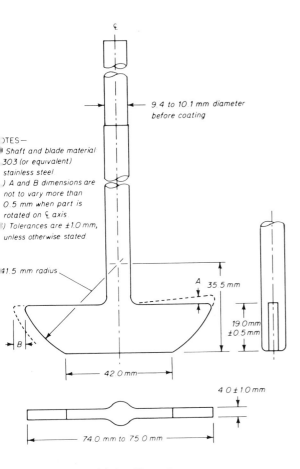

9.4 to 10.1 mm diameter
before coating

)TES—
Shaft and blade material
303 (or equivalent)
stainless steel
) A and B dimensions are
not to vary more than
0.5 mm when part is
rotated on ₵ axis
) Tolerances are ±1.0 mm,
unless otherwise stated

41.5 mm radius

A 35.5 mm

19.0 mm
±0.5 mm

42.0 mm

4.0 ± 1.0 mm

74.0 mm to 75.0 mm

Fig. 2. Paddle Stirring Element.

that its axis is not more than 2 mm at any point from the vertical axis of the vessel, and rotates smoothly without significant wobble. The blade passes through the diameter of the shaft so that the bottom of the blade is flush with the bottom of the shaft. The paddle conforms to the specifications shown in Figure 2. The distance of 25 ± 2 mm between the blade and the inside bottom of the vessel is maintained during the test. The metallic blade and shaft comprise a single entity that may be coated with a suitable inert coating. The dosage unit is allowed to sink to the bottom of the vessel before rotation of the blade is started. A small, loose piece of nonreactive material such as not more than a few turns of wire helix may be attached to dosage units that would otherwise float.

Apparatus Suitability Test—Individually test 1 tablet of the *USP Dissolution Calibrator, Disintegrating Type*[3] and 1 tablet of *USP Dissolution Calibrator, Nondisintegrating Type*,[3] according to the operating conditions specified. The apparatus is suitable if the results

[3]Available from USP-NF Reference Standards, 12601 Twinbrook Parkway, Rockville, Md. 20852.

obtained are within the acceptable range stated in the certificate for that calibrator in the apparatus tested.

Dissolution Medium—Use the solvent specified in the individual monograph. If the *Dissolution Medium* is a buffered solution, adjust the solution so that its pH is within 0.05 unit of the pH specified in the individual monograph. [NOTE—Dissolved gases can cause bubbles to form which may change the results of the test. In such cases, dissolved gases should be removed prior to testing.]

Time—Where a single time specification is given, the test may be concluded in a shorter period if the requirement for minimum amount dissolved is met. If two or more times are specified, specimens are to be withdrawn only at the stated times, within a tolerance of $\pm 2\%$.

Procedure for Capsules, Uncoated Tablets, and Plain Coated Tablets—Place the stated volume of the *Dissolution Medium* in the vessel of the apparatus specified in the individual monograph, assemble the apparatus, equilibrate the *Dissolution Medium* to $37 \pm 0.5°$, and remove the thermometer. Place 1 tablet or 1 capsule in the apparatus, taking care to exclude air bubbles from the surface of the dosage-form unit, and immediately operate the apparatus at the rate specified in the individual monograph. Within the time interval specified, or at each of the times stated, withdraw a specimen from a zone midway between the surface of the *Dissolution Medium* and the top of the rotating basket or blade, not less than 1 cm from the vessel wall. Perform the analysis as directed in the individual monograph. Repeat the test with additional dosage form units.

Where capsule shells interfere with the analysis, remove the contents of not less than 6 capsules as completely as possible, and dissolve the empty capsule shells in the specified volume of *Dissolution Medium*. Perform the analysis as directed in the individual monograph. Make any necessary correction. Correction factors greater than 25% of the labeled content are unacceptable.

Interpretation—Unless otherwise specified in the individual monograph, the requirements are met if the quantities of active ingredient dissolved from the units tested conform to the accompanying acceptance table. Continue testing through the three stages unless the results conform at either S_1 or S_2. The quantity, Q, is the amount of dissolved active ingredient specified in the individual monograph, expressed as a percentage of the labeled content; both the 5% and 15% values in the acceptance table are percentages of the labeled content so that these values and Q are in the same terms.

Acceptance Table

Stage	Number Tested	Acceptance Criteria
S_1	6	Each unit is not less than $Q + 5\%$.
S_2	6	Average of 12 units $(S_1 + S_2)$ is equal to or greater than Q, and no unit is less than $Q - 15\%$.
S_3	12	Average of 24 units $(S_1 + S_2 + S_3)$ is equal to or greater than Q, not more than 2 units are less than $Q - 15\%$, and no unit is less than $Q - 25\%$.

Two types of dissolution apparatus are officially recognized: Apparatus 1 (basket method), and Apparatus 2 (paddle method). For Apparatus 1, the basket containing the tablet or capsule is immersed in the dissolution fluid and rotated. For Apparatus 2, the dosage form is placed directly in the dissolution medium and the paddle is rotated. The dissolution fluid may be water, buffer solution, or dilute hydrochloric acid, maintained at 37°C. Samples of the fluid are removed at designated intervals and analyzed for drug content.

The U.S.P. monograph for aspirin tablets contains a dissolution test requiring the use of Apparatus 1 at 50 rpm with 500 ml of 0.05M acetate buffer (pH 4.5). Not less than 80% of the aspirin in each tablet must dissolve in 30 min. The dissolution test for digoxin tablets also calls for Apparatus 1, but the basket is rotated at 120 rpm and the dissolution fluid is dilute hydrochloric acid. Not less than 65% of the labeled amount of digoxin must dissolve in 60 min.

The tests described in the U.S.P. are but a few of the large number of dissolution methods proposed to reflect bioavailability. The type and intensity of agitation as well as the dissolution medium usually vary from method to method. There is general agreement that the dissolution medium should be aqueous and, where possible, should be of sufficient volume to easily dissolve the entire dose. It has been proposed that dissolution be studied at more than one pH, and at pH 1 and pH 7 to simulate the usual extremes of pH in the gastrointestinal tract. Others have suggested that small quantities of surface-active agents be added to the dissolution medium to facilitate wetting of the drug, for it is believed that bile salts and other constituents of bile act in this way in the small intestine. There is little agreement regarding the appropriate intensity of agitation and there is difficulty in equating intensities between methods. Many investigators believe that the tablet should be subjected to a minimum degree of abrasion and turbulence and that the agitation intensity of the dissolution test should be fixed accordingly.

Since 1960, there have been many examples of satisfactory correlations between absorption parameters and the results of in vitro dissolution tests. Rank order correlations of absorption data in man with in vitro dissolution data have been reported for different salts of tetracycline and tolbutamide, various commercial aspirin tablets, marketed tablets of spironolactone, and various tablet formu-

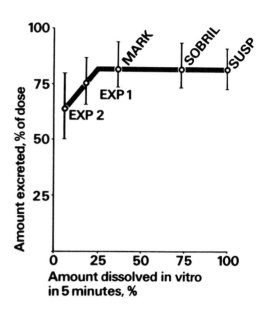

Fig. 5–8. In vivo–in vitro correlation for several formulations of oxazepam. EXP 1, EXP 2, MARK, and SOBRIL are tablets; SUSP is an aqueous suspension. When less than 25% of the dose is dissolved in vitro in 5 min, absorption is incomplete. (From Pilbrant, A., et al.[56])

lations of sulfamethazine and griseofulvin. Quantitative linear correlations between in vivo data and dissolution data have been found with different brands of prolonged-release amphetamine, aspirin tablets, different salts of penicillin V, different esters of erythromycin, and different dosage forms of salicylamide. These studies have been reviewed in detail by Wagner.[55]

Investigators in Sweden have studied the dissolution and bioavailability of oxazepam from different tablet formulations and an aqueous suspension.[56] Dissolution rates were determined by means of a paddle method using simulated gastric fluid. Absorption studies were carried out in healthy, fasting subjects. Absorption rate was assessed by determining the peak concentration of oxazepam in serum. The extent of absorption was evaluated from the sum of oxazepam and its conjugates excreted in the urine over 72 hr. An excellent linear correlation was observed between dissolution rate and peak concentration. When the amount excreted is plotted as a function of dissolution rate, a critical point is found for incomplete absorption corresponding to 25% dissolution in 5 min (Fig. 5–8).

These kinds of data are useful for establishing meaningful dissolution standards for quality control of tablet batches. Clearly, oxazepam tablets

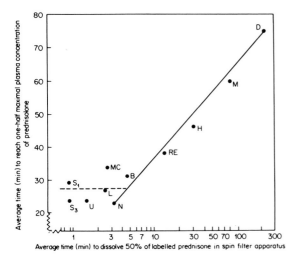

Fig. 5–9. In vivo–in vitro correlation of bioavailability and dissolution rate of different prednisone tablets. Prednisolone is the active metabolite of prednisone. Certain tablets (e.g., S_1, S_3, U, L, MC, B, and N) dissolve so rapidly that dissolution is not the rate-limiting step in absorption. (From Milsap, R.L., et al.[59] Copyright 1979. Reprinted by permission of John Wiley & Sons Ltd.)

Table 5–2. Influence of Dissolution Time on the Correlation Between Bioavailability and in vitro Dissolution of Digitoxin from Tablets*

Dissolution time (min)	Correlation coefficient
30	0.63
60	0.74
120	0.82

*Data from Cabana, B.E., and Prasad, V.K.[60]

from which less than 25% of the drug dissolves in 5 min should be rejected because incomplete absorption is likely.

Studies in Mexico compared the dissolution and absorption of five different brands of nitrofurantoin tablets.[57] A linear correlation ($r = 0.91$) was found between the cumulative amount excreted up to 10 hr after a single dose to healthy fasting subjects and the natural logarithm of the amount dissolved at 60 min using the USP dissolution test. Three of the products showed significantly lower bioavailability than the innovator's product.

Some investigators have proposed that in vitro–in vivo correlations should be based on a comparison of the log of the time required to dissolve 50% of the dose with the time required to reach one-half peak drug concentration in the plasma.[58,59] This type of plot, correlating the dissolution of prednisone from various commercial tablets with the plasma levels of prednisolone, its active metabolite, after a single dose of these tablets, is shown in Figure 5–9. Tablets S, U, L, B, MC, and N differed with respect to dissolution but gave similar in vivo (absorption) values. On the other hand, a linear relationship between plasma concentration and dissolution is found with the more slowly dissolving tablets.

These data indicate that there is some range of in vitro dissolution rates where in vivo measure-

ments will not differ significantly. For these rapidly dissolving tablets, the rate of absorption is independent of the in vitro dissolution rate, perhaps because dissolution is not rate limiting in the absorption of the drug. However, there is a critical value of the dissolution parameter; at this point, further decreases in dissolution will cause a progressive change in the absorption parameter. According to Figure 5–9, the critical time for 50% dissolution of prednisone in the particular apparatus is about 10 to 15 min. Whether this particular correlation applies to all tablet formulations of prednisone is unknown, but the development of a tablet from which at least 50% of the dose dissolves within 15 min would seem to be a desirable goal for a manufacturer wishing to minimize bioavailability problems.

There is some data to support the need for following the dissolution of more than 50% of the dose. Bioavailability and dissolution studies with digitoxin from different tablets have provided the correlations shown in Table 5–2.[60] The longer the dissolution time, the better is the correlation between dissolution and bioavailability. The investigators concluded that, under the stated conditions, 90% dissolution of digitoxin in 2 hr would give at least 90% of the bioavailability of a solution of the drug.[60]

The dissolution test has become an integral part of the control process for the manufacture of tablets, capsules, and other solid dosage forms, but it has also been imbued, by many, with a biologic significance or relevance. Whether or not this conclusion is justified is controversial. The U.S.P. tests and other dissolution methods have been criticized often on technical grounds. There are examples of drug products that failed to meet compendial standards for dissolution but provided adequate bioavailability.[61] On the other hand, there are no examples of a drug product that has met U.S.P. dissolution requirements but showed poor bioavailability characteristics.

Bioavailability studies are by definition clinical studies. Even if the in vitro test faithfully reflects the dissolution process in the gastrointestinal tract, dissolution is but one of several factors determining the bioavailability of a drug. Moreover, there is the reality of intra- and intersubject variability.[62] Nevertheless, dissolution is usually the most important factor in drug absorption, particularly for poorly water-soluble drugs, and carefully correlated in vitro dissolution tests can provide useful guidelines for bioavailability decisions.

REFERENCES

1. Wagner, J.G.: Design and data analysis of biopharmaceutical studies in man. Paper presented to the American Pharmaceutical Association National Meeting, Dallas, Texas, 1966.
2. Gantt, C.L., Gochman, N., and Dyniewicz, J.M.: Effect of a detergent on gastrointestinal absorption of a steroid. Lancet, 1:486, 1961.
3. Gantt, C.L., Gochman, N. and Dyniewicz, J.M.: Gastrointestinal absorption of spironolactone. Lancet, 1:1130, 1962.
4. Bauer, G., Rieckmann, P., and Schaumann, W.: Influence of particle size and dissolution rate on the gastrointestinal absorption of spironolactone. Arzneimittelforsch., 12:487, 1962.
5. Sjögren, J., Sölvell, L., and Karlsson, I.: Studies on the absorption rate of barbiturates in man. Acta Med. Scand., 178:553, 1965.
6. Serajuddin, A.T.M., et al.: Physicochemical basis of increased bioavailability of a poorly water-soluble drug following oral administration as organic solutions. J. Pharm. Sci., 77:325, 1988.
7. Wagner, J.G., Gerard, E.S., and Kaiser, D.G.: Effect of dosage form on serum levels of indoxole. Clin. Pharmacol. Ther., 7:610, 1966.
8. Langlois, Y., Gagnon, M.A., and Tétreault, L.: A bioavailability study on three oral preparations of the combination trimethoprim-sulfamethoxazole. J. Clin. Pharmacol., 12:196, 1972.
9. Putnam, L.E., et al.: Penicillin blood concentrations following oral administration of various dosage forms of penicillin V and comparison with penicillin G. Antibiot. Annu., 1965–1966, p. 483.
10. Neuvonen, P.J., Pentikäinen, P.J., and Elfving, S.M.: Factors affecting the bioavailability of phenytoin. Int. J. Clin. Pharmacol. Biopharm., 15:84, 1977.
11. Seager, H.: The effect of methylcellulose on the absorption of nitrofurantoin from the gastrointestinal tract. J. Pharm. Pharmacol., 20:968, 1968.
12. Bates, T.R., and Sequeira, J.A.: Bioavailability of micronized griseofulvin from corn oil-in-water emulsion, aqueous suspension, and commercial tablet dosage forms in humans. J. Pharm. Sci., 64:793, 1975.
13. Tannenbaum, P.J., et al.: The influence of dosage form on the activity of a diuretic agent. Clin. Pharmacol. Ther., 9:598, 1968.
14. Paikoff, M., and Drumm, G.: Method for evaluating dissolution characteristics of capsules. J. Pharm. Sci., 54:1693, 1965.
15. Lerk, C.F., et al.: In vitro and in vivo availability of hydrophilized phenytoin from capsules. J. Pharm. Sci., 68:634, 1979.
16. Boger, W.P., and Gavin, J.J.: Evaluation of tetracycline preparations. N. Engl. J. Med., 261:827, 1959.
17. Mallis, G.I., Schmidt, D.H., and Lindenbaum, J.: Superior bioavailability of digoxin solution in capsules. Clin. Pharmacol. Ther., 18:761, 1975.
18. Johnson, B.F., et al.: A completely absorbed oral preparation of digoxin. Clin. Pharmacol. Ther., 19:746, 1976.
19. Johnson, B.F., Smith, G., and French, J.: The comparability of dosage regimens of Lanoxin tablets and Lanoxicaps. Br. J. Clin. Pharmacol., 4:209, 1977.
20. O'Grady, J., et al.: Influence of soft gelatin on digoxin absorption. Br. J. Clin. Pharmacol., 5:461, 1978.
21. Lindenbaum, J.: Greater bioavailability of digoxin solution in capsules. Studies in the postprandial state. Clin. Pharmacol. Ther., 21:278, 1977.
22. Lloyd, B.L., et al.: Pharmacokinetics and bioavailability of digoxin capsules, solution and tablets after single and multiple doses. Am. J. Cardiol., 42:129, 1978.
23. Mellinger, T.J., and Bohorfoush, J.G.: Blood levels of dipyridamole (Persantin) in humans. Arch. Int. Pharmacodyn. Ther., 163:471, 1966.
24. Mellinger, T.J.: Serum concentrations of thioridazine after different oral medication forms. Am. J. Psychol., 121:1119, 1965.
25. Shaw, T.R.D., Howard, M.R., and Hamer, J.: Variation in the biological availability of digoxin. Lancet, 2:303, 1972.
26. Levy, G., and Gumtow, R.H.: Effects of certain tablet formulation factors on dissolution rate of the active ingredient. III. Tablet lubricants. J. Pharm. Sci., 52:1139, 1963.
27. Varley, A.B.: The generic inequivalence of drugs. JAMA, 206:1745, 1968.
28. Higuchi, T., Elowe, L.N., and Busse, L.W.: Physics of tablet compression. V. Studies on aspirin, lactose, lactose-aspirin, and sulfadiazine tablets. J. Am. Pharm. Assoc. (Sci. Ed.), 43:685, 1954.
29. Atkinson, R.M., et al.: Effect of particle size on blood griseofulvin levels in man. Nature, 193:588, 1962.
30. Barrett, W.E., and Bianchine, J.R.: The bioavailability of ultramicrosize griseofulvin (GRIS-PEG) tablets in man. Curr. Ther. Res., 18:501, 1975.
31. Schwartz, J.B., and Alvino, T.P.: Effect of thermal gelation on dissolution from coated tablets. J. Pharm. Sci., 65:572, 1976.
32. Lui, C.Y., et al.: Application of a radiotelemetric system to evaluate the performance of enteric coated and plain aspirin tablets. J. Pharm. Sci., 75:469, 1986.
33. Lappas, L.C., and McKeehan, W.: Polymeric pharmaceutical coating materials, II. In vivo evaluation as enteric coating. J. Pharm. Sci., 56:1257, 1967.
34. Rasmussen, S.: Intestinal absorption of quinine from enteric coated tablets. Acta Pharmacol. Toxicol., 24:331, 1956.
35. Lee, D.A.H., et al.: The effect of food and tablet formulation on plasma prednisolone levels following administration of enteric-coated tablets. Br. J. Clin. Pharmacol., 7:523, 1979
36. Day, R.O., et al.: Evaluation of an enteric coated aspirin preparation. Aust. N.Z. J. Med., 6:45, 1976.
37. Ryan, J.R., et al.: Enteric coating of fenoprofen calcium reduces gastrointestinal microbleeding. Clin. Pharmacol. Ther., 42:28, 1987.
38. Paull, P., et al.: Single-dose evaluation of a new enteric-coated aspirin preparation. Med. J. Aust., 1:617, 1976.
39. Mojaverian P., et al.: Effect of food on the absorption of enteric-coated aspirin: correlation with gastric residence time. Clin. Pharmacol. Ther., 41:11, 1987.
40. Fremstad, D., et al.: Absorption of quinidine from an en-

teric coated preparation. Eur. J. Clin. Pharmacol., *16*:107, 1979.

41. Green, D.M.: Tablets of coated aspirin microspherules—a new dosage form. J. New Drugs, 6:294, 1966.

42. Story, M.J.: Enteric-coated pellets: Theoretical analysis of effect of dispersion in the stomach on blood level profiles. J. Pharm. Sci., *66*:1495, 1977.

43. Bogentoft, C., et al.: Influence of food on the absorption of acetylsalicylic acid from enteric-coated dosage forms. Eur. J. Clin. Pharmacol., *14*:351, 1978.

44. Anslow, J.A., et al.: Minimization of gastric damage with enteric-coated aspirin granules compared to buffered aspirin. Pharmacol., *30*:40, 1985.

45. Rosenstein, G., and Belton, E.D.: The relation of potassium therapy to small-bowel lesions. Med. Ann. D.C., *38*:539, 1969.

46. Riley, S.A., et al.: Delayed-release mesalazine (5-aminosalicylic acid): coat dissolution and excretion in ileostomy subjects. Br. J. Clin. Pharmacol., *26*:173, 1988.

47. Asacol: mesalazine for ulcerative colitis. Drug Ther. Bull., *24*:38, 1986.

48. Schroeder, K.W., Tremaine, W.J., Ilstrup, D.M.: Coated oral 5-aminosalicylic acid therapy for mildly to moderately active ulcerative colitis. N. Engl. J. Med., *317*:1625, 1987.

49. Jacobsen, O., et al.: Effect of enterocoated cholestyramine on bowel habit after ileal resection: a double blind crossover study. Br. Med. J., *290*:1315, 1985.

50. Saffran, M., et al.: A new approach to the oral administration of insulin and other peptide drugs. Science, *233*:1081, 1986.

51. Wagner, J.G.: Biopharmaceutics and Relevant Pharmacokinetics. Hamilton, Ill., Drug Intelligence Publications, 1971, pp. 82–88.

52. Levy, G.: Comparison of dissolution and absorption rates of different commercial aspirin tablets. J. Pharm. Sci., *50*:388, 1961.

53. Levy, G., and Hollister, L.E.: Failure of U.S.P. disintegration test to assess physiologic availability of enteric coated tablets. N.Y. State J. Med., *64*:3002, 1964.

54. Wagner, J.G., et al.: Failure of U.S.P. tablet disintegration test to predict performance in man. J. Pharm. Sci., *62*:859, 1973.

55. Wagner, J.G.: Biopharmaceutics and Relevant Pharmacokinetics. Hamilton, Ill., Drug Intelligence Publications, 1971, pp. 125–147.

56. Pilbrant, A., et al.: Comparative bioavailability of oral dosage forms of oxazepam—correlation with in vitro dissolution rate. Acta Pharmacol. Toxicol., *40*:7, 1977.

57. Lopez, A.A., et al.: Bioequivalence study of nitrofurantoin tablets: in vitro-in vivo correlation. Int. J. Pharmaceutics, *28*:167, 1986.

58. Sullivan, T.J., Sakmar, E., and Wagner, J.G.: Comparative bioavailability: a new type of in vitro-in vivo correlation exemplified by prednisone. J. Pharmacokinet. Biopharm., *4*:173, 1976.

59. Milsap, R.L., et al.: Comparison of two dissolution apparatuses with correlation of in vitro-in vivo data for prednisone and prednisolone tablets. Biopharm. Drug Dispos., *1*:3, 1979.

60. Cabana, B.E., and Prasad, V.K.: Presentation at the APhA Academy of Pharm. Sci., 21st Nat. Meeting, Orlando, Fla., Nov. 16, 1976.

61. Ylitalo, P., Wilen, G., and Lundell, S.: Bioavailability of digoxin tablets in relation to their dissolution in vitro. J. Pharm. Sci., *64*:1264, 1975.

62. Huttenrauch, R., Speiser, P.: *In vitro-in vivo* correlation: an unrealistic problem. Pharmaceutical Research, *2*:97, 1985.

6

Nonoral Medication

The possible routes of drug administration are divided into two classes, enteral and parenteral. The enteral routes include sublingual or buccal, oral, and rectal administration. There are many parenteral routes. The most common are intravenous, intramuscular, and subcutaneous injections, inhalation, and topical applications to the skin, eyes, or certain mucous membranes. Drug absorption from these sites is determined by the physicochemical properties of the drug, the dosage form, and certain physiologic and anatomic factors. This chapter concerns some of the more important biopharmaceutic and pharmacokinetic principles that must be considered when a drug is administered by nonoral routes.

INTRAVENOUS INJECTION

Injection into a peripheral vein is the most common method of directly introducing a drug into the systemic circulation. Intravenous administration is used when a rapid clinical response is required, as in the treatment of epileptic seizures, acute asthmatic episodes, dangerously elevated or dangerously low blood pressure, or life-threatening arrhythmias. This route permits precise dosing that can result in predictable drug concentrations in the plasma.

Most drug solutions should be injected over a 1- to 2-min period or longer to avoid excessively high drug concentrations in the blood and other highly perfused tissues immediately following the injection. Although the initially high concentrations following a rapid iv injection are transient, they can produce local pain and undesirable cardiovascular and central effects. Serious clinical problems have resulted from too rapid injection of phenytoin. The usual intravenous loading dose (10 to 20 mg/kg) or maintenance dose (100 mg every

6 to 8 hr) of phenytoin sodium should be injected at a rate not exceeding 50 mg/min.

Insoluble materials, such as drug suspensions, cannot be given by intravenous injection because they may cause embolism. There may also be a danger of precipitation of a drug in the vein resulting in thrombophlebitis if a drug solution is injected too rapidly. Consequently, the manufacturer of injectable diazepam, which is used as an anticonvulsant in doses of 5 to 10 mg, directs that "when used intravenously the solution should be injected slowly, directly into the vein, taking at least one minute for each 5 mg given." Diazepam is poorly water-soluble. The injectable product contains the drug dissolved in 40% propylene glycol and 10% ethanol. When this solution is added to saline solution, a precipitate forms immediately. Even when this injection is given slowly there may be local pain due, at least in part, to the solvent.

An alternative solvent for intravenous administration of lipid soluble drugs such as diazepam has been described; the drug is dissolved in the soy bean oil phase of an emulsion. A clinical evaluation of diazepam emulsion given intravenously indicated that in 314 patients only 5% complained of discomfort and 0.3% of pain. In the control group of 63 patients treated with diazepam in the usual propylene glycol solvent, 43% complained of discomfort and 35% of pain after injection.[1]

Patients given repeated courses of cytotoxic drugs require central venous access when peripheral administration is ruled out by inadequate veins. Central access may also be useful for hyperalimentation and for patients with hemophilia and other hematological diseases. Access is usually achieved by using percutaneous catheters, such as the Hickman catheter. This is inconvenient and care is required to avoid sepsis. An alternative, consisting of a total implantable silicone catheter connected to a stainless steel chamber with a silicone injection port, has been described.[2]

Under general or local anesthesia, the catheter is inserted into a central vein through the arm, neck, or groin and connected by a subcutaneous tunnel to the chamber, which is implanted subcutaneously on the chest wall. The chamber must be flushed with heparinized saline solution after each use.

Some drugs, including lidocaine, theophylline, and certain antibiotics, are administered by means of intravenous infusion or drip. Continuous intravenous infusions of opiates are commonly used in intensive care units and for the management of postoperative pain. This method of administration is particularly useful with drugs having short half-lives or narrow therapeutic indices. Still more precise drug delivery can be achieved with an infusion pump. This controlled approach is needed with drugs like oxytocin, nitroglycerin, alfentanyl, esmolol, or dopamine which are rapidly metabolized.

To avoid the delay in reaching steady state, intravenous infusions are often preceded by a loading dose. Some of the dosing schemes are quite complicated. An example is found in a study concerned with the efficacy and safety of an intravenous dosage regimen of disopyramide in ventricular arrhythmias in patients with at least four premature ventricular contractions (PVCs) per minute.[3] Disopyramide was injected intravenously at a rate of 0.5 mg/kg over 5 min. Each patient received two or three additional loading doses during the first hour with at least 5-min intervals between them. Intravenous infusion was started with the first divided loading dose and continued at a rate of 1 mg/kg/hr for 3 hr and at 0.4 mg/kg/hr for an additional 15 hr. In 8 of 10 patients the frequency of PVCs fell by at least 70% and the response persisted during the continuous infusion.

A pharmacokinetic model of distribution and elimination, and the average drug concentration needed to maintain sleep were used to devise a dosing regimen for etomidate, a short-acting intravenous anesthetic agent.[4] The complex pharmacokinetic profile of etomidate (three-compartment open model) and its rapid elimination (clearance = 1200 ml/min) prompted the development of a three-step intravenous infusion regimen to satisfy the clinical requirements. Etomidate was given according to the following protocol: 0.1 mg/kg per min for 3 min, 0.02 mg/kg for 27 min, and 0.01 mg/kg for the remainder of the procedure.

The eyelid reflex disappeared about 2 min after the start of the first infusion. Anesthesia was considered clinically satisfactory in all cases and no important side effects were observed during maintenance or recovery. Nine of the 11 patients awoke within 10 min of stopping etomidate. A three-stage iv infusion dosing regimen to suppress ventricular ectopic depolarizations has also been described for flecainide.[5]

Sometimes, the administration of a drug as a continuous iv infusion appears to have clear advantages over intermittent treatment. For example, Hull et al.[6] compared continuous iv heparin with intermittent subcutaneous heparin (every 12 hr) in the initial treatment of patients with acute proximal deep-vein thrombosis. Intermittent subcutaneous treatment was inferior to continuous iv heparin in preventing recurrent venous thromboembolism. The incidence of recurrence was about 20% for the subcutaneous group and 5% for the iv infusion group.

Daily fluctuations in motor performance, frequently accompanied by dyskinesias, are one of the most common problems in patients with Parkinson's disease after long-term treatment with intermittent oral levodopa. Continuous iv infusions of levodopa have been found to correct random on-off fluctuations.[7] Constant plasma concentrations of levodopa produce a constant response for prolonged periods of time.

Patients with cancer treated with cisplatin are given metoclopramide to control nausea and vomiting. Substantial control of emesis (two episodes or fewer) was achieved in about 80% of the patients given continuous metoclopramide compared with about 50% of the patients receiving intermittent metoclopramide.[8]

Adoptive immunotherapy with bolus-dose recombinant interleukin-2 (IL-2) has been reported to induce tumor regression in some patients with cancer, but has been associated with severe fluid retention and other adverse effects. In an effort to preserve the efficacy but reduce the toxicity of this treatment, West et al.[9] used escalating doses of IL-2 as a constant iv infusion rather than as a bolus injection.

Response rate among the patients who could be evaluated was similar to the rates observed in earlier studies, which used bolus doses, suggesting that administration of IL-2 as a constant infusion preserved the antineoplastic activity of adoptive immunotherapy. At the same time, this mode of administration appears to substantially increase the safety and comfort of patients.

One study, using bolus doses of IL-2, found that 16 of 25 patients retained fluid in excess of 10% of total body weight, and 20 of the 25 patients experienced dyspnea. In the infusion study, severe fluid retention occurred in only 5 of 40 patients and pulmonary edema was observed in 6 patients. The investigators conclude that "by permitting the delivery of adoptive cellular therapy in a tolerable and safe manner, the administration of IL-2 as a constant infusion may . . . hasten the day when this form of biotherapy can be integrated into the combined-modality treatment of patients with cancer."

Intravenous infusions sometimes fail because of extravasation of infusate or development of phlebitis. This interferes with therapy, causes considerable patient discomfort, and increases workload for hospital staff. Extravasation and phlebitis may be initiated by venoconstriction in the region of the infusion site brought about by irritation of the endothelium. If this is the case, it may be possible to reduce the frequency of these events by keeping the veins dilated. This might be accomplished with topical nitroglycerin.

Nitroglycerin patches releasing 5 mg/day or placebo patches were applied to the skin of patients distal to intravenous infusion sites in a double-blind manner.[10] The frequency of infusion failure was much lower with the active patch than with placebo. Of the 103 infusions in the placebo group, 44 failed, compared with 15 failures among the 105 infusions in the nitroglycerin group.

When a drug is given intravenously, the amount administered and the rate of administration can be carefully controlled and bioavailability is ordinarily not an issue. The amount reaching the systemic circulation is the amount given. The iv administration of prodrugs, however, is an exception. Certain drugs are modified chemically to produce more water-soluble derivatives for injection. These derivatives frequently have little pharmacologic activity; clinical response depends on conversion to parent drug in the body. A slow rate of conversion could result in poor bioavailability of the active form of the drug.

Relatively few investigations have been directed to this problem. Studies in man indicate that dexamethasone phosphate (an ester prodrug) is rapidly and efficiently converted to dexamethasone after intravenous injection.[11] The overall conversion is approximately 90%, and the half-life of conversion is about 10 min. A different prodrug, dexamethasone sulfate, yields virtually no free dexamethasone in plasma or urine after intravenous injection.[12] About 60% of the dose is recovered in the urine in the form of unchanged dexamethasone sulfate. These results cast serious doubts on the clinical value of this prodrug.

Renal allograft rejections are often treated with large intravenous doses of prednisolone. The solubility of prednisolone, however, is poor and, in the US, it is usually given in the form of a freely soluble prodrug, either prednisolone sodium succinate or prednisolone disodium phosphate (prednisolone phosphate). In other countries, prednisolone tetrahydrophthalate (prednisolone phthalate) is also used.

The time course of hydrolysis of iv doses of prednisolone phosphate and phthalate (to form prednisolone) was studied in renal transplant patients.[13] In all patients, the hydrolysis of the prednisolone phosphate ester was faster than that of the prednisolone phthalate ester. The mean peak concentration of prednisolone was higher for the phosphate than the phthalate (18.5 μg/ml versus 2.9 μg/ml). The mean AUCs of prednisolone were 2341 μg/ml/min for the phosphate and 1299 μg/ml/min for the phthalate.

The phosphate ester appeared to be converted to prednisolone very efficiently. On the other hand, about 50% of the iv dose of the phthalate was metabolized and/or excreted before conversion. Therapeutic inequivalence must be expected when patients are treated with equimolar doses of these two prodrugs.

When chloramphenicol is required for intravenous therapy it is given in the form of a sodium salt of the succinate ester. Recent studies indicate that this ester prodrug may present bioavailability problems in certain patients. As much as 40% of the prodrug is recovered unchanged in the urine after intravenous injection to critically ill adult patients.[14] Similar results were found in sick children; bioavailability of chloramphenicol after injection of the succinate ester ranged from 55 to 92%.[15]

INTRA-ARTERIAL ADMINISTRATION

The principal application of this mode of drug administration is in the field of cancer chemotherapy. Liver involvement by metastatic cancer occurs frequently and is a major source of morbidity and mortality. With metastatic colorectal cancer, most of the tumor may reside in the liver. Infusion of chemotherapeutic agents directly into the hepatic artery can potentially expose the tumor to higher drug concentrations than are possible with conventional intravenous infusions.[16]

Theoretical advantages of intra-arterial drug administration have been described in considerable detail.[17,18] Only a small fraction of the dose of a drug given intravenously may reach the target organ if drug elimination by the lungs and other tissues is significant. Accordingly, drug selection for hepatic arterial administration should include agents with high extrahepatic clearance relative to hepatic blood flow. Under these conditions, exposure of the hepatic tumor to drug is increased relative to the exposure of such sensitive tissues as the bone marrow and gastrointestinal epithelium. Furthermore, if there is extraction of the drug by the liver, even less drug will be delivered systemically. In other words, for a given level of systemic exposure, more regional exposure can be obtained. The achievement of higher drug concentrations in the liver with lower systemic levels should increase local antitumor effects and decrease systemic toxic effects, thereby improving the therapeutic index of treatment.

In 1978, Ensminger et al.[19] evaluated the degree to which hepatic arterial infusion of floxuridine (FUDR) or fluorouracil produces higher hepatic and lower systemic drug concentrations than are achieved with corresponding peripheral venous infusions. Fifteen patients with primary or metastatic liver cancer were studied.

Both drugs are efficiently eliminated by the liver. On hepatic arterial infusion, 94 to 99% of FUDR and 19 to 51% of fluorouracil are extracted in one pass through the liver. The high hepatic extraction of these drugs suggests that infusion of these fluorinated pyrimidines directly into the hepatic artery should produce lower systemic drug concentrations than those obtained when equivalent doses are given by a peripheral vein. With FUDR, hepatic arterial infusion resulted in systemic levels of about 25% of corresponding systemic levels with intravenous infusion. Differences in systemic levels were less dramatic with fluorouracil; systemic levels with hepatic arterial infusion ranged from 50 to 77% of corresponding levels with peripheral vein infusion.

A principal objective of this investigation was to demonstrate higher drug concentrations in the liver and hepatic tumor after hepatic arterial administration than after intravenous administration of equivalent doses. Drug concentration in the hepatic vein was assumed to reflect the concentration prevailing proximally in the tumor blood supply. Hepatic arterial infusion produced hepatic vein levels that were about 2 to 6 times higher than those achieved when FUDR was given by a peripheral route. Hepatic vein levels of fluorouracil were also higher with hepatic arterial than peripheral vein administration, but differences were only in the order of 40 to 60%.

Hepatic tumors derive their blood supply primarily from the hepatic artery. Because only one-third of hepatic blood flow is derived from the hepatic artery, the actual tumor exposure to drug given via the hepatic artery may be two or three times higher than reflected in the hepatic vein levels.

These results generally support hepatic arterial infusion as a means to improve the therapeutic index of FUDR and fluorouracil in the treatment of liver cancer. This hypothesis was tested directly by Kemeny et al.,[20] who compared the efficacy of FUDR given by 14-day continuous infusion via the hepatic artery or cephalic vein in patients with liver metastases from colorectal cancer.

Intrahepatic therapy produced a significantly higher complete or partial response rate than systemic therapy (50% *versus* 20%). Patients randomized to systemic therapy who exhibited tumor progression were then given intrahepatic chemotherapy. About 25% of these patients had a partial response and 33% a minor response or stabilization of disease. The investigators concluded that hepatic arterial chemotherapy significantly increases response rate to FUDR for hepatic metastases from colorectal cancer and appears to be a more effective treatment than systemic chemotherapy.

Controlling Hepatic Blood Flow Rate

If the extrahepatic clearance of a drug is relatively high, the concentration of drug in the liver and hepatic tumor is dependent on the blood flow rate through the hepatic artery. A low arterial blood flow rate will ensure a high local drug level. Several methods have been evaluated to decrease hepatic arterial blood flow, including ligation of the hepatic artery, the use of balloon catheters, the infusion of vasoconstrictors such as epinephrine or vasopressin, and the use of biodegradable microspheres.[16]

Hepatic arterial injection of degradable starch microspheres, approximately 40-μm diameter, can produce transient, nearly complete blockage of blood through the hepatic arterial bed. Blood flow resumes in 15 to 30 min as the microspheres are digested by serum amylase. The hepatic arterial injection of a suspension of starch microspheres in a drug solution could temporarily retain the drug in the hepatic arterial capillary bed, resulting in higher drug concentrations in the surrounding tissue. When the antineoplastic drug carmustine (BCNU) is given with starch microspheres directly into the hepatic artery, systemic drug exposure is reduced up to 90% compared to the exposure when drug is injected alone, because of increased drug delivery to the liver and hepatic tumor.[16]

Gyves et al.[21] examined the potential for decreased systemic exposure to mitomycin by concurrent hepatic arterial injection of starch microspheres. Mitomycin was selected because it has activity against several tumors that metastasize to the liver, its dose is limited by myelosuppression when given systemically, and it has a high total body clearance.

Mitomycin (10 mg/m^2) was given via the hepatic artery to patients with incurable liver tumors, alone or with starch microspheres (36 or 90 million). Mitomycin concentrations were measured in plasma over the next 60 min.

Both doses of starch microspheres significantly reduced systemic exposure to mitomycin after hepatic arterial administration. At the lower dose, the microspheres reduced the average systemic exposure to mitomycin by 33%, with individual values ranging from 18 to 52%. At the higher dose of microspheres, the average reduction in systemic exposure was 40%, with a range of 17 to 72%.

The failure to observe a larger effect on mitomycin at the higher dose of microspheres than at the lower dose is surprising, but studies on hepatic blood flow distribution after administration of starch microspheres provide insight. In some patients, temporary arterial venous shunts develop within the liver during blockage of the arteriolar capillary bed by microspheres. The degree of intrahepatic shunting appears to be related to the dose of degradable starch microspheres. Arterial venous shunting reduces the effectiveness of the microspheres because drug in the shunted blood evades hepatic extraction and is available to the systemic circulation.

The effect of degradable starch microspheres on the pharmacokinetics of intrahepatic floxuridine and mitomycin was studied in patients with colon carcinoma metastatic to the liver.[22] The biodegradable microspheres decreased arterial blood flow to normal liver by about two-thirds and to hepatic tumor by nearly 80%. The microspheres reduced systemic (plasma) exposure to floxuridine by one-third and to mitomycin by 20%. The estimated increase in tumor exposure produced by the starch microspheres was nearly 4-fold for floxuridine and 3-fold for mitomycin.

The principal effect of degradable starch microspheres is a widening of the therapeutic window—the same degree of tumor exposure results in less systemic exposure. The investigators suggest that the search for agents that might lend themselves to the successful exploitation of this approach might best start with a re-examination of drugs that have demonstrated activity in pre-clinical trials but proved too toxic for clinical use.

Treating Brain Tumors—Some Potential Problems

Intra-arterial administration of antineoplastic drugs for the treatment of malignant gliomas, metastatic tumors, and primary lymphomas in the brain is also under investigation, but focal toxicity remains a problem. The most frequently reported local toxicity is retinal damage.

A possible cause of focal tissue damage is nonuniform drug delivery related to incomplete mixing. A key assumption underlying pharmacokinetic theory of arterial drug administration is that mixing is complete before the first distal arterial branch. This may not be the case, particularly if the infusion rate is much lower than blood flow rate.

According to Blacklock et al.,[23] at low infusion rates, the solution emerges from the catheter tip as a thin stream that remains stable for some distance and exits in variable concentrations into arterial branches. At higher infusion rates, the infused jet is unstable and tends to mix with the blood near the site of infusion.

These investigators studied brain distribution of labeled iodoantipyrine in monkeys after internal carotid artery infusion at slow infusion rates (1 to 2% of arterial blood flow) and fast infusion rates (20% of blood flow). The deposition of isotope in the infused hemisphere after slow infusion was strikingly heterogeneous, with as much as 13-fold differences in drug concentration in anatomically contiguous areas of the brain. Animals that were given fast intra-arterial infusions, designed to promote drug mixing, had much more uniform drug deposition in the perfused hemisphere.

Blacklock and his colleagues believe that the cause of heterogeneous distribution is drug streaming in the internal carotid artery and its branches. They note that "a variable delivery of antineoplastic agents to the perfused tissue . . . may result in subtherapeutic drug levels at sites containing tumor and toxic levels at other sites within the perfused hemisphere. Drug streaming during intraarterial infusion may be the cause of the focal cerebral toxicity currently being observed in patients who received intracarotid chemotherapy."

Dedrick[24] suggests that drug streaming may also be a problem for intrahepatic arterial administration. Hepatic arterial infusion of floxuridine has produced considerable local toxicity (e.g., intestinal ulcers, biliary sclerosis) not seen with systemic administration. This may due to drug streaming. Dedrick concluded that "it would be prudent to consider suitable techniques, such as pulsing or jetting the infusate, to attempt to eliminate or reduce the potential problem." The efficacy and safety of intra-arterial chemotherapy cannot be evaluated until intravascular drug streaming is eliminated as a confounding factor in clinical trials.

SPINAL ADMINISTRATION

Many drugs do not easily penetrate the blood-brain barrier; systemic administration results in low and ineffective drug concentrations in cerebrospinal fluid (CSF). An alternative route for the administration of antibiotics, antifungals, or antineoplastics, which may be required for life-threatening situations, is direct injection into the CSF. This is usually accomplished by lumbar puncture and injection into the subarachnoid space. A comprehensive review of intrathecal drug therapy was published in 1978.[25]

Spinal administration of opiates was first considered about 10 yr ago. Opioid receptors are present at several sites in the spinal cord. An intrathecal injection of morphine 0.5 mg delivers far more drug to these spinal receptors than does a much larger, probably lethal, dose of morphine given by iv injection. Disappointingly, this does not result in a more profound degree of analgesia but does provide a more persistent effect. A single dose of intrathecal morphine produces analgesia for 12 to 24 hr in patients who have not previously received opiates. Intrathecal morphine is often used in conjunction with local anesthetics in spinal anesthesia.

Epidural administration of opiates provides a major advantage over intrathecal administration in that the use of an epidural cannula allows for repeat injections or continuous infusion to sustain analgesia.[26] The most important distinction between the epidural and intrathecal routes is the extent to which drug in the epidural space is transferred to the intrathecal rather than the systemic circulation. Several studies have found that morphine but not other opiates is preferentially transferred to the cerebrospinal fluid after subdural administration.

Nordberg et al.[27] investigated the pharmacokinetics of epidural morphine in plasma and cerebrospinal fluid (CSF) in patients undergoing elective thoracotomy for pulmonary tumor. Patients received 2, 4, or 6 mg of morphine administered epidurally (at the lumbar level) within 3 hr after surgery. Morphine was absorbed rapidly from the epidural space; peak plasma concentrations were 20 to 40 ng/ml, comparable to the levels found after intramuscular injection of morphine, and occurred within 15 min after administration. The half-life of morphine in plasma averaged about 3 hr. Cerebrospinal fluid concentration of morphine was 50 to 200 times higher than morphine concentration in plasma throughout the 5-hr period of study. Because of the high CSF/plasma concentration ratio, CSF morphine levels were substantial even 20 hr after epidural injection.

The mean duration of analgesia (the time interval between the epidural morphine dose and the first intramuscular injection of meperidine) increased with increasing epidural doses, ranging from 8.6 hr after the 2-mg dose to 15.6 hr after the 6-mg dose. In the group receiving the 6-mg dose, the respiratory rate tended to decrease after injection.

In another study, 33 patients were randomly assigned to two groups to study the analgesic potency, duration of action, and side effects of epidurally and intramuscularly administered morphine after hip surgery.[28] An epidural injection of 10 ml of normal saline solution containing 2 mg morphine was given to one group, and a 10-mg intramuscular injection of morphine was given to the other.

There was a more rapid onset of action after intramuscularly injected morphine (less than 15 min in all patients) than after epidurally injected morphine (15 to 60 min). However, the degree of pain relief was substantially greater and the duration of action markedly longer after epidurally administered morphine than after intramuscularly administered morphine. On the average, an additional

21 mg of intramuscularly administered morphine was required to maintain analgesia in the first group during the 15-hr observation period, whereas only an additional 1.6 mg of epidurally administered morphine was required in the second group. Five of 15 patients who received morphine epidurally required no additional analgesia after the initial dose, compared with only 1 of 18 patients given morphine intramuscularly.

Carmichael et al.[29] carried out a randomized, double-blind, placebo-controlled study of the efficacy, duration, and safety of epidurally administered morphine for the management of pain after cesarean section. Three groups of patients received either 0, 4, or 8 mg morphine sulfate in 10 ml of normal saline solution through an epidural catheter at the completion of the operation.

Compared with the saline solution controls, both groups receiving morphine epidurally had significantly greater pain relief, a longer time to the first administration of additional analgesic, and a decreased amount of supplemental analgesia required in the first 36 hr after surgery. The average time to the first administration of an additional analgesic drug was 2.8 hr for the group receiving saline solution, 22.5 hr for the group receiving 4 mg of morphine, and 26.5 hr for the group receiving 8 mg of morphine. The average numbers of supplemental analgesic doses over the 36-hr period were 11.5 for the group receiving saline solution, 2.6 for the group receiving 4 mg of morphine and 1.8 for the group receiving 8 mg of morphine.

Some clinicians have found that the duration of analgesia from a single dose of epidural morphine is insufficient and have favored continuous epidural infusion. El-Baz et al.[30] evaluated postoperative pain relief and the incidence of side effects in patients given either intermittent epidural injection of morphine as needed or continuous epidural morphine supplemented with iv morphine on request. Postoperative pain relief was similar with both methods.

Intermittent epidural injection of morphine relieved pain for an average of 5.8 hr per injection, but was associated with urinary retention in all 30 patients, with pruritus in 12, and with respiratory depression in 8. Continuous epidural infusion of morphine, with occasional iv morphine supplementation, was associated with minimal adverse effects. One patient complained of pruritus and two patients developed urinary retention.

There is also interest in the use of continuous

epidural morphine in conjunction with patient-controlled or on-demand analgesia. In one study,[31] patients who underwent abdominal surgery were given 2 mg morphine through an epidural catheter. Following this bolus, a 0.25% solution of morphine HCl was infused at a basal rate of 0.06 ml/hr (equivalent to 0.16 mg morphine per hr). This basal infusion was tapered to zero over several days.

Mean morphine consumption was 4.8 mg on the day of surgery, 1.9 mg on the first postoperative day, and 0.6 mg on the second postoperative day. Satisfactory analgesia was obtained in all patients. A fixed regimen of morphine probably would have required more drug and produced less satisfactory analgesia.

INTRAPERITONEAL ADMINISTRATION

The poor response to chemotherapy in patients with malignant disease of the gastrointestinal tract has prompted efforts to develop alternative techniques for administering therapy. Direct delivery of drug into an area of the body with cancer (regional therapy) is one such approach. The idea behind regional chemotherapy is to provide a pharmacokinetic advantage through high local concentrations of drug, with substantially lower systemic exposure to the drug. Intrahepatic artery treatment of carcinoma of the colon metastatic to the liver, described earlier, is an example of regional therapy.

Another example is the intraperitoneal (IP) administration of antineoplastic drugs as therapy for tumors principally confined to the abdominal cavity.[32] Pharmacokinetic theory predicts that a large and potentially advantageous difference in drug concentration occurs between the peritoneal cavity and the plasma after certain anticancer drugs are given intraperitoneally in large volume.[33]

The rate of removal of a drug from the abdominal cavity will greatly influence the difference in exposure between the cavity and the systemic circulation. Large, water-soluble, and ionized molecules will exit more slowly than smaller, lipid-soluble molecules and demonstrate larger differentials in concentration.

Dedrick[33] points out that when mannitol is given to rats intraperitoneally, the drug concentration in the peritoneal cavity falls with time, while the plasma concentration increases transiently, reaches a peak, and then begins to fall more or less in parallel with the peritoneal concentration, but at about a 10-fold lower value of concentration. This pattern may be expected with any hydrophilic drug given intraperitoneally.

A major exit mechanism for drugs from the peritoneal cavity is by way of the portal circulation. Systemic exposure after IP administration of drugs subject to extensive first-pass hepatic metabolism will be much lower than predicted by diffusion theory alone. 5-Fluorouracil (5-FU), the most useful drug in the treatment of malignant disease of the GI tract, is extensively metabolized in the liver during its first passage through this organ.

A constant intraperitoneal 5-FU infusion by means of a totally implanted pump system has also been described.[34] In this study, 5 patients received one or more courses of 5-day continuous IP therapy. In each course, a 100 to 1,000 concentration differential in favor of the peritoneal cavity was maintained. Steady-state venous plasma 5-FU concentrations averaged 0.34 μM, whereas steady-state peritoneal levels average 697 μM.

A clinical study at the National Cancer Institute compared continuous intravenous 5-FU with IP 5-FU in patients undergoing surgical resections for carcinoma of the colon and at risk of tumor recurrence.[35] Although survival rates were not significantly different between the two groups, the total amount of 5-FU that was tolerated was significantly greater in the patients treated with IP 5-FU. Furthermore, the risk of local peritoneal cavity recurrence was significantly less in patients receiving IP therapy.

INTRAMUSCULAR INJECTION

The delivery of exact quantities of drug is usually assured by intramuscular (IM) administration, but the rate of drug absorption may vary widely. Factors that influence absorption rate include the vascularity of the injection site, the degree of ionization and lipid solubility of the drug, the volume of the injection, and the osmolality of the solution.[36]

The site of injection seems to be a particularly important determinant of the absorption rate of drugs after intramuscular administration. Drugs are usually injected into the arm (deltoid), thigh (vastus lateralis), or buttocks (gluteus maximus).

In one investigation, lidocaine plasma levels in patients with proven or suspected myocardial infarctions were determined after administration of 200 mg of the drug intramuscularly.[37] Injection sites were deltoid, lateral thigh, or buttocks. Injection into the deltoid muscle gave higher levels than in-

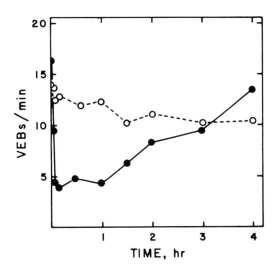

Fig. 6–1. Occurrence of ventricular ectopic beats (VEBs/min) after injection of lidocaine, 4.5 mg/kg, into the vastus lateralis (○) or the deltoid muscle (●). (Data from Schwartz, M.L., et al.[38])

jection into the lateral thigh, which in turn gave higher levels than injection into the buttocks. In a resting patient, the deltoid muscle has the greatest vascularity of the three sites studied. This may account for the more rapid absorption of lidocaine from this site. The generally low plasma levels obtained after injection into the buttocks may reflect the high affinity of lidocaine for fatty tissue and the poor vascularity of this tissue.

Injection of 4.5 mg/kg lidocaine into the deltoid muscle of patients with ventricular ectopic beats (VEBs) has been found to give peak concentrations exceeding 2 μg/ml within 10 min. The rapid attainment of therapeutic blood levels is accompanied by a clinically significant reduction in VEBs. Considerably slower absorption and lower peak concentrations of lidocaine were found after injection into the vastus lateralis muscle. These lower levels did not produce a significant reduction in VEBs.[38] Clinical effect data are shown in Figure 6–1.

Intravenous lidocaine is widely used to prevent ventricular fibrillation among patients who are admitted to hospital during the early stages of acute myocardial infarction (MI). The real threat of ventricular fibrillation, however, is not after hospitalization but before admission—waiting for the ambulance or on the way to the hospital. Intervention by early administration of lidocaine by paramedics or others outside the hospital requires consideration of intramuscular rather than intravenous administration.

To determine whether IM lidocaine before hospital admission is effective in preventing ventricular fibrillation, Koster and Dunning[39] undertook a controlled community study in the Netherlands. About 6000 patients with suspected MI were randomized to either a lidocaine group or a control group. Paramedics used an automatic injector to give a 400-mg dose of lidocaine into the patient's deltoid muscle. All subsequent events were documented by electrocardiographic (ECG) monitoring. The goal of the trial was to reduce the incidence of primary ventricular fibrillation in the 60-min period after lidocaine administration.

The diagnosis of acute MI was made in about one-third of the patients. Ventricular fibrillation occurring within 60 min after randomization was observed in 8 lidocaine-treated patients and in 17 control patients. A greater difference was observed during the 15 to 60 min period after injection. During this period 12 patients in the control group compared with only 2 in the lidocaine group developed ventricular fibrillation. The results suggest that early administration of lidocaine is useful but that patients have little protection from arrhythmias in the 15-min period after injection, perhaps related to slow absorption of the drug.

Initial evaluation of the hepatitis B vaccine under controlled conditions indicated a level of immunogenicity far higher than has been seen in actual use. This unexpectedly poor response may be related to the site of injection. For example, the combined seroconversion rate was 94% among 20 hemodialysis centers that vaccinated staff members in the arm but only 81% in 23 centers using buttock injection.[40] People who lack antibody to hepatitis B surface antigen after vaccination remain susceptible to hepatitis B infection.

In another investigation,[41] the standard three-injection series of hepatitis B vaccine given to 133 community hospital workers by buttock injection produced detectable levels of antibody in only 77 (58%). The next 50 workers to receive the vaccine were given the series of injections in the arm; antibody to hepatitis B surface antigen was found 1 month after the third dose in 87% of this group.

Ukena et al.[41] also gave a complete series of 3 doses by arm injection to 20 hospital workers who had not responded to the initial series given in the buttock; an antibody response was detected in 85% of them. The authors note that "this rate far exceeds the approximately 30 percent response rate among healthy persons revaccinated after nonresponse to arm injection." It is likely that the site of injection may influence the antibody response to hepatitis B vaccine and that healthy adults who do not respond to buttock injection have a good chance of responding when revaccinated in the arm.

Weber et al.[42] administered a series of 3 doses of hepatitis B plasma vaccine to 194 healthy hospital workers, largely female (88%) and relatively young (average age about 35 yr), by intramuscular buttock injection using a 1-inch, 23-gauge needle. Overall, only 56% of the subjects developed detectable antibody to hepatitis B surface antigen in serum after immunization. Logistic regression analysis revealed that the most important predictor for lack of antibody response to the vaccine was the weight-height index, computed as follows:

WEIGHT-HEIGHT INDEX

$$= [\text{weight (kg)}] \, [\text{height (m)}]^{-p},$$

where p equals 2 for males and 1.5 for females. According to Weber et al., "the weight-height index is highly correlated with obesity as determined by skin-fold measurements and has been found to be the most satisfactory relative weight index."

Only 30% of employees with a weight-height index greater than the sex-adjusted 75th percentile for the US population developed significant postimmunization antibodies, compared with 63% of those employees under the 75th percentile. Inadvertent deposition of vaccine into fat may be responsible for the lower response rate following buttock injection.

Cockshott et al.[43] have estimated that buttock injection using a 3.5-cm needle results in deposition into fat rather than muscle in 85% of men and 95% of women. Undoubtedly, the problem is exacerbated in obese subjects and when a shorter needle is used.

Administration of human diploid-cell rabies vaccine in the gluteal area also results in lower neutralizing antibody titer than vaccination in the deltoid area.[44] In adults, the vaccine should always be given in the deltoid muscle; in children the anterolateral aspect of the thigh is also acceptable.

Serum levels and urinary excretion of cephacetrile, cephaloridine, and gentamicin were measured in healthy subjects after intramuscular injection

Table 6–1. Peak Cephradine Concentrations (μg/ml) in Plasma after Intramuscular Injections* at Different Sites to Male and Female Subjects†

Injection site	Males	Females
Gluteus maximus	11.1	4.3
Deltoid	11.7	10.2
Vastus lateralis	9.8	9.4

*Injected doses = 475 mg.
†Data from Vukovich, R.A. et al.[46]

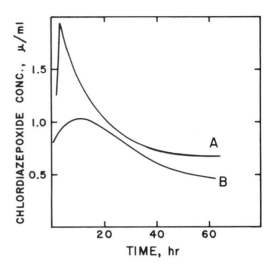

Fig. 6–2. Chlordiazepoxide concentrations in blood after oral (A) or intramuscular (B) administration of a 50-mg dose. (Data from Greenblatt, D.J., Shader, R.I., and Koch-Weser, J.[48])

into the thigh or buttocks.[45] Significantly faster absorption of cephacetrile was noted after injection into the thigh. Similar trends were apparent after injection of gentamicin and cephaloridine.

Male and female subjects each received a single intramuscular injection of cephradine, a cephalosporin antibiotic, once weekly for 3 consecutive weeks. The drug was injected into the gluteus maximus, vastus lateralis, or deltoid muscle.[46] Comparable cephradine concentrations in the serum were observed in males, irrespective of the injection site. Serum levels similar to those produced in males were observed in females after deltoid or vastus lateralis injection. Much lower levels, however, were found in females after injection into the gluteus maximus muscle; peak cephradine concentrations in the serum were less than half those observed after deltoid or vastus lateralis injection (Table 6–1). These findings provide an interesting example of sex differences in the intramuscular absorption of drugs.

Drugs are often given by intramuscular injection to patients who are unable to receive oral medication. This route is also used for drugs that are poorly absorbed from the gastrointestinal tract. Intramuscular injections are usually considered less hazardous and easier to administer than intravenous injections. On the other hand, they are often more painful. Intramuscular injections are routinely administered by nurses, other nonphysician medical personnel, or even by patients to themselves. The popularity of intramuscular injections is reflected in the results of a survey of more than 18,000 hospitalized patients monitored over a 10-yr period. More than half the patients received at least 1 intramuscular injection during their hospital stay.[47]

Many physicians assume that the intramuscular route is as reliable as the intravenous route and results in equal bioavailability of the injected drug. This is not always the case and there is now considerable evidence that intramuscular injection of drugs does not always assure rapid or complete absorption.

Chlordiazepoxide is commonly given by intramuscular injection when rapid sedation is needed. However, some clinicians have observed that large doses of intramuscular chlordiazepoxide appear, at times, to be slowly effective or ineffective. Comparison of chlordiazepoxide concentrations in the blood after oral or intramuscular administration of 50-mg doses in healthy subjects indicates more rapid absorption after oral administration. On the average, peak concentrations of chlordiazepoxide were about 75% greater after the oral dose.[48] These data are shown in Figure 6–2. The time course of chlordiazepoxide concentration in blood in most subjects after intramuscular administration suggests that drug precipitates at the injection site.[49]

Similar results have been observed with pentobarbital.[50] Oral administration results in considerably higher pentobarbital levels in plasma than does intramuscular injection. This study also shows that giving the drug according to a specified injection technique (i.e., a defined needle size and site of injection) results in higher plasma levels than does routine, uncontrolled injections (Fig. 6–3).

There is little appreciation of the thickness of gluteal fat, particularly in female patients. Few female patients and less than 15% of male patients do in fact receive an intramuscular injection when a needle of the usual size is inserted into the but-

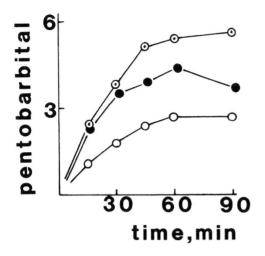

Fig. 6–3. Average pentobarbital concentrations (μg/ml) in plasma following a 100-mg dose. Key: (⊙) oral administration; (●) intramuscular injection, defined needle size and injection site; (○) intramuscular injection, unspecified. (Data from Nair, S.G., et al.[50])

tocks; most patients receive an intralipomatous injection.[43] If deposition into the muscle is desired, we need to choose needles whose length is appropriate for the site of injection and the patient's deposits of fat.

The use of intramuscular diazepam to provide rapid preanesthetic sedation and amnesia is also controversial. Several studies suggest that the absorption of diazepam after intramuscular injection is slow and erratic.[44–52] In contrast, diazepam absorption appears to be rapid, uniform, and complete after oral administration.

Clinical studies to evaluate diazepam as a pediatric premedication show that an oral dose with scopolamine provides satisfactory hypnosis and amnesia; intramuscular diazepam with the same dose of oral scopolamine is considerably less effective.[52] Studies in adults suggest that a 10 mg oral dose of diazepam fails to provide adequate sedation in only 12% of the patients whereas the same dose given intramuscularly shows a failure rate of 37%.[51,53]

Oral administration of thyroid hormone is satisfactory for most patients with hypothyroidism but there is some interest in an injection dosage form for patients with severe hypothyroidism complicated by other diseases, or for those in myxedematous coma. Unfortunately, studies in healthy adults indicate that intramuscular injection of triiodothyronine results in exceedingly slow absorption

of the drug. Only 50% of the dose is absorbed 8 hr after injection. Absorption persists for more than 1 day after administration. It has been suggested that the medication be given intravenously if rapid onset of thyroid-hormone effect is desired.[55]

The slow absorption of some drugs after intramuscular administration is probably a result of precipitation at the injection site. The pH of phenytoin solution for injection is about 12; rapid precipitation is observed if the pH is adjusted to about 7. The dissolution of the crystalline precipitate of phenytoin in the muscle is slow, and absorption is unusually prolonged.

There is occasional need to switch from oral to intramuscular phenytoin because of medical or surgical emergencies. However, several studies have demonstrated that intramuscular administration of phenytoin in doses equal to previous oral doses results in a considerable decrease in plasma phenytoin levels and a potential loss of seizure control.[56,57] With the return to oral phenytoin, phenytoin concentrations in the plasma rise and attain levels significantly higher than steady-state levels before intramuscular therapy.[58] This transient "overshoot," which may last for several days, is the result of slow but continuous phenytoin absorption from the muscle depot during the re-initiation of oral therapy. The elevated phenytoin concentrations in the plasma during this period may be associated with adverse neurologic effects. A typical plasma phenytoin concentration versus time profile in epileptic patients during sequential oral, intramuscular, and oral dosing periods is shown in Figure 6–4.

A method for shifting from oral to intramuscular phenytoin administration in patients requiring parenteral therapy for as long as 2 wk has been proposed.[58] Based on the results of clinical studies, it has been recommended that the usual dose of phenytoin be increased by 50% when switching from oral to intramuscular administration. When a patient is switched back from intramuscular to oral therapy, a dose equal to one half of the original oral dose should be given for the same period of time the patient received intramuscular phenytoin. This dosing scheme seems to avoid significant changes in plasma phenytoin levels when switching from one route to the other.

Digoxin also precipitates at the injection site on intramuscular administration, resulting in slow and incomplete absorption as well as considerable local pain and tissue necrosis.[59] Although intramuscular

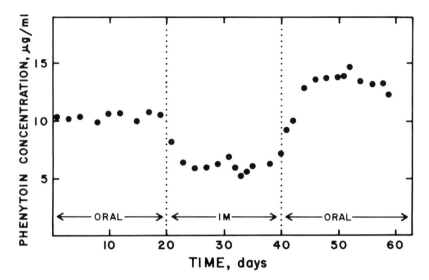

Fig. 6–4. Phenytoin levels in plasma during sequential oral, intramuscular, and oral dosing (4.7 mg/kg per day) in epileptic patients. (Data from Wilder, B.J., et al.[58])

digoxin produces adequate serum digoxin levels in some patients, it should be avoided.

Untoward local effects of intramuscular injections can be due to the mechanical aspects of the injection, or the properties of the drug or its solvent. Propylene glycol, a commonly used solvent, is a particular problem. These effects can develop immediately on injection or have a delayed onset. The release of creatine phosphokinase (CPK) from muscle cells into the blood is a common consequence of the trauma of intramuscular injections. Elevations in serum CPK tend to be greater when large volumes are injected, when the pH or tonicity of the injected solution is far from the physiologic range, or when the solution is intrinsically irritating.[60,61] Studies with intramuscular chlordiazepoxide indicate that the rise in CPK after injection is due largely to the solvent.[60]

Although local adverse effects of intramuscular injections are of concern for certain drugs, the overall incidence of clinically important local complications is low. Among some 26,000 hospitalized medical patients, 46% of whom received at least one intramuscular injection, local complications were reported in a total of only 48 patients (0.4% of all intramuscular recipients).[62] The most common adverse reactions were abscess formation at the injection site, local induration, erythema or wheal formation, and persistent pain. Injections of cephalothin and tetracycline presented the most frequent problems. Local complications were reported in 9 of the 83 patients (10.8%) receiving intra-

muscular cephalothin. The use of intramuscular injections of these high risk drugs needs to be reassessed.

There has been interest for some time in using the slow absorption of insoluble material in a muscle depot as a means of achieving prolonged drug effects. This aspect of parenteral therapy is considered in Chapter 7.

SUBCUTANEOUS INJECTION

Absorption of drugs from subcutaneous tissues is influenced by the same factors that determine the rate of absorption from intramuscular sites. Generally, it is held that the blood supply to this region is poorer than to muscle tissue and, consequently, drug absorption may be slower. Absorption may be hastened by massage, application of heat to increase blood flow to the injected area, local co-administration of vasodilators, or inclusion of the enzyme hyaluronidase in the drug solution. This enzyme breaks down the hyaluronic acid of the connective tissue matrix, allowing the drug solution to spread over a wider area. Absorption can be slowed by adding a vasoconstrictor such as epinephrine to the injection solution. This is commonly done to prolong the effects of local anesthetics.

The most important drug that is routinely administered subcutaneously is insulin. Studies in diabetic children show that with either subcutaneous or intramuscular injection, the absorption rate of insulin is about 50% faster when injected into the

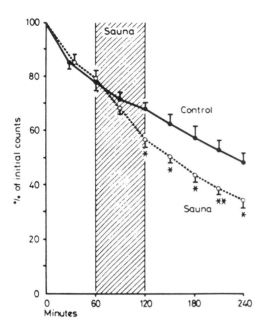

Fig. 6–5. Effect of sauna treatment on the disappearance of ^{125}I-insulin from subcutaneous injection site. (From Koivisto, V.A.[66])

arm rather than the thigh.[63] This difference could constitute a potential source of variability in diabetic control. These investigators also found that insulin injected either intramuscularly or subcutaneously is absorbed at about the same rate. This observation is contrary to the general impression that absorption from subcutaneous sites is slower than from intramuscular sites.

Studies in insulin-dependent diabetics show that exercise and local heating increase both adipose tissue blood flow and insulin absorption after a subcutaneous injection into the anterior thigh.[64] Local cooling decreased blood flow and insulin absorption. A strong correlation (r = 0.97) was observed between adipose tissue blood flow and the first-order absorption rate constant for insulin. These findings help explain why acute exercise in insulin-dependent diabetics is frequently associated with metabolic complications.[65] Studies in Finland indicate that sauna treatment can also accelerate insulin absorption (Fig. 6–5) and lead to hypoglycemia.[66] Such an effect might be prevented by taking a snack or reducing the insulin dose. Cigarette smoking causes peripheral vasoconstriction and may substantially reduce the rate of insulin absorption from subcutaneous tissues.

The duration of action of insulin after injection is controlled largely by its crystallinity. Insulin forms a poorly water-soluble complex when reacted with zinc chloride. Depending on the pH, it may precipitate either as an amorphous or a crystalline solid. Prompt Insulin Zinc Suspension (Semilente insulin) consists of amorphous insulin zinc complex. The drug is readily absorbed upon injection and has a relatively short duration of action (12 to 16 hr). Extended Insulin Zinc Suspension (Ultralente insulin) is made up predominantly of crystalline complex. It is slowly absorbed and has a longer duration of action (36 hr) than prompt insulin zinc suspension. Insulin Zinc Suspension (Lente insulin) is a mixture containing about 7 parts of crystalline to 3 parts of amorphous insulin zinc complex. It is intermediate in duration of action (24 to 28 hr). Another difference in the 3 formulations is their particle size. Prompt insulin consists of small particles; extended insulin is made up of relatively large particles.

EXTERNAL AND IMPLANTABLE PUMPS FOR CONTINUOUS PARENTERAL THERAPY

Until rather recently, the patient requiring continuous parenteral drug therapy had to be hospitalized and tethered to an intravenous drip system. The need to have more accurate delivery of various intravenous solutions and medications, however, has fostered the development of infusion pumps and regulators for bedside use in hospitalized patients to replace the traditional iv drip. Further developments in infusion pump technology, notably in the areas of electronic control and miniaturization, have now made continuous parenteral drug therapy available to ambulatory patients, thereby reducing costs, discomfort, and hospital time—and offering the promise of better treatment of disease.

There are several established portable infusion pumps that are intended to be worn externally. An example is the Auto Syringe (Travenol Labs, Chicago, IL), a battery-driven device that employs standard syringe reservoirs for drug delivery. Several models are available, weighing from 10 to 16 oz, and designed to hang vertically from a belt on the patient's hip. The device has an alarm system to indicate when the battery runs down or the catheter is plugged or kinked. Portable infusion pumps have been used largely for the continuous administration of insulin, but they may be useful for the delivery of antibiotics, cancer chemotherapeutic agents, and other drugs.

The Food and Drug Administration (FDA) has recently approved an implantable drug delivery system (Infusaid; Infusaid Corp., Norwood, MA) for patients who require the continuous administration of heparin or cytotoxic agents. This disc-shaped device weighs about 200 g. It is usually implanted in a subcutaneous pocket in the upper chest or the lower abdominal wall and attached to a Silastic catheter surgically placed to deliver drug solution to a desired artery or vein. The pump consists of two chambers, separated by titanium bellows. The outer chamber contains a fluorocarbon that exerts a vapor pressure of several hundred millimeters of mercury at body temperature. This vapor pressure is the power source, compressing the bellows and forcing drug solution in the inner compartment into the catheter. Periodically, the drug chamber is refilled by percutaneous injection through a central injection port with a self-sealing septum. A side injection port is available on some models to permit bolus injections. The Infusaid pump can hold up to 50 ml of drug solution; flow rate may be varied, but must be factory-calibrated.

Insulin Administration

Patients with type I (insulin-dependent) diabetes mellitus, formerly called juvenile diabetes, do not respond to oral hypoglycemic agents and require exogenous insulin. Many forms of insulin are commercially available; they differ in concentration, time of onset, duration of action, purity, and source. The earliest use of regular insulin in patients with diabetes required at least four injections per day, associated with meals to reduce postprandial serum glucose concentrations. Today, combinations of slow- and intermediate-acting and regular insulin are used, and most patients require two injections daily, one before breakfast and the other before the evening meal. Although this regimen provides acceptable regulation in the majority of patients, all but the most fastidious in observing dietary restrictions and monitoring blood glucose for dosage adjustment will show large swings in serum glucose concentrations during the course of a day and average glucose concentrations well above normal limits.

Hyperglycemia may be a risk factor in the development of diabetic nephropathy, neuropathy, and retinopathy, and stricter control of blood glucose concentrations is now considered desirable to slow or prevent the progression of diabetic complications. The development of portable infusion pumps has been one element in this effort. Continuous administration of insulin in conjunction

with glucose monitoring at home to adjust dosage is being widely investigated as a means of normalizing blood glucose in diabetic patients. These open-loop systems are typically designed to deliver insulin subcutaneously at a constant basal rate interrupted when necessary for before-meal bolus doses of regular insulin. Initial evaluation of this new approach to the treatment of diabetes is encouraging with respect to control of blood glucose, but more study is required to determine long-term benefits.

Mecklenburg et al.[67] compared the metabolic control achieved by glucose monitoring at home and the insulin-infusion pump with that previously obtained with conventional insulin therapy in a series of 100 patients with type I diabetes; the patients in the study were followed up for up to 15 months. The target range of capillary-blood glucose concentration was between 60 and 140 mg/dl. Fasting blood glucose decreased from a mean level of 201 mg/dl before insulin-pump therapy was begun to 158 mg/dl after 30 days, and to less than 140 mg/dl after 3 months on the pump. Statistically significant improvement in metabolic control was found in 71 of the 100 patients. Of the patients receiving insulin-pump therapy for at least 6 months, 62% had mean blood glucose values of 140 mg/dl or lower.

Similarly encouraging results have been observed by Rudolf et al.[68] in pregnant diabetic patients. An improvement in glucose control was achieved within the first month of treatment with the insulin pump and sustained to term. Prevention of maternal hyperglycemia may be important in minimizing the risks for the infant of the diabetic mother. Even modest elevations of maternal glucose levels during the third trimester of pregnancy have been associated with increased risk of perinatal mortality.

Continuous subcutaneous insulin infusion has resulted in improved glucose control in most insulin-dependent diabetics, but it has been much less successful in patients with brittle diabetes. This condition occurs in a small proportion of type I diabetics; it is characterized by unpredictable swings in blood glucose concentration, apparent changes in daily insulin requirement, and an increased number of hospital admissions for ketoacidosis or hypoglycemic coma. Poor glucose control in brittle diabetics may be related to irregular insulin absorption from subcutaneous tissue; therefore, these patients may benefit from an alternative site of insulin administration.

Pickup et al.[69] found little improvement in metabolic control when brittle diabetics were switched from conventional insulin therapy to subcutaneous insulin-pump therapy. Significant improvements, however, were observed in 5 patients when insulin was infused continuously into the deltoid muscle rather than subcutaneously. One patient's disease could be controlled only by intravenous insulin.

The authors ascribe the poor effectiveness of subcutaneous insulin in these patients to erratic absorption. They note that factors such as variation in local subcutaneous blood flow and enzymatic destruction of insulin under the skin may contribute to the problem. Insulin absorption from muscle seems to be more predictable. Pickup et al., however, do not recommend continuous intramuscular insulin infusion as a routine outpatient treatment for brittle diabetes because of serious technical difficulties such as the insertion and long-term securing of the intramuscular cannula.

Pozza et al.[70] describe a patient with brittle diabetes in whom adequate metabolic control could not be achieved by continuous subcutaneous, intramuscular, or intravenous administration of insulin. Appreciable improvement in mean glucose concentration and mean amplitude of glycemia excursions was attained, however, by continuous intraperitoneal administration of insulin through a permanently inserted catheter. The authors suggest that "the intraperitoneal approach has the advantage of delivering insulin at a more physiological site, since the hormone reaches the liver before entering the peripheral circulation."

Infusion Pumps for Other Drugs

Outpatient treatment of severe congestive heart failure remains a problem because of the limited availability of orally effective inotropic agents. Berger and McSherry[71] have described a totally implantable infusion system (Infusaid) to administer dobutamine on an ambulatory basis to patients with refractory congestive heart failure.

Another Infusaid implantable pump has been approved by the FDA to deliver the aminoglycoside antibiotic amikacin directly to the site of infection in patients with osteomyelitis. Osteomyelitis infections are notoriously difficult to treat; severe cases may be incurable and require amputation. Pump treatment with targeted delivery may produce much higher antibiotic levels at the site of infection and thereby be more effective than conventional treatment. Furthermore, the device allows discharge of the patient from the hospital far earlier than the 8 to 10 wk period required to eradicate the infection because the patient receives continuous antibiotic treatment at home.

Both implantable and external infusion pumps have been used with success for the continuous delivery of heparin in the treatment of clotting disorders. Hattersley et al.[72] have described the use of continuous-pump heparin therapy in the treatment of patients with venous thrombosis or pulmonary embolism. The following protocol was used: *(a)* intravenous bolus of 50 units/kg heparin; *(b)* constant heparin infusion of 15 to 25 units/kg per hour; *(c)* modify infusion rate if necessary to maintain an activated coagulation time of 150 to 190 sec.

Efforts have also been directed to continuous-infusion cancer chemotherapy, through an arterial line for organ-specific treatment or through a venous line for systemic therapy; external, portable, and implanted pumps have been evaluated.[73] The rationale for arterial infusion to a specific organ is attainment of high drug concentration at the tumor site and reduced systemic exposure and toxicity. The basis for continuous venous administration is to overcome the short half-life of many cytotoxic drugs and ensure drug exposure to tumor cells during a growth phase.

Lokich et al.[74] described the use of subclavian vein catheterization and a portable infusion pump for continuous delivery of fluorouracil and other antineoplastic drugs to patients with metastatic malignancy. Phillips et al.[75] described the use of a totally implantable system for continuous intra-arterial delivery of antitumor drugs to 6 patients with malignant gliomas. The core of the system is an Infusaid pump, implanted in the infraclavicular subcutaneous pocket, that infused drug solution directly in the internal carotid artery. The Infusaid pump has also been used for direct delivery of antineoplastic drugs to the liver via the hepatic artery in patients with hepatic metastases.[73,76]

Gyves et al.[77] determined fluorouracil concentration in peritoneal fluid and plasma during a 5-day course of continuous intraperitoneal infusion of the drug at a dose of 1 g/day in 5 patients with colonic or gastric cancer. Drug administration involved an infusion pump connected to a peritoneal dialysis catheter implanted in the abdominal cavity and attached to an injection port.

Fluorouracil concentration in plasma ranged from 0.13 to 1.1 μM, whereas drug levels in peritoneal fluid ranged from 0.12 to 2.3 mM. This large difference in concentration was maintained over the 5-day period in each patient. The selective regional advantage of intraperitoneal infusion of fluorouracil, calculated from the ratio of steady-state concentration of drug in peritoneal fluid to that in plasma, ranged from 550 to 7852 in individual patients and averaged 2559.

Although the effectiveness of intraperitoneal infusion of antineoplastic drugs in the treatment of intraperitoneal and hepatic cancer remains to be demonstrated, the availability of implantable devices for convenient access to the peritoneal cavity and developments in infusion pump technology should facilitate further clinical investigation in this area.

Pain associated with advanced cancer is usually well controlled with oral medication. For those unable to take drugs by mouth, continuous subcutaneous infusion has become an established technique. Jones and Hanks[78] described a new portable infusion device that can be set to deliver opioid analgesics for more than 1 month.

INHALATION

The lungs are remarkably efficient organs for the transport of gases; the large surface area of the alveoli, the high permeability of the alveolar epithelium, and the rich blood supply perfusing the lungs facilitate rapid exchange between blood and inspired air. These characteristics are equally important for drug absorption and ensure the rapid uptake of drugs given by inhalation. An additional advantage of this route of administration is that the drug is not subject to first-pass hepatic metabolism; drug is absorbed directly into the bloodstream. Gaseous or volatile anesthetics are the most important examples of drugs routinely given by this route. Inhalation of amyl nitrate has been used in the past to abort attacks of angina. Nicotine, morphine, and tetrahydrocannibinol are rapidly absorbed following inhalation of tobacco, opium, or marijuana smoke.

There have been many investigations on the absorption of gases from the lungs, but relatively few concerning pulmonary absorption of drugs presented in the form of solid or liquid particulates. Useful information is available from a series of studies involving tracheal instillation of drug solutions in rats.[79] These studies indicate many similarities between gastrointestinal and pulmonary absorption. Most compounds seem to be absorbed by passive diffusion across a lipid-pore membrane. Large polar molecules like heparin are slowly absorbed.[80] Absorption of weak electrolytes like p-amino-salicylic acid, procainamide, or sulfisoxazole is a function of pH.[81] The absorption of lipid-soluble molecules is rapid.

Schanker et al.[82,83] compared the rates of pulmonary absorption of aerosolized *versus* intratracheally injected drug solutions in several animal species. At various times after drug administration, the lungs were removed and assayed for unabsorbed drug. The twelve drugs studied had widely different absorption rates. In the rat, after aerosol administration, absorption half-lives ranged from 0.3 min for antipyrine to 44 min for inulin. In all cases, however, the drug was absorbed approximately 2 times more rapidly when inhaled as an aerosol than when given by intratracheal instillation.

Therapeutic aerosols are usually produced by metered-dose inhalers, which provide unit doses of medication from fluorocarbon-pressurized canisters. An alternative approach involves continuously or intermittently generated wet aerosols from ultrasonic or jet nebulizers containing drug solutions; patients usually inhale the medication by tidal breathing.

Although, in principle, any drug intended for systemic effect may be given by way of the lungs, in practice, aerosol administration has been essentially limited to those drugs that affect pulmonary function. An exception is Medihaler Ergotamine, an aerosol device used to abort migraine and other vascular headaches. Aerosolized drugs used in the treatment of asthma and other reversible airflow obstructions include adrenocorticoid steroids (e.g., beclomethasone), bronchodilators (e.g., metaproterenol, albuterol), and antiallergics (e.g., cromolyn).[84]

One reason for the limited use of aerosols for inhalation is the relatively poor efficiency of the dosage form with respect to delivery of drug to the respiratory tract. A large fraction of an aerosolized dose impacts in the mouth and throat and is eventually swallowed rather than inhaled. Considerable variability may be observed in the amount of drug actually reaching the pulmonary tree. Therefore, despite the rapid absorption that can take place from the lungs, aerosol administration cannot be viewed as a routine alternative to intravenous injection. Nevertheless, this route of administration is an important one for many drugs used in respiratory disorders.

At one time, there was controversy as to the best route of administration of bronchodilators. Inhaled bronchodilators are delivered directly to the target organ and minimize the risk of systemic effects. On the other hand, some argue for the intravenous route, particularly in the presence of increasing airways obstruction, because aerosol penetration is limited. The few comparative studies that have been carried out favor aerosol therapy. One study showed that intravenous and inhaled terbutaline provide equivalent benefit in chronic asthma, but that the inhalation route is preferred because it avoids systemic side effects.[85]

Pentamidine is one of few drugs effective in the prophylaxis and therapy of *Pneumocystis carinii* pneumonia (PCP) in patients with acquired immunodeficiency syndrome (AIDS), but the effectiveness of parenterally administered pentamidine is severely limited by serious side effects. Aerosolized pentamidine may be able to eradicate and prevent PCP without these adverse effects.

One report concerned the successful treatment of first episodes of PCP in 13 patients with AIDS by giving 600 mg of aerosolized pentamidine for 20 min daily for 21 days.[86] The only reported side effect was a cough in all but 1 patient.

The particle size of the aerosolized droplets or particulates, although difficult to control, is a critical factor in the efficacy of the dosage form. Large particles (20 μm) impact in the mouth, throat, and upper respiratory tract. Small particles (0.6 μm) penetrate more efficiently into the periphery of the pulmonary tree, from which absorption is most rapid, but total retention is poor and a large fraction of the dose is exhaled.

The condition of the patient may limit the penetration of aerosolized drug into the respiratory tract. The lack of effect of bronchodilator aerosols in severe asthma appears to be related to the patient's inability to inhale an adequate amount rather than to an intrinsic resistance to the drug.[87]

The development of the drug cromolyn and its aerosol dosage form has been particularly well documented. This compound is indicated for the prophylactic treatment of bronchial asthma; the drug is classified as an antiallergic, and is poorly absorbed from the gastrointestinal tract. After deposition in the lungs of various laboratory animals, the drug is well absorbed.[88] Studies in healthy sub-jects indicate about 5 to 10% of the administered dose is deposited in the lungs.[89] Poorer deposition has been observed in asthmatic patients.[90]

Cromolyn is administered by means of an inhalation device called a Spinhaler, designed to deliver the drug as a powder aerosol into the lungs when the device is actuated by the inspiratory effort. The drug for inhalation has a particle size range in which more than 50% by weight is between 2 and 6 μm.

The breath-actuated aerosol dosage form used for cromolyn may have some advantages over the conventional pressurized metered-dose inhaler; the conventional device requires synchronization of the release of the metered dose with the beginning of a deep inspiration to achieve good penetration of the lungs. This synchronization is not required for the breath-actuated device because release of the drug is automatically coordinated with the inspiratory phase of respiration.

A recent comparison of conventional versus breath-actuated aerosols of cromolyn in asthmatic children showed that the breath-actuated device was significantly more effective in reducing symptoms and bronchodilator intake.[91] Another clinical study compared the efficacy of isoproterenol from a breath-actuated inhaler and from a conventional inhaler.[92] The results indicated that both devices give an equally satisfactory degree of relief from bronchospasm, but there is a significant reduction in the number of doses of isoproterenol used during treatment with the breath-actuated device.

Unfortunately, the breath-actuated device is neither ideal nor suitable for all patients. Some patients are irritated by powder inhalation. The powder may be hygroscopic, making its use in humid conditions difficult. Some children are unable to inspire vigorously enough to activate the device.

A new powder inhaler, called a Turbuhaler, has been developed and is claimed to overcome most of the major problems associated with the Spinhaler.[93] It is described as a multidose system that is free of propellants, carriers, and other drug additives and that does not demand coordination between activation and inhalation.

There is convincing evidence that many patients who do not benefit from corticosteroid or bronchodilator aerosol therapy may fail to respond because they do not use the pressurized inhaler correctly. A report from the United Kingdom concerning treatment of asthmatic children with corticosteroid therapy concluded with the following:[94] "Failure to respond to BDA (beclomethasone dipropionate aerosol) was frequently associated with low social status, crowded homes and the communication difficulties associated with immigrants to this country. It is likely that failure to inhale the corticosteroid aerosol properly and regularly is often responsible for a poor response." Another study found that 45 of 321 asthmatic patients used their inhalers incorrectly in spite of careful instruction. All but two of the patients who were unable to inhale correctly from a pressurized canister could use a breath-actuated device efficiently.[95]

Metered-dose inhalers (MDIs) are not easy to use, and patients usually receive little or no instruction in their use. Newman and Clarke[96] recommended that the patient "breathe out fully; hold both the head and the canister upright; place the mouthpieces between the lips; fire the inhaler while inhaling slowly and deeply; hold the breath for 10 seconds, or if less for as long as possible."

Lengthening the pathway between the actuator of the MDI and the mouth may reduce problems of coordination by introducing a delay between actuation and inhalation.[97] This idea is the basis for the development of spacers or cylinders that have a mouthpiece at one end and a fitting at the other to accommodate the mouthpiece of a conventional MDI. Spacers are claimed to reduce the need for optimal coordination and thereby to improve delivery of drugs to the lungs.

There is convincing evidence that spacers decrease oropharyngeal deposition of oral aerosols. As such, they may be particularly useful in reducing the topical side effects of inhaled corticosteroids. An inhalation aerosol formulation of triamcinolone acetonide with a spacer device is commercially available for treatment of asthma in children and adults; the product has been associated with a lower incidence of fungal colonization in the mouth.[98]

Evidence to support the use of spacers to improve the efficacy of bronchodilator aerosols is less convincing. Roughly, an equal number of studies have found a significant improvement when a spacer device was used and have failed to find an important difference. An example of a positive outcome is a study in children with exercise-induced asthma treated with placebo or terbutaline delivered by a conventional aerosol or an aerosol with a tube spacer.[99]

Both terbutaline treatments resulted in a signif-icant increase in forced expiratory volume compared with placebo, but treatment with the device using a spacer produced significantly more improvement than did treatment with the conventional inhaler. The number of errors in inhalation technique was reduced when the spacer was used and this may account for the greater improvement.

Konig[97] concluded his review of MDI spacers as follows: "It seems that spacer devices are neither a breakthrough of such magnitude that their use should be made mandatory for users of MDIs nor a useless gimmick, but they definitely have a value somewhere between these extremes." Spacers may not improve the effects of aerosolized bronchodilator drugs in older children and adults with an adequate technique of inhalation, but may be useful in patients with problems of coordination and in young children. Spacers seem to be indicated in patients who develop oral candidiasis and other topical side effects during treatment with inhalation corticosteroids and in children unable to use the conventional MDI.

Nebulizers

A nebulizer makes an aerosol by blowing air or oxygen through a drug solution. Many inhaled drugs including albuterol, ipratropium, cromolyn sodium, and beclomethasone can be delivered in this way. Nebulization is effective because it allows high doses of drugs to be inhaled without any special effort to coordinate breathing. The aerosol is delivered through a face mask or a mouthpiece. Nebulized bronchodilators are particularly helpful in the acutely breathless patient both at home and in hospital. They can be used in young children and in patients on ventilators.[100]

Although the efficacy of nebulization is widely accepted, there are non-drug related complications associated with its use. Factors such as osmolality, acidity, preservatives, and bacterial contamination must be taken into consideration. Beasley et al.[101] suggest that nebulizer solutions be formulated as isotonic solutions with a pH > 5. Chemical preservatives should be avoided if possible. Solutions should be prepared under sterile conditions in unit dose vials, ready to use. Special attention must be paid to cleaning the nebulizer unit on a regular basis.

TOPICAL APPLICATION TO THE EYE

Drugs are administered to the eye for local effects such as miosis, mydriasis, anesthesia, or reduction of intraocular pressure. Steroids and anti-infective drugs are also frequently used in the eye.

Drugs may be applied in the form of sterile aqueous solutions, aqueous suspensions, solutions or suspensions in oil, ointments, or inserts intended to reside in the conjunctival cul-de-sac. After application, a drug penetrates the cornea, a barrier with both hydrophilic and lipophilic characteristics, to the aqueous humor bathing the lens. Penetration to the vitreous humor occurs through the ciliary bodies and iris.

The biphasic nature of the cornea suggests that the chemical form of a drug may influence the drug's penetration to the aqueous humor. This has been observed with dexamethasone.[104] In both the inflamed and uninflamed rabbit eye with intact corneal epithelium, the acetate derivative produced higher concentrations in the cornea and aqueous humor than did either the more polar phosphate derivative or the less polar free alcohol. The presence of intraocular inflammation increased the ability of the free alcohol to penetrate the cornea, but had little effect on the penetration of the acetate ester.

Based on the usual theories of drug absorption, one would expect the pH of the tear film to influence the ocular absorption of weak electrolytes. There is some evidence for this with pilocarpine, a cholinergic drug used in the treatment of glaucoma. Pilocarpine is a weak base (pKa 7.1); the drug is a more effective ocular hypotensive agent when administered at pH 6.5 (22% un-ionized) than at pH 5 (1% un-ionized).[105] The commercial preparation consists of an acid salt of pilocarpine buffered to about pH 4 to 5 for maximum chemical stability. Upon instillation of solutions of pilocarpine hydrochloride or nitrate in the eye, tear film pH is reduced by 1.1 to 1.6 pH units and remains below pretreatment pH for up to 1 hr.[106] These are not optimal conditions for the absorption of pilocarpine.

The pH-dependent ocular absorption of pilocarpine has been confirmed in more recent studies, but these investigators found a similar pH effect on the absorption of glycerin, a nonelectrolyte.[107] Sieg and Robinson concluded that although a pH-partition mechanism may play a small role, the overriding effect is pH-induced lacrimation. Over a pH range of 5 to 8, the lacrimation response decreases with increasing pH. Thus, at a higher pH less drug is washed away by nonspecific lacrimation, and bioavailability is improved. All drugs

should show an improved absorption as pH is elevated within an acceptable range.

An important problem accompanying the instillation of eye drops is the immediate loss that occurs by drainage. The fraction of the drop lost increases as the instilled volume increases. Studies in the rabbit with pilocarpine show a marked dependence of miotic effect on drop size.[108] A 5-μl drop of pilocarpine produces about twice the peak intensity of effect and about 4 times the total miotic effect (determined from the area under the change in pupillary diameter versus time curve) as does a 75-μl drop containing the same amount of drug. A 5-fold decrease in volume from 25 to 5 μl, results in a 3-fold increase in fraction absorbed.[109]

Under normal conditions, the human eye can hold about 10 μl of fluid. The normal dropper used in commercial ophthalmic preparations delivers approximately 50 to 75 μl. The use of smaller drops (5 to 10 μl) of somewhat higher concentration would reduce costs and might decrease side effects. This suggestion is reinforced by the observation that instillation of 10 μl of a 2% epinephrine solution to rabbits gave the same pupillary response as did 50 μl of a 1% solution and produced less pain and lacrimation.[108]

Some patients are directed to instill more than 1 drop of an ophthalmic preparation at a time. Others require more than 1 preparation and administer them at the same time. The limited ability of the eye to accommodate fluid in excess of tear volume requires reconsideration of these practices because bioavailability and effectiveness may be compromised.[110] The change of pupillary diameter in the rabbit eye as a function of time after instillation of 25 μl of pilocarpine nitrate, followed by 25 μl of saline solution at various time intervals, is shown in Figure 6–6. The second drop reduces the activity of the first drop unless spaced about 5 min apart in rabbits and probably a slightly shorter time in man.[110] Rather than instilling 2 drops of a drug solution, it is advisable to raise the drug concentration and use a single smaller drop. There also appears to be a strong argument for a combination product, where possible, rather than separate solutions, when 2 or more drugs are required routinely for therapy.

It is generally believed that the inclusion of viscosity-increasing agents in an ophthalmic solution will increase ocular bioavailability by prolonging the contact time of drug in the eye. Studies in rabbits with pilocarpine in methylcellulose solu-

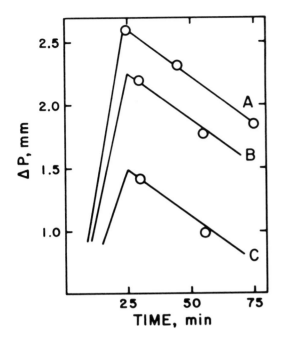

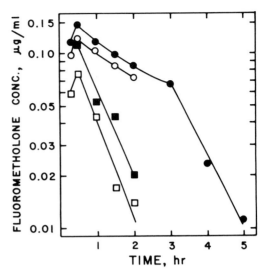

Fig. 6–6. Change in pupillary diameter (ΔP) after a 25-μl drop of pilocarpine (A) or the pilocarpine drop followed 2 min (B) or 30 sec (C) later by a drop of saline solution. (Data from Chrai, S.S., et al.[110])

Fig. 6–7. Fluorometholone concentrations in aqueous humor after topical administration of 50 μl of a saturated solution (□), and 50 μl of a 0.01% (■), 0.05% (○), or 0.1% (●) suspension. (Data from Sieg, J.W., and Robinson, J.R.[112])

tions of different viscosity generally support this premise, but improvements in miotic activity were modest.[111] The investigators suggest that still smaller effects would be noted with smaller drops.

Studies with steroids have shown that the dosage form can have pronounced effects on drug concentrations in the eye. Steroid concentrations in the aqueous humor after topical application of fluorometholone suspensions and a saturated solution of the drug are shown in Figure 6–7. Peak concentrations occurred after 30 min, irrespective of the dosage form, but were higher after instillation of the suspensions than after administration of the saturated solution. The 0.1% and 0.05% suspensions produced a considerably longer effect compared to that observed with the more dilute suspension and the solution.[112]

Corneal and aqueous humor steroid concentrations resulting from topical application of 0.125% and 1.0% suspensions of prednisolone acetate have also been determined.[113] The 1.0% preparation produced much higher steroid levels at both sites in normal and inflamed rabbit eyes. These studies suggest that particles present in an ophthalmic suspension are retained within the cul-de-sac of the

eye and once dissolved contribute significantly to the amount of steroid penetrating the cornea.

Many drugs are available in the form of sterile ophthalmic ointments. The major advantage of an ointment over an aqueous suspension or solution is the possibility of increased contact time and prolonged effect. The major disadvantage is the mixing problem between the ointment vehicle and the tears, which may limit the penetration rate. These characteristics of ophthalmic ointments are illustrated in the results of studies that determined steroid concentrations in the aqueous humor after application of a fluorometholone ointment to rabbit eye.[112] Peak concentrations were not reached until 3 hr after dosing, but drug levels persisted for far longer than observed after instillation of suspensions or a solution of the drug. The delay in attaining high drug levels may be overcome by instilling a drop of drug solution before applying the ointment.

Aqueous gels appear to have the same advantages as traditional oleaginous ophthalmic ointments. Much higher and more persistent levels of radioactivity were found in rabbit cornea and aqueous humor after administration of tritiated prednisolone acetate or tritiated prednisolone sodium phosphate in an aqueous gel than in the respective reference preparation, a suspension in the case of

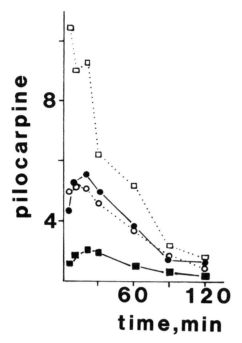

Fig. 6–8. Aqueous humor levels of pilocarpine (μg/ml) after topical dosing with 0.01 M ointment (●,○) or solution (■,□) in intact (●,■) or abraded (○,□) rabbit eyes. (Data from Sieg, J.W., and Robinson, J.R.[107])

the acetate and a solution in the case of the phosphate.[112]

Incorporation of pilocarpine into a petrolatum-based ointment vehicle resulted in increased drug levels in the aqueous humor of normal rabbit eyes compared to those produced by an equivalent dose of aqueous solution.[107] A different picture emerged when the rabbit's eyes were abraded. Abrasion markedly increased the bioavailability of pilocarpine from the aqueous solution, but had no effect on drug absorption from the ointment. The net result is that under these conditions bioavailability is greater from the solution than the ointment (Fig. 6–8).

The use of ophthalmic drug solutions or suspensions in oil has been limited, but there may be some advantage to this dosage form. One report noted that in healthy subjects pilocarpine dissolved in castor oil has a greater degree and duration of effect on the pupil than the same amount of drug given in aqueous solution.[115] Statistically significant drug effects were noted for as long as 24 hr after administration of the oil-based drops. Other approaches to prolonging the effects of drugs used in the eye are considered in Chapter 7.

Distinctions are rarely made in topical ophthal-

mic drug therapy between age groups. Generally, the same dose of an ophthalmic solution, suspension, or ointment is given to infants and adults. Recent experimental work challenges this lack of discrimination. Identical doses of 25 μl tritiated pilocarpine solution were instilled into the eyes of 20- and 60-day-old rabbits. Drug concentrations in the aqueous humor were always higher in the young rabbits. The total area under the drug concentration versus time curves differed by a factor of two.[116] These studies suggest that lower doses of eye medication may be appropriate in young children.

Despite the many problems that have been enumerated, topical application is an efficient way of delivering drug to various parts of the eye. This is seen clearly in a study on the ocular penetration of chloramphenicol.[117] Chloramphenicol concentrations were determined in the aqueous humor after administration of the drug as an ophthalmic ointment, subconjunctival injection, or intravenous injection. A 1% ointment produced peak chloramphenicol concentrations of 20 μg/ml; a 100 mg/kg intravenous dose of chloramphenicol resulted in peak levels of only 2 μg/ml. In all cases, the ointment was the most efficient means of drug delivery, providing the highest chloramphenicol concentration in the aqueous humor per mg of administered drug.

Although the eye is not a route for systemic drug administration, systemic absorption can occur. Systemic effects have been observed in laboratory animals after repetitive administration of certain eye drops, including those containing steroids. Systemic absorption probably results from entry of the drug into the lacrimal duct, which drains lacrimal fluid into the nasal cavity and ultimately into the gastrointestinal tract.

One study has shown that ordinary doses of phenylephrine eye drops significantly raised blood pressure in patients with insulin-dependent diabetes and in patients who had been taking reserpine or guanethidine.[118] Systolic and diastolic blood pressure rose by about 30 and 15 mm Hg, respectively, in these patients after 3 or 4 doses given over a 2-hr period before ocular surgery. There have been several reports of aplastic anemia in patients using chloramphenicol in eye drops or ophthalmic ointment.[119]

Finnish investigators measured atropine plasma levels and monitored blood pressure, heart rate, and salivary secretion in eight patients after application of 40 μl of 1% atropine ophthalmic solution to the lower cul-de-sac of one eye in connection with ocular surgery.[120] Atropine plasma levels were determined by means of a sensitive radioreceptor assay.

An average peak plasma atropine concentration of 860 pg/ml was reached within 8 min in all patients. No effects on heart rate or blood pressure were observed when compared with placebo but 30 min after administration of atropine eye drops, salivary secretion was reduced.

The approval of timolol, a beta adrenergic antagonist, for the topical treatment of glaucoma has raised concerns over possible systemic absorption and adverse effects. Studies in the United States and Sweden indicate that routine use of timolol ophthalmic solution in healthy subjects results in detectable drug concentrations in blood and urine.[121,122] Small effects on exercise tachycardia were observed, but no effects on pulmonary function were noted. However, clinical reports of respiratory embarrassment and death in asthmatic patients taking ophthalmic timolol have prompted the United States Food and Drug Administration to contraindicate its use in such patients.[66] A review of the systemic side effects associated with the ophthalmic administration of timolol has been presented.[124] Caution should be used when ophthalmic timolol is given to elderly patients or those patients with contraindications to systemic beta-blockers, such as restrictive airway disease.

In 1986, two new beta-adrenergic-receptor blocking drugs, betaxolol and levobunolol, were approved by the US FDA for ophthalmic use in the treatment of chronic open-angle glaucoma. Betaxolol is a relatively selective beta blocker, blocking beta$_1$ receptors in the heart at concentrations below those required to block beta$_2$ receptors in the bronchi. At low doses, betaxolol is probably less likely to precipitate bronchospasm in patients with asthma than timolol or levobunolol.

As noted, drugs applied to the eye appear to be absorbed via the nasolacrimal duct, which drains lacrimal fluid into the nasal cavity, and ultimately into the GI tract. Zimmerman et al.[125] have evaluated two techniques to reduce nasolacrimal drainage and improve the therapeutic index of topically applied ophthalmic drugs: simple eyelid closure and nasolacrimal occlusion (NLO). Nasolacrimal occlusion involves pressing a fingertip to the inside corner of the eye after application of the medication.

Plasma concentrations of timolol were deter-mined in healthy subjects 1 hr after instillation of 1 drop of 0.5% timolol maleate in the lower cul-de-sac of each eye, followed by NLO for 5 min, eyelid closure for 5 min, or no intervention. The same design was used to evaluate the penetration of topically applied fluorescein in the anterior chamber of the eye. Each person received 1 μl of 10% fluorescein in the lower cul-de-sac of each eye, and fluorophotometric readings were taken at intervals for up to 3 hr after administration.

Timolol concentration in plasma 1 hr after application of the drug to the eyes was about 1.3 ng/ml when there was no intervention and <0.5 ng/ml when eyelid closure or NLO was applied. On the other hand, relative fluorescein concentrations in the anterior chamber of the eye were significantly higher when eyelid closure or NLO followed administration of the marker.

The simple procedures of nasolacrimal occlusion or eyelid closure appear to reduce the systemic absorption of topical timolol. Furthermore, these procedures increase the concentration of fluorescein in the anterior chamber, presumably by increasing corneal contact time. Zimmerman et al.[125] suggest that ''although only timolol and fluorescein were used in these experiments, theoretically, all topically applied drugs should manifest similar behavior. Generally, decreasing the amount of drug presented to the nasopharyngeal mucosa will decrease the systemic blood concentration of that drug. Similarly, prolonged corneal contact time will probably elevate intraocular concentration of a drug.'' These techniques may prove to be particularly useful in the treatment of asthmatic patients with ophthalmic beta blockers and in the treatment of hypertensive patients with ophthalmic epinephrine or phenylephrine where caution is required to avoid adverse effects.

INTRAVAGINAL APPLICATION

A large number of products are available for the intravaginal administration of various drugs in the form of tablets, creams, ointments, douches, and suppositories. Virtually all are intended to act locally in the treatment of bacterial or fungal infections or atrophic vaginitis, or to prevent conception.

Dinoprostone, the naturally occurring prostaglandin E$_2$, is available in the form of vaginal suppositories as a uterine stimulant to induce fetal abortion. This form of the drug also provides a safe and effective noninvasive method for inducing labor. There is considerable interest in the development of long-acting intravaginal dosage forms of progestational agents or other contraceptive drugs. These dosage forms are considered in greater detail in Chapter 7. It is well recognized that drugs applied to the vagina may be absorbed, but there is little information available on specific drugs or on the biopharmaceutics of vaginal dosage forms.

The systemic absorption of metronidazole by the oral and vaginal routes was compared in healthy adult subjects.[126] Each subject received single 500-mg doses of metronidazole in the form of an oral, vaginal insert, or vaginal cream preparation on three occasions. Bioavailability from both vaginal products was about 20% compared with the oral preparation. Mean peak plasma concentrations were 15.6 μg/ml for the oral form and about 1.9 μg/ml for both the cream and the insert.

The data indicate that some vaginal absorption occurs from both the cream and insert preparations of metronidazole. These results underscore the concerns regarding the administration of vaginal metronidazole to pregnant patients. There are serious reservations as to the use of metronidazole in pregnancy; these reservations are not eliminated if the drug is given intravaginally.

INTRANASAL APPLICATION

Drugs are usually administered intranasally for the alleviation of local symptoms. These products typically contain decongestants, antihistamines, and corticosteroids. There is also interest in the intranasal route for the systemic administration of drugs. The nasal mucosa appears to be more permeable to drugs than the gastrointestinal mucosa, no local metabolism is known, and drugs absorbed through the nasal mucosa go directly to the blood stream and are not subject to first-pass hepatic metabolism.

The advantages of intranasal administration were demonstrated with propranolol, a drug subject to considerable presystemic metabolism and a low bioavailability after oral administration.[127] The time course of propranolol in serum and the total area under the serum level-time curve after intranasal administration of the drug in an aqueous gel were almost identical to those observed after intravenous administration, indicating rapid and complete absorption of therapeutic doses of propranolol after intranasal application. In contrast, the total area under the curve after oral administration was only 25% of that found after intravenous propranolol.

Nitroglycerin provides another example. Laryngoscopy and tracheal intubation produce increases in arterial pressure and heart rate that, in some patients, can provoke left ventricular failure, myocardial ischemia, and cerebral hemorrhage. Nitroglycerin (NTG) solution given intranasally before laryngoscopy and intubation can minimize these changes.[128]

Female patients undergoing breast surgery were randomized to either an NTG or control group. The NTG group received 2 ml of an NTG solution (60 mg), instilled intranasally 1 min before inducing anesthesia. The control group received no NTG. No change in arterial pressure was found in patients who received NTG before tracheal intubation. In the control group, an abrupt increase in arterial pressure (from 136 to 182 mm Hg) was observed immediately after intubation. NTG is rapidly absorbed when given intranasally; peak blood levels are reached within two minutes.[128] When NTG is given in this manner, it provides a safe, simple, and effective method to attenuate the hypertensive response to laryngoscopy and tracheal intubation.

Huang et al.,[129] using an in situ perfusion method in the rat, have determined that nasal absorption does not appear to be restricted to the nonionized form of the compound; the ionized species was absorbed about 25% as fast as the nonionized species. They also studied the effect of lipid solubility on the extent of nasal absorption using a small series of barbiturates, and found that absorption was dependent on the chloroform/water partition coefficient of the barbiturate.

The drug characteristics needed for good nasal absorption seem to be similar to those required for good absorption from the GI tract, but the membranes of the nasal mucosa appear to be more permeable than those of the gut. In general, peptides are not well absorbed after intranasal application but absorption can be promoted with certain additives such as surface-active agents. The nasal membranes may also be more sensitive than those of the gut; local toxicity may require attention for clinical application.

Some drugs have been found to affect the movement of nasal cilia. Cilia move in a well-organized and coordinated manner to propel the overlying mucus layer toward the back of the throat. In this way, inspired dust, allergens, and bacteria trapped in the mucus are removed. Chronic ciliary stasis may lead to recurrent infection.

Hermens and Merkus[130] have reviewed the effects of drugs on nasal ciliary movement. They observed that "drugs in nasal preparations for local use as well as for systemic use, should not interfere with the self-cleaning capacity of the nose, effectuated by the ciliary epithelium. Many drugs and additives, however, have a negative effect on nasal ciliary function." Propranolol has a particularly profound effect on ciliary movement. Bile salts, widely evaluated as promoters of intranasal absorption, are also ciliotoxic. "The feasibility of nasal drug administration will depend in large part on the effects on the ciliated epithelium. These effects will determine the acceptability of the formulation by the patient and thus the success of long-term nasal drug delivery."

In an effort to better understand nasal absorption, particularly the effects of surfactants, Hersey and Jackson[131] described an *in vitro* model using nasal mucosa excised from dogs or rabbits to study permeability. The nasal mucosa was mounted as a flat sheet between two lucite half-chambers. Permeability was evaluated by measuring the unidirectional flux of several water-soluble compounds: water, sucrose, polyethylene glycol (mol wt 5000), and cholecystokinin octapeptide. In both these preparations, permeability coefficients decreased with increasing molecular weight.

The addition of 0.5% sodium deoxycholate to the mucosal bathing solution resulted in a threefold increase in permeability to sucrose. Similar increases in permeability were observed with cholecystokinin octapeptide. The increase in permeability was not reversible and was accompanied by histological evidence of extensive loss of the surface epithelial layer. These findings suggest that bile salts enhance nasal permeability by removing the epithelial cells, which constitute a major permeability barrier, and argue for extreme caution in using bile salts as adjuvants for intranasal administration of therapeutic agents.

Useful animal models to study nasal absorption have been developed. These models have been used to analyze the effect of molecular size and to elucidate structural requirements for absorption. Fisher et al.[132] measured nasal absorption in the rat of several radiolabeled water-soluble compounds ranging in molecular weight from about 200 to 70,000 daltons. The compounds were instilled into the nasal cavities of anesthetized animals and sim-

ilar doses were given intravenously for comparison; serial samples of bile and urine were collected.

Nasal absorption of two organic acids (4-oxo-4H-l-benzopyran-2-carboxylic acid and p-aminohippuric acid) with molecular weights of about 200 daltons was complete or nearly complete; nasal absorption was about 15% for insulin (MW = 5,200), and 3% for dextran (MW = 70,000). An earlier study with the same methodology found that about 50% of a dose of sodium cromoglycate (MW = 512) was absorbed from the nasal cavity.

Applying these data, the investigators found a strong linear correlation between the log of the percentage of dose absorbed and the log of the molecular weight (r = 0.996). For these compounds, the proportion of an intranasal dose absorbed is largely a function of molecular weight, suggesting an aqueous channel mechanism for the absorption of water-soluble compounds.

McMartin et al.[133] used the same animal model to study the nasal absorption of an octapeptide (MW = 800) and a protein (horseradish peroxidase, MW = 30,000) and found bioavailabilities of 73% and 0.6% respectively. These findings were combined with published data for 23 other, mostly water-soluble compounds to examine the relationship between extent of absorption and molecular properties such as size, charge, or polarity.

The strongest correlation was with molecular weight. A log-log plot of nasal absorption versus molecular weight showed good bioavailability for all molecules up to about 1000 daltons molecular weight; the mean nasal absorption of the 15 compounds of MW <1000 was 70%. Absorption falls off sharply at higher molecular weights. A similar analysis of data on gastrointestinal absorption suggests a much lower molecular weight cutoff of about 200 daltons.

McMartin and his colleagues suggest that there are two mechanisms of drug transport from the nasal cavity. "A fast rate that is dependent on lipophilicity, and a slower rate that is dependent on molecular weight; the slower rate is nevertheless fast enough to give a high degree of absorption for low molecular weight polar compounds."

The first example of intranasal administration for systemic effects was the use of posterior pituitary hormones and related compounds such as oxytocin and desmopressin. Oxytocin (MW = 1007) is available as a nasal solution (40 units/ml) indicated to stimulate lactation. The usual dose is one spray or three drops applied to one or both nostrils 2 to 3 min before nursing or pumping of breasts.

Desmopressin is a synthetic polypeptide (MW = 1183) structurally related to arginine vasopressin (antidiuretic hormone). Desmopressin acetate nasal solution (0.1 mg/ml) is indicated for the prevention or control of polydipsia, polyuria, and dehydration associated with diabetes insipidus caused by insufficient antidiuretic hormone.

Intranasal therapy has now been extended to anterior pituitary hormones, notably to luteinizing hormone-releasing hormone (LHRH) agonists, which, paradoxically, act pharmacologically as antagonists. These compounds are under investigation for the treatment of endometriosis and prostatic cancer. The best studied are leuprolide, buserelin, and nafarelin.

A randomized trial comparing buserelin with orchidectomy in patients with prostatic cancer concluded that the LHRH agonist was a safe and effective alternative to orchidectomy.[134] A randomized trial of subcutaneous leuprolide versus diethylstilbestrol (DES) in patients with prostate cancer and distant metastases found that leuprolide was "therapeutically equivalent to and causes fewer side effects than DES."[135]

More recently, Falkson and Vorobiof[136] reported on the efficacy, safety, and tolerability of daily intranasal administration of buserelin in the treatment of patients with metastatic prostatic cancer. Buserelin was used in the form of a nasal spray delivering 100 μg of drug per inhalation.

Twenty-five patients (80%) responded to treatment, 2 with complete remission, 12 with partial remission, and 11 who improved. The median baseline value for testosterone was 14.4 nmol/l, compared with values of 10.8 nmol/l after 1 month of treatment with buserelin.

Falkson and Vorobiof concluded that "intranasal buserelin is an effective, simple, and safe way to achieve androgen deprivation in the treatment of advanced prostatic cancer. This treatment neither causes the psychological problems of castration nor is it associated with the morbidity of estrogen administration." Furthermore, the nasal spray provides a method of administration that is more acceptable to patients than daily subcutaneous injections.

Intranasal administration of LHRH agonists has also been found to be effective in the treatment of endometriosis. Henzl et al.[137] randomized 213 patients with confirmed endometriosis to either na-

farelin by nasal spray (400 or 800 μg/day) or oral danazol (800 mg/day) for 6 months of treatment. More than 80% of the patients in each treatment group had objective improvements as assessed by laparoscopy. The investigators concluded that nafarelin administration by nasal spray is an effective agent for treating endometriosis and has few side effects other than hypoestrogenism.

Do local inflammation and congestion associated with the common cold or hay fever modify the bioavailability of drugs administered intranasally? This interesting question was considered by Larsen et al.[138] who investigated the influence of experimental rhinitis on the intranasal absorption of buserelin, assessed by the gonadotropin response, in 24 healthy subjects. Each subject was treated with 200 μg buserelin in one nostril on each of two occasions. On one occasion, the drug was given 15 min after induction of inflammation by histamine; on the other occasion, the drug was given 15 min after saline solution treatment.

Treatment with histamine induced a significant increase in nasal airway resistance. After each dose of buserelin, serum luteinizing hormone (LH) concentrations rose steeply during the first 30 min after spraying, reaching a maximum at 3 to 4 hr followed by a gradual decline. The mean peak LH concentration was 17.7 mU/ml when the drug was preceded by saline and 19.8 mU/ml when buserelin followed pretreatment with histamine. The average AUC over 6 hours was 82 mU × hr/ml for the control arm and 84 mU × hr/ml for the experimental rhinitis arm. This study shows that the response to buserelin administered intranasally using a metered-dose pump spray was not affected by histamine-induced rhinitis.

The nasal absorption of other hormones such as insulin and calcitonin has also been studied. There is great interest in developing a dosage form of insulin that does not require injection. Intranasal administration results in measurable blood levels of insulin and a hypoglycemic response, but absorption is limited and not sufficiently reproducible. Nasal administration of insulin with a "promoter" such as bile salts improves bioavailability.

Aungst et al.[139] compared the absorption of insulin from different sites of application in adult male rats and also determined the effects of sodium glycocholate on absorption. Rectal insulin was more effective in lowering plasma glucose than was nasal, buccal, or sublingual insulin. The bioavailability of rectal insulin, after a dose of 10 U/kg body weight, was estimated at about 20%, compared with a value of less than 1% for intranasal insulin.

Administration of insulin in a solution containing 5% sodium glycocholate increased absorption by each route of administration. Under these conditions, nasal and rectal insulin had similar bioavailability and were about half as effective as intramuscular insulin in reducing plasma glucose levels. Oral insulin at five times the dose (with or without bile salt) had no hypoglycemic effect.

Despite these promising studies in laboratory animals, a 5% solution of bile salt is clinically unacceptable. A more dilute and better tolerated preparation is unlikely to yield clinically adequate absorption of insulin. Most investigators have abandoned the notion that intranasal insulin could replace insulin injections. Interest persists, however, in combining intranasal insulin with injections to improve glycemic control in insulin-dependent diabetics and in supplementing drug therapy with intranasal insulin in non-insulin-dependent diabetic (NIDD) patients.

El-Etr et al.[140] reported on the efficacy of an insulin nasal spray administered before meals in eight NIDD patients. All hypoglycemic agents were stopped one week before testing. Insulin was administered as a calibrated spray twice in each nostril 20 min before a standardized lunch. Four sprays delivered a total dose of 1 U/kg body weight. The insulin solution contained 1% sodium deoxycholate as an absorption promoter. In the control study, insulin administration was omitted.

Plasma glucose increased from 12.7 mmol/l at baseline to 14.6 mmol/l, 1 hr after the standardized meal when no insulin was given. When intranasal insulin was administered, plasma glucose decreased from 12.3 mmol/l at baseline to 10.5 mmol/l, 1 hr after lunch. Differences in plasma glucose between drug and control studies persisted for up to 3 hr after the meal. The insulin level peaked at 10 min after insulin spray; the minimum glucose value was observed at 30 min after administration. The investigators concluded that "an insulin spray before lunch not only prevented the increase but also induced a decrease in the postprandial blood glucose in all patients tested without side-effects, apart from a slight nasal irritation for 1 to 2 minutes."

There is considerable interest in the use of calcitonin for the prevention or treatment of osteoporosis. Widespread use, however, will be im-

practical until a method of administration more suitable than subcutaneous injection can be developed. Addressing this point, Reginster et al.[141] evaluated the effectiveness of intranasal calcitonin in the prevention of early postmenopausal bone loss.

Seventy-nine women who had been menopausal for under 3 yr and who had not been specifically treated to prevent bone loss were randomized to a 12-month course of either calcium (500 mg/day) or calcium plus intranasal salmon calcitonin (50 IU/day). At the end of the study, bone mineral density had decreased in the calcium-only group by an average of 3.2% but had increased in the calcium plus calcitonin group by 1.4%. The decrease in bone mineral density in the calcium-only group confirms its lack of effectiveness in the prevention of osteoporosis. Intranasal salmon calcitonin, on the other hand, when given with calcium, appeared to counteract early postmenopausal bone loss.

APPLICATION TO THE SKIN

Dermatologic preparations are usually intended to act locally in the treatment of skin disorders. Application of drugs to the skin minimizes systemic exposure. This is exemplified by the safe and effective topical use of 5-fluorouracil to treat premalignant and malignant skin lesions. Systemic administration of 5-fluorouracil often results in serious adverse effects.

Systemic administration of glucocorticoids gives excellent results in clearing inflammatory skin lesions, but their adverse effects are considerable. Many of these diseases can be controlled by topical application of glucocorticoids with a dramatic decrease in the incidence of adverse effects. This advantage of topical drug therapy must be viewed as a relative rather than absolute one, because some systemic absorption occurs with almost all drugs.

Human skin consists of three distinct layers: the epidermis, the dermis, and the subcutaneous fat. The epidermis is the nonvascular, multilayered, outer region of the skin. The most superficial layer of the epidermis is the stratum corneum, which is composed of several layers of dead keratinized cells. The stratum corneum is generally recognized as the principal skin barrier to loss of water and to entry of foreign substances. The dermis or true skin is a highly vascular region. Drugs penetrating to this region are likely to reach the systemic circulation.

In principle, the vascularity of the dermis should produce a "sink" condition such that drug concentration is very much less than that present on the skin surface. Accordingly, further penetration of drug to tissues below the dermis is considered unlikely. Surprisingly, a review of the literature reveals several reports showing that deeper penetration can take place and that much higher subcutaneous drug levels can be achieved after topical application than after oral or parenteral administration.[142]

One study found that salicylate levels in the muscle adjacent to the site of topical application of labeled triethanolamine salicylate were 20 times higher than after oral administration of a dose of aspirin that produced blood levels 10 to 100 times greater than those after topical dosing. These results suggest that topical application of analgesics may provide relief of local pain and discomfort without systemic side effects.

The site of application and the state of the skin plays an important role in percutaneous absorption of drugs. Considerable regional variation in the percutaneous penetration of hydrocortisone has been observed in man.[143] Absorption is rapid in regions with large or numerous hair follicles. Hydrocortisone penetrates the scalp and forehead much more readily than it penetrates the ventral surface of the forearm. Absorption is decreased in some regions of skin having thickened stratum corneum (e.g., the foot). On the other hand, absorption from the palm, which has a fairly thick stratum corneum and no hair follicles, is comparable to that from the forearm. The scrotum provides almost no barrier to the absorption of hydrocortisone.

A more recent study examined the percutaneous absorption of sodium benzoate, caffeine, benzoic acid, and aspirin applied to different sites.[144] Skin permeability varied substantially, depending both on the properties of the drug and on the site of application. Whatever the compound applied, the forehead was about twice as permeable as the arm or abdomen. Application behind the ear produced intermediate results.

Cuts, diaper rash, inflammation, mild burns, or any other condition in which the stratum corneum is damaged or destroyed promotes the absorption of drugs through the skin.[145,146] Studies in patients with mycosis fungoides indicate that the percutaneous absorption of the antineoplastic drug carmustine through affected skin is much greater than through uninvolved skin.[147]

Stripping the skin with cellophane tape until it glistens removes the stratum corneum and causes damage to the upper layers of epidermis. This procedure is often used as a model for damaged and diseased skin. Stripped skin showed a fourfold increase in the penetration of hydrocortisone compared with intact skin.[148]

Hydration of the skin, by soaking in water or by occluding the skin surface with an impermeable material such as a plastic film, alters the barrier characteristics of the stratum corneum and promotes drug absorption. The enhancement of biologic activity of topical steroids by occlusion is well documented.[149] An occlusive dressing increases the absorption of hydrocortisone through normal human skin about tenfold.[146] The greatest percutaneous absorption of hydrocortisone was obtained by stripping the skin followed by a 24-hr occlusion. Penetration under these conditions was about 20 times the value for normal skin.[148] Occlusion also increases the percutaneous absorption of testosterone.[150] Certain lipophilic ointment bases may retard water loss from skin and promote hydration and drug absorption.

Aging and environmental factors that lead to dehydration of the skin can retard drug absorption. Environmental temperature can affect the hydration of the stratum corneum as well as the local blood flow. The absorption of a topically applied cholinesterase inhibitor from the cheek in normal male subjects increased 8-fold when the subjects were exposed to increasing temperatures ranging from $-18°C$ to $46°C$.[151]

The chemical form of the drug and the vehicle in which the drug is incorporated can have an important influence on percutaneous absorption.[152] For example, the efficacy of fluocinolone acetonide in inflammatory dermatoses (eczema and psoriasis) strongly depends on the vehicle.[153] An ointment formulation of 0.025% fluocinolone acetonide dissolved in propylene glycol and dispersed in soft paraffin was compared with 0.025% microcrystalline drug suspended in soft paraffin. The preparation containing drug dissolved, rather than suspended, in the ointment was significantly more effective in both eczema and psoriasis patients.

A human bioassay system was used to compare formulations of topically applied corticosteroids.[154] The test is based on the local vasoconstriction and skin blanching produced by penetration of the steroid through the stratum corneum. The degree of blanching is used as an index of bioavailability.

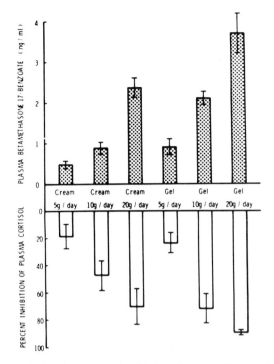

Fig. 6–9. Average levels of betamethasone 17-benzoate in plasma and inhibition of plasma cortisol after repeated applications of a cream or a gel base. (From Mizuchi, A., et al.[156] Copyright 1969, Baltimore, Williams & Wilkins.)

Examples of large differences between products containing the same amount of drug were common. In another study, using the same methodology, a proprietary cream containing 0.1% hydrocortisone was found to be substantially more effective than several other commercial formulations containing 1% hydrocortisone.[155]

The percutaneous absorption of betamethasone 17-benzoate has been studied in patients with skin disorders following application of either a gel or a cream.[156] Betamethasone concentrations in plasma and inhibition of plasma cortisol were significantly greater following the use of the gel rather than the cream (Fig. 6–9). The results of these studies and others convincingly demonstrate that dermatologic products are not necessarily therapeutically interchangeable.

The incorporation of certain chemicals such as dimethyl sulfoxide (DMSO) into topical formulations has been advocated to enhance penetration. In vitro and in vivo studies suggest that DMSO enhances the percutaneous absorption of many drugs, possibly by producing structural changes in the skin, such as swelling of the stratum corneum, and possibly by replacement of water as the con-

tinuous membrane phase of the skin barrier.[157] The use of DMSO in dermatologic products, however, remains controversial; questions of both safety and efficacy persist.

Other agents have also been studied as potential ''penetration enhancers.'' One report presents the results of the vasoconstrictor assay following application of betamethasone 17-benzoate with different enhancing agents.[158] Propylene glycol with oleic acid, propylene glycol with azone, and dimethylformamide, among other agents, increased steroid bioavailability. The investigators caution, however, that irritant effects may make some penetration enhancers unacceptable for clinical use.

Despite the importance of biopharmaceutics in the development of drug products intended to be applied to the skin, surprising little work has been carried out to quantitatively define dose-response relationships. An important exception is the work of Wester and Maibach.[159] Carbon-14 labeled testosterone, hydrocortisone, and benzoic acid in organic solvent were applied to a uniform area of skin of human male subjects; absorption was estimated by measuring urinary excretion of total ^{14}C. With testosterone, concentration was increased from 3 to 400 $\mu g/cm^2$ in 3 steps. Although the total amount absorbed increased with dose, the percent absorbed decreased from 11.8 to 2.8%. Similar decreases in the efficiency of percutaneous absorption with increasing drug concentration were observed with hydrocortisone and benzoic acid. The data are summarized in Table 6–2. The reason for this dose-dependency is not clear; whether or not it will be observed with more complex formulations of drug remains to be determined.

These investigators used a similar approach in monkeys to determine if the percutaneous absorption of hydrocortisone changes with repeated applications.[160] Radiolabeled hydrocortisone was applied to the forearm on day 1, followed by 7 days of application of nonradioactive drug. On day 8, the labeled drug was again applied. The absorption of hydrocortisone increased considerably during repeated administration, whether it was applied in an acetone vehicle or an emulsion ointment base. About 0.5% of the applied dose was absorbed after the first dose of ointment. This increased to about 2% after the last dose (Fig. 6–10). Long-term application of hydrocortisone may alter the percutaneous barrier, resulting in enhanced penetration. Similar results have been observed with salicylic

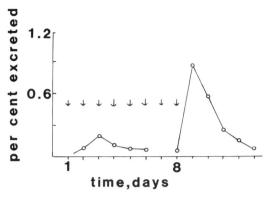

Fig. 6–10. Percutaneous absorption of ¹⁴C-hydrocortisone (estimated from urinary excretion data) on day 1 and day 8; nonradioactive drug was applied on days 2 through 7. The ointment containing hydrocortisone was applied to the same site each day. (Data from Wester, R.C., Noonan, P.K., and Maibach, H.I.[160])

acid,[161] but these findings are less surprising because of the keratolytic effects of the drug.

The unexpected results following repeated application of hydrocortisone in monkeys were not reproduced in a more recent study in human subjects that compared the penetration of hydrocortisone, testosterone, and estradiol following repeated administration with that observed after a single dose.[162] The drugs were applied to the ventral forearm skin once a day for 14 days. The first and eighth dose were radiolabeled.

The mean % dose absorbed for testosterone and estradiol were nearly the same for both test doses. Urinary excretion of labeled hydrocortisone was about 30% greater following the eighth dose than after the first dose, but the difference was not statistically significant. More work is needed because many questions pertaining to the effect of repeated application on percutaneous absorption in humans remain unanswered.

Measuring radioactivity in urine following topical application of a labeled compound is a standard method for determining percutaneous absorption.[148] In an attempt to find an easier way to assess absorption after topical administration, Rougier et al.[144] compared urinary excretion of radioactivity

following topical application of labeled sodium benzoate, caffeine, benzoic acid, or aspirin, to four different sites, with the amount of radioactivity in the stratum corneum at these sites shortly after administration.

Subjects were studied on two different occasions. The first study involved urinary excretion of labeled drug and the second concerned skin penetration. Thirty minutes after the second application, and after washing, the stratum corneum of the treated area was removed by 15 successive strippings with cellophane tape and the radioactivity contained therein was measured.

A strong linear correlation was observed between the amount of drug present in the stratum corneum shortly after application and urinary excretion of radioactivity. The investigators concluded that the stripping method can be used to make predictions of percutaneous absorption of different agents, irrespective of site of application, by measuring the quantity present in the stratum corneum after application. For many drugs it may be possible to carry out this determination with unlabeled compound because of the relatively high drug concentration in the stratum corneum.

In vitro techniques to estimate percutaneous absorption usually involve placing a piece of excised skin in a diffusion chamber, applying radioactive compound to one side of the skin, and then assaying for radioactivity in the collection vessel on the other side. Excised human cadaver skin and animal skin have been used; the skin may be intact or separated into epidermis or dermis. These methods are probably of value to the extent that they distinguish compounds with low permeability from those with high permeability.

Live animal models have also been used to study percutaneous absorption. In general, percutaneous absorption in the pig, rhesus monkey, and squirrel monkey is usually similar to that in man, whereas in the rat and rabbit skin penetration is greater than that observed in man.[148]

The idea of bioavailability as applied to drugs that are intended to act locally in the skin is a

Table 6–2. Percutaneous Absorption of Different Doses of Hydrocortisone and Benzoic Acid in Man*

	Hydrocortisone (μg/cm²)		Benzoic acid (μg/cm²)		
	4	40	3	400	2000
Amount absorbed (μg)	0.06	0.24	1.1	102.8	288
% Absorbed	1.6	0.6	37	25.7	14.4

*Data from Wester, R.C., and Maibach, H.I.[159]

confusing one. We wish to have maximum penetration of the drug into the skin; yet, we wish to minimize systemic absorption, to avoid adverse effects. Unfortunately, this delicate balance is not always achieved. Life-threatening systemic toxicity has been observed following liberal application of boric acid preparations to damaged skin of human infants. Substantial absorption, high blood levels, and clinical toxicity requiring forced diuresis were observed in a patient using a 12% salicylic acid ointment applied to 85 to 90% of the body surface for treatment of hyperkeratosis.[162]

Hexachlorophene bathing of infants had been widely advocated as effective prophylaxis against nursery epidemics of staphylococcal skin infections. However, clinical studies in newborn infants bathed daily with 3% hexachlorophene lotion showing measurable blood levels of the drug (as high as 0.6 μg/ml)[164] and toxicologic studies in newborn monkeys bathed for 90 days with this product showing blood levels of about 2 μg/ml and brain lesions,[165] have challenged the safety of this practice. A more recent paper reported that of 18 children with normal skin, accidentally intoxicated by a talc powder containing 6% hexachlorophene, 4 died and 2 remained paraplegic.[166]

Systemic toxicity of topically applied drugs is of particular concern in infants because they appear to absorb drugs through the skin as efficiently as do adults and the ratio of surface area to body weight in the newborn is 3 times that in adults.[150] The same strength formulation applied to the same relative area may result in much higher blood levels of drug in the infant than in the adult.

Although hexachlorophene is no longer used in over-the-counter products in the United States, it continues to be used by surgical staffs in hospitals. An important study in Sweden has revealed that among 460 children born to nurses who had been using soap containing 1 to 3% hexachlorophene, 25 had severe congenital defects, 3 had Down's syndrome, and another 46 had minor deformities.[167] These figures represent a birth defect rate 5 times that expected in the general population. The National Institute of Child Health and Human Development has recommended that women working in hospitals not use hexachlorophene-containing products.

Another drug that has had extensive use in dermatologic products but is now under scrutiny is gamma benzene hexachloride (lindane).[160] This compound is effective for the treatment of scabies and lice (pediculosis). Experimental studies have demonstrated that gamma benzene hexachloride can be absorbed from the skin and convulsions and death occur in animals after topical application of large amounts of the drug. Convulsions have also been reported in children after excessive topical application of commercial products. The Medical Letter on Drugs and Therapeutics cautions against prolonged or excessive use and suggests that alternative therapy such as sulfur in petrolatum may be safer for infants and children.[168]

Preparations designed to be applied to the skin to repel insects have been widely used for many years. The most effective topical insect repellent known is diethyltoluamide, commonly called "deet." Deet is absorbed through the skin into the systemic circulation and has caused serious toxic effects in children and adults, especially when used in high concentrations. Prolonged or excessive application of any insect repellent should be avoided.[169]

Although topical steroids are far safer in treating skin disease than systemically administered steroids, percutaneous absorption may lead to suppression of pituitary ACTH production and to reduced cortisol production by the adrenal cortex. The degree to which this occurs depends on the potency of the steroid, the amount used, the area of skin to which it is applied, the duration of treatment, and the amount of occlusion.

As a general rule, little effect on cortisol production is likely to occur with up to 50 g weekly for an adult or 15 g weekly for a child of a potent steroid ointment used without occlusion.[170] Frequent repeat prescriptions of potent topical steroids should be dispensed only after re-examination and consideration of possible alternative treatments.

A 2% topical formulation of minoxidil, a potent vasodilator used in severe hypertension, is now available for treatment of male pattern baldness. Franz[171] has estimated that 2 to 4% of a dose applied to the scalp is absorbed. Based on these findings, application of a 2% lotion twice a day to the entire scalp may provide a systemic dose of about 2 mg/day. This is less than the recommended oral adult antihypertensive dose of 10 to 40 mg/day. Short-term use of minoxidil has resulted in minimal decreases in blood pressure in normotensive patients; whether topical minoxidil has a hypotensive effect on patients with hypertension is not clear.[172]

There is now considerable interest in the topical application of drugs intended for systemic effects.

This route of administration may be useful for drugs with low bioavailability after oral administration due to first-pass metabolism. It may be particularly useful for short-acting drugs since percutaneous absorption tends to be slow, and prolonged effects may be realized. Most attention has been given to topical preparations of nitroglycerin, a compound with low oral bioavailability and a short duration of action, but one that remains important in the prevention and treatment of angina pectoris.

Nitroglycerin ointment has been available for more than 20 years, but only recently has its advantage been realized. Comparative studies of the effects of nitroglycerin ointment and placebo in 14 patients with angina pectoris have shown that nitroglycerin ointment produces a significant increase in exercise capacity, which persists for at least 3 hr.[173] The effects of the ointment are comparable to those produced by sublingual nitroglycerin, but of far longer duration. The effects of buccal nitroglycerin are usually dissipated in 30 min or less. Other studies have confirmed and extended these findings.[174-176] The ointment, however, has a slower onset of action than buccal medication and is never used for acute angina.

Nitroglycerin ointment is available in a 2% strength in a lanolin-petrolatum base. Each inch squeezed from the tube contains 15 mg nitroglycerin. The patient is titrated in 1/2-in. increments until a satisfactory dose is found. The ointment is usually applied every 4 to 6 hr to the anterior chest and covered with an occlusive wrap fixed with adhesive. The amount of nitroglycerin absorbed after topical application is a function of both the dose and the surface area over which it is applied.[177] Applying twice the dose (32 mg vs 16 mg) over a fixed area of skin resulted in almost twice the area under the nitroglycerin concentration in blood versus time curve for a 90-min period following administration. Increasing the skin surface area over which a fixed dose (16 mg) of nitroglycerin ointment is applied by a factor of 4, results in a 2-fold increase in the area under the curve.

Other lipid-soluble potent drugs may also yield clinically useful blood levels after topical application to the skin. A hydroalcoholic gel containing estradiol 0.6 mg/g, applied on the lower part of the abdomen, was used for cyclic (3 weeks on, 1 week off) replacement therapy in postmenopausal women. Increased serum concentrations of estradiol and estrone were observed during six months

of treatment. Therapy was effective in abolishing hot flushes in most women.[178]

Lichen sclerosus, a chronic cutaneous disorder that most commonly occurs on the vulva in postmenopausal women and that is characterized by decreased levels of dihydrotestosterone, free testosterone, and androstenedione, was treated with topical testosterone.[179] All patients were given 2% testosterone propionate in white petrolatum for application to the vulva twice a day. After several months of treatment, dihydrotestosterone and testosterone levels rose and exceeded normal values. This was accompanied by clinical improvement in most cases.

Prolonged-release dosage forms of drugs intended to be applied to the skin for systemic effects are considered in Chapter 7.

BUCCAL OR SUBLINGUAL ADMINISTRATION

Certain tablets are intended to be placed beneath the tongue or in the cheek pouch and retained in the mouth. These regions are vascular and allow rapid absorption of certain drugs in a manner consistent with pH-partition theory. The buccal or sublingual route appears ideal for lipid-soluble drugs that are metabolized in the gastrointestinal tract or liver during absorption, because the blood supply draining the buccal cavity empties directly into the systemic circulation and bypasses the liver. In general, buccal or sublingual tablets are designed to disintegrate and dissolve slowly in the mouth to minimize the possibility of swallowing part of the dose. Exceptions include nitroglycerin and isosorbide dinitrate, which should dissolve within seconds to provide prompt relief for acute anginal episodes.

This mode of therapy is most frequently used for the administration of nitrates and certain hormones such as methyltestosterone, testosterone, and oxytocin, but buccal absorption of many drugs including estradiol, sympathomimetic amines, methadone, meperidine, buprenorphine, lidocaine, chlorpheniramine, imipramine, desipramine, and barbiturates has been demonstrated.[180-184] The pH of saliva is usually about 6. Increasing the pH of fluids in the buccal cavity promotes the absorption of weak bases but reduces the absorption of weak acids.[180-182]

The buccal absorption of flurbiprofen, a nonsteroidal anti-inflammatory drug, was studied in human subjects by delivering a solution of the drug buffered to pH 5.5 or 7.0 through a flow cell in contact with the buccal membrane of the mouth.[185] Flurbiprofen is a weak acid. Consequently, absorption was greater at pH 5.5 where the acid was less dissociated than at pH 7.0. The investigators concluded that the buccal membrane was essentially lipoidal, showing no evidence of aqueous pores.

Although similarities exist between gastrointestinal and buccal absorption of drugs, some important differences must also exist. Clindamycin, which is known to be well absorbed from the gastrointestinal tract, is absorbed poorly, if at all, from the buccal cavity over the pH range of 4.0 to 8.5.[186] A higher degree of lipid solubility may be required for good absorption from the buccal cavity than from the gastrointestinal tract.

Other differences between buccal and gastrointestinal absorption have been identified in recent studies with β-blockers.[187,188] At least for some drugs, loss of drug from the oral cavity is not synonymous with systemic absorption; a storage compartment in the buccal membrane appears to exist. Once a drug is in the storage compartment, it may repartition into the oral cavity or be slowly absorbed into the systemic circulation. This phenomenon may be responsible for the slow absorption of buprenorphine after buccal administration.[184] A 2-fold difference between loss of drug from the oral cavity and appearance of drug in the systemic circulation has been observed with morphine.[189] At pH 6.5, 82% of a dose of morphine sulfate was recovered from the mouth after a 10-min exposure, suggesting that 18% of the dose was absorbed. A second study comparing the total area under the morphine concentration in plasma versus time curve after buccal and intramuscular administration indicated that the relative bioavailability of morphine from the oral cavity was only 9%.

Sublingual nitroglycerin remains the treatment of choice in the acute management of angina pectoris. Its advantages are thought to include a lack of tolerance, ease of administration, and rapid, consistent, and almost complete absorption. Some of these ideas have been challenged by recent studies.[190] Sublingual nitroglycerin tablets (0.4 mg) were given to healthy subjects and blood samples were collected for 3 hours to determine nitroglycerin levels. The tablet was placed under the subject's tongue and moistened with water; all subjects were asked to maintain the tablet in place and to avoid swallowing. After 8 min, they were in-

structed to spit out the remains of the tablets; the mouth was then rinsed with water and the rinsings added to the first collection. This material was assayed for residual nitroglycerin. All subjects also received intravenous nitroglycerin, so absolute bioavailability could be calculated.

Nitroglycerin levels were variable after sublingual administration. Bioavailability ranged from 3 to 113%, with an average value of about 40%. The mean time to peak concentration was about 5 min but in some subjects the peak was not observed until 10 min after administration. On the average, about 30% of the dose was recovered from the mouth rinsings taken at 8 min after administration. The rest of the dose presumably was swallowed and metabolized in the GI tract and liver.

The low and variable absorption of sublingual nitroglycerin may be related to the patient's inability to maintain the dose in the mouth without swallowing and to inadequate moisture in the mouth. A dry mouth has been cited as a factor in patients who appear resistant to nitroglycerin. Dry mucous membranes in patients experiencing anginal pain are expected. One investigator proposed that it should be routine practice to ensure that the sublingual mucosa is sufficiently moist to facilitate the dissolution of sublingual tablets of nitroglycerin.[191]

Nicotine gum was developed as substitution therapy to help people stop smoking. The preparation consists of nicotine bound to an ion exchange resin and incorporated into a gum base. The resin is expected to release almost all its nicotine over 20 to 30 min of chewing. The gum also contains a bicarbonate buffer to enhance the buccal absorption of nicotine.

Nicotine levels in the blood were compared after cigarette smoking and chewing nicotine gum.[192] In the first phase of the study, subjects abstained from cigarette smoking and chewed gum containing either 2- or 4-mg nicotine every hour from 9 AM to 8 PM. Subjects were asked to chew the gum slowly and steadily for 20 min. In the next phase of the study, subjects smoked cigarettes without restriction and without the use of gum. An average of nearly two packs of cigarettes per day were consumed.

The cigarettes provided a total of about 34 mg nicotine per day and steady-state concentrations in blood of 25 to 30 ng/ml nicotine. Average blood nicotine concentrations for subjects chewing 2- and 4-mg gum were only 29% and 42%, respectively, of that observed while smoking cigarettes. Complete delivery of nicotine in the gum would have provided a daily intake of either 24 mg (2-mg gum) or 48 mg (4-mg gum). The relative blood levels observed in this study suggest that delivery of nicotine from gum is less than complete.

The first problem is the release of nicotine from the gum. Extraction of nicotine, the difference between the dose and the amount remaining in the gum after chewing for 20 min, was only 53% for the 2-mg gum and 72% for the 4-mg gum. The difference in extraction between dosage strengths may be related to the fact that the 4-mg gum tends to cause more salivation than the 2-mg gum.

Even at this degree of extraction the 4-mg gum should deliver about 34 mg nicotine per day or about the same amount of nicotine as derived from smoking, unless other losses are incurred. The investigators found that in addition to an unextracted residue of about 28% of the dose, another 25% was expectorated, and an additional 25% was swallowed. Nicotine is rapidly absorbed from the gastrointestinal tract but is subject to a large first-pass effect.

Assuming complete absorption (and no first-pass effect) from the oral cavity of extracted nicotine and a 70% first-pass effect for swallowed material, one may calculate that only 1.2 mg of the 4 mg in the gum is available to the systemic circulation. This corresponds to an effective daily dose of only 14-mg nicotine or less than half that derived from smoking cigarettes. These calculations are consistent with the relative blood level data. Despite the relatively poor absorption characteristics of the dosage form, nicotine gum is helpful to people who are trying to stop smoking.[193]

An interesting technique for the administration of a bronchodilator aerosol, fenoterol, in children with asthma, ranging in age from 3 months to 9 years, has been described.[194] Rapid and effective bronchodilation was obtained in most patients simply by directing the jet of the aerosol onto the buccal mucosa. This technique could prove useful in the treatment of young children who cannot use an aerosol dosage form in the recommended manner.

The idea of a buccal spray has been applied to nitroglycerin.[195] An oral nitroglycerin aerosol spray is marketed in the US for prevention and treatment of angina pectoris. The oral spray is available in canisters dispensing 200 metered aerosolized doses of 0.4 mg nitroglycerin. It is sprayed onto or under the tongue. Significant effects on exercise tolerance and heart rate were detected at 2 min after use of the spray.

Some patients may find it easier to use the spray than to open a bottle and remove a small sublingual tablet. Because a dry mouth can delay the dissolution of sublingual nitrate tablets, the aerosol droplets may be better absorbed in some patients. The 3-yr shelf-life of the spray is also an advantage over sublingual tablets, which have a shelf-life of 1 yr under ideal conditions and can lose potency rapidly if they are not kept tightly capped in dark glass containers.

Preliminary findings suggesting that lorazepam is more rapidly absorbed after sublingual administration than after IM injection prompted investigators to compare the efficacy of lorazepam as a preanesthetic agent when given by these two routes.[196] Women admitted for dilatation and curettage participated in the study. Two hr before the procedure each patient received a sublingual tablet and an IM injection, one of which was a placebo.

Irrespective of the route of administration, lorazepam produced significant drowsiness and reduced anxiety within 30 min. Patients in the group receiving active sublingual medication, however, were more drowsy at 60 and 90 min after dosing, as compared with the IM group. Furthermore, lack of recall was significantly greater with sublingual lorazepam than with intramuscular lorazepam. Sublingual lorazepam may be superior to IM lorazepam with the additional advantage of no pain or discomfort on administration.

Alprazolam is widely prescribed as an anxiolytic agent and is under investigation for the treatment of panic disorders. Sublingual administration may be a useful alternative for panic disorder patients who cannot swallow tablets or for those who do not have access to water or some other liquid to facilitate swallowing.

Healthy human subjects received alprazolam on two occasions in random sequence. On one occasion a tablet was swallowed with 100–200 ml water; on the other occasion, the tablet was placed under the tongue and held there for 15 min. The peak plasma concentration of alprazolam after sublingual administration was slightly higher than after oral administration (17 versus 15 ng/ml) and the time to peak was reached earlier after the sublingual dose (1.2 versus 1.7 hr). The mean total area under the plasma concentration curve for sublingual administration was about the same as that following oral dosage.

Alprazolam absorption following sublingual administration is at least as rapid as after oral administration on an empty stomach, and completeness of absorption is comparable. The two routes appear to be bioequivalent. Sublingual administration, however, may prove to be preferable to oral administration of alprazolam after a meal, when gastric emptying is prolonged and the rate of absorption is reduced.[197]

Hypertensive emergencies require immediate reduction in blood pressure. Most often they are treated with parenteral drugs such as nitroprusside, diazoxide, or labetalol. Effective drugs that can be self-administered would be advantageous. Oral clonidine and captopril have been found useful in this respect, and both oral and buccal nifedipine have been reported to lower blood pressure within 1 hr in patients with dangerously elevated pressures.

Although buccal nifedipine appears to be useful for reducing elevated blood pressure, doubts have been raised as to whether its effects are the result of buccal absorption or, alternatively, the result of swallowing the material contained in the soft gelatin capsule followed by gastrointestinal absorption. To clarify this question, the sublingual absorption of nifedipine was investigated in healthy human subjects and compared with oral administration.[198]

The subjects bit a capsule containing 10 mg nifedipine in solution and were instructed to keep the capsule in the mouth and to avoid swallowing. After 20 min, the material remaining in the mouth was recovered and the mouth was rinsed thoroughly. On a second occasion, the participants bit another capsule of nifedipine, but this time they swallowed the capsule and its contents with water.

After biting the capsule and not swallowing for 20 min, nearly 90% of the dose was recovered from the mouth. Absorption was slow and led to low plasma levels of nifedipine. Median peak plasma concentration after sublingual administration was 10 ng/ml, reached at 45 min after biting the capsule. After biting and swallowing the capsule, the median peak plasma concentration was 71 ng/ml. The relative bioavailability of nifedipine after sublingual compared with oral administration was only 17%.

The favorable therapeutic results obtained with sublingual administration of nifedipine are proba-

bly due to swallowing the drug. If a fast onset of action of nifedipine is desired, the patient should be instructed to bite a capsule and to swallow the contents with water. This will ensure rapid absorption and high levels of the drug.

Relatively few bioavailability studies have been reported for drugs in sublingual dosage forms. The peripheral vasoconstriction effects of ergotamine, 0.25 mg intramuscularly and 2 mg sublingually, and a sublingual placebo were compared by means of plethysmography in normal subjects.[199] There were no significant differences between the ergotamine preparations; both were significantly more active than placebo. Winsor concludes that the two forms at the appropriate doses should be equally effective in the treatment of migraine.

The absorption of methyltestosterone was compared in healthy subjects after administration of 10- and 25-mg tablets and an aqueous solution containing 10 mg of methyltestosterone, all of which were swallowed, as well as after administration of 5 and 10 mg sublingual tablets.[200] The extent of absorption per mg of dose for 25-mg tablets, 10-mg tablets, 10 mg sublingual tablets, and 5 mg sublingual tablets, relative to the oral solution, was 0.90, 0.95, 1.42, and 1.63, respectively. The sublingual tablets produced significantly higher methyltestosterone levels in the serum per mg of dose than did the other dosage forms. These results clearly demonstrate the potential advantage of sublingual administration and the avoidance of presystemic metabolism.

Similar findings have been reported with isosorbide dinitrate.[201] Peak concentrations following 5 mg sublingual or oral doses of the drug were 8.9 and 3.1 mg/ml, respectively (Fig. 6–11).

RECTAL ADMINISTRATION

Certain drugs are given rectally, usually in the form of enemas or suppositories, for local therapy or for systemic effect. The rectal administration of drugs intended for systemic effect is usually limited to those situations in which oral administration is difficult or contraindicated. Suppositories are used more frequently in children than in adults and are a far more important dosage form in Europe than in the United States. Drugs that are administered by this route include aspirin, acetaminophen, indomethacin, theophylline, chlorpromazine, prochlorperazine, cyclizine, promethazine, and certain barbiturates and other anticonvulsive drugs.

Absorption across the rectal mucosa occurs in

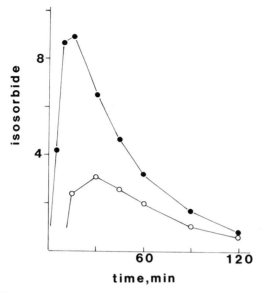

Fig. 6–11. Isosorbide concentrations in plasma following a 5-mg sublingual (●) or oral (○) dose. (Data from Assinder, D.F., Chasseaud, L.F., and Taylor, T.[201])

the same manner as in other parts of the alimentary tract. Although the rectum has a good blood supply, it is devoid of villi and has a relatively small surface area. Hence, drug absorption from the rectum is often slow. Wagner has proposed the following general principles with respect to drug absorption following rectal administration to man:[202] (1) Absorption from the rectum is usually more rapid and more efficient when drugs are given in solution form (microenemas) than in suppository form. (2) Absorption is generally more variable when drugs are administered in solution form rectally than in solution form orally. (3) The presence of fecal matter in the rectum retards absorption. Absorption is more rapid and efficient if a cleansing enema precedes drug administration. (4) Some suppository bases, such as polyethylene glycols (PEG), are irritating to the human rectum and tend to promote defecation and loss of the drug. (5) Bioavailability from suppositories may be poor because the drug is not released or is slowly released.

The pH of a rectal solution may also influence absorption. A dramatic improvement in the rectal absorption of morphine was reported in going from a rectal solution at pH 4.5 to one at pH 7.4.[203] The peak concentration of morphine went from 10 ng/ml to 24 ng/ml and the area under the concentration-time curve increased by about 50%. Side effects, including nausea and sedation, were observed after the more alkaline solution but not after

the rectal solution buffered to pH 4.5. These findings are consistent with pH-partition theory.

Rectal administration of theophylline suppositories in the treatment of children with bronchial asthma is questionable. Several studies have concluded that rectal absorption of theophylline from suppositories is slow and erratic.[204,205] Better success has been found with retention enemas of the drug.[206] A clinical study in asthmatic children indicated that adequate serum levels, comparable to those found after a 20-min intravenous infusion of theophylline, can be obtained after a single rectal dose of the drug in aqueous solution.[207] A comparative bioavailability study of oral and rectal solutions of theophylline found that the drug was more rapidly absorbed from oral solutions, as indicated by the peak concentration (7.3 vs 4.9 μg/ml) and the time to peak (1 hr vs 2 hr). On the other hand, the extent of absorption of theophylline after rectal administration was very good, about 90% that found after oral administration. These findings suggest that rectal solutions of theophylline are a reasonable alternative when oral dosing is not possible or desirable.[208]

Attempts to develop rectal dosage forms of tetracycline or penicillin G have been unsuccessful because of the intrinsically poor absorption of these drugs across the rectal mucosa. Studies in healthy subjects indicate that the absorption of tetracycline hydrochloride and sodium penicillin G after rectal administration of aqueous solutions is only about 10% that observed after oral administration of drug solutions to fasting subjects.[209]

The rectal absorption of the antibiotic lincomycin has been studied in children and adults.[210] The extent of absorption of lincomycin in children after rectal administration of an aqueous solution was only 50% that observed after oral administration of a syrup form of the drug and was considerably more variable.

The absorption of lincomycin after rectal administration of an aqueous solution to adults who were given an enema to cleanse the lower colon and rectum the night before was comparable to that observed after oral administration of a capsule of the drug. The bioavailability of lincomycin from the rectal solution in subjects who had not received an enema was only 70% relative to the oral capsule. The absorption of the drug from polyethylene glycol suppositories was poor and erratic. The bioavailability of lincomycin from the suppository was only about one third that found with the capsule given orally.

The polyethylene glycol suppositories used in these studies were apparently irritating; 4 of 12 subjects had bowel movements within 2 hr after administration. Moreover, a linear correlation was found in 11 of the 12 subjects between the area under the serum concentration-time curve of lincomycin (relative bioavailability) and time from insertion of suppository to first bowel movement (retention time).

Attaining an adequate retention time may be a problem in some patients, regardless of the suppository base. Studies in children with a commercially available cocoa butter suppository containing 5 grains of aspirin produced retention times ranging from 2 to 44 hr.[211] The availability of aspirin in 4 children who retained the suppository for 5 hr or less ranged from 54 to 64% of the dose. More than 80% of the dose of rectal aspirin was absorbed in 4 children who retained the suppository for 10 hr or more. Slow absorption of aspirin from this product was also found in adults. Attempts to improve the absorption of aspirin from rectal suppositories have been frustrated because of the strong association between rapid absorption of aspirin from the rectum and the incidence of local side effects.[212] The investigators concluded that it is difficult to formulate a rectal dosage form of aspirin combining good tolerance with acceptable bioavailability.

There is continued interest in the development of rectal dosage forms of other antipyretic and/or analgesic drugs. Studies in patients with elevated rectal temperature find that rectal acetaminophen suppositories are significantly more effective in reducing fever than placebo, but only 60% as potent as the oral form of the drug.[213] Other studies in febrile children, ranging in age from 3 months to 6 years, indicate that rectal suppositories containing a dose of 15 to 20 mg/kg acetaminophen produce an antipyretic effect almost equal to an oral elixir of the drug and offer an alternative in those children for whom oral administration is not possible.[214]

The absorption of the nonsteroidal anti-inflammatory and analgesic drug naproxen after rectal suppository is almost as rapid and complete as after the commercial oral tablet.[215] The bioavailability of the drug in the suppositories was 95% that of the tablets. When indomethacin is given orally as capsules or rectally as suppositories, 100 mg nightly doses are equally effective in relieving morning symptoms in patients with rheumatoid arthritis.[216] The mean plasma indomethacin concentration was 200 ng/ml during the oral dosing, and 220 ng/ml during the rectal dosing. No differences were seen in side effects or patient preference of the dosage forms.

Rectal suppositories of oxymorphone have been compared with intramuscular injections of the drug in patients with postoperative pain.[217] Rectal administration resulted in lower and delayed peak analgesia and a slightly longer duration of effect than intramuscular administration. When total effect was considered, rectal oxymorphone was found to be one tenth as potent as the intramuscular form.

Allopurinol lowers uric acid levels and is used for the treatment of gout. More recently, allopurinol has also been used prophylactically in patients who are going to receive cytotoxic drugs, to prevent the development of hyperuricemia and consequent uric acid nephropathy. Although allopurinol is usually administered orally, the development of nausea and vomiting among patients undergoing cancer chemotherapy frequently precludes the use of oral tablets. Several cancer centers have used extemporaneously prepared suppositories containing allopurinol to overcome this problem.

Investigators measured allopurinol and oxipurinol, an active metabolite, concentrations in plasma after intravenous, oral, and rectal administration of allopurinol.[218] The rectal dosage form was a suppository prepared by grinding the oral tablets into a fine powder and incorporating the powder into cocoa butter. The bioavailability of the tablet given orally was about 67% but no measurable plasma levels of allopurinol or oxipurinol were found in any subject after rectal administration. The use of rectal suppositories of allopurinol as an adjunct in cancer chemotherapy should be re-examined.

Another example of poor bioavailability after the administration of an extemporaneously prepared suppository has been reported with tamoxifen, a drug used in the management of breast cancer.[219] The mean bioavailability of the suppositories was less than 30% relative to oral tablets of tamoxifen. Whether the findings with allopurinol and tamoxifen reflect poor absorption in the lower bowel or slow release from the formulation is not clear. Under any circumstances, however, extemporaneously prepared suppository formulations must be evaluated with regard to bioavailability before they are widely used in the institution as an alternate dosage form.

There has been substantial interest in the development of rectal dosage forms of anticonvulsants, particularly diazepam, for children and adults. The bioavailability of diazepam from rectal suppositories is better than from intramuscular injections but not comparable to oral administration.[220,221] On the other hand, diazepam absorption from rectal solutions is far better than from suppositories, and the rate of absorption of the drug from rectal solutions is greater than from oral tablets.[221] Rectal administration of diazepam solution may be a suitable alternative to intravenous injection in young children with convulsive disorders, but additional efficacy studies are required before this approach can be recommended.[222,223] Although high, possibly anticonvulsant, blood levels are achieved after rectal solutions, considerable variability is observed, perhaps related to difficulties in administration.

A more recent report concerned the absorption of single doses of diazepam in adult epileptic subjects following intravenous, oral, and rectal administration.[224] No dosage form produced diazepam concentrations comparable to those found after rapid intravenous injection, concentrations known to be effective in the treatment of status epilepticus. Diazepam oral tablets and rectal solution produced similar peak levels after delays of 15–90 min; the levels were, on average, about half those observed after intravenous administration. Serum diazepam levels above 400 ng/ml, thought to be necessary for a satisfactory anticonvulsant effect, were reached in only a few subjects after rectal administration.

Another study examined the absorption of diazepam after rectal administration in children with epilepsy.[225] When given as a rectal solution, diazepam was rapidly absorbed, resulting in serum concentrations above 200 ng/ml within 10 min in most children. The investigators suggest that this route of administration and dosage form may be an effective alternative to intravenous administration. A commercial suppository formulation of diazepam, on the other hand, was absorbed slowly and not recommended for urgent treatment of seizures.

The results of a clinical trial of single dose rectal and oral administration of diazepam 20 mg for the prevention of serial seizures in adult epileptic patients has also been reported.[226] Diazepam was given rectally as a new suppository formulation with rapid release characteristics immediately after a seizure and was effective in preventing recurrent seizures within a 24-hour observation period. The suppository produced a wide range of diazepam levels in serum; the mean serum concentration at 60 min was 190 µg/ml. In a similar study, oral administration of diazepam also reduced the incidence of serial seizures compared with a placebo. The mean 60 min serum diazepam level was 273 ng/ml.

Intravenous secobarbital has been used in the emergency treatment of acute convulsive conditions. Some epilepsy centers have explored the use of rectal secobarbital as adjunct therapy in poorly controlled epileptic children. Sodium secobarbital suppositories were prescribed for home use in children who frequently had prolonged seizures. Parents were instructed to administer the suppository when their child had a seizure that lasted more than 15 min. The availability of this dosage form offered the possibility of aborting seizures and obviating the need to bring the child to the hospital emergency room.

The absorption of rectal secobarbital was studied in epileptic children.[227] Some subjects received a rectal solution of secobarbital and the others were given secobarbital suppositories. The peak serum concentration of secobarbital was consistently higher and occurred earlier in children given the solution rather than the suppository. The extent of absorption, however, was about the same for both dosage forms. If rectal secobarbital is considered for treatment of prolonged seizures, a rectal solution may offer a more rapid and consistent onset of effect than a suppository.

Clinical studies suggest that rectal valproate may also be useful in the treatment of epilepsy. The bioavailability of sodium valproate after repeated administrations of rectal suppositories was studied in epileptic children and adolescents on chronic valproic acid therapy.[228] Some patients were treated with repeated doses of an oral solution and others with an enteric coated tablet of valproate. Serum levels of valproic acid were determined at steady state. Thereafter, suppositories were given regularly instead of the oral dosage forms; serum levels were again measured after several days of dosing.

Average steady-state concentrations of valproic acid were about the same for all three dosage forms, suggesting bioequivalence with respect to extent of absorption. Serum level-time profiles were nearly identical for the oral and rectal solutions. Steady-state serum levels during oral administration of enteric-coated tablets showed less fluctuation than those measured after the oral or rectal solution, suggesting slower absorption.

Intravenous metronidazole is widely used for prophylaxis and therapy of anaerobic infections in abdominal and gynecologic surgery, but the cost of this therapy is high; equally effective but less expensive alternative dosage forms are sought. Clinical investigators in Australia have reported that rectal administration of metronidazole suppositories provides adequate therapeutic plasma levels of the drug after surgery; they suggest that use of suppositories could result in a significant decrease in drug costs.[229] An earlier study indicated that the bioavailability of metronidazole from a rectal suppository was about 90% relative to an oral tablet of the drug.[230]

Rectal solutions of corticosteroids are used in the treatment of inflammatory bowel disease, but there is controversy as to whether their effect is local or systemic. The idea of a local effect has gained favor because early studies claimed poor absorption of corticosteroids after rectal instillation. More recent investigations challenge this idea. Prednisolone appears in the plasma of patients with ulcerative colitis after administration of prednisolone-21-phosphate retention enemas.[231] Blood levels of prednisolone are similar after oral or rectal administration of the drug. These findings suggest that 20 mg prednisolone given by retention enema may exert systemic effects. About 50 to 90% of a dose of hydrocortisone is absorbed from a rectal solution of the drug, if the retention time exceeds 8 hr.[232] On the other hand, the relative bioavailability of methylprednisolone is only 14% after a rectal solution of methylprednisolone acetate, suggesting that the drug may act locally rather than systemically (Fig. 6–12).[233]

An enema containing mesalamine (5-aminosalicylic acid) is available for treatment of mild to moderate distal ulcerative colitis.[234] Severe ulcerative colitis is treated with systemic corticosteroids and less severe disease is usually treated with oral sulfasalazine and/or corticosteroid enemas. Sulfasalazine, a prodrug hydrolyzed to sulfapyridine and mesalamine in the lower bowel, is effective but many patients must discontinue the drug because of adverse effects.

Most authorities believe that the active component of sulfasalazine is mesalamine and that most

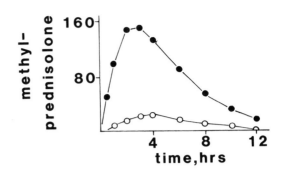

Fig. 6–12. Methylprednisolone concentrations in plasma (ng/ml) following single oral (●) or rectal (○) dose of methylprednisolone acetate. (Data from Gary, D.C., et al.[233])

or all of its toxicity is due to sulfapyridine. Oral mesalamine, however, is rapidly absorbed in the small intestine and little if any of the dose reaches the colon. Accordingly, dosage forms designed to deliver mesalamine to the lower bowel are under investigation. Mesalamine enema is the first of these products to be approved in the US.

It is generally appreciated that the formulation can markedly affect the absorption of drugs from rectal suppositories. Accordingly, there is a potential for clinically important differences in bioavailability among commercially available products. Unfortunately, few clinical studies on this question have been reported. The bioavailability of salicylate from 5 brands of aspirin rectal suppositories was compared to oral administration of the drug in a tablet.[235] When the products were retained for longer than 10 hr, absorption was essentially complete; however, when retention was limited to 2 hr, the absorption of aspirin from one product was 40% of the dose whereas only 20% of the dose was absorbed from the others. Thus, substantial differences in the rate of aspirin absorption exist among marketed rectal suppositories.

The bioavailability of acetaminophen after rectal administration of three acetaminophen suppository formulations obtained from hospital and commercial sources was compared to that after oral administration of a tablet dosage form.[236] The absorption of acetaminophen from the three rectal products ranged from 68 to 88% relative to the tablet. As shown in Figure 6–13, the absorption rate varied markedly among products. The acetaminophen in one formulation was so slowly absorbed that the clinical value of the product is questionable.

There has been renewed interest in the rectal

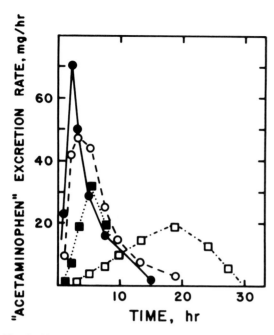

Fig. 6–13. Urinary excretion of unchanged and metabolized acetaminophen ("acetaminophen") after oral administration of a tablet (●) or after rectal administration of different suppositories (○,■,□). (Data from Feldman, S.[236])

administration of drugs with the realization that it may result in improved bioavailability by avoiding first-pass hepatic metabolism. Parts of the rectum are perfused by the inferior and middle hemorrhoidal veins, which do not drain into the portal system. On the other hand, the superior hemorrhoidal vein enters the hepatic portal circulation by way of the inferior mesenteric vein.

Rectal administration of the investigational analgesic meptazinol in healthy subjects resulted in more rapid and complete absorption than after oral administration.[237] The more rapid absorption may be the result of avoiding the delayed gastric emptying seen after oral administration of the drug. The more complete absorption suggests that at least part of the rectal dose was absorbed directly into the systemic circulation and not subject to presystemic hepatic metabolism.

Blood levels of lidocaine were determined in healthy subjects following 200 mg intravenous, 300 mg oral, and 300 mg rectal doses of the drug. The mean bioavailability of lidocaine was considerably higher after rectal than after oral administration (63% vs 31%). Analysis of the data suggests that about half of the rectal dose bypasses the liver during absorption.[238] These findings suggest that,

in principle, it is possible to partially avoid first-pass hepatic metabolism by giving a drug rectally.

In another study, investigators found that rectal propranolol resulted in a different metabolite pattern than that observed after oral or intravenous administration of the drug.[239] The ratio of metabolite to parent drug in plasma after rectal propranolol was always larger than after intravenous administration but smaller than after oral dosing. This suggests partial avoidance of first-pass metabolism by the rectal route, consistent with earlier results.

REFERENCES

1. Von Dardel, O., Mebius, C., and Mossberg, T.: Diazepam in emulsion form for intravenous usage. Acta Anaesthesiol. Scand., 20:221, 1976.
2. Young, A.E., et al.: Totally implantable vascular access for long term chemotherapy. Br. Med. J., 291:1608, 1985.
3. Reddy, C.P., Benes, J., and Beck, B.: Intravenous disopyramide: safety and efficacy of a new dosage regimen. Clin. Pharmacol. Ther., 35:610, 1984.
4. Fragen, R.J., et al.: A pharmacokinetically designed etomidate infusion regimen for hypnosis. Anesth. Analg., 62:654, 1983.
5. Wang, T., et al.: The development and testing of intravenous dosing regimens: application to flecainide for the suppression of ventricular arrhythmias. Clin. Pharmacol. Ther., 43:499, 1988.
6. Hull, R.D., et al.: Continuous intravenous heparin compared with intermittent subcutaneous heparin in the initial treatment of proximal-vein thrombosis. N. Engl. J. Med., 315:1109, 1986.
7. Obeso, J.A., Luquin, M.R., and Martinez-Lage, J.M.: Lisuride infusion pump: a device for the treatment of motor fluctuations in Parkinson's disease. Lancet, 1:467, 1986.
8. Warrington, P.S., et al.: Optimising antiemesis in cancer chemotherapy: Efficacy of continuous versus intermittent infusion of high dose metoclopramide in emesis induced by cisplatin. Br. Med. J., 293:1334, 1986.
9. West, W.H., et al.: Constant-infusion recombinant interleukin-2 in adoptive immunotherapy of advanced cancer. N. Engl. J. Med., 316:898, 1987.
10. Wright, A.M., Hecker, J.F., and Lewis, G.B.H.: Use of transdermal glyceryl trinitrate to reduce failure of intravenous infusion due to phlebitis and extravasation. Lancet, 2:1148, 1985.
11. Hare, L.E., et al.: Bioavailability of dexamethasone. II. Dexamethasone phosphate. Clin. Pharmacol. Ther., 18:330, 1975.
12. Miyabo, S., et al.: A comparison of the bioavailability and potency of dexamethasone phosphate and sulphate in man. Eur. J. Clin. Pharmacol., 20:277, 1981.
13. Frey, B.M., Seeberger, M., and Frey, F.J.: Pharmacokinetics of 3 prednisolone prodrugs. Evidence of therapeutic inequivalence in renal transplant patients with rejection. Transplantation, 39:270, 1985.
14. Slaughter, R.L., et al.: Chloramphenicol sodium succinate kinetics in critically ill patients. Clin. Pharmacol. Ther., 28:69, 1980.
15. Nahata, M.C., and Powell, D.A.: Bioavailability and clearance of chloramphenicol after intravenous chloramphenicol succinate. Clin. Pharmacol. Ther., 30:368, 1981.
16. Ensminger, W.D., and Gyves, J.W.: Clinical pharma-

cology of hepatic arterial chemotherapy. Semin. Oncol., *10*:176, 1983.

17. Eckman, W.W., Patlak, C.S., and Fenstermacher, J.D.: A critical evaluation of the principles governing the advantages of intra-arterial infusions. J. Pharmacokinet. Biopharm., 2:257, 1974.

18. Øie, S., and Huang, J-D.: Influence of administration route on drug delivery to a target organ. J. Pharm. Sci., *70*:1344, 1981.

19. Ensminger, W.D., et al.: A clinical pharmacological evaluation of hepatic arterial infusions of 5-fluoro-2'-deoxyuridine and 5-fluorouracil. Cancer Res., *38*:3784, 1978.

20. Kemeny, N., et al.: Intrahepatic or systemic infusion of fluorodeoxyuridine in patients with liver metastases from colorectal carcinoma. Ann. Intern. Med., *107*:459, 1987.

21. Gyves, J.W., et al.: Improved regional selectivity of hepatic arterial mitomycin by starch microspheres. Clin. Pharmacol. Ther., *34*:259, 1983.

22. Pfeifle, C.E., et al.: Pharmacologic studies of intra-hepatic artery chemotherapy with degradable starch microspheres. Cancer Drug Delivery, *3*:1, 1986.

23. Blacklock, J.B., et al.: Drug streaming during intra-arterial chemotherapy. J. Neurosurg., *64*:284, 1986.

24. Dedrick, R.L.: Arterial drug infusion: pharmacokinetic problems and pitfalls. J. Natl. Cancer. Inst., *80*:84, 1988.

25. Allinson, R.R., and Stach, P.E.: Intrathecal drug therapy. Drug Intell. Clin. Pharm., *12*:347, 1978.

26. Slattery, P.J., and Boas, R.A.: Newer methods of delivery of opiates for relief of pain. Drugs, *30*:539, 1985.

27. Nordberg, G., et al.: Pharmacokinetic aspects of epidural morphine analgesia. Anesthesiol., *58*:545, 1983.

28. Reiz, S., et al.: Epidural morphine for postoperative pain relief. Acta Anaesth. Scand., *25*:111, 1985.

29. Carmichael, F.J., Rolbin, S.H., and Hew, E.M.: Epidural morphine for analgesia after Caesarean section. Can. Anaesth. Soc. J., *29*:359, 1982.

30. El-Baz, N.M.I., Faber, L.P., and Jensik, R.J.: Continuous epidural infusion of morphine for treatment of pain after thoracic surgery: a new technique. Anesth. Analg., *63*:757, 1984.

31. Bullingham, R.E.S.: Optimum management of postoperative pain. Drugs, *29*:376, 1985.

32. Markman, M.: Intraperitoneal chemotherapy for malignant diseases of the gastrointestinal tract. Surg. Gynecol. Obstet., *164*:89, 1987.

33. Dedrick, R.L.: Theoretical and experimental bases of intraperitoneal chemotherapy. Semin. Oncol., Vol. 12, Suppl. 4, pp 1–6.

34. Gyves, J.W., et al.: Constant intraperitoneal 5-fluorouracil infusion through a totally implanted system. Clin. Pharmacol. Ther., *35*:83, 1984.

35. Sugarbaker, P.H., et al.: Prospective, randomized trial of intravenous versus intraperitoneal 5-fluorouracil in patients with advanced primary colon or rectal cancer. Surgery, *98*:414, 1985.

36. Greenblatt, D.J., and Koch-Weser, J.: Intramuscular injection of drugs. N. Engl. J. Med., *295*:542, 1976.

37. Cohen, L.S., et al.: Plasma levels of lidocaine after intramuscular administration. Am. J. Cardiol., *29*:520, 1972.

38. Schwartz, M.L., et al.: Antiarrhythmic effectiveness of intramuscular lidocaine: Influence of different injection sites. Clin. Pharmacol. Ther., *14*:77, 1974.

39. Koster, R.W., and Dunning, A.J.: Intramuscular lidocaine for prevention of lethal arrhythmias in the prehospitalization phase of acute myocardial infarction. N. Engl. J. Med., *313*:1105, 1985.

40. Suboptimal response to hepatitis B vaccine given by injection into the buttock. MMWR, *34*:105, 1985.

41. Ukena, T., et al.: Site of injection and response to hepatitis B vaccine. N. Engl. J. Med., *313*:579, 1985.

42. Weber, D.J., et al.: Obesity as a predictor of poor antibody response to hepatitis B plasma vaccine. JAMA, *254*:3187, 1985.

43. Cockshott, W.P., et al.: Intramuscular or intralipomatous injections? N. Engl. J. Med., *301*:356, 1982.

44. Fishbein, D.B., et al.: Administration of human diploid-cell rabies vaccine in the gluteal area. N. Engl. J. Med., *318*:124, 1988.

45. Reeves, D.S., Bywater, M.J., and Wise, R.: Availability of three antibiotics after intramuscular injection into thigh and buttock. Lancet, 2:1421, 1974.

46. Vukovich, R.A., et al.: Sex differences in the intramuscular absorption and bioavailability of cephradine. Clin. Pharmacol. Ther., *18*:215, 1975.

47. Miller, R.R., and Greenblatt, D.J. (eds.): Drug Effects in Hospitalized Patients: Experiences of the Boston Collaborative Drug Surveillance Program. 1966-1975. New York, John Wiley and Sons, 1976.

48. Greenblatt, D.J., Shader, R.I., and Koch-Weser, J.: Slow absorption of intramuscular chlordiazepoxide. N. Engl. J. Med., *291*:1116, 1974.

49. Greenblatt, D.J., et al.: Absorption of oral and intramuscular chlordiazepoxide. Eur. J. Clin. Pharmacol., *13*:267, 1978.

50. Nair, S.G., et al.: Plasma pentobarbitone levels. Anaesthesia, *31*:1037, 1976.

51. McCaughey, W., and Dundee, J.W.: Comparison of the sedative effects of diazepam given by the oral and intramuscular routes. Br. J. Anaesth., *44*:901, 1972.

52. Root, B., and Loveland, J.P.: Pediatric premedication with diazepam or hydroxyzine: Oral versus intramuscular route. Anesth. Analg., *52*:717, 1973.

53. Assaf, R.A.E., Dundee, J.W., and Gamble, J.A.S.: The influence of the route of administration on the clinical action of diazepam. Anaesthesiology, *30*:152, 1975.

54. Gamble, J.A.S., Dundee, J.W., and Assaf, R.A.E.: Plasma diazepam levels after single dose oral and intramuscular administration. Anaesthesiology, *30*:164, 1975.

55. DeGroot, L.J., Pretell, E., and Garcia, M.E.: Absorption of intramuscularly administered tri-iodothyronine. N. Engl. J. Med., *274*:133, 1966.

56. Dam, M., and Olesen, V.: Intramuscular administration of phenytoin. Neurology, *16*:288, 1966.

57. Serrano, E., et al.: Plasma diphenylhydantoin values after oral and intramuscular administration of diphenylhydantoin. Neurology, *23*:311, 1973.

58. Wilder, B.J., et al.: A method for shifting from oral to intramuscular diphenylhydantoin administration. Clin. Pharmacol. Ther., *16*:507, 1974.

59. Steiness, E., Svendsen, O., and Rasmussen, F.: Plasma digoxin after parenteral administration: local reaction after intramuscular injection. Clin. Pharmacol. Ther., 16:430, 1974.

60. Sidell, F.R., Culver, D.L., and Kaminskis, A.: Serum creatine phosphokinase activities after intramuscular injection: the effect of dose, concentration, and volume. JAMA, *229*:1894, 1974.

61. Greenblatt, D.J., Shader, R.I., and Koch-Weser, J.: Serum creatine phosphokinase concentrations after intramuscular chlordiazepoxide and its solvent. J. Clin. Pharmacol., *16*:118, 1976.

62. Greenblatt, D.J., and Allen, M.D.: Intramuscular injection-site complications. JAMA, *240*:542, 1978.

63. Nora, J.J., Smith, D.W., and Cameron, J.R.: The route of insulin administration in the management of diabetes mellitus. J. Pediatr., *64*:547, 1964.

64. Kølendorf, K., Bojsen, J., and Nielsen, S.L.: Adipose

tissue blood flow and insulin disappearance from subcutaneous tissue. Clin. Pharmacol. Ther., 25:598, 1979.

65. Berger, M., et al.: Pharmacokinetics of subcutaneously injected tritiated insulin: effects of exercise. Diabetes, 28(Suppl. 1):53, 1979.

66. Koivisto, V.A.: Sauna-induced acceleration in insulin absorption from subcutaneous injection site. Br. Med. J., 280:1411, 1980.

67. Mecklenberg, R.S., et al.: Clinical use of the insulin infusion pump in 100 patients with type I diabetes. N. Engl. J. Med., 307:514, 1982.

68. Rudolf, M.C.J., et al.: Efficacy of the insulin pump in the home treatment of pregnant diabetics. Diabetes, 30:891, 1981.

69. Pickup, J.C., et al.: Management of severely brittle diabetes by continuous subcutaneous and intramuscular insulin infusions: evidence for a defect in subcutaneous insulin absorption. Br. Med. J., 282:347, 1981.

70. Pozza, G., et al.: Long-term continuous intraperitoneal insulin treatment in brittle diabetes. Br. Med. J., 286:255, 1983.

71. Berger, M., and McSherry, C.K.: Outpatient dobutamine infusion using a totally implantable infusion pump for refractory congestive heart failure. Chest, 88:295, 1985.

72. Hattersley, P.G., Mitsuoka, J.C., and King, J.H.: Heparin therapy for thromboembolic disorders. A prospective evaluation of 134 cases monitored by the activated coagulation time. JAMA, 250:1413, 1983.

73. Lokich, J., and Ensminger, W.: Ambulatory pump infusion devices for hepatic artery infusion. Semin. Oncol., 10:183, 1983.

74. Likich, J., et al.: The delivery of cancer chemotherapy by constant venous infusion. Ambulatory management of venous access and portable pump. Cancer, 50:2731, 1982.

75. Phillips, T.W., et al.: New implantable continuous administration and bolus dose intracarotid drug delivery system for the treatment of malignant gliomas. Neurosurg., 11:213, 1982.

76. Cohen, A.M., et al.: Treatment of hepatic metastases by transaxillary hepatic artery chemotherapy using an implanted drug pump. Cancer, 51:2013, 1983.

77. Gyves, J.W., et al.: Constant intraperitoneal 5-fluorouracil infusion through a totally implanted system. Clin. Pharmacol. Ther., 35:83, 1984.

78. Jones, V.A., and Hanks, G.W.: New portable infusion pump for prolonged subcutaneous administration of opioid analgesics in patients with advanced cancer. Br. Med. J., 292:1496, 1986.

79. Enna, S.J., and Schanker, L.S.: Absorption of drugs from the rat lung. Am. J. Physiol., 223:1227, 1972.

80. Schanker, L.S., and Burton, J.A.: Absorption of heparin and cyanocobalamin from the rat lung. Proc. Soc. Exp. Biol. Med., 152:377, 1976.

81. Schanker, L.S., and Less, M.J.: Lung pH and pulmonary absorption of nonvolatile drugs in the rat. Drug Metab. Dispos., 5:174, 1977.

82. Schanker, L.S., Mitchell, E.W., and Brown, R.A., Jr.: Species comparison of drug absorption from the lung after aerosol inhalation or intratracheal injection. Drug Metabol. Dispos., 14:79, 1986.

83. Schanker, L.S., Mitchell, E.W., and Brown, R.A., Jr.: Pulmonary absorption of drugs in the dog: comparison with other species. Pharmacol., 32:176, 1986.

84. Newhouse, M.T., and Dolovich, M.B.: Control of asthma by aerosols. N. Engl. J. Med., 315:870, 1986.

85. Pierce, R.J., et al.: Comparison of intravenous and inhaled terbutaline in the treatment of asthma. Chest, 79:506, 1981.

86. Merz, B.: Aerosolized pentamidine promising in *pneumocystis* therapy, prophylaxis. JAMA, 259:3223, 1988.

87. Murray, A.B., et al.: The effect of pressurized isoproterenol and salbutamol in asthmatic children. Pediatrics, 54:746, 1974.

88. Moss, G.F., and Ritchie, J.T.: The absorption and clearance of disodium cromoglycate from the lung in rat, rabbit and monkey. Toxicol. Appl. Pharmacol., 17:699, 1970.

89. Moss, G.F., et al.: Plasma levels and urinary excretion of disodium cromoglycate after inhalation by human volunteers. Toxicol. Appl. Pharmacol., 20:147, 1971.

90. Walker, S.R., et al.: The fate of (^{14}C) disodium cromoglycate in man. J. Pharm. Pharmacol., 24:252, 1972.

91. Robson, R.A., Taylor, B.J., and Taylor, B.: Sodium cromoglycate: spincaps or metered dose aerosol. Br. J. Clin. Pharmacol., 11:383, 1981.

92. Keidan, S.: Comparison of a breath-actuated pressurized inhaler and a conventional pressurized inhaler. Practitioner, Mar. 1974, p. 2.

93. Wetterlin, K.: Turbuhaler: A new powder inhaler for administration of drugs to the airways. Pharm. Res., 5:506, 1988.

94. Gwynn, C.M., and Smith, J.M.: Long-term results with beclomethasone dipropionate aerosol in children with bronchial asthma: why does it fail? Br. J. Clin. Pharmacol., 4:269S, 1977.

95. Paterson, I.C., and Crompton, G.K.: Use of pressurized aerosols by asthmatic patients. Br. Med. J., 1:76, 1976.

96. Newman, S.P., and Clarke, S.W.: The proper use of metered dose inhalers. Chest, 86:342, 1984.

97. Konig, P.: Spacer devices used with metered-dose inhalers: breakthrough or gimmick? Chest, 88:277, 1985.

98. Corticosteroid aerosols for asthma. Med. Lett. Drugs Ther., 27:5, 1985.

99. Pedersen, J.Z., and Bundgaard, A.: Comparative efficacy of different methods of nebulising terbutaline. Eur. J. Clin. Pharmacol., 25:739, 1983.

100. Nebulisers in the treatment of asthma. Drug Ther. Bull., 25:101, 1987.

101. Beasley, R., Rafferty, P., and Holgate, S.T.: Adverse reactions to the nondrug constituents of nebuliser solutions. Br. J. Clin. Pharmacol., 25:283, 1988.

102. Hodges, I.G.C., Milner, A.D., and Stokes, G.M.: Assessment of a new device for delivering aerosol drugs to asthmatic children. Arch. Dis. Child., 56:787, 1981.

103. Sackner, M.A., Brown, L.K., and Kim, C.S.: Basis of an improved metered aerosol delivery system. Chest, 80S:915S, 1981.

104. Kupferman, A., et al.: Topically applied steroids in corneal disease. III. Role of drug derivative in stromal absorption of dexamethasone. Arch. Ophthalmol., 91:373, 1974.

105. Anderson, R.A., and Cowle, J.B.: Influence of pH on the effect of pilocarpine on aqueous dynamics. Br. J. Ophthalmol., 52:607, 1968.

106. Longwell, A., et al.: Effect of topically applied pilocarpine on tear film pH. J. Pharm. Sci., 65:1654, 1976.

107. Sieg, J.W., and Robinson, J.R.: Vehicle effects on ocular drug bioavailability. II: Evaluation of pilocarpine. J. Pharm. Sci., 66:1222, 1977.

108. Chrai, S.S., et al.: Lacrimal and instilled fluid dynamics in rabbit eyes. J. Pharm. Sci., 62:1112, 1973.

109. Patton, T.F.: Pharmacokinetic evidence for improved ophthalmic drug delivery by reduction of instilled volume. J. Pharm. Sci., 66:1058, 1977.

110. Chrai, S.S., et al.: Drop size and initial dosing frequency problems of topically applied ophthalmic drugs. J. Pharm. Sci., 63:333, 1974.

111. Chrai, S.S., and Robinson, J.R.: Ocular evaluation of

methylcellulose vehicle in albino rats. J. Pharm. Sci., *63*:1218, 1974.

112. Sieg, J.W., and Robinson, J.R.: Vehicle effects on ocular drug bioavailability. I.: Evaluation of fluorometholone. J. Pharm. Sci., *64*:931, 1975.

113. Kupferman, A., and Leibowitz, H.M.: Topically applied steroids in corneal disease. IV. The role of drug concentration in stromal absorption of prednisolone acetate. Arch. Opthalmol., *91*:377, 1974.

114. Schoenwald, R.D., and Boltralik, J.J.: A bioavailability comparison in rabbits of two steroids formulated as high-viscosity gels and reference aqueous preparations. Invest. Ophthalmol. Vis. Sci., *18*:61, 1979.

115. Smith, S.A., Smith, S.E., and Lazare, R.: An increased effect of pilocarpine on the pupil by application of the drug in oil. Br. J. Ophthalmol., *62*:314, 1978.

116. Friedman, T.S., and Patton, T.F.: Differences in ocular penetration of pilocarpine in rabbits of different ages. J. Pharm. Sci., *65*:1095, 1976.

117. George, F.J., and Hanna, C.: Ocular penetration of chloramphenicol. Effects of route of administration. Arch. Ophthalmol., *95*:879, 1977.

118. Kim, J.M., Stevenson, C.E., and Mathewson, H.S.: Hypertensive reactions to phenylephrine eyedrops in patients with sympathetic denervation. Am. J. Ophthalmol., *85*:862, 1978.

119. Abrams, S.M., Degnan, R.J., and Vinciguerra, V.: Marrow aplasia following topical application of chloramphenicol eye ointment. Arch. Intern. Med., *140*:576, 1980.

120. Lahdes, K., et al.: Systemic absorption of topically applied ocular atropine. Clin. Pharmacol. Ther., *44*:310, 1988.

121. Affrime, M.B., et al.: Dynamics and kinetics of ophthalmic timolol. Clin. Pharmacol. Ther., *27*:471, 1980.

122. Alvan, G., et al.: Absorption of ocular timolol. Clin. Pharmacokinet., *5*:95, 1980.

123. Anon.: Additions to Timoptic contraindications. FDA Drug Bull., *11*:17, 1981.

124. Munroe, W.P., Rindone, J.P., and Kershner, R.M.: Systemic side effects associated with the ophthalmic administration of timolol. Drug Intell. Clin. Pharm., *19*:85, 1985.

125. Zimmerman, T.J., et al.: Improving the therapeutic index of topically applied ocular drugs. Arch. Ophthalmol., *102*:551, 1984.

126. Alper, M.M., et al.: Systemic absorption of metronidazole by the vaginal route. Obstet. Gynecol., *65*:781, 1985.

127. Hussain, A., et al.: Nasal absorption of propranolol in humans. J. Pharm. Sci., *69*:1240, 1980.

128. Fassoulaki, A., and Kaniaris, P.: Intranasal administration of nitroglycerine attenuates the pressor response to laryngoscopy and intubation of the trachea. Br. J. Anaesth., *55*:49, 1983.

129. Huang, C.H., et al.: Mechanism of nasal absorption of drugs I: physicochemical parameters influencing the rate of in situ nasal absorption of drugs in rats. J. Pharm. Sci., *74*:608, 1985.

130. Hermens, W.A.J.J., and Merkus, W.H.M.: The influence of drugs on nasal ciliary movement. Pharm. Res., *4*:445, 1987.

131. Hersey, S.J., and Jackson, R.T.: Effect of bile salts on nasal permeability in vitro. J. Pharm. Sci., *76*:876, 1987.

132. Fisher, A.N., et al.: The effect of molecular size on the nasal absorption of water-soluble compounds in the albino rat. J. Pharm. Pharmacol., *39*:357, 1987.

133. McMartin, C., et al.: Analysis of structural requirements from the nasal cavity. J. Pharm. Sci., *76*:535, 1987.

134. Koutsilieris, M., et al.: Objective response and disease outcome in 59 patients with stage D2 prostatic cancer treated with either buserelin or orchiectomy. Urology, *27*:221, 1986.

135. The Leuprolide Study Group: Leuprolide versus diethylstilbestrol for metastatic prostate cancer. N. Engl. J. Med., *311*:1281, 1984.

136. Falkson, G., and Vorobiof, D.A.: Intranasal buserelin in the treatment of advanced prostatic cancer: a phase II trial. J. Clin. Oncology, *5*:1419, 1987.

137. Henzl, M.R., et al.: Administration of nasal nafarelin as compared with oral danazol for endometriosis. A multicenter double-blind comparative trial. N. Engl. J. Med., *318*:485, 1988.

138. Larsen, C., et al.: Influence of experimental rhinitis on the gonadotropin response to intranasal administration of buserelin. Eur. J. Clin. Pharmacol., *33*:155, 1987.

139. Aungst, D.J., Rogers, N.J., and Shefter, E.: Comparison of nasal, rectal, buccal, sublingual and intramuscular insulin efficacy and the effects of a bile salt absorption promoter. J. Pharmacol. Exp. Ther., *244*:23, 1988.

140. El-Etr, M., Slama, G., and Desplanque, N.: Preprandial intranasal insulin as adjuvant therapy in type II diabetics. Lancet, *2*:1085, 1987.

141. Reginster, J.Y., et al.: 1-Year controlled randomized trial of prevention of early postmenopausal bone loss by intranasal calcitonin. Lancet, *2*:1481, 1987.

142. Guy, R.H., and Maibach, H.I.: Drug delivery to local subcutaneous structures following topical administration. J. Pharm. Sci., *72*:1375, 1983.

143. Feldmann, R.J., and Maibach, H.I.: Regional variation in percutaneous penetration of ^{14}C-cortisol in man. J. Invest. Dermatol., *48*:181, 1967.

144. Rougier, A., Lotte, C., and Maibach, H.I.: In vivo percutaneous penetration of some organic compounds related to anatomic site in humans: predictive assessment by the stripping method. J. Pharm. Sci., *76*:451, 1987.

145. Washitake, M., et al.: Studies on percutaneous absorption of drugs. III. Percutaneous absorption of drugs through damaged skin. Chem. Pharm. Bull., *21*:2444, 1973.

146. Feldmann, R.J., and Maibach, H.I.: Penetration of ^{14}C-hydrocortisone through normal skin. The effect of stripping and occlusion. Arch. Dermatol., *91*:661, 1965.

147. Zackheim, H.S., et al.: Percutaneous absorption of 1,3-bis (2-chloroethyl)1-nitrosourea (BCNU, carmustine) in mycosis fungoides. Br. J. Dermatol., *97*:65, 1977.

148. Wester, R.C., and Maibach, H.I.: Cutaneous pharmacokinetics: 10 steps to percutaneous absorption. Drug Metabol. Revs., *14*:169, 1983.

149. Montagna, W., Stoughton, R.B., and VanScott, E.J.: Pharmacology and the Skin. New York, Appleton-Century-Crofts, 1972, pp. 535–545.

150. Wester, R.C., et al.: Percutaneous absorption of testosterone in the newborn rhesus monkey: comparison to the adult. Pediatr. Res., *11*:737, 1977.

151. Craig, F.N., Cummings, E.G., and Sim, V.M.: Environmental temperature and the percutaneous absorption of a cholinesterase inhibitor. J. Invest. Dermatol., *68*:357, 1977.

152. Katz, M., and Poulsen, B.J.: Corticoid, vehicle, and skin interaction in percutaneous absorption. J. Soc. Cosmet. Chem., *23*:565, 1972.

153. Portnoy, B.: The effect of formulation on the clinical response to topical flucinolone acetonide. Br. J. Dermatol., *77*:579, 1965.

154. Stoughton, R.B.: Bioassay system for formulations of

topically applied glucocorticosteroids. Arch. Dermatol., *106*:825, 1972.

155. Barry, B.W., and Woodford, R.: Proprietary hydrocortisone creams. Vasoconstrictor activities and bioavailabilities of six preparations. Br. J. Dermatol., *95*:423, 1976.

156. Mizuchi, A., et al.: Percutaneous absorption of betamethasone 17-benzoate measured by radioimmunoassay. J. Invest. Dermatol., *67*:279, 1976.

157. Kligman, A.M.: Topical pharmacology and toxicology of dimethyl sulfoxide. Part I. JAMA, *193*:140, 1965; Part II. JAMA, *193*:151, 1965.

158. Bennett, S.L., Barry, B.W., and Woodform, R.: Optimization of bioavailability of topical steroids: non-occluded penetration enhancers under thermodynamic control. J. Pharm. Pharmacol., *37*:298, 1985.

159. Wester, R.C., and Maibach, H.I.: Relationship of topical dose and percutaneous absorption in rhesus monkey and man. J. Invest. Dermatol., *67*:518, 1976.

160. Wester, R.C., Noonan, P.K., and Maibach, H.I.: Percutaneous absorption of hydrocortisone increases with long-term administration. Arch. Dermatol., *116*:186, 1980.

161. Roberts, M.S., and Horlock, E.: Effect of repeated skin application on percutaneous absorption of salicylic acid. J. Pharm. Sci., *67*:1685, 1978.

162. Bucks, D.A., Maibach, H.I., and Guy, R.H.: Percutaneous absorption of steroids: effect of repeated application. J. Pharm. Sci., *74*:1337, 1985.

163. Davies, M.G., Vella Briffa, D., and Greaves, M.W.: Systemic toxicity from topically applied salicylic acid. Br. Med. J., *1*:661, 1979.

164. Curley, A., et al.: Dermal absorption of hexachlorophene in infants. Lancet, 2:296, 1971.

165. Anon.: Hexachlorophene and newborns. FDA Drug Bull., Dec. 1971.

166. Goutieres, F., and Aicardi, J.: Accidental percutaneous hexachlorophene intoxication in children. Br. Med. J., 2:663, 1977.

167. Gunby, P.: New study shows hexachlorophene is teratogenic in humans. JAMA, *240*:513, 1978.

168. Anon: Kwell and other drugs for treatment of lice and scabies. Med. Lett. Drugs Ther., *19*:17, 1977.

169. Insect repellants. Med. Lett. Drugs Ther., *27*:61, 1985.

170. Hazards of topical steroid therapy. Adverse Drug Reaction Bull, December 1985, No. 115, pp. 428–431.

171. Franz, T.J.: Percutaneous absorption of minoxidil in man. Arch. Dermatol., *121*:202, 1985.

172. Topical minoxidil for baldness. Med. Lett. Drugs. Ther., *29*:87, 1987.

173. Reichek, N., et al.: Sustained effects of nitroglycerin ointment in patient with angina pectoris. Circulation, *50*:348, 1974.

174. Davidov, M.E., and Mroczek, W.J.: The effect of nitroglycerin ointment on the exercise capacity in patients with angina pectoris. Angiology, *27*:205, 1976.

175. Armstrong, P.W., et al.: Nitroglycerin ointment in acute myocardial infarction. Am. J. Cardiol., *38*:474, 1976.

176. Francis, G.S., and Hagan, A.D.: Nitroglycerin ointment: a review. Angiology, *28*:873, 1977.

177. Sved, S., McLean, W.M., and McGilveray, I.J.: Influence of the method of application on pharmacokinetics of nitroglycerin from ointment in humans. J. Pharm. Sci., *70*:1368, 1981.

178. Holst, J., et al.: Percutaneous estrogen replacement therapy. Effects on circulating estrogens, gonadotropins and prolactin. Acta Obstet. Gynecol. Scand., *62*:49, 1983.

179. Friedrich, E.G., Jr., and Kalra, P.S.: Serum levels of sex hormones in vulvar lichen sclerosus, and the effect of topical testosterone. N. Engl. J. Med., *310*:488, 1984.

180. Beckett, A.H., and Triggs, E.J.: Buccal absorption of basic drugs and its application as an *in vivo* model of passive drug transfer through lipid membranes. J. Pharm. Pharmacol., *19*:315, 1967.

181. Bickel, M.H., and Weder, H.J.: Buccal absorption and other properties of pharmacokinetic importance of imipramine and its metabolites. J. Pharm. Pharmacol., *21*:160, 1969.

182. Beckett, A.H., and Moffat, A.C.: The buccal absorption of some barbiturates. J. Pharm. Pharmacol., *23*:15, 1971.

183. Burnier, A.M., et al.: Sublingual absorption of micronized 17 β-estradiol. Am. J. Obstet. Gynecol., *140*:146, 1981.

184. Bullingham, R.E.S., et al.: Sublingual buprenophine used postoperatively: clinical observations and preliminary pharmacokinetic analysis. Br. J. Clin. Pharmacol., *12*:117, 1981.

185. Barsuhn, C.L., et al.: Human buccal absorption of flurbiprofen. Clin. Pharmacol. Ther., *44*:225, 1988.

186. Taraszka, M.J.: Absorption of clindamycin from the buccal cavity. J. Pharm. Sci., *59*:873, 1970.

187. Schürmann, W., and Turner, P.: A membrane model of the human oral mucosa as derived from buccal absorption performance and physicochemical properties of the β-blocking drugs atenolol and propranolol. J. Pharm. Pharmacol., *30*:127, 1978.

188. Henry, J.A., et al.: Drug recovery following buccal absorption of propranolol. Br. J. Clin. Pharmacol., *10*:61, 1980.

189. Weinberg, D.S., et al.: Sublingual absorption of selected opioid analgesics. Clin. Pharmacol. Ther., *44*:335, 1988.

190. Noonan, P.K., and Benet, L.Z.: Incomplete and delayed bioavailability of sublingual nitroglycerin. Am. J. Cardiol., *55*:184, 1985.

191. Rasler, F.E.: Ineffectiveness of sublingual nitroglycerin in patients with dry mucous membranes. N. Engl. J. Med., *314*:181, 1986.

192. Benowitz, N.L., Jacob, P., III, and Savanapridi, C.: Determinants of nicotine intake while chewing nicotine polacrilex gum. Clin. Pharmacol. Ther., *41*:467, 1987.

193. Tonnesen, P., et al.: Effect of nicotine chewing gum in combination with group counseling on the cessation of smoking. N. Engl. J. Med., *318*:15, 1988.

194. Shore, S.C., Weinberg, E.G., and Durr, M.H.: Buccal administration of fenoterol aerosol in young children with asthma. S. Afr. Med. J., *50*:1362, 1976.

195. Oral nitroglycerin spray. Med. Lett. Drugs Ther., *28*:59, 1986.

196. Gale, G.D., Galloon, S., and Porter, W.R.: Sublingual lorazepam: a better premedication? Br. J. Anaesth., *55*:761, 1983.

197. Scavone, J.M., Greenblatt, D.J., and Shader, R.I.: Alprazolam kinetics following sublingual and oral administration. J. Clin. Psychopharmacol., *7*:332, 1987.

198. van Harten, J., et al.: Negligible sublingual absorption of nifedipine. Lancet, 2:1363, 1987.

199. Winsor, T.: Plethysmographic comparison of sublingual and intramuscular ergotamine. Clin. Pharmacol. Ther., *29*:94, 1981.

200. Alkalay, D., et al.: Sublingual and oral administration of methyltestosterone. A comparison of drug bioavailability. J. Clin. Pharmacol., *13*:142, 1973.

201. Assinder, D.F., Chasseaud, L.F., and Taylor, T.: Plasma isosorbide dinitrate concentrations in human subjects after administration of standard and sustained release formulations. J. Pharm. Sci., *66*:775, 1977.

202. Wagner, J.G.: Biopharmaceutics and Relevant Pharma-

cokinetics. Hamilton, Ill., Drug Intelligence Publications, 1971, p. 215.

203. Moolenaar, F., et al.: Drastic improvement in the rectal absorption profile of morphine in man. Eur. J. Clin. Pharmacol., 29:119, 1985.

204. Brodwall, E.K.: The resorption of theophylline: Blood concentrations after intravenous, peroral, rectal, and intramuscular administration. Acta Med. Scand., 146:123, 1953.

205. Truitt, E.B., Jr., McKusick, V.A., and Krantz, J.C.: Theophylline blood levels after oral, rectal and intravenous administration and correlation with diuretic action. J. Pharmacol. Exp. Ther., 100:309, 1950.

206. Yunginger, J.W., et al.: Serum theophylline levels and control of asthma following rectal theophylline. Ann. Allergy, 24:469, 1966.

207. Pedersen, S., and Sommer, B.: Rectal administration of theophylline in aqueous solution. Acta Paediatr. Scand., 70:243, 1981.

208. Mason, W.D., et al.: Bioavailability of theophylline following a rectally administered concentrated aminophylline solution. J. Allergy Clin. Immunol., 66:119, 1980.

209. Wagner, J.G., Leslie, L.G., and Gove, R.S.: Relative absorption of both tetracycline and penicillin G administered rectally and orally in aqueous solution. Int. J. Clin. Pharmacol. Ther. Toxicol., 2:44, 1969.

210. Wagner, J.G., Carter, C.H., and Martens, I.J.: Serum concentrations after rectal administration of lincomycin hydrochloride. J. Clin. Pharmacol., 8:154, 1968.

211. Nowak, M.M., Grundhofer, B., and Gibaldi, M.: Rectal absorption from aspirin suppositories in children and adults. Pediatrics, 54:23, 1974.

212. Borg, K.O., et al.: Bioavailability and tolerance studies on acetylsalicylic acid suppositories. Acta Pharm. Suec., 12:491, 1975.

213. Maron, J.J., and Ickes, A.C.: The antipyretic effectiveness of acetaminophen suppositories versus tablets: a double blind study. Curr. Ther. Res., 20:45, 1976.

214. Vernon, S., Bacon, C., and Weightman, D.: Rectal paracetamol in small children with fever. Arch. Dis. Child., 54:469, 1979.

215. Desager, J.P., Vanderbist, M., and Harvengt, C.: Naproxen plasma levels in volunteers after single dose administration by oral and rectal routes. J. Clin. Pharmacol., 16:189, 1976.

216. Baber, N., et al.: Indomethacin in rheumatoid arthritis: comparison of oral and rectal dosing. Br. J. Clin. Pharmacol., 10:387, 1980.

217. Beaver, W.T., and Feise, G.A.: A comparison of the analgesic effect of oxymorphone by rectal suppository and intramuscular injection in patients with postoperative pain. J. Clin. Pharmacol., 17:276, 1977.

218. Appelbaum, S.J., et al.: Allopurinol kinetics and bioavailability: intravenous, oral and rectal administration. Cancer Chemother. Pharmacol., 8:93, 1982.

219. Tukker, J.J., Blankenstein, M.A., and Nortier, J.W.R.: Comparison of bioavailability in man of tamoxifen after oral and rectal administration. J. Pharm. Pharmacol., 38:888, 1986.

220. Kanto, J.: Plasma concentrations of diazepam and its metabolites after peroral, intramuscular, and rectal administration. Int. J. Clin. Pharmacol. Ther. Toxicol., 12:427, 1975.

221. Moolenaar, F., et al.: Biopharmaceutics of rectal administration in man. IX. Comparative biopharmaceutics of diazepam after single rectal, oral, intramuscular, and intravenous administration in man. Int. J. Pharmaceut., 5:127, 1980.

222. Langslet, A., et al.: Plasma concentrations of diazepam and N-desmethyldiazepam in newborn infants after intravenous, intramuscular, rectal and oral administration. Acta Paediatr. Scand., 67:699, 1978.

223. Dulac, O., et al.: Blood levels of diazepam after single rectal administration in infants and children. J. Pediatr., 93:1039, 1978.

224. Dhillon, S., Oxley, J., and Richens, A.: Bioavailability of diazepam after intravenous, oral and rectal administration in adult epileptic patients. Br. J. Clin. Pharmacol., 13:427, 1982.

225. Dhillon, S., Ngwane, E., and Richens, A.: Rectal absorption of diazepam in epileptic children. Arch. Dis. Childhood, 57:264, 1982.

226. Milligan, N.M., et al.: A clinical trial of single dose rectal and oral administration of diazepam for the prevention of serial seizures in adult epileptic patients. J. Neurol. Neurosurg. Pyschiatry, 47:235, 1984.

227. Levine, H.L., et al.: Rectal absorption and disposition of secobarbital in epileptic children. Ped. Pharmacol., 2:33, 1982.

228. Issakainen, J., and Bourgeois, B.F.D.: Bioavailability of sodium valproate suppositories during repeated administration at steady state in epileptic children. Eur. J. Pediatr., 146:404, 1987.

229. Ioannides, L., et al.: Rectal administration of metronidazole provides therapeutic plasma levels in postoperative patients. N. Engl. J. Med., 305:1569, 1981.

230. Bergan, T., and Arnold, E.: Pharmacokinetics of metronidazole in healthy adult volunteers after tablets and suppositories. Chemotherapy, 26:231, 1980.

231. Powell-Tuck, J., et al.: Plasma prednisolone levels after administration of prednisolone-21-phosphate as a retention enema in colitis. Br. Med. J., 1:193, 1976.

232. Lima, J.J., et al.: Bioavailability of hydrocortisone retention enemas in normal subjects. Clin. Pharmacol. Ther., 28:262, 1980.

233. Gary, D.C., et al.: Rectal and oral absorption of methylprednisolone acetate. Clin. Pharmacol. Ther., 26:232, 1979.

234. Mesalamine for ulcerative colitis. Med. Lett. Drugs Ther., 30:53, 1988.

235. Gibaldi, M., and Grundhofer, B.: Bioavailability of aspirin from commercial suppositories. J. Pharm. Sci., 64:1064, 1975.

236. Feldman, S.: Bioavailability of acetaminophen suppositories. Am. J. Hosp. Pharm., 32:1173, 1975.

237. Franklin, R.A., Southgate, P.J., and Coleman, A.J.: Studies on the absorption and disposition of meptazinol following rectal administration. Br. J. Clin. Pharmacol., 4:163, 1977.

238. deBoer, A.G., et al.: Rectal bioavailability of lidocaine in man: partial avoidance of "first-pass" metabolism. Clin. Pharmacol. Ther., 26:701, 1979.

239. de Leede, L.G., et al.: Rectal and intravenous propranolol infusion to steady state: kinetics and beta-receptor blockade. Clin. Pharmacol. Ther., 35:148, 1984.

7

Prolonged-Release Medication

PHARMACOKINETIC THEORY

The duration of drug effect is a function of the pharmacokinetics of the drug molecule in an individual patient. The clearance and apparent volume of distribution of a drug determine the degree of persistence of the molecule in the body. This persistence is characterized in terms of half-life or mean residence time (MRT). Because the duration of drug action is related to the distribution and elimination kinetics of a drug, the frequency of dosing must also bear some relationship to the drug's half-life or MRT.

We often find that the frequency of dosing needed to maximize the benefit-to-risk ratio of a drug is unreasonable. For example, in most patients, procainamide must be given every 3 to 4 hr around the clock to assure continuous suppression of irregular cardiac rhythms. The same dosing requirements apply to the use of the bronchodilator theophylline in children. The optimum use of idoxuridine eye drops for herpetic keratitis calls for hourly administration.

A particularly conscientious patient may be able to comply with these requirements during the waking hours, but even he is confounded during the sleep period. Excessively frequent dosing requirements do not encourage compliance to the prescribed drug regimen, particularly when the drug is used prophylactically or to treat a silent disease such as hypertension.

The alternative solutions to this important therapeutic problem include giving the drug less frequently and accepting a less favorable therapeutic outcome, seeking new drugs with similar pharmacologic effects but more favorable pharmacokinetic characteristics, or developing a prolonged-release dosage form. In most cases, experience

dictates that the pharmaceutical solution be examined first.

Drug Absorption and Duration of Effect

Prolonged-release medication is a dosage form containing more drug than a conventional dosage form but releasing the drug far more slowly, over a period of hours or even days rather than seconds or minutes. In essence, we seek a situation where the duration of drug action is substantially determined by the duration of drug release from the dosage form rather than the drug molecule's pharmacokinetic properties.

This idea can be expressed mathematically by considering the intravenous and oral administration of a drug that distributes rapidly from the bloodstream. After intravenous bolus administration, drug concentration in the blood is given by:

$$C = C_o \exp(-kt) \qquad (7\text{--}1)$$

where C_o is the initial drug concentration and k is the first-order elimination rate constant. Under these conditions, MRT is given by:

$$MRT_{iv} = 1/k \qquad (7\text{--}2)$$

The persistence of drug in the body and the duration of drug effect is a function of drug elimination kinetics.

Following oral administration of the drug, assuming first-order absorption, concentration in the blood is given by:

$$C = C^*F[\exp(-kt) - \exp(-k_a t)] \quad (7\text{--}3)$$

where C^* is a complex constant, F is the fraction of the oral dose reaching the systemic circulation, and k_a is the first-order absorption rate constant. The MRT is given by the following equation:

$$MRT_{oral} = MRT_{iv} + 1/k_a \qquad (7\text{--}4)$$

The time course of drug concentration in the blood is affected by the absorption process, i.e., MRT_{oral} > MRT_{iv}. But, for most drugs, absorption from conventional dosage forms is so rapid that MRT_{oral} is not substantially greater than MRT_{iv}. Accordingly, even after oral administration the duration of effect is largely a function of the elimination kinetics of the drug.

However, if the release rate of drug from the dosage form is decreased (i.e., decrease k_a), we simultaneously increase MRT_{oral}. The MRT becomes more dependent on the release rate and less dependent on the drug molecule's kinetics. Using this approach, a situation is reached where the MRT and the duration of effect are largely controlled by the release rate of drug from the dosage form.

Frequency of Dosing and Therapeutic Index

The *therapeutic index* of a drug is most usefully defined in man as the ratio of the maximum drug concentration in blood that can be tolerated to the minimum drug concentration needed to produce a satisfactory clinical response. Therapeutic concentration ranges for certain drugs in man have been identified. In some cases, these ranges are narrow, resulting in small therapeutic indices.

The average therapeutic range of theophylline concentration in blood is about 8 to 20 $\mu g/ml$; the therapeutic index of theophylline is 2.5. Estimates of therapeutic index for other drugs are 2.0 for digoxin and valproic acid, 2.7 for procainamide, and 4.0 for lidocaine. We seek to maintain drug concentrations in blood well within the therapeutic range during drug therapy. This requires not only the selection of an appropriate daily dose; the drug must also be given with sufficient frequency so as to minimize the range of blood concentrations that are produced. The ratio of maximum to minimum drug concentrations at steady state should not exceed the therapeutic index of the drug. This concentration ratio is a function of the half-life of a drug and the frequency of dosing.

For drugs that are both absorbed and distributed rapidly, Theeuwes and Bayne[1] have demonstrated the following relationship:

$$\tau < t_{1/2} \, (\ln TI)/(\ln 2) \qquad (7\text{--}5)$$

where τ is the dosing interval, $t_{1/2}$ is the half-life, and TI is the therapeutic index. A drug with a therapeutic index of 2 and a half-life of 3 hr must be given no less frequently than every 3 hr to avoid excessive or subtherapeutic concentrations. A drug with a similar half-life but a therapeutic index of 4 may be given every 6 hr.

When drug effects are directly related to concentration in blood but distribution is slow, the drug must be given even more frequently than suggested by Equation 7–5. In such cases, a better estimate of dosing interval may be obtained by replacing $t_{1/2}$ with 0.693(MRT) where MRT is the mean residence time.

Steady-State Concentrations and Release Rate

Dosing regimens for rapidly absorbed drugs are a function of the pharmacodynamic and pharmacokinetic characteristics of the drug molecule; they must be based on the therapeutic index and half-life or MRT of the drug itself. Reducing the absorption rate of a drug by controlling its release rate from the dosage form, however, can dramatically affect drug concentrations at steady state. For a given dosage regimen, the slower the release rate of drug, the smaller is the ratio of maximum to minimum drug concentrations at steady state. Under these conditions, we can give larger doses at less frequent intervals and still stay within the therapeutic concentration range of the drug; this is the rationale for prolonged-release medication.

Prolonged-release medication offers obvious advantages for drugs with short half-lives and small therapeutic indices. These specialized dosage forms permit such drugs to be given at more reasonable intervals throughout the day; implications include more optimal therapy, patient convenience, and improved patient compliance with the prescribed regimen. The application of prolonged-release medication, however, is not limited to such drugs. Since these dosage forms offer the potential of reducing the peak-to-trough drug concentration ratio, they may be useful for many more drugs.[2]

Reducing the peak-to-trough concentration ratio has been found to improve the benefit-to-risk ratio of some drugs. The potassium-depleting effect of hydrochlorothiazide disappears, while its diuretic effect is slightly enhanced, when the drug is given every 3 hr rather than once a day.[3] The nephrotoxicity of gentamicin is substantially reduced when steady-state concentrations are maintained in a narrow range of about 1 to 4 $\mu g/ml$.[4] The safety of certain anticancer drugs, including bleomycin[5] and methotrexate,[6] is increased when given continuously by infusion rather than intermittently.

By minimizing fluctuations in blood levels we may be able to reduce the dosage required, improve the effectiveness, and decrease the adverse effects of a drug. For instance, pilocarpine administered continuously by an ocular insert reduces elevated intraocular pressure in patients with glaucoma without the marked myopia commonly seen in patients using pilocarpine eyedrops every six hours.

White[7] compared intraoperative and postoperative effects of fentanyl and ketamine administered by continuous intravenous infusion with those produced by intermittent iv bolus doses. Continuous infusion minimized the peaks and valleys of drug concentration in blood and, presumably, brain that ordinarily result from intermittent dosage.

Women scheduled for elective outpatient gynecologic surgery received either fentanyl or ketamine as an intravenous adjunct to nitrous oxide for maintenance of general anesthesia after induction with thiopental. The drugs were given either by continuous iv infusion or intermittent iv bolus. The method of drug administration resulted in important differences.

Only about one-half the dosage of fentanyl or ketamine was needed to maintain anesthesia when the drugs were given by continuous infusion rather than by intermittent bolus. The use of less drug resulted in more rapid recovery from anesthesia and in substantially less postoperative sedation, and minimized postoperative psychomotor dysfunction. Excessive sedation was noted in about 50% of the patients in the bolus groups but in less than 10% of the patients in the infusion groups.

Continuous infusion also improved intraoperative conditions. Respiratory depression and muscular rigidity occurred less frequently with continuous rather than intermittent administration of fentanyl. Hypertension and tachycardia occurred less frequently with continuous rather than intermittent ketamine.

Zero-Order Release

Continuous, constant-rate intravenous infusion leads to constant blood levels. Under these conditions, blood levels are invariant with time; there are no peaks or troughs. Provided that the constant drug concentration is within the therapeutic range, this is an ideal situation for many drugs. The only way to achieve constant blood levels is to administer the drug at a constant (zero-order) rate over the entire dosing interval. The concentration of drug at steady state is given by the following equation:

$$C_{ss} = k_o/Cl \qquad (7\text{--}6)$$

where k_o is the zero-order delivery or release rate of drug, and Cl is the clearance of the drug. Fluctuations in blood levels do occur under these conditions, because of temporal variations in clearance or in the delivery rate, but they are usually small.

Until recently, constant rate intravenous infusion, by means of a carefully controlled drip or mechanical pump, was the only way to attain constant blood or tissue levels of drug. Today, there are dosage forms intended for oral, ocular, intravaginal, or intramuscular administration that release drug in a zero-order or near zero-order fashion. These dosage forms are discussed in other sections of this chapter.

ORAL MEDICATION

Most prolonged-release dosage forms are intended for oral administration. A prolonged-release dosage unit contains more drug than a conventional dosage unit but is intended to be given less frequently. A drug that is ordinarily given at a dose of 250 mg 4 times a day in a conventional tablet or capsule may be given at a dose of 500 mg twice a day, or 1 g once a day, in a prolonged-release dosage form. The ultimate criteria for evaluating such dosage forms are: (1) the amount of drug intended to be absorbed is indeed absorbed in a predictable and consistent manner; and (2) the steady-state ratio of maximum to minimum drug concentrations is no greater than or, optimally, less than that produced by the more frequently administered conventional dosage form.

The early history of the prolonged-release oral dosage form is probably best forgotten. Products were developed empirically, often with little rationale, and bioavailability problems were common. Many people viewed these dosage forms as little more than marketing inducements. Today, the situation has improved; many of the available products are well designed drug delivery systems and have a defined therapeutic goal. In some cases, the prolonged-release dosage form is the most important and most frequently used form of the drug.

A wide variety of techniques have been used to develop prolonged-release oral dosage forms. These techniques include the use of drug substances of decreased solubility or dissolution rate, accomplished by increasing particle size or substituting less soluble salts or complexes, ion exchange resins to bind the drug substance, porous, nondisintegrating, inert carriers as matrices for the drug, slowly eroding coatings or matrices, and coatings that serve as membranes for drug diffusion.

Most oral prolonged-release dosage forms can be characterized as either subdivided or single units. Subdivided prolonged-release dosage forms, exemplified by the hard gelatin capsule containing numerous drug-impregnated beads, present the drug to the gastrointestinal tract in the form of many slowly-dissolving particles or granules. Often, several kinds of beads are found in the capsule, some releasing the drug rapidly, others releasing the drug over a period of several hours, still others releasing the drug at intermediate rates. Spansule is a trade name historically associated with this dosage form. More details of these and other formulations can be found in a recent review by Longer and Robinson.[8] Phenothiazines, antihistamines, iron, and many other drugs are available in this kind of dosage form. In general, the release and absorption of drugs from slow-release beads can be described by first-order kinetics.

The single-unit prolonged-release dosage form remains more or less intact throughout the gastrointestinal tract, releasing the drug continuously during its passage down the tract. An example of this dosage form is the inert plastic matrix, a dosage form that has been used widely in Europe. The drug is mixed with inert, insoluble, powdered matrix material consisting of plastic resins and other ingredients and compressed. In the gastrointestinal tract, drug particles from the surface of the matrix system dissolve and leave pores through which drug from within the tablet leaches out. The matrix retains its shape during the leaching process and is eliminated in the feces. The release rate of drug decreases with time and, in this sense, resembles a first-order process.[9]

The steady-state plasma levels and pharmacologic effects of a daily dose of 0.2-g metoprolol, a cardioselective β-blocker, in a prolonged-release matrix tablet and in regular 0.1-g tablets were studied in healthy subjects. The following dosing regimens were used: (1) one prolonged-release tablet once a day; (2) two 0.1-g regular tablets once a day; and (3) one 0.1-g regular tablet every 12 hr. The peak-to-trough concentration ratio of metoprolol was, on the average, about 10 for the matrix tablet and the twice-a-day regimen and about 40 for the once-a-day administration of the regular tablets (Fig. 7–1). Metoprolol in the matrix tablet produced a more uniform effect on heart rate and systolic blood pressure during exercise than the corresponding daily dose of metoprolol given as two 0.1-g tablets once daily or as one 0.1-g tablet twice a day.[10] Although metoprolol has a relatively short half-life, about 3 hr, a once-a-day regimen can be developed with a prolonged-release dosage form. The same is true for propranolol.[11]

Some pharmaceutical scientists judge subdivided prolonged-release dosage forms to be potentially safer than intact or single-unit dosage forms because a mechanical failure of the coating or matrix would result in the immediate release of only a small fraction of the entire dose. Mechanical failure is unlikely to occur with the matrix tablet, but it may occur in those single-unit dosage forms that rely on a continuous membrane to control release. A failure in this case may result in the immediate dumping of the entire dose, a quantity of drug that is 2 or 3 times the amount given as a single dose in a conventional dosage form.

Because prolonged-release products are complex dosage forms, substantial differences in performance among different products of the same drug may occur. Although the prolonged-release matrix tablet of metoprolol, previously described, has a longer duration of effect than the same dose of the drug given as regular tablets,[12] this is not true for a different prolonged-release product of metoprolol.[13,14] One product shows a significant improvement over conventional metoprolol whereas the other does not.

Considerable differences among prolonged-release products of theophylline have also been reported. Studies in adult subjects indicate that theophylline is slowly but completely and consistently absorbed from three of six prolonged-release formulations. Theophylline absorption from the other three products is more erratic and less complete.[15] In another study, theophylline absorption from three commercial products labeled as prolonged-release was compared to the absorption from a standard uncoated tablet. Two of the prolonged-release products showed considerably slower absorption of theophylline than did the regular tablet, but the third product did not.[16]

To determine whether clinically important changes in serum theophylline concentrations occur when patients switch their brand of prolonged-release theophylline, 10 subjects with asthma were given the same dose of four different

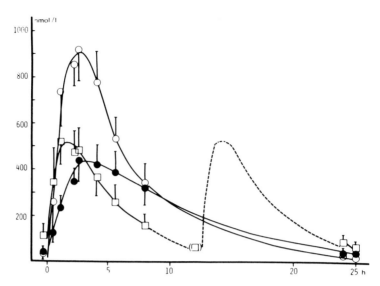

Fig. 7–1. Mean steady-state plasma concentrations of metoprolol after repetitive dosing of a prolonged-release tablet (0.2 g) once a day (●), two 0.1 g regular tablets once a day (○), and one 0.1 g regular tablet every 12 hr (□). (From Johnsson, G., et al.[10])

commercially available products for 2-week periods in a random, double-blinded, crossover fashion.[17]

On at least one occasion in every subject, switching between brands of theophylline resulted in serum theophylline levels outside the accepted therapeutic range, and this was associated with toxic symptoms in 5 of the subjects. Worsening pulmonary function was observed in two subjects when switching resulted in lowered theophylline levels. Many of the changes in theophylline concentrations on switching from one brand to another could not be predicted by the bioavailability differences between the products. The investigators concluded that "these results argue against the open substitution of these formulations and suggest that if patients are switched between different brands of SR theophylline, their serum theophylline concentration needs to be closely monitored."

Much has been published concerning prolonged-release theophylline during the past 10 years. The drug has a relatively short half-life, particularly in children, and a small therapeutic index. Clinical studies suggest that 40% of all children receiving conventional products of theophylline in the usual every 6-hr manner will have excessive or subtherapeutic blood levels of the drug.[18]

Although no well-controlled clinical trials have been published showing that prolonged-release theophylline preparations are more effective than plain theophylline tablets or solutions, many clinicians report that the long-acting formulations are more effective in controlling symptoms, especially during the night. Furthermore, compliance is likely to improve when patients take medication only twice a day, rather than 3 or 4 times a day. On the other hand, some clinicians have found that when adverse effects occur with prolonged-release theophylline, they persist longer. Some patients taking the long-acting preparations complain of insomnia, a known adverse effect of theophylline.

Adult smokers and children, who metabolize theophylline rapidly, may benefit most from treatment with prolonged-release preparations. In many patients, it may be necessary to individualize the daily dose and, in some patients, it may be necessary to give the product more frequently than twice a day.

Individual variability in dosing requirements is clearly seen in the results of a study evaluating one of the more commonly prescribed prolonged-release theophylline preparations, Theodur.[19] In a panel of 20 asthmatic patients, 6 to 18 years of age, receiving the long-acting theophylline product twice a day, the daily doses needed to produce an average blood level of about 15 μg/ml ranged from 6.1 to 16.3 mg/kg. The blood levels resulting from these individualized regimens, as estimated from 4 to 5 blood samples taken over the course of each of 2 consecutive steady-state dosing intervals, showed surprisingly little fluctuation. Peak and trough values and peak-to-trough ratios for the 20

Table 7–1. Peak and Trough Serum Concentrations of Theophylline During 24 hr at Steady State in Children Receiving, on the Average, 10 mg/kg Twice a Day in a Prolonged-Release Product.*

Patient	Peak concn. (μg/ml)	Trough concn. (μg/ml)	Peak-to-trough ratio
1	17.6	10.3	1.7
2	22.7	12.7	1.8
3	17.0	12.0	1.4
4	22.9	14.8	1.5
5	16.4	11.2	1.5
6	18.9	12.4	1.5
7	17.2	7.0	2.5
8	21.8	16.3	1.3
9	13.7	8.7	1.6
10	15.5	12.6	1.2
11	20.3	16.6	1.2
12	18.5	9.0	2.1
13	18.4	10.6	1.7
14	19.7	12.1	1.6
15	17.6	10.5	1.7
16	20.3	15.4	1.3
17	17.5	11.8	1.5
18	23.5	16.7	1.4
19	14.5	7.6	1.9
20	16.8	10.4	1.6

*Data from Kelly, H.W., and Murphy, S.[19]

patients are shown in Table 7–1. Average blood levels are shown in Figure 7–2. If twice-a-day doses of regular theophylline, sufficient to produce average levels of about 15 μg/ml, were given to these patients we would expect to find peak-to-trough concentration ratios of about 10.

A circadian variation in theophylline levels in serum is quite evident during treatment with certain twice-a-day slow-release theophylline products. Steady-state theophylline concentrations for the 12-hr period following the morning dose are different from those following the evening or night dose. In one study, peak concentration at steady state after an 11 AM dose occurred at about 3 hr after dosing, whereas peak level was observed at about 9 hr following the 11 PM dose, which was taken immediately before retiring.[20] The area under the concentration-time curve during a dosing interval at steady state was also smaller after the night dose than following the morning dose. These differences reflect a circadian variation in theophylline absorption rather than in theophylline metabolism.

A change in posture could be a simple explanation of the circadian variation in theophylline pharmacokinetics.[21] This was examined in healthy human subjects who took 450 mg slow-release aminophylline orally at the same time of day on two separate occasions. On one day the subjects remained standing and on the other, they lay supine throughout the study. Theophylline levels in plasma were measured hourly for 6 hr after the dose.

At each sampling time, theophylline levels were higher during the standing experiment than during the supine study. Peak concentration of theophylline with the subjects standing occurred at 5 hr and was 6.4 mg/L. Theophylline levels were ascending for the entire 6-hr study period in the supine group;

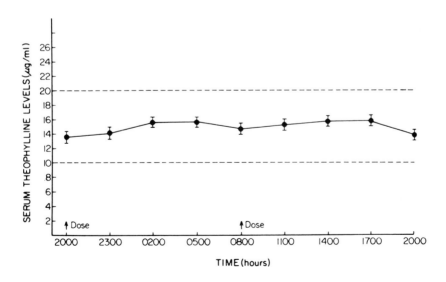

Fig. 7–2. Mean steady-state serum concentrations of theophylline in children receiving an average dosage of 10 mg/kg in a prolonged-release product every 12 hr. (From Kelly, H.W., and Murphy, S.: Efficacy of a 12-hour sustained-release preparation in maintaining therapeutic serum theophylline levels in asthmatic children. Pediatrics, 66:100, 1980. Copyright American Academy of Pediatrics 1980.)

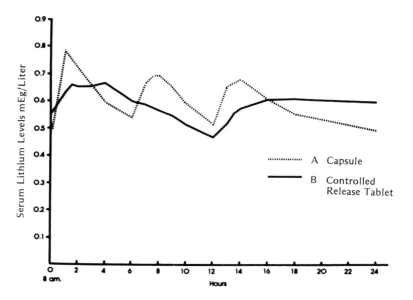

Fig. 7–3. Mean steady-state serum levels of lithium in healthy subjects who received a 300-mg capsule 3 times a day or a 450-mg prolonged-release tablet twice a day. (From Caldwell, H.C., et al.[24])

mean concentration at 6 hr was 5.4 mg/L. The investigators concluded that the supine position assumed at bedtime may be an adequate explanation for the diurnal variation seen with twice-a-day prolonged-release theophylline products.

Theophylline is widely used in children, so it is not surprising that slow-release tablets are sometimes chewed or crushed to facilitate swallowing. This practice may result in a loss of the prolonged-release characteristic of the product. To examine this question, Theo-Dur, a widely used formulation, was given to healthy adult subjects on three occasions, at least 1 week apart.[22] On the first day, subjects were randomly allocated to either swallow intact or chew, and then swallow, a 300 mg tablet. Subjects were then crossed over for the second dose. The effects of crushing the tablet prior to ingestion were studied at the third dose. Swallowing the tablets intact resulted in a significantly longer time to peak concentration compared with chewing or crushing (i.e., 6 hr *vs* about 3 hr) and the peak concentration was somewhat lower, 35.6 μmol/L, compared with chewing (43.1 μmol/L) or crushing (41.9 μmol/L). Area under the curve, however, was about the same for all three modes of administration. Chewing or crushing Theo-Dur tablets does not appear to have a substantial effect on the bioavailability characteristics of the product, suggesting that it may be a suitable preparation for use in young children.

A prolonged-release liquid theophylline prepa-

ration, aimed at the pediatric population and designed for twice-daily administration, is under investigation.[23] The suspension was compared with aminophylline solution (administered every 8 hr) in 27 asthmatic children less than 12 years of age. Average steady-state levels of theophylline were about 10% lower during treatment with the suspension than with the solution. Peak levels were also lower (11.2 vs 14.2 μg/ml) and the difference between C_{max} and C_{min} was smaller (6.9 vs 10.0 μg/ml) with the suspension. The investigators concluded that the slow-release suspension should prove to be useful in patients who require maintenance theophylline therapy, but who cannot take solid oral dosage forms.

Lithium carbonate is the drug of choice in treating certain phases of manic depression. Although the drug has a long half-life, about 24 hr, it also has a narrow therapeutic index and must be given 3 or 4 times a day. Steady-state serum level fluctuations of lithium were compared following regular capsules (300 mg 3 times a day) or prolonged-release tablets (450 mg every 12 hr) of lithium carbonate.[24] Average blood levels are shown in Figure 7–3. The degree of fluctuation (Fl) of serum levels was assessed by the following equation:

$$Fl = (C_{max} - C_{min})/\overline{C} \qquad (7\text{--}7)$$

where C_{max} and C_{min} are the maximum and minimum drug concentrations over the 24-hr steady-state dosing cycle, and $\overline{C}$ is the mean concentration over the cycle. $\overline{C}$ is estimated from the ratio of area under the curve to dosing interval. This fluctuation index is analogous to the coefficient of variation; small values are desired for the prolonged-release preparation. This index may be more stable than the peak-to-trough concentration ratio, which could be highly unstable in the presence of error for small values of C_{min}. In this study, the index was 0.46 for the prolonged-release tablet regimen and 0.66 for the regular capsule regimen, suggesting that the regular product produces about 40% more fluctuation in serum lithium levels than the slow-release formulation.

Fluctuations in serum levels are related not only to the release rate of drug from the dosage form and the frequency of administration (dosage interval), but also vary with drug elimination rate. Steady-state studies with a prolonged-release theophylline product found a linear relationship between percent fluctuation and theophylline clearance in individual subjects.[25]

Weinberger and Hendeles[26] also calculated the percent fluctuation in steady-state serum levels of theophylline for different products. With one prolonged-release product, percent fluctuation was 57% in slow metabolizers of theophylline (half-life = 7.7 hr) but increased to 154% in rapid metabolizers (half-life = 3.7 hr).

Several antiarrhythmic drugs are plagued with the undesirable characteristics of short half-life and narrow therapeutic index. Procainamide is an example; its half-life is about 3 hr. Therapeutic and toxic effects have been related to drug concentrations in plasma. The therapeutic range is 4 to 8 µg/ml but can often extend to 10 µg/ml without toxicity. To maintain safe, adequate blood levels, the regular tablet form of the drug must be given every 3 to 4 hr.

Steady-state levels of procainamide were determined in patients receiving about 20 mg/kg per day in the form of prolonged-release matrix tablets of the drug every 8 hr.[27] Mean procainamide blood levels are plotted in Figure 7–4. In 17 of the 26 patients, blood levels were maintained above a level of 4 µg/ml for at least 75% of the time. Of the 9 patients showing blood levels below the minimum level for more than 25% of the time, 8 would have benefited from an increased daily dose or improved compliance with the regimen. In 4 of the 26 patients, blood levels were above 10 µg/ml for more than 10% of the time. All 4 patients required a lower daily dose and, possibly, more frequent administration. The results suggest that this prolonged-release form of procainamide, given every 8 hr, would benefit most patients if the daily dose were individualized.

Disopyramide is another orally effective antiarrhythmic; its electrophysiologic properties are similar to those of quinidine and procainamide. A therapeutic range of 2 to 4 µg/ml has been suggested for the drug. Because of its short half-life, disopyramide must be given 4 times a day to maintain safe and effective concentrations in plasma. Disopyramide concentrations were determined in plasma following repeated doses of regular capsules (150 mg every 6 hr) or prolonged-release matrix tablets (300 mg every 12 hr) to patients with various kinds of arrhythmia.[28] A level of 4 µg/ml with regular capsules was exceeded by 2 patients, and 1 patient exceeded this level with the matrix tablet. None of the patients had a level below 2 µg/ml. The average steady-state peak-to-trough concentration ratio was 1.4 for the capsules and 1.6 for the prolonged-release tablets. The average fluctuation index was 0.36 for the regular product and 0.43 for the prolonged-release preparation. Although the matrix tablet was given only half as frequently as the regular capsules, little difference in blood levels of disopyramide was noted between products. The matrix tablet of disopyramide appears to be a useful prolonged-release form of the drug.

Drugs absorbed by specialized, capacity-limited transport processes are ordinarily not good candidates for prolonged-release dosage forms. Facilitated absorption is often site-specific and drug released beyond this site in the intestine is usually poorly absorbed. Iron may be an exception. A prolonged-release preparation containing 100 mg of ferrous iron, given twice daily, was compared to a conventional tablet containing 50 mg of ferrous sulfate, given 4 times daily. In patients with iron deficiency anemia, more iron was absorbed from the slow-release preparation.[29]

Prolonged-release forms of drugs such as nitrofurantoin[30] or lithium[31] have been investigated for reducing the incidence of nausea and vomiting resulting from gastrointestinal irritation or high blood concentration peaks. Studies with lithium in human subjects show that rapidly disintegrating tablets generally produce more nausea than do prolonged-release tablets. The incidence of this side effect appears to correlate with high concentrations of lithium in the stomach and proximal intestine.

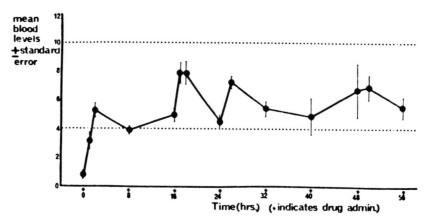

Fig. 7–4. Mean levels of procainamide during repetitive dosing of a prolonged-release tablet every 8 hr. (From Cunningham, T., Sloman, G., and Nyberg, G.[27])

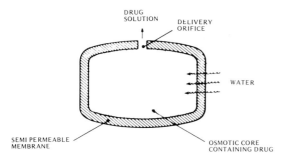

Fig. 7–5. Cross section of an elementary osmotic pump (EOP) designed to release drug in a zero-order (constant-rate) manner. (From Theeuwes, F.[33] Reproduced with permission of the copyright owner.)

On the other hand, the slower the release of lithium from a dosage form, the higher is the incidence of diarrhea. This adverse effect seems to be related to high concentrations of lithium in the distal intestine, a situation found only with prolonged-release products.[31] More recent studies confirm these results.[32]

Zero-Order Release

The ideal approach to minimizing blood level fluctuations of a drug is to have zero-order release from the dosage form. A system, termed the elementary osmotic pump (EOP), is now available to achieve this goal. Figure 7–5 shows a diagram of this dosage form, which resembles a coated tablet. The EOP tablet contains a solid core of drug and adjuvants coated with a polymer membrane, permeable to water and interrupted only by a single small orifice with a diameter of 0.1 to 0.4 mm.[33] After the tablet is swallowed, the membrane se-

lectively admits water from the gastrointestinal tract; drug within the membrane is gradually dissolved. The internal pressure produced by entry of the water forces the drug solution out of the orifice. Since the volume of the system is fixed, constant-rate release is achieved. Typically, 60 to 80% of drug content is delivered at a constant rate; the rest of the dose is released in a pseudo-first-order fashion. The depleted membrane sac is excreted intact. Release rates as high as 60 mg/hr may be achieved with this dosage form. Drug release is independent of pH or motility.

The duration of drug delivery is controlled by the permeability of the membrane and the composition of the core. At a given rate of drug delivery, the duration of controlled release is determined by the amount of drug in the core. In practice, however, the duration of release is limited by intestinal transit time and probably cannot exceed 8 to 12 hr without compromising the extent of absorption.

The hemodynamic effects and plasma levels of metoprolol have been determined after single and multiple doses of EOP tablets or more conventional prolonged-release tablets of the drug.[37] Both dosage forms were given once a day for 8 days to healthy subjects. The prolonged-release tablets contained 200 mg metoprolol tartrate; the EOP tablets contained 190-mg metoprolol fumarate (equivalent to 200 mg of the tartrate) with a 19 mg/hr zero-order release rate. Both formulations reduced exercise heart rate and exercise systolic blood pressure for the entire 24-hr steady-state dosing interval, but the EOP tablets elicited a more uniform response. Mean steady-state plasma profiles of me-

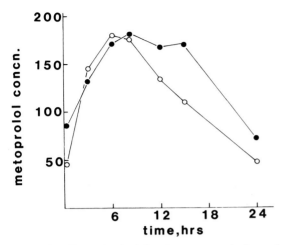

Fig. 7–6. Mean steady-state plasma concentrations of metoprolol (ng/ml) in healthy subjects after repetitive dosing of an EOP prolonged-release product (●) or a more conventional prolonged-release product (○), once a day. (Data from Kendall, M.J., et al.[34])

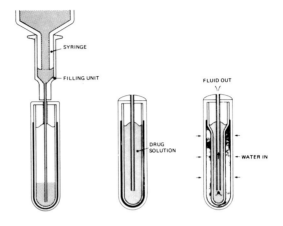

Fig. 7–7. Schematic representation of the filling and operation of the osmotic pump. (From Eckenhoff, B., and Yum, S.I.[38] By permission of the publishers, Butterworth & Co. Ltd. Copyright 1981.)

toprolol are shown in Figure 7–6. Peak-to-trough concentration ratios were 4.5 for the conventional prolonged-release tablets and 2.6 for the EOP tablets. Fluctuation indices were 1.31 for the prolonged-release tablets and 0.88 for the EOP tablets. Both hemodynamic and pharmacokinetic criteria support the superiority of the EOP tablet.

The steady-state metoprolol levels produced by the EOP tablets show considerable fluctuation over the dosing interval even though release rate approximated zero-order. This occurs because release took place over a relatively small fraction (10 out of 24 hr) of the dosing interval. To obtain constant blood levels, there must be constant-rate release over the entire dosing interval. This situation was more closely approximated in studies with acetazolamide, a drug that reduces intraocular pressure, in EOP tablets.[35] Relatively constant blood levels of acetazolamide were obtained by dosing every 12 hr with EOP tablets that release the drug over an 8-hr period, or about three quarters of the dosing interval.

Bayne et al.[36] described the evaluation of constant release rate dosage forms of indomethacin, based on the elementary osmotic pump principle and intended to be taken twice a day. Indomethacin is usually given 3 or 4 times a day in the treatment of rheumatoid arthritis and osteoarthritis.

Steady-state levels of indomethacin were determined in plasma of healthy subjects who had received 150 mg/day for 5 days according to the

following regimens: (a) controlled-release tablet delivering drug over 8 hr, given twice a day; (b) controlled-release tablet delivering drug over 11 hr, given twice a day; (c) regular capsules of indomethacin given 4 times a day; (d) regular capsules given 3 times a day.

Average indomethacin levels in plasma at steady state were similar for all four regimens, but subjects taking the prolonged-release dosage forms showed much less fluctuation in plasma levels of drug than subjects taking regular capsules. Also, trough levels of indomethacin before the morning dose were significantly higher during treatment with controlled-release tablets than with regular capsules. This difference may be important for the relief of morning stiffness often seen in arthritics.

Generic osmotic pumps are also available as experimental tools for animal or clinical studies. They are useful for, but not limited to, oral administration.[9,37,38] A diagram of this dosage form is shown in Figure 7–7. The reservoir is filled with a drug solution. The wall of the reservoir is inert, impermeable, and flexible. A sleeve of osmotically active agent is placed between the reservoir wall and the rigid semipermeable membrane.

Water from the surroundings is imbibed through the outer membrane into the osmotic sleeve at a rate controlled by the permeability of the membrane and the osmotic pressure difference across the membrane. The incoming water squeezes the reservoir and drug solution is expelled in a constant-volume per-unit-time fashion. Delivery of drug solution continues at a constant rate until the drug reservoir is completely collapsed.

Limitations of Prolonged-Release Medication

A factor that circumscribes the use of oral prolonged-release medication is the limited residence time of the dosage form in the small intestine. Absorption from the colon may be poor or unpredictable. Hence, small intestine transit time is often of paramount importance in determining the bioavailability of the drug from this dosage form.

The gastrointestinal transit of a radiolabeled osmotic tablet (elementary osmotic pump) has been monitored in groups of young and elderly healthy human subjects.[39] Gastric emptying and small intestine transit were similar for both groups of subjects. Gastric emptying of the tablet when given after a light breakfast (orange juice, cornflakes, and milk) averaged about 3 hr; the tablets arrived at the cecum, on average, about 7 hr after dosing.

In another study, the position in the gastrointestinal tract of an orally administered osmotic tablet containing a radiolabel and oxprenolol, a beta-blocker available in Europe, was followed in fasted subjects by gamma scintigraphy.[40] Gastric emptying times (about 1 hr) and the time to arrival in the colon (about 4 hr) were relatively consistent from one subject to another.

On the other hand, there were wide individual variations in colonic transit with values ranging from 2.5 to 27.5 hr. Accordingly, total transit time ranged from 6 to 32 hr. In the individual with the most rapid colonic transit and total transit, the bioavailability of oxprenolol was only 14%, and 79% of the administered dose was recovered in the stool. In the two individuals with the slowest colonic transit, bioavailability was 40% and 54%.

External gamma scintigraphy was also used to monitor the gastrointestinal transit of radiolabeled prolonged-release tablets containing 800 mg ibuprofen in fasted healthy subjects.[41] The tablet was formulated using an erodible polymer matrix system.

The gastric retention time of the tablets ranged from 10 to 60 min, with a mean value of 35 min. Transit time of a tablet through the small intestine was calculated by subtracting gastric residence time from the time at which the tablet was observed to enter the large bowel. Small bowel transit time ranged from about 2 to 8 hr, with a mean value of 4.7 hr. Again, total transit time was variable (8 to 18 hr) and largely dependent on large bowel residence time, which ranged from 6 to 14 hr.

A statistically significant correlation (r = 0.89) was observed between the area under the curve for 24 hr after administration of ibuprofen and total gastrointestinal transit time. Area under the curve for the subject with the most rapid total transit time (8 hr) was only 94 μg-hr/ml compared with a mean value for the group of 180 μg-hr/ml.

For dosage forms like the matrix tablet or the elementary osmotic pump, which remain intact in the gastrointestinal tract, we usually assume an average effective absorption time of 9 to 12 hr after administration. The release rate of drug from the dosage form must be programmed accordingly. Slower release rates run the risk of poor bioavailability. For dosage forms with similar transit times that release drugs in an apparent first-order manner, release half-lives should not exceed 3 to 4 hr.

Since there is a limit to how much we can reduce the release rate of a drug from certain prolonged-release dosage forms without compromising bioavailability, there is also a limit as to how much we can prolong the duration of drug action by these oral dosage forms. Mathematical simulations of the time course of drug in the blood on multiple dosing of slow-release dosage forms suggest that ordinarily drugs with relatively short half-lives (i.e., less than or equal to 6 hr), and low therapeutic indices (i.e., less than or equal to 3) should be given no less frequently than every 12 hr.[2]

Prolonged-release dosage forms that consist of beads, pellets, or particulates, or that disintegrate into particulates, may be retained in the small intestine for longer periods. The small intestine transit time of pellets depends on size, density, and composition. One study found that increasing the density of standardized pellets from 1.0 to 1.6 increased the average transit time from 7 to 25 hr,[42] but these results could not be confirmed.[43]

We still cannot predict the effect of food on the bioavailability of drugs given in prolonged-release dosage forms. Investigators recently studied the effect of food-related changes in gastric emptying on the absorption of procainamide from a nondisintegrating wax-matrix sustained-release tablet. Gastric residence time was greater in fed than in fasted subjects (3.5 vs 1 hr), but food had no effect on the time required to detect procainamide in plasma, on the time to reach peak concentration of procainamide, or on the extent of absorption of procainamide.[44] A standard meal also had little effect on the absorption of pseudoephedrine from a slow-release capsule formulation based on a system using both ion exchange technology and a wax coating.[45]

The effect of food on drug absorption kinetics may differ markedly from one prolonged-release formulation to another. Theophylline is a case in point. Food has little effect on the absorption profile for theophylline after administration of Theo-Dur, a well-absorbed and widely prescribed slow-release theophylline product.[46] The pediatric version of this product, Theo-Dur Sprinkle, is also completely absorbed in fasting subjects but less than half the dose is absorbed when it is taken after breakfast.[47]

Scandinavian scientists reported the results of a study with children and adults who were given a single dose of a prolonged-release theophylline preparation (Theolair-SR) after an overnight fast and later after a standardized breakfast.[48] Food dramatically reduced the absorption rate of theophylline (see Fig. 7–8), particularly in the children, but it had no effect of the extent of absorption.

About two-thirds of the dose of theophylline is absorbed after administration of Uniphyl, another slow-release product, to fasted subjects, whereas 85% of the dose is absorbed when it is given after a meal.[49] Although there is an increase in bioavailability with food, there is little effect on the rate of absorption of theophylline. Theo-24, a once-a-day theophylline product, is also incompletely absorbed in fasting subjects. With this product, however, food not only increases the extent of absorption, but also greatly increases the rate of absorption with about half the daily dose absorbed in a 4-hr period, giving rise to excessively high blood levels of theophylline.[50]

Exposure of the distal small intestine and colon to drug is far more likely when a prolonged-release formulation rather than a conventional tablet or capsule is taken. In some cases, this may result in a higher incidence of lower bowel toxicity. Microorganisms in the lower bowel may enzymatically reduce a drug, leading to metabolites that are not ordinarily seen after administration of the drug in conventional dosage forms. Bacterial metabolism may decrease bioavailability or result in toxic metabolites.

Drugs that are metabolized and inactivated by the gastrointestinal mucosa during absorption may show a higher availability after administration in conventional dosage forms than in slow-release forms, because of capacity-limited biotransformation. This may explain why the apparent bioavailability of chlorpromazine in man is significantly less after administration of a prolonged-release capsule than after administration of a liquid or tablet dosage form of the drug.[49]

Drugs that are efficiently absorbed only in the proximal intestine should not be administered in a prolonged-release product. The consequence of this approach would be incomplete absorption.

PARENTERAL MEDICATION
Intramuscular Injections

There has been interest for many years in using the slow absorption of insoluble material in a muscle depot as a means of attaining prolonged drug

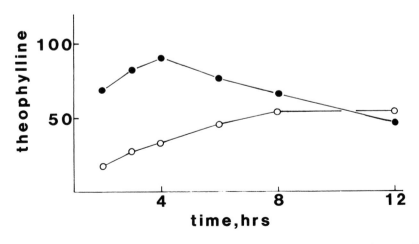

Fig. 7–8. Theophylline concentrations in serum (μmol/L) after a single dose of a prolonged-release product to fasted (●) and fed (○) children. (Data from Pedersen, S.[48])

action. Unlike oral prolonged-release dosage forms, parenteral therapy is not restricted in frequency of administration to once or twice a day. Therefore, these dosage forms can be administered weekly, monthly, or even less frequently. Sterile aqueous suspensions of insoluble salts of penicillin G, such as procaine penicillin G and benzanthine penicillin G, are available for intramuscular injection. These preparations are administered less frequently than injectable solutions of potassium penicillin G. Another long-acting intramuscular penicillin preparation consists of procaine penicillin G suspended in peanut or sesame oil, thickened with aluminum monostearate. Poorly water-soluble esters of prednisolone, testosterone, estradiol, medroxyprogesterone, and fluphenazine are also given as intramuscular injections in the form of aqueous suspensions.

Desoxycorticosterone (DOC) is a mineralocorticoid used as replacement therapy in chronic primary adrenocortical insufficiency. Therapy is initiated with intramuscular DOC acetate (DOCA). Once the maintenance dosage is established, a long-acting, microcrystalline, aqueous suspension of DOC pivalate may be used. The usual intramuscular dose of the pivalate is 25 mg for each mg of the daily maintenance dose of DOCA, repeated at 4-week intervals.

Dexamethasone is a fluorinated derivative of prednisolone used primarily in inflammatory or allergic conditions. Dexamethasone acetate is available as a long-acting repository suspension for intramuscular injection. Long-acting intramuscular formulations of methylprednisolone acetate, prednisolone acetate, triamcinolone acetonide, and triamcinolone diacetate are also available.

Androgens are used for replacement therapy in hormone-deficiency states in men and for certain gynecologic conditions and metastatic breast cancer in women. Androgens or anabolic steroids are also used in certain cases to increase growth.

Testosterone itself is not suitable for therapeutic use, except perhaps topically or by means of subcutaneous implants, because it is subject to rapid hepatic metabolism. This problem is overcome by using testosterone esters that are hydrolyzed to testosterone in the body. The esters are dissolved in oil and injected intramuscularly.

In general, the longer the hydrocarbon chain of the ester substituent, the more slowly is testosterone released into the systemic circulation. The most common esters of testosterone are the pro-

prionate, cypionate, and enanthate. Testosterone propionate is usually injected several times a week, but the longer-acting cypionate and enanthate esters need be given every 2 to 4 weeks. These longer-acting esters are drugs of choice for hypogonadism, which requires long-term therapy.

A slow-release intramuscular preparation of a luteinizing-hormone releasing-hormone (LHRH) agonist, formulated in microcapsules designed to release 100 μg/day, has also been described.[52] This preparation, administered once a month, was effective in patients with advanced ovarian and advanced prostatic carcinoma.

Failure to take medication frequently complicates the management of chronic schizophrenia. Fluphenazine decanoate and enanthate are injectable phenothiazine esters that can be administered at intervals of 1 to 3 weeks or longer for treatment of schizophrenia. In contrast, fluphenazine hydrochloride is given orally, 1 to 4 times a day. These poorly water soluble esters are prodrugs and are converted to fluphenazine upon dissolution in the body. The times required, after intramuscular injection in the dog, for 50% of the dose to be excreted in the urine and feces is 7.8 days for the enanthate ester and 22.6 days for the decanoate ester.[53] Dogs were protected against the emetic effects of a 40 μg/kg iv dose of apomorphine for 46 days after being given fluphenazine enanthate and for 105 days after a single dose of the decanoate.[53] Studies in human subjects indicate that absorption from the muscle depot occurs with a half-life of about 3 to 4 days for the decanoate ester.[54] Clinical studies with fluphenazine decanoate indicate that long-acting antipsychotic medication significantly reduces the tendency of chronic psychotic patients to discontinue treatment.[55]

The usual practice of giving fluphenazine decanoate every 2 weeks is primarily based on custom; several lines of evidence suggest that it may be given less frequently. Investigators have studied the persistence of fluphenazine levels in plasma in patients stabilized for at least 1 year on fluphenazine decanoate, 12.5 mg intramuscularly every 2 weeks.[56] Patients were randomized to either continued treatment or placebo injections every 2 weeks for 12 weeks.

No patient relapsed during the study. Mean plasma fluphenazine at baseline for all subjects was 0.86 ng/ml. For the first 6 weeks after withdrawal of the depot medication there was no statistically significant difference in fluphenazine levels between the continued treatment and placebo groups. The investigators suggested that 2-week intervals between injections of fluphenazine decanoate are excessive and that wider intervals (e.g., 3 to 4 weeks) may achieve similar clinical results.

Haloperidol decanoate, a depot form of the most widely used antipsychotic drug, is also available. The preparation is a sesame oil solution containing the equivalent of 50 mg haloperidol per ml. It is administered by deep injection into the gluteus muscle, usually at monthly intervals. After injection there is slow transfer of the ester from the lipid carrier to the aqueous medium of the tissue. Esterases in muscle tissue and plasma split the ester, releasing haloperidol.

The apparent half-life of haloperidol after depot injection is about 3 weeks. Half-life in this case reflects the release rate of the drug from the muscle depot rather than the rate of metabolism of haloperidol. Steady state occurs after 3 to 4 months of treatment. Short periods of oral haloperidol supplementation may be needed to treat reemergent psychotic symptoms until steady state is reached.

Haloperidol decanoate is intended to be used in patients stabilized on oral haloperidol. An important issue is the relationship between the intramuscular dose and the daily oral dose. As with all neuroleptics, the lowest effective dose is sought to avoid extrapyramidal side effects.

After oral administration, haloperidol is subject to first-pass metabolism; bioavailability is estimated at 60 to 70%. The bioavailability of the intramuscular depot form is probably complete. Based on relative bioavailability and frequency of dosing, a 20-fold conversion is appropriate when switching from oral haloperidol (daily dose) to haloperidol decanoate (dosed every 28 days). Clinical studies suggest that the depot form of the drug may allow even greater dose sparing.[57]

Patients with chronic schizophrenia, stabilized on oral halperidol, were switched to haloperidol decanoate, administered every 4 weeks. The first dose was determined by psychiatric history and the oral dose of haloperidol needed to stabilize the patient. Thereafter, the patient's dose could be adjusted upward or downward at 4-week intervals. For the 30 patients completing the study, the ratio of haloperidol decanoate to oral haloperidol required to achieve equal efficacy ranged from 10:1 to 15:1, lower than the 20:1 ratio needed to maintain equivalent blood levels of haloperidol. These results suggest that by reducing the variability in blood level of a drug, we may be able to achieve equal efficacy with less drug.

Estrogens and progestins are prescribed to mimic or accentuate the biologic effects of endogenous hormones: to supplement inadequate endogenous production, to correct hormonal imbalance, to reverse an abnormal process, and for contraception. Estradiol is the principal and most biologically potent ovarian estrogenic hormone. It is usually given intramuscularly in the form of an ester (benzoate, cypionate, or valerate) in oil or in an aqueous suspension. Duration of effect varies from several days to several weeks depending on the ester and formulation.

Intramuscular progestin products include a sesame-oil solution of hydroxyprogesterone caproate, used for menstrual disorders (duration of action is about 9 to 17 days), and an aqueous suspension of medroxyprogesterone acetate (MPA), used for endometriosis and injected every 3 months.

Several intramuscular depot preparations are under investigation for use as contraceptives. One preparation that is widely used throughout the world (but not in the U.S.) is depot MPA. The contraceptive use of depot MPA has been controversial for more than a decade. The drug is used in 80 countries and its use in developing nations is endorsed by scientific panels of the World Health Organization and other international agencies. The U.S. Food and Drug Administration has repeatedly denied approval of a 3-month depot MPA product for use as a contraceptive, concluding that the potential adverse effects (carcinogenicity and teratogenicity) of the drug outweigh its benefits.

Another depot progestin, norethindrone enanthate, is also used outside the U.S. for contraceptive purposes. An injection schedule calling for the first four injections to be given at 8-week intervals and subsequent injections to be given at 12-week intervals produced no pregnancies in 295 women over about 1,600 women months.[58]

Implants

The technology supporting the use of drug implants is well established but commercially successful clinical applications have been slow in coming. Numerous devices have been described for the diffusion of steroids through silicone rubber. For example, contraceptive devices in the form of silicone-rubber capsules containing progesterone have been implanted subcutaneously. Silicone-rubber capsules containing ethinyl estradiol have been used in the treatment of patients with prostate cancer. Certain disorders of male reproductive function can be treated with long-acting implants of testosterone.

Many investigators are now applying the principles of prolonged release from silicone rubber and other polymers for long-term drug treatment. Examples include systems for narcotic antagonists, such as naloxone, in the treatment of opiate addiction, chemotherapeutic agents for the treatment of cancer, and heparin in the treatment of abnormal blood clotting.

A subdermal silastic implant containing levonorgestrel has been described. The capsules are implanted into a woman's upper or lower arm with a hypodermic needle. Within 24 hr, enough drug is released from the invisible yet palpable implant to prevent pregnancy. The capsules are said to be effective for 5 years. They can be removed if the woman wishes to become pregnant.

The generic osmotic pump, described earlier in this chapter, is a particularly useful implant for experimental drug studies in animals. The device can be implanted in the subcutaneous tissue, muscle, or peritoneal cavity. A catheter can be attached for localized administration to areas remote from the site of implantation. Commercially available pumps permit constant-rate drug delivery over 1 or 2 weeks. Publications to date have illustrated the use of the generic osmotic pumps for delivering many drugs and chemicals in various animals including mice, rats, rabbits, dogs, monkeys, sheep, and cows.[9]

Refillable implants have also been described.[59] These devices have been used in patients prone to thrombophlebitis and pulmonary embolism who require heparin. Ordinarily, heparin is given to outpatients by subcutaneous injection 4 to 6 times a day. One refillable implant delivers heparin solution continuously over 45 days before refilling is necessary. These implants have also been used to provide an intra-arterial infusion of 5-fluorouracil for the treatment of hepatoma and primary liver cancer. Recent reports describe refillable implants for the delivery of insulin[60] and antiarrhythmic drugs.[61]

A patient with refractory congestive heart failure was treated, on an outpatient basis, with intermittent dobutamine using a totally implantable infusion pump. Dobutamine was infused for 48 hr every week and resulted in sustained clinical improvement.[62]

The Food and Drug Administration has approved the use of an implantable pump to deliver the aminoglycoside antibiotic amikacin directly to the site of an osteomyelitis infection.

Battery-powered pumps were implanted in patients for phase I and II trials of low-dose continuous-infusion doxorubicin or vinblastine. The median duration of pump function was 145 days. The systems infused drugs for about 60% of their patient implant time. During 27.5 patient-years of implantation, no failure of pump mechanism was observed and pump accuracy was within 2% of stated standards. Complications requiring a second surgical procedure occurred in 24% of the patients.[63]

Remote-controlled insulin pumps were implanted into insulin dependent type I diabetics for a 1-year feasibility trial in four centers.[64] The total observation time was about 18 patient-years. Only 3 of 20 pumps had to be removed prematurely. Patients self-monitored blood glucose levels with a mean of 5.5 measurements per day. About 63% of these measurements were in the normal range. On the average, 3.25 glucose measurements per patient-month were in the hypoglycemic range and 2.6 episodes of hypoglycemia with symptoms were reported per patient-month, but very few of these episodes required medical attention. The investigators concluded that despite some technical and clinical problems, the pump, when used with a stable insulin preparation, was an effective means of treating insulin-dependent patients.

OCULAR MEDICATION

Drug effects in the eye tend to be short-lived because of the eye's efficient mechanisms to maintain homeostasis. Ocular inserts intended to release drug slowly, in a controlled fashion, offer the potential benefits of a dramatic decrease in the frequency of dosing, more uniform clinical response, and a decrease in adverse effects.

One device, called the Ocusert, containing pilocarpine, is used for lowering elevated ocular pressure. The patient places the insert under the eyelid, where it remains for 7 days, slowly and continuously delivering pilocarpine. In contrast, pilocarpine eye drops are usually instilled 3 or 4 times daily; high concentrations of the drug after dosing may produce blurring or dimming of vision for as long as 1 hr.

The Ocusert consists of the drug enclosed by a dense membrane. The detailed physical chemistry of this system is described elsewhere.[65] Pilocarpine dissolves in the membrane and diffuses slowly to the eye. The total dosage delivered by a single Ocusert system over its 7-day lifetime is about one eighth of the amount provided by the usual 2% eye drops of pilocarpine.

Studies in the rabbit show that pilocarpine levels in ocular tissue rise and fall within each 6-hr interval between eye drops but remain relatively constant over a 2- to 8-day period with the Ocusert system (Fig. 7–9).[66] Clinical studies comparing pilocarpine eye drops with the Ocusert found comparable reductions in intraocular pressure, but 36 of the 40 patients preferred the Ocusert.[67] Another comparative study concluded that the Ocusert pilocarpine system presents many advantages and is a desirable method of therapy in selected cases of glaucoma.[68] Advantages of the device include therapeutic effectiveness, less effect on accommodation, less miosis, and convenience for the patient. Some disadvantages were the need for instruction and encouragement of the patient, retention difficulties, occasional discomfort, and higher cost.

INTRAUTERINE DEVICES

Intrauterine devices (IUDs) for contraceptive purposes are available in medicated and unmedicated forms. Medicated devices contain a diffusible contraceptive agent and are claimed to provide greater efficacy than an unmedicated device of the same size and design.

A device containing progesterone (Progestasert) releases small quantities of hormone at a uniform rate (65 μg/day) into the endometrial cavity, resulting in glandular atrophy and a chronic decidual reaction that is unfavorable for implantation; progesterone may also directly inhibit sperm. The device requires yearly replacement but devices containing a larger amount of progesterone have been found to produce effective contraception for 2 years or more.[49] Progestasert contains an amount of progesterone equivalent to the progestational agent contained in merely a half a dozen birth control pills. The product clearly illustrates the principle of using controlled-release technology to determine duration of drug effect; progesterone itself has a half-life of less than 1 hour.

TRANSDERMAL MEDICATION

Transdermal medication is intended to be applied to the skin but to elicit systemic effects. Compared to oral drug therapy, transdermal therapy has the potential advantages of avoiding biochemical degradation in the gastrointestinal tract and presystemic metabolism in the gut wall and liver, and of being able to provide long periods of drug action for relatively short-acting drugs.

Certain factors limit the application of rate-controlled transdermal drug delivery. The most im-

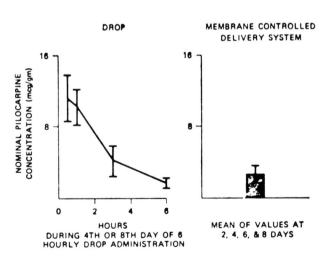

Fig. 7–9. Pilocarpine concentrations in cornea with eye-drop administration of 2% pilocarpine nitrate every 6 hr (left panel) or with a 20 μg/hr membrane-controlled pilocarpine delivery system (right panel). (From Sandelbeck, L., Moore, D., and Urquhart, J.[66] Published with permission from The American Journal of Ophthalmology, 80:274–283, 1975. Copyright by the Ophthalmic Publishing Company.)

portant one is the need for potent drugs. Existing technology is limited to drugs active at daily parenteral doses of 15 mg or less.

Transdermal scopolamine was the first transdermal system approved in the U.S. with label specifications of rate-controlled delivery. It is indicated for the prevention of motion sickness. The transdermal system is contained in a thin disk that the patient places on intact skin, usually behind the ear. The unit has multiple layers including a backing membrane, a drug reservoir consisting of solid drug suspended in a liquid vehicle, a microporous rate-controlling membrane, and a skin contact adhesive.

Scopolamine is a well-known antiemetic drug; however, it causes undesirable side effects when given in conventional tablets. These side effects appear to be related to the wide fluctuations in scopolamine concentrations in blood that occur between doses. The transdermal scopolamine system is applied only once every 3 days and provides relatively constant blood levels of scopolamine over this period.

The transdermal product delivers 0.5-mg scopolamine over 3 days. A priming quantity of 140 μg of drug is released at an asymptomatically declining rate over 6 hr, stabilizing at a maintenance rate of 5 μg/hr for the remainder of the 3-day period.

Efficacy of transdermal scopolamine has been compared with oral dimenhydrinate and placebo.[70] The transdermal device was applied 13.5 to 15 hr before exposure to motion; oral medication was given 1.5 hr before motion, and again 2.5 hr after motion began. In one study, directly comparing transdermal scopolamine with oral dimenhydrinate, the transdermal medication protected 79% of the subjects from motion sickness, whereas the oral drug protected 58%; in a second study, protection rates of 68% and 41% were found for the scopolamine and dimenhydrinate therapy, respectively. No patient was protected by the placebo.

Another study examined the influence of the time between application and exposure to motion on the efficacy of the transdermal system. Application 16 hr before motion resulted in a 100% protection rate; application 4 hr before motion protected 74% of the participants. Dry mouth, drowsiness, and blurred vision, typical side effects of scopolamine, were minimal with the transdermal system.

Other investigators have found that transdermal scopolamine is significantly more effective in preventing motion sickness induced by a ship-motion simulator than is placebo or orally administered meclizine (25 mg), a commonly used antihistamine/antinauseant.[71] A patch containing either placebo or active drug was applied behind the ear 12 hr before exposure to the simulator, and meclizine or placebo tablet was taken 2 hr before exposure. The trial lasted 90 min or until vomiting was imminent.

About two-thirds of the patients receiving transdermal scopolamine had no symptoms compared with 33% given oral meclizine and 39% given placebo. Dryness of mouth was reported more frequently with scopolamine than with meclizine or placebo. No other side effects were notable. Transdermal scopolamine may be the treatment of choice for motion sickness, but the patch must be applied at least several hours before motion to obtain optimal effect.

Several transdermal nitroglycerin systems have been marketed for the treatment of angina pectoris. These systems are more convenient to use than nitroglycerin ointment, permit more precise dosing, and need be applied less frequently than the ointment. All are intended to be applied to the upper arm or chest once a day. They should not be applied to the distal part of the extremities because bioavailability may be decreased.

Chien et al.[72] applied three commercially available nitroglycerin patches to freshly excised abdominal skin from young hairless mice and determined skin-penetration kinetics. They found that the amount of nitroglycerin delivered through the skin over 24 hr was similar for each transdermal system, ranging from 3.3 to 3.5 mg.

Other investigators measured the bioavailability of nitroglycerin from a reformulated transdermal system (Nitro-Dur II) relative to the original product (Nitro-Dur) in healthy male subjects.[73] The apparent dose of nitroglycerin delivered to each subject by each formulation was calculated from the difference between the original content of the patch and the residual nitroglycerin content after 24 hr of skin contact.

The mean total amounts of nitroglycerin delivered by the original product (I) and Nitro-Dur II were similar, 9.8 mg and 10.7 mg, respectively. Large differences in delivery, however, were observed in individual subjects; only 2.5 mg nitroglycerin was delivered from the original formulation in one subject, whereas in another subject the same formulation delivered 19.3 mg. The new formulation in the same two subjects delivered 7.4 and 14.4 mg nitroglycerin, respectively. Transport through the skin rather than release from the dosage form is the rate-limiting step in the transdermal absorption of nitroglycerin. Differences among subjects reflect differences in skin permeability.

Transdermal nitroglycerin was conditionally approved by the Food and Drug Administration for the prevention and treatment of angina pectoris due to coronary artery disease. Blood level measurements demonstrating nitroglycerin concentrations in plasma similar to concentrations produced by nitroglycerin ointment, a product with established efficacy, was largely the basis for approval. According to the FDA, conditional approval reflects a determination that the drug may be marketed, while further investigations of its effectiveness are undertaken. At this time, the FDA has not made a final determination.

The evidence to date suggests rather serious shortcomings of the once-a-day nitroglycerin patch mostly related to nitrate tolerance, a well-known phenomenon. Many studies using transdermal nitroglycerin in patients with angina or congestive heart failure that have demonstrated effectiveness within several hours of application of the transdermal system, have also documented the attenuation or absence of effects within 12 to 24 hr. Other studies have suggested that complete tolerance may develop in a short time during continuous once-a-day administration of a nitroglycerin patch.[74]

A comprehensive analysis of the published clinical literature on transdermal nitroglycerin systems for the treatment of angina concluded that the patch delivering 10 mg per 24 hr is not effective at 24 hr after application.[75] This conclusion supports the hypothesis that nitroglycerin's effect on exercise tolerance is attenuated by nitrate tolerance even though blood levels persist.

A randomized controlled trial in more than 400 men with chronic stable angina showed that continuous use of transdermal nitroglycerin 5 mg/24 hr had no advantage over placebo in terms of efficacy (anginal attack rates and sublingual nitroglycerin consumption) or quality of life (as measured by a sickness impact profile and a health index of disability).[76] Patients receiving nitroglycerin reported headaches more frequently than patients on placebo and a higher proportion of them withdrew from the trial for this reason.

The future of transdermal nitroglycerin is uncertain. Current trends suggest that the dosage form will continue to be used but in doses of 10 mg/24 hr or higher, applied intermittently with a nitrate-free period (e.g., 12 hr on, 12 hr off) rather than continuously. A rest period between applications may restore sensitivity and overcome tolerance. Several studies have produced results supporting this hypothesis.[74]

Clonidine is an effective centrally-acting antihypertensive drug, but oral therapy requires administration 2 to 4 times a day and is associated with a relatively high incidence of adverse effects. Transdermal clonidine was developed with the aim of reducing frequency of administration to once weekly and with the hope of reducing side effects.

One multicenter trial evaluated weekly application of transdermal clonidine patches in patients with mild essential hypertension (diastolic blood pressure in the range of 91 to 104 mm Hg).[77] Of the 85 patients completing the trial, 54 responded (diastolic pressure < 90 mm Hg or a decrease in diastolic pressure of at least 10 mm Hg). Among the responders, 31% required one patch (releasing clonidine at a rate of 0.1 mg/day), 54% required two patches, and the other 19% needed three.

Dry mouth and drowsiness, typical side effects of clonidine, occurred in about one-third of the patients, but these symptoms were usually mild and only two subjects had to be dropped because of side effects. Of far greater concern, erythematous skin reactions were observed in 8 patients. This report and others suggest a frequency of skin reactions considerably higher than that encountered with oral clonidine. This problem may limit the use of transdermal clonidine.[78]

Most postmenopausal women who require estrogen-replacement therapy use oral medication. With this approach, however, the liver is exposed to relatively high concentrations of estrogen; increased production of coagulation factors, renin substrate, and bile acids may occur. These changes may account for the increased incidence of venous thrombosis and pulmonary embolism, hypertension, and gallstones in women treated with estrogens. This concern stimulated interest in the administration of estrogens in a way that minimizes hepatic exposure and led to the development of transdermal estradiol.

A patch releasing either 50 or 100 μg estradiol per day was approved in the U.S. for the treatment of postmenopausal symptoms but not for the prevention of osteoporosis. Transdermal estradiol may be useful in this regard but the evidence is not yet available. The advantages claimed for the patch over oral estrogens are that estradiol goes directly to the blood (avoiding gastrointestinal effects, first-pass hepatic metabolism, and stimulation of hepatic enzymes), doses are much lower, and serum concentrations more closely resemble those found naturally before menopause.[79]

The dosage unit consists of a drug reservoir, a rate-controlling membrane, and an adhesive layer. It is intended to be applied to the trunk (but not the breasts) twice weekly. Like other estrogens for postmenopausal symptoms, the patches are generally used in cycles such as 3 weeks on and 1 week off and require the additional administration of a progestin to reduce the risk of endometrial hyperplasia and subsequent complications.

Transdermal estradiol appears to be as effective as much higher doses of oral estrogen in treating postmenopausal vasomotor symptoms, but whether the patches will be safer remains to be determined. The most common adverse effect observed with transdermal therapy has been mild to moderate erythema at the application site. This may be related to the formulation rather than to the drug itself because the problem occurs with both active and placebo patches.

BUCCAL MEDICATION

A transmucosal controlled-release formulation, containing 1, 2, or 3 mg of nitroglycerin, is available in the U.S. for both acute treatment and long-term control of angina pectoris. The product contains nitroglycerin impregnated in an inert cellulose polymer matrix. When the tablet is placed in the buccal cavity between the upper lip and gum, or between the cheek and gum, a gel forms that makes the tablet adhere to the mucosal surface, and drug slowly diffuses from the formulation to saliva and across the mucosal membranes to the systemic circulation.[80]

Onset of effects occurs in minutes and nitroglycerin continues to be absorbed as long as the tablet remains intact, usually about 4 to 5 hours. Treadmill studies in patients with angina found beneficial effects for up to 5 hours when the tablet remained intact for 5 to 6 hours. If continuous nitroglycerin therapy is desired, the next tablet should be taken within 1 hour after the previous tablet dissolves. Tolerance has not been reported with up to 2 weeks' use of transmucosal nitroglycerin, possibly because intermittent use pro-

duces a rapid rise and fall in plasma and tissue nitroglycerin levels with a nitrate-free interval at night when no medication is taken.[80]

The analgesic effects of buccal and intramuscular morphine were compared in patients who experienced pain after elective orthopedic surgery.[81] Each patient simultaneously received a buccal tablet and an injection, only one of which contained morphine. Tablets were moistened, to facilitate adherence to the mucosa, and placed between the upper lip and gum. They dissolved slowly, over about 6 hr. Efficacy was evaluated over an 8-hr period.

Seven of the 20 patients given buccal morphine required a second dose within 8 hours of the first dose; 10 of the 20 patients receiving intramuscular morphine required a second dose. As judged by the reduction in pain score, both preparations produced a similar degree of postoperative analgesia. Concentrations of morphine in plasma were lower after buccal morphine but persisted for a longer time than morphine levels after injection. The investigators suggested that this may be a useful dosage form in the management of postoperative pain.

RECTAL MEDICATION

No prolonged-release rectal dosage forms are commercially available. The generic osmotic pump, described earlier in this chapter, however, has been administered rectally in several pharmacokinetic studies in human subjects.

In one study,[82] healthy subjects inserted an osmotic pump containing antipyrine. The system remained in place in the lower rectum with a small thread attached to it and fixed to the buttock, unless there was a need to defecate. In this case, the system was pulled out, cleaned, and reinserted immediately after defecation. After 38 hr, the first system was replaced by a second which stayed in the rectum for an additional 60 hr. The constant-release rate from the osmotic pump gave rise to constant blood levels of antipyrine over a 24- to 90-hr period. This approach may be an alternative to constant rate intravenous infusion for steady state studies.

The effects of relatively constant plasma levels of triazolam, a rapidly eliminated benzodiazepine, were studied in young healthy male subjects to determine whether tolerance to certain effects may develop over a relatively short period of time.[83] The drug was given over a period of 30 hr (2 days and 1 night) at a zero-order rate using a rectal osmotic pump. The investigators concluded that the experimental design might prove useful in the study of tolerance to drugs.

The utility of an osmotic rectal drug delivery system as a tool in steady-state pharmacokinetic interaction studies has been investigated using the cimetidine-antipyrine interaction.[84] Antipyrine was given by means of a rectal osmotic pump releasing the drug at a zero-order rate of 15 mg/hr for about 30 hr. By consecutive use of three of these systems, antipyrine was administered for 90 hr. Forty-eight hr after the start of the study, when steady state had been achieved, 400 mg cimetidine was given orally followed by three consecutive 200-mg cimetidine doses every 2 hr. The investigators concluded that the osmotic rectal drug delivery system is a useful tool in pharmacokinetic interaction studies because it provides constant steady-state concentrations, permitting investigation of the time course of drug interactions.

REFERENCES

1. Theeuwes, F., and Bayne, W.: Dosage form index: An objective criterion for evaluation of controlled-release drug delivery systems. J. Pharm. Sci., 66:1388, 1977.
2. Gibaldi, M., and McNamara, P.J.: Steady-state concentrations of drugs with short half-lives when administered in oral sustained release formulations. Int. J. Pharmacol., 2:167, 1979.
3. Murphy, J., Casey, W., and Lasagna, L.: The effect of dosage regimen on the diuretic efficacy of chlorothiazide in human subjects. J. Pharmacol. Exp. Ther., 134:286, 1961.
4. Trollfors, B., et al.: Quantitative nephrotoxicity of gentamicin in nontoxic doses. J. Infect. Dis., 141:306, 1980.
5. Sikic, B.I., et al.: Improved therapeutic index of bleomycin when administered by continuous infusion in mice. Cancer Treat. Rep., 62:2011, 1978.
6. Bleyer, W.A.: The clinical pharmacology of methotrexate: new applications of an old drug. Cancer, 41:36, 1978.
7. White, P.F.: Use of continuous infusion versus intermittent bolus administration of fentanyl or ketamine during outpatient anesthesia. Anesthesiol., 59:294, 1983.
8. Longer, M.A., and Robinson, J.R.: Sustained-release drug delivery systems. In Remington's Pharmaceutical Sciences. Easton, Pa., Mack Publishing, 1985, pp. 1644–1661.
9. Theeuwes, F.: Drug delivery systems. Pharmacol. Ther., 13:149, 1981.
10. Johnsson, G., et al.: Plasma levels and pharmacological effects of metoprolol administered as controlled release (Durules) and ordinary tablets in healthy volunteers. Int. J. Clin. Pharmacol. Ther. Toxicol., 18:292, 1980.
11. Leahey, W.J., et al.: Comparison of the efficacy and pharmacokinetics of conventional propranolol and a long acting preparation of propranolol. Br. J. Clin. Pharmacol., 9:33, 1980.
12. Harron, D.W.G., and Shanks, R.G.: Comparison of the duration of effect of metoprolol and a sustained release formulation of metoprolol (Betaloc-SA). Br. J. Clin. Pharmacol., 11:518, 1981.
13. Quarterman, C.P., Kendall, M.J., and Welling, P.G.: Plasma levels and negative chronotropic effect of metoprolol following single doses of a conventional and sustained-release formulation. Eur. J. Clin. Pharmacol., 15:97, 1979.
14. Kendall, M.J., et al.: A single and multiple dose pharmacokinetic and pharmacodynamic comparison of conventional and slow-release metoprolol. Eur. J. Clin. Pharmacol., 17:87, 1980.
15. Weinberger, M., Hendeles, L., and Bighley, L.: The relation of product formulation to absorption of oral theophylline. N. Engl. J. Med., 299:852, 1978.
16. Upton, R.A., et al.: Evaluation of the absorption from some commercial sustained-release theophylline products. J. Pharmacokinet. Biopharm., 8:131, 1980.
17. Baker, J.R., et al.: Clinical relevance of the substitution of different brands of sustained-release theophylline. J. Allergy Clin. Immunol., 81:664, 1988.
18. Ginchansky, E., and Weinberger, M.: Relationship of theophylline clearance to oral dosage in children with chronic asthma. J. Pediatr., 91:655, 1977.
19. Kelly, H.W., and Murphy, S.: Efficacy of a 12-hour sustained-release preparation in maintaining therapeutic serum theophylline levels in asthmatic children. Pediatrics, 66:97, 1980.
20. Jackson, S.H.D., et al.: Circadian variation in theophylline absorption during chronic dosing with a slow release theophylline preparation and the effect of clock time on dosing. Br. J. Clin. Pharmacol., 26:73, 1988.
21. Warren, J.B., Cuss, F., and Barnes, P.J.: Posture and theophylline kinetics. Br. J. Clin. Pharmacol., 19:707, 1985.
22. MacKintosh, D.A., Baird-Lambert, J., and Buchanan, N.: Theo-Dur: no loss of sustained-release effect with chewing or crushing. Aust. N.Z. J. Med., 15:351, 1985.
23. Guill, M.F., et al.: Clinical and pharmacokinetic evaluation of a sustained-release liquid theophylline preparation. J. Allergy Clin. Immunol., 82:281, 1988.
24. Caldwell, H.C., et al.: Steady-state lithium blood level fluctuations in man following administration of a lithium carbonate conventional and controlled-release dosage form. J. Clin. Pharmacol., 21:106, 1981.
25. Jackson, S.H.D., and Wright, J.M.: Sustained serum theophylline concentrations during chronic twice daily administration of a slow release preparation. Eur. J. Clin. Pharmacol., 24:205, 1983.
26. Weinberger, M., and Hendeles, L.: Slow-release theophylline. Rationale and basis for product selection. N. Engl. J. Med., 308:760, 1983.
27. Cunningham, T., Sloman, G., and Nyberg, G.: Procainamide blood levels after administration of a sustained-release preparation. Med. J. Aust., 1:370, 1977.
28. Forssell, G., et al.: Comparative bioavailability of disopyramide after multiple dosing with standard capsules and controlled-release tablets. Eur. J. Clin. Pharmacol., 17:209, 1980.
29. Nielson, J.B., et al.: Absorption of iron from sustained release and rapidly disintegrating tablets. Influence of daily numbers of administrations. Acta Med. Scand., 194:123, 1973.
30. Kalowski, S., Radford, N., and Kincaid-Smith, P.: Crystalline and macrocrystalline nitrofurantoin in the treatment of urinary-tract infections. N. Engl. J. Med., 240:385, 1974.
31. Borg, K.O., Jeppsson, J., and Sjögren, J.: Influence of the dissolution rate of lithium tablets on side effects. Acta Pharm. Suec., 11:133, 1974.
32. Edström, A., and Persson, G.: Comparison of side effects with coated lithium carbonate tablets and lithium sulphate

preparations giving medium-slow and slow-release. Acta Psychiatr. Scand., *55*:153, 1977.

33. Theeuwes, F.: Elementary osmotic pump. J. Pharm. Sci., *64*:1987, 1975.

34. Kendall, M.J., et al.: Comparison of the pharmacokinetic and pharmacodynamic profiles of single and multiple doses of a commercial slow-release metoprolol formulation with a new Oros® delivery system. Br. J. Clin. Pharmacol., *13*:393, 1982.

35. Theeuwes, F., Bayne, W., and McGuire, J.: Gastrointestinal therapeutic system (acetazolamide) 15/125: efficacy and side effects. Arch. Ophthalmol., *96*:2219, 1978.

36. Bayne, W., et al.: Kinetics of osmotically controlled indomethacin delivery systems after repeated dosing. Clin. Pharmacol. Ther., *32*:270, 1982.

37. Theeuwes, F., and Yum, S.I.: Principles of the design and operation of generic osmotic pumps for the delivery of semisolid or liquid drug formulations. Ann. Biomed. Eng., *4*:343, 1976.

38. Eckenhoff, B., and Yum, S.I.: The osmotic pump: novel research tool for optimizing drug regimens. Biomaterials, *2*:89, 1981.

39. Wilson, C.G., and Hardy, J.G.: Gastrointestinal transit of an osmotic tablet drug delivery system. J. Pharm. Pharmacol., *37*:573, 1985.

40. Davis, S.S., et al.: Relationship between the rate of appearance of oxprenolol in the systemic circulation and the location of an oxprenolol Oros 16/260 drug delivery system within the gastrointestinal tract as determined by scintigraphy. Br. J. Clin. Pharmacol., *26*:435, 1988.

41. Parr, A.F., et al.: Correlation of ibuprofen bioavailability with gastrointestinal transit by scintigraphic monitoring of [171]Er-labeled sustained-release tablets. Pharm. Res., *4*:486, 1987.

42. Bechgaard, H., and Ladefoged, K.: Distribution of pellets in the gastrointestinal tract: The influence on transit time exerted by the density and diameter of pellets. J. Pharm. Pharmacol., *30*:690, 1978.

43. Bechgaard, H., et al.: Gastrointestinal transit of pellet systems in ileostomy subjects and the effect of density. J. Pharm. Pharmacol., *37*:718, 1985.

44. Rocci, M.L., et al.: Food-induced gastric retention and absorption of sustained-release procainamide. Clin. Pharmacol. Ther., *42*:45, 1987.

45. Wecker, M.T., et al.: Influence of a standard meal on the absorption of controlled-release pseudoephedrine capsules. J. Pharm. Sci., *76*:29, 1987.

46. Welling, P.G.: Interactions affecting drug absorption. Clin. Pharmacokin., *9*:404, 1984.

47. Pederson, S., and Moeller-Petersen, J.: Erratic absorption of a slow-release theophylline product caused by food. Pediatrics, *74*:534, 1984.

48. Pederson, S., and Moeller-Petersen, J.: Influence of food on the absorption rate and bioavailability of a sustained release theophylline preparation. Allergy, *37*:531, 1982.

49. Milavetz, G., et al.: Relationship between rate and extent of absorption of oral theophylline from Uniphyl brand of slow-release theophylline and resulting serum concentrations during multiple dosing. J. Allergy Clin. Immunol., *80*:723, 1987.

50. Hendeles, L, et al.: Food-induced dose-dumping from a once-a-day theophylline product as a cause of theophylline toxicity. Chest, *87*:758, 1985.

51. Hollister, L.E., et al.: Studies of delayed-action medication. V. Plasma levels and urinary excretion of four different dosage forms of chlorpromazine. Clin. Pharmacol. Ther., *11*:49, 1970.

52. Parmar, H., et al.: Randomised controlled study of orchid-

ectomy vs long-acting D-trp-6-LHRH microcapsules in advanced prostatic carcinoma. Lancet, 2:1201, 1985.

53. Dreyfuss, J., et al.: Release and elimination of ^{14}C-fluphenazine enanthate and decanoate esters administered in sesame oil to dogs. J. Pharm. Sci., *65*:505, 1976.

54. Curry, S.H., et al.: Kinetics of fluphenazine after fluphenazine dihydrochloride, enanthate and decanoate administration to man. Br. J. Clin. Pharmacol., *7*:325, 1979.

55. Devito, R.A., et al.: Fluphenazine decanoate vs oral antipsychotics. A comparison of their effectiveness in the treatment of schizophrenia as measured by a reduction in hospital readmissions. J. Clin. Psychiatry, *39*:26, 1978.

56. Gitlin, M.J., et al.: Persistence of fluphenazine in plasma after decanoate withdrawal. J. Clin. Psychopharmacol., *8*:53 1988.

57. Nair, N.P.V., et al.: A clinical trial comparing intramuscular haloperidol decanoate and oral haloperidol in chronic schizophrenic patients: efficacy, safety, and dosage equivalence. J. Clin. Psychopharmacol., *6*:30S, 1986.

58. Giwa-Osagie, O.F., Savage, J., and Newtar, J.R.: Norethisterone oenanthate as an injectable contraceptive: use of a modified dose schedule. Br. Med. J., *1*:1660, 1978.

59. Blackshear, P.J.: Implantable drug-delivery systems. Sci. Am., *241*:66, 1979.

60. Rupp, W.M., et al.: The use of an implantable insulin pump in the treatment of Type II diabetes. N. Engl. J. Med., *307*:265, 1982.

61. Anderson, J.L., et al.: Long-term intravenous infusion of antiarrhythmic drugs using a totally implanted drug delivery system. Am. J. Cardiol., *49*:1954, 1982.

62. Berger, M., and McSherry, C.K.: Outpatient dobutamine infusion using a totally implantable infusion pump for refractory congestive heart failure. Chest, *88*:295, 1985.

63. Vogelzang, N.J., et al.: A programmable and implantable pumping system for systemic chemotherapy: a performance analysis in 52 patients. J. Clin. Oncol., *5*:1968, 1987.

64. Point Study Group: One-year trial of a remote-controlled implantable insulin infusion system in Type I diabetic patients. Lancet, 2:866, 1988.

65. Chandrasekaran, S.K., Benson, H., and Urquhart, J.: Methods to achieve controlled drug delivery: The biomedical engineering approach. *In* Sustained and Controlled Release Drug Delivery Systems. New York, Marcel Dekker, 1978, pp. 557–593.

66. Sandelbeck, L., Moore, D., and Urquhart, J.: Comparative distribution of pilocarpine in ocular tissues of the rabbit during administration by eyedrop or by membrane-controlled delivery systems. Am. J. Ophthalmol., *80*:274, 1975.

67. Worthen, D.M., Zimmerman, T.J., and Wind, C.A.: An evaluation of the pilocarpine Ocusert. Invest. Ophthalmol., *13*:296, 1974.

68. Pollack, I.P., Quigley, H.A., and Harbin, T.S.: The Ocusert pilocarpine system: advantages and disadvantages. South. Med. J., *69*:1296, 1976.

69. Mishell, D.R., Jr., and Martinez-Mannautou, J. (eds.): Proceedings of the Symposium on Clinical Experience with the Progesterone Uterine Therapeutic System, Acapulco, Oct. 15–16, 1976. Amsterdam, Excerpta Medica, 1978.

70. Price, N.M., et al.: Transdermal scopolamine in the prevention of motion sickness at sea. Clin. Pharmacol. Ther., *29*:414, 1981.

71. Dahl, E., et al.: Transdermal scopolamine, oral meclizine, and placebo in motion sickness. Clin. Pharmacol. Ther., *36*:116, 1984.

72. Chien, Y.W., Keshary, P.R., Sarpotdar, P.P.: Comparative controlled skin permeation of nitroglycerin from marketed transdermal delivery systems. J. Pharm. Sci., *72*:968, 1983.

73. Noonan, P.K., et al.: Relative bioavailability of a new transdermal nitroglycerin delivery system. J. Pharm. Sci., *75*:688, 1986.

74. Gibaldi, M.: Drug administration: tolerance. Persp. Clin. Pharm., *6*:57, 1988.

75. Colditz, G.A., Halvorsen, K.T., and Goldhaber, S.Z.: Randomized clinical trials of transdermal nitroglycerin systems for the treatment of angina: a meta-analysis. Am. Heart J., *116*:174, 1988.

76. Fletcher, A., McLoone, P., and Bulpitt, C.: Quality of life on angina therapy: a randomised controlled trial of transdermal glyceryl trinitrate against placebo. Lancet, *2*:4, 1988.

77. Weber, M.A., et al.: Transdermal administration of clonidine for treatment of high blood pressure. Arch. Intern. Med., *144*:1211, 1984.

78. Transdermal antihypertensive drugs. Lancet, *1*:79, 1987.

79. Transdermal estrogen. Med. Lett. Drugs Ther., *28*:119, 1986.

80. Transmucosal controlled-release nitroglycerin. Med. Lett. Drugs Ther., *29*:39, 1987.

81. Bell, M.D.D., et al.: Buccal morphine—a new route for analgesia? Lancet, *1*:71, 1985.

82. deLeede, L.G.J., deBoer, A.G., and Breimer, D.D.: Rectal infusion of the model drug antipyrine with an osmotic delivery system. Biopharm. Drug Dispos., *2*:131, 1981.

83. Breimer, D.D., et al.: Central effects during the continuous osmotic infusion of a benzodiazepine (triazolam). Br. J. Clin. Pharmacol., *19*:807, 1985.

84. Teunissen, M.W.E., et al.: Influence of cimetidine on steady state concentration and metabolite formation from antipyrine infused with a rectal osmotic mini pump. Eur. J. Clin. Pharmacol., *28*:681, 1985.

8

Bioavailability

The time course of a drug in the body depends on how the drug is given. Blood levels are likely to be different after a single oral dose compared with the same dose given by rapid intravenous injection. There are two reasons for this difference: one is related to the completeness of absorption and the other to the rate of absorption of the drug. These two characteristics of drug absorption are called the *bioavailability* of the drug.

In most cases, we are particularly concerned with the fraction of the oral dose that actually reaches the bloodstream, because this amount is the *effective dose* of a drug. In some cases, notably those involving drugs used as a single dose for acute purposes, such as sedation or pain, we are also concerned with the rate of absorption of the drug.

Many drugs are not completely available after oral administration. Some drugs have low permeability and are slowly absorbed even when given in solution; examples include cromolyn, neomycin, and riboflavin. Since the residence of a drug at absorption sites in the gastrointestinal tract is limited by motility, there may be insufficient time for complete absorption. The availability of these compounds may be increased by administering them with food or with drugs that decrease motility, or by developing more lipid-soluble prodrugs.

Other drugs are so poorly water soluble that dissolution may be incomplete during the period of time available for absorption; some examples are phenytoin, griseofulvin, and isotretinoin. The availability of these drugs may be increased, in some cases dramatically, by dosage form changes, such as particle size reduction, or by means of water-soluble prodrugs.

A large number of drugs demonstrate incomplete bioavailability because of chemical degradation in the stomach (e.g., penicillin G), preabsorptive metabolism by enzymes in the proximal small intestine (e.g., aspirin) or bacteria in the distal small intestine and colon (e.g., digoxin), or presystemic metabolism in the gut wall (e.g., isoproterenol) or liver (e.g., propranolol) during absorption. A drug subject to presystemic metabolism may be completely absorbed but incompletely available, because part of the dose is metabolized to other products during the drug's passage from the gut lumen to the systemic circulation.

The availability of drugs subject to acid hydrolysis in the stomach may be improved by the use of enteric-coated dosage forms. Few strategies are available to improve the availability of drugs subject to preabsorptive or presystemic metabolism.

ESTIMATING THE BIOAVAILABILITY OF A DRUG

The fraction or percent of an administered dose that actually reaches the systemic circulation is called the *absolute* or *systemic bioavailability* of a drug. Systemic bioavailability is determined from blood level or urinary excretion data after oral administration, with reference to similar data after intravenous administration.

The total area under the drug level in blood or plasma versus time curve (AUC), after a single dose, reflects the amount of drug reaching the bloodstream. For most drugs, if we double the amount injected intravenously, we double the AUC. It follows that if we compare the AUC after oral administration with that obtained after intravenous administration, we can determine the fraction (F) of the oral dose available to the systemic circulation. In other words,

$$F = (AUC)_{oral}/(AUC)_{iv} \qquad (8\text{--}1)$$

If only 60% of an oral dose reaches the bloodstream, then F = 0.60; if the entire dose is available, then F = 1.0

As noted in Chapter 1, the usual bioavailability study is terminated before drug concentrations in blood return to negligible levels. The AUC beyond the last concentration data point (C* at t*) is estimated from the equation:

$$\text{Area from } t^* \text{ to } \infty = C^*/k \qquad (8\text{--}2)$$

where k is the first-order elimination rate constant. This partial area is added to the area from t = 0 to t = t*, calculated by means of the trapezoidal rule (see Appendix I), to determine AUC.

We sometimes recognize, from preliminary data, that the intravenous dose must be smaller than the oral dose to achieve comparable blood levels. In this case, for purposes of safety, different oral and intravenous doses are used for estimating systemic availability. Under these conditions,

$$F = (AUC)_{oral}D_{iv}/(AUC)_{iv}D_{oral} \qquad (8\text{--}3)$$

where D refers to the dose.

For some drugs, urinary excretion data can also be used to estimate availability. After intravenous administration of a drug, a fraction of the dose is excreted unchanged in the urine; the rest of the dose is subject to nonrenal elimination. In some cases, this fraction is so small as to represent a negligible amount or an amount too small to measure with precision. Under these conditions, urinary excretion data will not be useful. On the other hand, there are drugs for which evaluation of urinary excretion data is the method of choice for estimating availability. The thiazide class of diuretics is an example.[1]

For most drugs, the same fraction of the dose is excreted in the urine regardless of the size of the intravenous dose. Accordingly, by comparing the total amount of drug excreted unchanged (A_u) after a single oral and intravenous dose of a drug, we can determine the fraction (F) of the oral dose available to the bloodstream. In other words,

$$F = (A_u)_{oral}/(A_u)_{iv} \qquad (8\text{--}4)$$

When different oral and intravenous doses are used, the following equation applies:

$$F = (A_u)_{oral}D_{iv}/(A_u)_{iv}D_{oral} \qquad (8\text{--}5)$$

Absolute bioavailability has been determined for comparatively few drugs. The principal reason for this lack of information is that most drugs are not approved for intravenous use. Intramuscular administration may be an alternative absolute standard, particularly for soluble drugs, but again, relatively few drugs are approved for intramuscular administration. Because of this, the bioavailability of a drug is usually determined against a relative standard, one that does not assure complete availability.

A commonly used relative standard is an aqueous oral solution of the drug. Blood levels or urinary excretion data are compared after a single dose of the drug administered as the test product or the oral solution. To determine the availability of the drug from the test dosage form *relative* to that from the standard dosage form (F_{rel}), the following equations apply:

$$F_{rel} = (AUC)_{test}/(AUC)_{standard} \qquad (8\text{--}6)$$

and

$$F_{rel} = (A_u)_{test}/(A_u)_{standard} \qquad (8\text{--}7)$$

It can be debated that the maximum availability of a drug from an oral dosage form can never exceed that found from an aqueous oral solution. This is probably true in most instances; however, it may not be true for drugs that are poorly soluble in acid and precipitate in the form of coarse crystals in the stomach on swallowing the aqueous solution, or for drugs that are subject to acid hydrolysis and for which the test dosage form provides protection not afforded by the solution. In these cases, F_{rel} may exceed unity.

Some drugs defy formulation as aqueous solutions and one must resort to other relative standards; these include nonaqueous oral solutions, oral suspensions, or other solid oral dosage forms.

The physicochemical basis for using a nonaqueous solution of a drug as a bioavailability standard has been considered by Serajuddin et al.,[2] who studied the absorption of an investigational drug coded REV 5901. The drug existed in both solid and metastable liquid forms, had a pK_a of 3.7, and low water solubility (0.002 mg/ml at 37°). Appreciable solubility was observed only at pH values of 2 or less. Dissolution rate at pH >3 was practically zero.

REV 5901 was quite soluble in several nonaqueous solvents approved for oral use. The bioavailability of some of these nonaqueous solutions as well as an aqueous suspension was compared. Bioavailability was 76% after administration of a solution in polysorbate 80 (Tween 80), 61% when given as a solution in peanut oil, and 35% as an aqueous suspension, relative to an oral solution of polyethylene glycol 400 (PEG 400), which provided the highest blood levels.

The investigators observed that on dilution of the water-miscible organic solutions (PEG 400 and Tween 80) with aqueous media, the drug immediately formed saturated solutions and the excess drug separated as emulsified oily globules. The dispersability of the globules improved when surfactants were present in the aqueous media. The average globule size was 1.6 μM, compared with a particle size of 5 to 10 μM when the drug was suspended in water. Therefore, a considerably larger surface area was available when the drug was ingested as a solution in Tween or PEG 400, rather than as an aqueous suspension.

Although the investigational drug was practically insoluble at the pH of the small intestine, its solubility was increased dramatically when bile salts and lecithin were added to the aqueous media. Serajuddin et al. concluded that the large surface area of the drug separating from organic solutions would facilitate dissolution in the presence of biological surfactants and increase bioavailability.

The innovator's dosage form, regardless of its availability, is often used as a relative standard, because presumably its efficacy is established. When a relative standard, other than an aqueous oral solution, is used, it is not uncommon to find that $F_{rel} > 1.0$.

Figure 8–1 shows blood levels of the antihypertensive drug prazosin after oral administration of 5 mg by capsule or hydroalcoholic solution.[3] The mean AUC for the test capsule was 174 ng/hr per ml whereas that for the solution was 199.0 ng/hr per ml. According to Equation 8–6, the relative availability of prazosin from the capsule is 0.87 or 87%.

A relative availability of 1.0 does not imply complete availability; we can only conclude from this information that the availability of drug from the test dosage form is equal to that from the standard. Propoxyphene gives almost the same blood levels after oral administration of commercial capsules or aqueous solution,[4] but the systemic availability of the drug after either dosage form is only about 20% because of presystemic metabolism.[5]

Most bioavailability studies are carried out by giving a single dose of drug to ambulatory, healthy subjects, after an overnight fast. There is concern that, in some instances, this kind of study does not

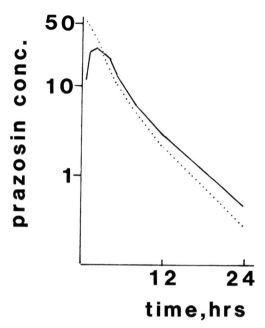

Fig. 8–1. Semilogarithmic plot of prazosin concentrations in plasma (ng/ml) following a 5-mg oral dose by capsule (—) or solution (···). (Data from Hobbs, D.C., Twomey, T.M., and Palmer, R.F.[3])

reflect the general use of the drug and may provide misleading information. This concern is particularly evident for the evaluation of prolonged-release dosage forms. We have learned enough about drug absorption to recognize that, in some cases, food, activity (sleeping vs awake), and disease may have differential effects on drug availability from oral dosage forms. Two dosage forms that differ in their release rates of drug may show equivalent AUC values in normal subjects but different values in a population with above average gastrointestinal motility. Differences between fed and fasted populations may also occur.

Oral administration of two 0.25 mg digoxin tablets and two 0.2 mg digoxin capsules containing a water-miscible solution of the drug yields similar values for AUC, indicating bioequivalence. The area under the curve following the tablets is 103% relative to the capsules. When either dosage form is given with propantheline, an anticholinergic that slows stomach emptying and decreases gastrointestinal motility, there is an increase in AUC but the change is larger for the tablets than for the capsules—24% versus 13%. Consequently, under conditions of hypomotility, digoxin AUC after administration of the tablets is 113% relative to the capsules.[6]

The oral absorption of digoxin in tablet form has been reported to be reduced after cancer chemotherapy and radiation therapy. Bjornsson et al.[7] studied possible differences in the effect of high-dose cancer chemotherapy on the relative bioavailability of digoxin given in tablet form and in solution-in-capsule form. Each subject received a single oral dose of either 0.5 mg tablets or 0.4 mg capsules before and after chemotherapy.

Before chemotherapy, the AUC following the tablets was 104% relative to the capsules. Chemotherapy reduced the average AUC after tablet administration by nearly 50%, compared with a reduction of only 15% with the capsules. Consequently, after chemotherapy, digoxin AUC following the tablets was only 74% relative to the capsules.

These concerns have led to increasing interest in steady-state studies for the evaluation of relative availability. When a constant dose of a drug is given at constant dosing intervals (e.g., 150 mg every 12 hr), the AUC during a single dosing interval at steady state (AUC_{ss}) is equal to the total AUC after a single dose (AUC). It follows from Equation 8–6 that:

$$F_{rel} = (AUC_{ss})_{test}/(AUC_{ss})_{standard} \quad (8–8)$$

We can also show that:

$$F_{rel} = (A_{u,ss})_{test}/(A_{u,ss})_{standard} \quad (8–9)$$

where $A_{u,ss}$ is the amount of drug excreted unchanged in the urine during a single dosing interval at steady state. Since the average drug concentration in blood or plasma at steady state, $\overline{C}_{ss}$, is equal to the ratio of AUC_{ss} to the dosing interval, τ, it follows that:

$$F_{rel} = (\overline{C}_{ss})_{test}/(\overline{C}_{ss})_{standard} \quad (8–10)$$

By obtaining blood levels or urinary excretion data at steady state for a relatively short period of time (one dosing interval), we can determine the relative availability of a drug. Moreover, this assessment takes into account the general conditions of use of the drug, particularly when patients rather than healthy subjects are studied.

Dickerson and co-workers[8] determined the steady-state levels of pseudoephedrine after multiple dosing of two prolonged-release capsules given every 12 hr; one capsule (A) contained 120-mg pseudoephedrine and the other (B) contained 150 mg of the drug. The mean steady-state concentrations, $\overline{C}_{ss}$, were 447 ng/ml for capsule A and

510 ng/ml for capsule B. Adjusting these data for the difference in dose (120 mg vs 150 mg), we can calculate that the bioavailability of pseudoephedrine from capsule A relative to capsule B is 110%. Therefore, the dosage forms are nearly bioequivalent.

An advantage of steady state over single dose evaluation of availability is evident in the results of studies with the anticonvulsant drug carbamazepine.[9] Figure 8–2 shows serum concentrations of carbamazepine after single 200-mg doses of two different commercial tablets. It is difficult to determine from these data whether the higher serum levels resulting from product A are the result of greater availability of carbamazepine or merely faster absorption. Steady-state concentrations, shown in Figure 8–3, resulting from multiple dosing of each product at equal daily doses in each patient, clearly indicate that the products are bioequivalent.

Bioavailability studies are typically of a crossover design; each person in a panel of subjects receives each treatment. This design avoids the problem of intersubject variability in drug elimination, which could obscure comparisons of AUC or A_u; all dosage forms are compared in each individual. The cross-over design, however, does not account for intrasubject variability (i.e., variability in drug elimination in the same subject from one administration to another). Drugs that show a high degree of intrasubject variability require large panels of subjects to differentiate dosage forms or to conclude that dosage forms are bioequivalent with an adequate degree of certainty.

When two products are given to the same individual on separate occasions and result in different AUC values, the dissimilarity may either be due to different bioavailability characteristics or to variability in drug clearance from one occasion to the other. In a two-period crossover study, we may incorrectly interpret the variation in clearance as reflecting a difference in bioavailability. Therefore, we would like to correct for the variability in clearance to improve our evaluation of bioavailability.

Some investigators have suggested that if half-lives are different between two treatments, this might reflect a difference in clearance. The equation for this correction is as follows:

$$F = (AUC)_{test}(t_{1/2})_{standard}/(AUC)_{standard}(t_{1/2})_{test}$$

$$(8–10a)$$

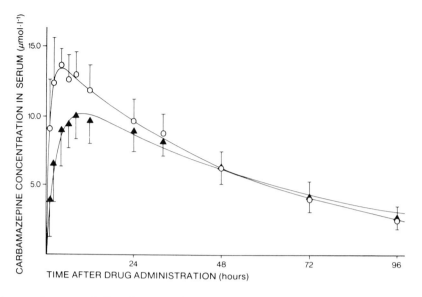

Fig. 8–2. Carbamazepine concentrations in serum after single 200-mg oral doses in 2 different tablet products. (Data from Anttila, M., et al.[9])

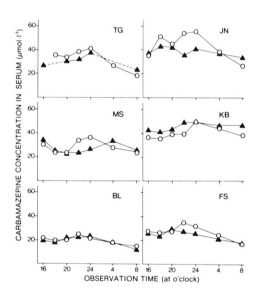

Fig. 8–3. Carbamazepine concentrations in serum at steady state in different subjects after repetitive oral dosing with 2 different tablet products. (Data from Anttila, M., et al.[9])

If half-life estimates are randomly distributed for test and reference treatments, then half-life correction is warranted, if the variance of the corrected bioavailability (F) value is less than for uncorrected values. In those situations where half-life estimates are not randomly distributed across treatments (i.e., the half-life for one treatment is consistently larger than for another), then prolonged absorption

of the drug rather than variation in clearance may be causing the apparent half-life change. In this circumstance, half-life correction is not appropriate.

A more rigorous correction can be applied by administering simultaneously the oral dosage form and an intravenous solution of labeled drug. In this manner, clearance can be calculated independently for each leg of the study. Alternatively, an oral solution containing labeled drug can be given at the same time as the test dosage form. Interest in reducing the effect of intrasubject variability on bioavailability studies by correcting for differences in clearance has been stimulated by increased availability of stable isotopes (e.g., drug molecules containing ^2H or ^{13}C atoms), which are considered safer than radioactive isotopes, and the advances in gas chromatography-mass spectrometry (GC-MS).[10]

One report describing the use of stable isotopes was concerned with the bioavailability of maprotiline, a tetracyclic antidepressant.[11] Six subjects were given simultaneous single 50-mg oral doses of tablets containing maprotiline HCl and an aqueous solution containing trideuterated maprotiline HCl. The mean AUC values for the solution and tablet had coefficients of variation (CVs) of about 65%, whereas the mean value for relative bioavailability (AUC_{tab}/AUC_{soln}) had a CV of only 5%.

More recently, Shinohara et al.[12] used stable isotopes to determine the bioavailability of methyltestosterone (MT) tablets in 8 subjects. The study was carried out in a crossover manner in order to compare the stable isotope method with the conventional crossover method. Each subject was given a 10-mg MT tablet with a reference solution containing 10 mg trideuterated methyltestosterone (MT3D) on one occasion, and a solution containing 10 mg MT with the MT3D reference solution on another. Serum samples were analyzed for MT and MT3D by GC-MS.

When the tablet and reference solution were given at the same time, the peak concentration of MT3D (reference solution) was almost twice as great as that for MT (tablet), but the average AUC values were nearly identical. Mean relative bioavailability for the tablet was 101%. The mean AUCs for the reference solution and tablet had CVs of 42% and 45%, respectively. The mean relative bioavailability had a coefficient of variation of only 18%.

Relative bioavailability was also determined from AUC values for MT after administration of tablet and solution on separate occasions. The mean was 97%, similar to the results in the stable-isotope study, but the coefficient of variation was 38%, more than twice that observed in the isotope study. The investigators concluded that the assumption of a constant clearance in individual subjects on different occasions may be a poor one, certainly for methyltestosterone, and probably for most drugs.

Shinohara et al. also made theoretical calculations to estimate the number of subjects required to detect (with a probability of 0.8) a difference of 20% between the tablet and solution. They estimated that 40 subjects were required for a conventional crossover study, whereas only 12 subjects would be needed for the stable-isotope method.

In 1979, investigators from the FDA and other laboratories reported a new approach to comparative bioavailability testing.[13] They proposed the usual crossover design but added that each formulation would be taken with a solution containing a stable isotope of the drug. They used this approach to compare the bioavailability of two brands of imipramine tablets.

A solution containing 25 mg dideuterated imipramine (IMP2D) was taken each time an imipramine (IMP) tablet was administered. Blood samples were collected after drug administration and plasma was analyzed for IMP and IMP2D. Crossover studies were run 1 week apart.

The data were analyzed in the conventional way by comparing the AUC resulting from each tablet, as well as in a new way by comparing relative parameters. The AUC for IMP from tablet A relative to the AUC for IMP2D from the reference solution given at the same time was compared with the corresponding values for tablet B relative to its reference solution.

Although both methods of comparison suggested that the two imipramine tablets were bioequivalent, statistical power differed remarkably. This is readily seen when the data set is used to calculate the number of subjects needed to detect (with a probability of 0.8) a difference in AUC of 20% between the two tablets. The conventional crossover study was found to require 20 subjects, whereas the relative crossover study (using a stable isotope as an internal standard) would require only 4 subjects.

ESTIMATING THE ABSORPTION RATE OF A DRUG

Rigorous methods are available to evaluate the kinetics of drug absorption after administration of a test dosage form, but these methods require concentration-time data after rapid intravenous injection of the drug in the same individual.[14] Unfortunately, an intravenous reference curve is not available for most drugs.

At this time there are no completely satisfactory methods to evaluate absorption kinetics solely from data obtained after oral administration. Despite the limited methodology, there is keen interest in some quarters for comparative absorption rate data. Regulatory agencies often ask for a quantitative evaluation of absorption kinetics as part of the pharmacokinetic characterization of new drugs; this is considered particularly important for those drugs where rapid absorption is needed for clinical response and for drugs in prolonged-release dosage forms.

The pharmaceutical industry has an additional interest in the evaluation of absorption rate, to establish in vivo-in vitro correlations. Quantitative correlations between gastrointestinal absorption and in vitro dissolution rates may permit rapid screening of new dosage forms and serve as a quality control tool to quickly assess the potential effects of small changes in processing or composition

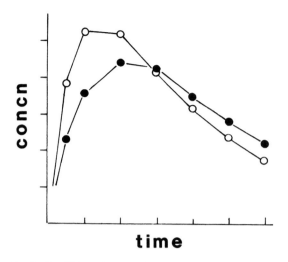

Fig. 8–4. Effect of absorption rate on the time course of drug in the plasma after a single oral dose. The faster the absorption, the higher is the peak concentration and the shorter is the time to peak.

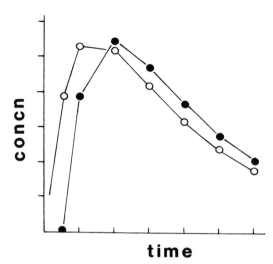

Fig. 8–5. Effect of a delay in gastric emptying or drug release from the dosage form on the time course of drug in the plasma after a single oral dose. The peak concentrations after each dose are similar but there is a difference in the time to peak.

or of product age on the bioavailability of drug from the dosage form.

For clinical purposes, most investigators find it sufficient to compare peak concentrations of drug in blood or plasma and the time required to reach the peak after a single dose of the drug in different dosage forms. The faster the absorption of a drug, the larger is the peak concentration, and the shorter is the time to peak (Fig. 8–4). Sometimes, one may find two dosage forms that release drug at about the same rate but differ in their dependence on gastric emptying or in the time for onset of drug release. The latter may be observed when a film-coated tablet is compared with an uncoated tablet. When this occurs, the peak concentrations will be about the same, but the time to peak will differ, because of the difference in lag time before absorption begins (Fig. 8–5).

Precise definition of the time to peak is often difficult because of limited opportunities to take blood samples. Ronfeld and Benet have shown that, with normal biological and experimental variability, it may be impossible to differentiate, on the basis of peak times, two dosage forms that differ in their release rates of drug by a factor of two.[15] Accordingly, this method for comparing absorption rates may be insufficiently sensitive for some needs. Furthermore, estimates of relative times to peak or peak concentrations are of little use in the evaluation of prolonged release dosage

forms, which may produce no well defined peak concentration.

The statistical moments theory offers an attractive alternative for the evaluation of absorption data. As noted in Chapter 2, the difference between the mean residence time (MRT) after administration of a test dosage form (MRT_{test}) and the MRT after rapid intravenous injection (MRT_{iv}) is the mean absorption time (MAT):

$$MAT = MRT_{test} - MRT_{iv} \qquad (8\text{–}11)$$

If absorption is first-order, then:

$$MAT = 1/k_a \qquad (8\text{–}12)$$

where k_a is the first-order absorption rate constant.

Even in the absence of intravenous data, MAT is useful. For example, the relative ranking of MRT values following several dosage forms mirrors the relative ranking of the dosage forms with respect to drug release and absorption.

Riegelman and Collier proposed that the difference in MRT after a test oral dosage form and an aqueous solution, (MRT_{soln}) is equivalent to the mean dissolution time (MDT) or mean release rate of drug from the dosage form in the gastrointestinal tract:[16]

$$MDT = MRT_{test} - MRT_{soln} \qquad (8\text{–}13)$$

This approach has the potential to be a useful tool in the biopharmaceutic evaluation of dosage forms.

The absorption of furosemide has been studied by means of moment analysis.[17] The mean residence time after an intravenous bolus of furosemide, MRT_{iv}, was 51 min. After oral administration of a furosemide tablet to fasting subjects MRT was 135 min. The difference (MAT) is 84 min. The mean absorption time for oral furosemide was significantly greater than MRT_{iv}, indicating absorption rate-limited elimination kinetics.

The mean absorption time for furosemide tablets given immediately after a meal was 144 min, considerably longer than the mean value calculated when the tablets were given to fasting subjects. The difference in MAT values for the tablet given to fasted and fed subjects, 60 min in this case, is a representation of the delay in absorption resulting from the meal. It might be looked upon as the mean increase in gastric emptying time.

When an oral solution of furosemide was given after a meal, MAT was 109 min. The difference between MAT for the tablet and solution given after a meal was 35 min, representing the mean postprandial dissolution time for furosemide tablets.

PREABSORPTIVE HYDROLYSIS AND METABOLISM

The principal sites of chemical or biochemical (metabolic) conversion of a drug in the gut lumen are the stomach (acid), small intestine (esterases and other enzymes), and distal small intestine and colon (gut bacteria). These conversions can take place in parallel with or precede drug absorption and result in reduced availability.

Some drugs are not chemically stable at the low pH of the stomach; examples include penicillin G, methicillin, erythromycin, and digoxin. After oral administration, they are subject to acid hydrolysis in the stomach to form inactive products; less than 100% of the administered dose is available for absorption. This problem can usually be predicted from in vitro chemical stability studies.

The availability of drugs subject to acid hydrolysis in the stomach is a function of the rate of dissolution and the residence time of the drug in the stomach. Minimizing the dissolution of the drug in the stomach leads to increased availability. Factors that promote gastric emptying or increase gastric pH also result in improved bioavailability.

The importance of enzymatic hydrolysis in the fluids of the small intestine in determining the availability of drugs is unknown. Esterases are certainly ubiquitous in the body and could, in principle, degrade drugs like aspirin or ester prodrugs like pivampicillin or chloramphenicol palmitate before or in competition with the absorption process. In general, however, the gut wall is likely to be a more important site for the enzymatic hydrolysis of esters than is the gut lumen. If pivampicillin, for example, is subject to hydrolysis in the fluids of the small intestine, this surely must represent only a small fraction of the dose because the blood levels of ampicillin are much higher after a dose of the prodrug than after an equivalent dose of ampicillin. This means that a significant fraction of the pivampicillin dose must be absorbed (penetrate the gut wall) as such and thereby evade preabsorptive metabolism.

Many different kinds of microorganisms are normal residents of the lower intestine. These bacteria, which constitute the intestinal microflora, can carry out a variety of metabolic processes, but they are particularly adept at reduction, including the reduction of double bonds, azo groups, aldehydes, ketones, and alcohols.[18]

Most drugs are absorbed before reaching the ileum and are not subject to metabolism by intestinal microorganisms. On the other hand, a substantial fraction of an oral dose of a slowly absorbed drug or a drug given in a prolonged-release dosage form may reach the lower intestines. When this occurs, preabsorptive metabolism by the intestinal microflora may affect the availability of the drug. This situation applies to digoxin.

In certain patients, about 10% of the population taking the drug, the availability of digoxin is unusually low. These patients also excrete large amounts of digoxin reduction products or DRPs in the urine. Moreover, there is a tendency in the general population to greater excretion of DRPs when poorly absorbed preparations are taken (Fig. 8–6). There is convincing evidence that digoxin is extensively inactivated by intestinal microorganisms in a minority of those receiving the drug and that this problem is more widespread with slowly absorbed preparations of the drug.[19,20]

The proposition that metabolism by intestinal microflora is more important for slowly-absorbed than for rapidly-absorbed drug products was tested by determining the effect of metoclopramide on digoxin absorption after a 0.5-mg dose of digoxin tablets or a 0.4-mg dose of a digoxin solution encapsulated in soft gelatin.[21] Digoxin is more rapidly and more completely absorbed from the soft gelatin capsules than from the tablets. Metoclopramide de-

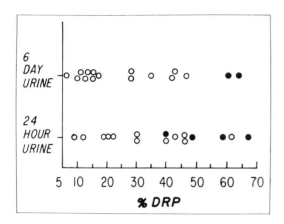

Fig. 8–6. Percent of drug-related material in the urine present as digoxin reduction products after a single oral dose of digoxin. ○: solutions or tablets with high dissolution rates. ●: tablets with low dissolution rates. (From Lindenbaum, J., et al.[19])

creased the bioavailability of digoxin tablets by about 25%, on the average, but had no effect on the bioavailability of digoxin following administration of soft gelatin capsules.

Another example is seen with acenocoumarol, an oral anticoagulant used outside the U.S. Acenocoumarol is converted by gut flora in vitro to amino and amido metabolites. Under typical clinical conditions, however, bacterial metabolism is of little importance because acenocoumarol is rapidly absorbed from its dosage form. Studies with commercial tablets indicate no measurable levels of reduced metabolites in plasma and less than 1% of the oral dose is excreted in urine as reduced metabolites. Administration of slowly-dissolving capsules containing relative coarse, crystalline acenocoumarol produced measurable plasma levels of both the amido and amino metabolites. Urinary recovery of reduced metabolites accounted for 6 to 12% of the dose.[22]

Certain oral antibiotics, including tetracycline and erythromycin alter the bacterial flora and decrease the inactivation of digoxin. Steady-state serum levels of digoxin in some patients have been found to increase 2-fold during oral antibiotic treatment, presenting the risk of toxicity.[24]

Other reports indicate that changes in gut bacteria as a result of treatment with antibiotics affect the disposition of sulfasalazine and oral contraceptives. Bacterial metabolism reduces the azo linkage in sulfasalazine to liberate sulfapyridine and 5-aminosalicylic acid (mesalamine) in the lower bowel.

A 5-day course of oral ampicillin, 250 mg 4 times daily, significantly reduced gut bacteria-mediated conversion of sulfasalazine to sulfapyridine. AUC values for sulfapyridine after a single oral dose of sulfasalazine decreased from 370 μg-hr/ml under control conditions to 239 μg-hr/ml after ampicillin.[23]

PRESYSTEMIC METABOLISM

After oral administration, a drug must pass sequentially from the gastrointestinal lumen, through the gut wall, then through the liver before reaching the systemic circulation (Fig. 8–7). This sequence is an anatomic requirement because blood perfusing the entire length of the gastrointestinal tract, with the exception of the buccal cavity and lower rectum, drains into the liver by way of the hepatic portal vein. Since the gut wall and liver are sites of drug metabolism, a fraction of the amount absorbed may be eliminated (metabolized) before reaching the bloodstream. Therefore, an oral dose of a drug may be completely absorbed but incompletely available to the systemic circulation because of presystemic or *first-pass* metabolism in the gut wall or liver.

Criteria have been developed to identify and quantify the extent of presystemic metabolism and to indicate where it is occurring. Its detection requires only that systemic availability is less than the fraction of the dose absorbed. The fraction absorbed may be determined from the urinary excretion of drug and metabolites, usually as total radioactivity, after oral administration of the drug (in a radiolabeled form), relative to that after intravenous administration. Many drugs undergoing presystemic metabolism in man have been identified on the basis of this type of information. Differentiation of the gut wall and liver as the site of presystemic metabolism is relatively simple in animals, but more difficult in man.

The theory and our understanding of hepatic presystemic metabolism is relatively advanced; our knowledge of gut wall metabolism is less well developed. Because an understanding of the hepatic first-pass effect is often useful in differentiating the sites of presystemic elimination, we will first consider the liver as the site of presystemic metabolism.

Hepatic Presystemic Metabolism

The liver is the most important site of presystemic elimination because of its high level of drug

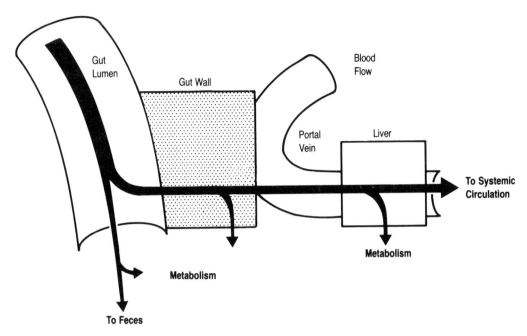

Fig. 8–7. After oral administration, a drug must pass sequentially from the gut lumen through the gut wall, then through the liver, before reaching the systemic circulation. Metabolism may occur in the lumen before absorption, in the gut wall during absorption, and/or in the liver after absorption but before reaching the systemic circulation. (From Rowland, M., and Tozer, T.N.[24])

metabolizing enzymes, its ability to rapidly metabolize many different kinds of drug molecules, and its unique anatomic location. A large number of drugs are subject to considerable hepatic first-pass metabolism; examples include β-blockers (propranolol and metoprolol), analgesics (propoxyphene, meperidine, and pentazocine), antidepressants (imipramine and nortriptyline), and antiarrhythmics (lidocaine and verapamil).

Hepatic presystemic metabolism is most easily understood when the liver is the sole organ of drug elimination. Under these conditions, the clearance of a drug, as determined after intravenous administration from the ratio of dose to area (AUC), is equal to hepatic clearance (Cl_H), which is given by:

$$Cl_H = Q_H ER_H \qquad (8\text{–}14)$$

where Q_H is hepatic blood flow and ER_H is the hepatic extraction ratio (see Chap. 2). Hepatic blood flow in man ranges from about 1.1 to 1.8 L/min, with an average of about 1.5 L/min. Hepatic extraction ratio may range from 0 to 1, depending on the liver's ability to metabolize the drug. The maximum clearance of a drug eliminated exclu-

sively by hepatic metabolism is equal to hepatic blood flow; this occurs when $ER_H = 1.0$.

The fraction of drug eliminated from portal blood during absorption is given by the hepatic extraction ratio, ER_H; the remainder $(1 - ER_H)$ escapes into the systemic circulation, and is then cleared from the circulation by the liver, according to Equation 8–14. If a fraction (f) of the oral dose (D_o) is absorbed and then subjected to hepatic presystemic metabolism, the AUC after oral administration (AUC_o) is given by:

$$AUC_o = fD_o(1 - ER_H)/Q_H ER_H \qquad (8\text{–}15)$$

Since $Q_H ER_H$ is equal to hepatic clearance, which, under these conditions, is given by the ratio of intravenous dose (D_{iv}) to area (AUC_{iv}), we may rewrite Equation 8–15 as follows:

$$AUC_o/AUC_{iv} = fD_o(1 - ER_H)/D_{iv} \qquad (8\text{–}16)$$

The ratio of areas after oral and intravenous administration of equal doses of a drug is equal to its systemic availability (F). If we also assume that absorption is complete (f = 1), then:

$$F = (1 - ER_H) \qquad (8\text{–}17)$$

Equation 8–17 shows that systemic availability

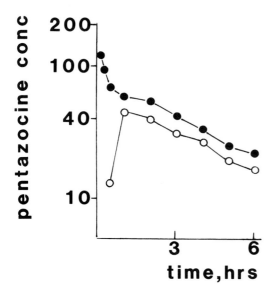

Fig. 8–8. Pentazocine concentrations in plasma (ng/ml) after administration of 100 mg orally (○) or 30 mg intravenously (●). (Data from Ehrnebo, M., Boréus, L.O., and Lönroth, U.[29])

Table 8–1. Relationship Between Steady-State Concentration of Alprenolol on 200 mg Twice a Day and Single Dose Data After Oral or Intravenous Administration*

Rank No.	Steady-state concn. (ng/ml)	Bioavailability (oral)	Clearance (iv)
1	37.0	0.15	0.71
2	32.1	0.13	0.52
3	14.1	–	1.37
4	13.2	0.07	0.94
5	12.0	0.05	0.78
6	3.9	0.03	0.41
7	2.7	0.01	2.03

*Data from Alván, G., et al.[30]

depends on the hepatic extraction ratio. Drugs with low extraction ratios, such as antipyrine, warfarin, and tolbutamide, undergo little presystemic metabolism.

An estimate of the hepatic extraction ratio may be made by determining the clearance of the drug after intravenous administration and comparing this value to a mean value for liver blood flow, according to a rearrangement of Equation 8–14:

$$ER_H = Cl_H/Q_H \qquad (8–18)$$

The intravenous clearance of propranolol is about 1.05 L/min in man. Assuming an average liver blood flow of 1.5 L/min, we can calculate that $ER_H = 0.7$ and $F = 0.3$. Although propranolol is well absorbed, only 30% of an oral dose is available to the systemic circulation. This kind of information, in conjunction with experimental estimates of F, has been used to substantiate the predominantly hepatic presystemic elimination of several drugs, including propranolol,[25] lidocaine,[26] imipramine,[27] papaverine,[28] and pentazocine.[29]

Plasma concentrations of pentazocine after administration of 100 mg orally and 30 mg intravenously are shown in Figure 8–8. Although the intravenous dose is smaller, it results in higher plasma levels. The systemic availability of pentazocine after oral administration, calculated after taking into account the difference between intravenous

and oral doses in 5 subjects, varied from 11 to 32%, with a mean value of 18%. This low systemic availability of pentazocine is consistent with its high hepatic clearance, in the order of 1.2 L/min.[29]

With many drugs, presystemic metabolism and systemic availability vary markedly from one person to another. The variability contributes to the interindividual differences in steady-state concentrations of the drug. Studies with the β-blocker alprenolol show a 14-fold range in steady-state concentrations in healthy subjects taking oral doses of 200 mg twice a day. Intravenous studies in the same subjects indicate only a 4-fold range of clearance values.

Additional studies reveal that the rank order for individual steady-state plasma concentrations of alprenolol is the same as that for the relative bioavailability of the 200-mg oral dose; no correlation is found between steady-state levels and individual clearance values (Table 8–1). These results demonstrate that differences in first-pass metabolism contribute substantially to interindividual variability in steady-state plasma concentrations of a drug with a high hepatic extraction ratio.[30]

Presystemic metabolism after oral administration of a drug results in the formation of a bolus of metabolites during the drug's first pass through the liver. Accordingly, we would expect to see higher peak levels of metabolites after oral administration of a drug with a high hepatic extraction ratio than after parenteral administration. Figure 8–9 shows mean plasma concentrations of nortriptyline (NT) and its 10-hydroxy metabolite after oral and intramuscular administration of the same dose of NT. Lower concentrations of NT occur after oral than after intramuscular administration. In contrast, initial plasma concentrations of the metabolite (up to 10 hr) are much higher after oral than after intramuscular doses.[31]

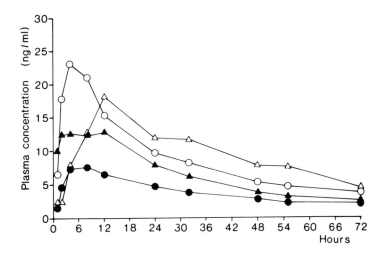

Fig. 8–9. Nortriptyline (▲,●) and 10-hydroxynortriptyline (△,○) concentrations in plasma after oral (●,○) and intramuscular injection (▲,△) of a 40-mg dose of nortriptyline. (From Alván, G., et al.[31])

Gut Wall Presystemic Metabolism

Presystemic metabolism in the gut wall and liver can be differentiated in animals by comparing drug concentration after oral and intraportal administrations to assess the contribution of the gut wall, and after intraportal and intravenous administrations to assess the contribution of the liver.

Glucuronidation of morphine, naloxone, and buprenorphine by the liver and intestine has been compared in rats.[32] The drugs were given by peripheral intravenous (iv) and hepatic portal vein (hpv) injection, and instilled into the duodenum (id). AUC decreased in the following order: iv > hpv > id. The results suggest that these related compounds are subject to presystemic metabolism, in both the gastrointestinal wall and the liver. For each drug, hepatic extraction was more efficient than intestinal extraction.

Another experimental model was developed to determine the site of first-pass metabolism of midazolam, a benzodiazepine with high presystemic extraction after oral administration.[33] Domestic pigs received single intravenous and oral doses of the drug. Multiple blood samples were simultaneously drawn from the portal vein and from a systemic vein during the first 8 hr after the dose. Differences in AUC at the two sampling sites after oral administration indicate hepatic extraction; differences after iv administration indicate gut wall extraction.

After iv administration, midazolam had a high systemic clearance value, suggesting the likelihood of first-pass metabolism. AUC values for systemic vs portal sites were nearly identical, suggesting little, if any, metabolism in the gut wall. After oral administration the systemic/portal AUC ratio averaged only 0.15, suggesting a high degree of hepatic extraction. The portal AUC after oral administration was similar to the systemic AUC after iv administration, again suggesting little gut wall metabolism. The investigators concluded that the extensive presystemic extraction of oral midazolam is largely the result of hepatic biotransformation rather than metabolism either within the gastrointestinal tract or during absorption into the portal circulation.

Despite the importance of understanding the site of presystemic extraction of drugs, human studies are limited by the necessarily invasive experimental techniques. Sampling of portal blood is generally possible only in patients in whom portal catheterization is otherwise clinically indicated.

An example is found in a report on the concentrations of phenacetin and its metabolite, acetaminophen, in portal and hepatic venous blood after intragastric or intraduodenal administration of phenacetin to patients with portal hypertension.[34] The concentration ratio of metabolite to drug in portal blood soon after drug administration was low, ranging from 0.01 to 0.11. Furthermore, at each sampling time, the concentration ratio in the portal vein was much lower than in the hepatic vein or in peripheral blood. The hepatic extraction ratio of phenacetin was estimated to be about 0.6 to 0.8, consistent with the low bioavailability of the drug.[35]

These results indicate that O-dealkylation of phenacetin occurs mainly in the liver and only to a limited extent in the gut wall.

A similar study in patients with portal hypertension was carried out with flurazepam.[36] High concentrations of the mono- and didesethyl metabolites of flurazepam were found in portal vein blood soon after intraduodenal administration of the drug, consistent with intestinal wall metabolism. Efficient hepatic extraction of both flurazepam and its metabolites, however, was also observed. The results suggest that presystemic metabolism of flurazepam in man occurs in the gut wall as well as in the liver.

More direct evidence of gut wall metabolism in man is found in a report on the concentrations of ethinyl estradiol and its conjugated metabolite in portal and peripheral vein blood following oral administration to postsurgical patients.[37] In each patient, for about 40 to 50 min after administration, the concentration of conjugated ethinyl estradiol in the portal vein was considerably higher than in the peripheral vein. Back and co-workers calculated that about 44% of the absorbed dose undergoes presystemic metabolism in the gut wall;[37] an additional 25% of the dose is subjected to hepatic first-pass metabolism.

In vitro studies show that ethinyl estradiol is extensively metabolized by human jejunal mucosa, obtained by biopsy from healthy subjects, to form the sulfate conjugate.[38] The degree of conjugation of mestranol and levonorgestrel, two other contraceptive steroids, was much lower than for ethinyl estradiol. The results with levonorgestrol are consistent with the high systemic availability of the steroid.[39]

Changes in metabolite excretion patterns may provide indirect evidence for gut wall metabolism. Intravenous isoproterenol is excreted largely unchanged in man. On the other hand, the sulfate conjugate accounts for 80% of the drug in the urine after oral administration. No sulfate conjugate is found after intravenous administration. The results suggest that the presystemic metabolism of isoproterenol in man is confined to the mucosal surface of the gut wall.[40]

Albuterol (salbutamol), a potent beta-adrenergic agonist used widely in the treatment of bronchial asthma, is subject to substantial presystemic metabolism after oral administration. Morgan et al.[41] studied the kinetics of albuterol and its sulfate conjugate metabolite, in plasma and urine, after intravenous and oral administration.

After iv administration, total plasma clearance was 480 ml/min and the elimination half-life was about 4 hr. Urinary excretion of unchanged albuterol accounted for 64% of the dose and the sulfate metabolite accounted for 12%. After oral administration, systemic availability was only 50%, and urinary excretion of unchanged drug and metabolite accounted for 32% and 48% of the dose, respectively.

Total urinary recovery of drug-related material was similar after each route of administration, indicating that although oral albuterol has a low bioavailability, it is well absorbed from the gastrointestinal tract. The data also indicate that the fraction of the dose of albuterol eliminated on the first pass could be accounted for entirely as sulfate conjugate formed, presumably, in the gut wall.

Commonly, the existence of gut wall metabolism is inferred when the degree of presystemic metabolism of drug exceeds the hepatic extraction ratio. For example, the hepatic extraction ratio of terbutaline, determined after intravenous administration, is only about 0.08. This means that if the entire oral dose were absorbed, a systemic availability of 92% should result. In fact, the availability of terbutaline is only 10%. Determination of free terbutaline in the feces suggests that only 55% of the drug is absorbed. Under these conditions, we expect a systemic availability of 0.55 × 0.92 or 51%. Clearly, incomplete absorption and hepatic presystemic metabolism cannot account for the low systemic availability of terbutaline. We must conclude that a large fraction of the dose of terbutaline is metabolized by another presystemic route, most likely the gut wall.[42]

REGULATORY AND CLINICAL CONSIDERATIONS

Both biopharmaceutic and metabolic factors influence the bioavailability of drugs. Although there is usually little we can do to alter unfavorable metabolic characteristics, this is not true for biopharmaceutic factors that limit the availability of a drug. During the last decade there has been a heightened awareness of the role of the dosage form on the bioavailability and clinical efficacy of drugs; the general result has been better dosage forms.

For some time now, the U.S. Food and Drug Administration has required some degree of characterization of bioavailability for all new drugs intended for oral use. Some attention has also been given to dosage forms intended for other routes of administration. These requirements have established a standard of performance.

More recently, the FDA has required secondary (or generic) manufacturers who are interested in marketing a drug after a patent or period of exclusive-use has lapsed to demonstrate bioequivalence (comparable bioavailability) with the innovator's dosage form before approval to market is granted. The Congress directed the FDA to apply these criteria to generic products through the passage of the Drug Price Competition and Patent Restoration Act in 1984. Before this landmark legislation, the only way a secondary manufacturer could market a drug was to carry out clinical trials demonstrating comparable efficacy to the innovator's product.

A bioequivalence trial generally consists of a comparison of the area under the drug concentration-time curve, peak concentration, and time to peak concentration after a single dose of the generic and "standard" product using a randomized, two-way crossover design. Urinary excretion data may also be useful, particularly for drugs that are substantially excreted unchanged. The FDA bioequivalence guidance for hydrochlorothiazide recommends a urinary excretion study.

Panels of healthy human subjects are almost always used in bioequivalence studies. The FDA recognizes the possibility that some conditions found only in special populations (patients, elderly, etc.) could affect bioavailability and is prepared to modify its guideline calling for the use of normal subjects if the need is adequately documented for a given drug.

The Agency also requires the determination of metabolite kinetics if the drug is metabolized to a clinically important biotransformation product. This requirement is controversial. Some scientists believe that a metabolite should be followed only as an alternative when it is difficult to measure unchanged drug in the plasma.

Can dissolution testing assure bioequivalence? This question has been widely debated. The FDA and most pharmaceutical scientists believe that there is not yet evidence to show that a dissolution test will assure bioequivalence. Dissolution testing is important in assuring lot-to-lot uniformity of a drug product and supporting minor changes (e.g., a change in color) in the product. Also, it is FDA policy that if a product meets in vivo bioequivalence requirements at one dosage strength and the formulations of other strengths are proportional to the strength tested and meet dissolution require-

ments, then no further in vivo studies are needed for approval.

The usual criteria for bioequivalence calls for the mean AUC and C_{max} values for the two products to be within 20%, but the FDA also applies a 90% confidence interval test based on the two one-sided t-test approach,[43] one test to verify that the bioavailability of the test product is not too low, and the other to show that it is not too high. The entire 90% confidence interval must also lie within the limits of plus-or-minus 20%.

This confidence interval requirement ensures that the difference in mean values for AUC and C_{max} will be much less than 20%. The experience to date in reviewing bioequivalence studies with generic products indicates that 80% of the approvals had AUC values within 5% of the reference product. In view of this experience, some scientists believe that the FDA should be more stringent, requiring the mean values for AUC to be within 10% rather than 20%. On the other hand, some believe that the current requirements for C_{max} values are too stringent, considering the difficulty in accurately estimating this value, and the typical finding for most products (generic or brand name) that C_{max} values are more variable than AUC values.

The approval process for generic products has worked remarkably well for conventional oral dosage forms. Almost no documented examples of clinically important differences between generic and original products have been reported. The one class of drugs that continues to be put forward (often with scant evidence) as a challenge to the sufficiency of bioequivalence studies to assure the performance of a generic product is the anticonvulsants.

A case for bioinequivalence of a generic drug product has been made in a report concerning a 16-year-old girl with severe cerebral palsy and seizures since birth.[44] During treatment with primidone and other medication, her usual seizure frequency was one to two seizures per week. Serum levels of both primidone and phenobarbital, its metabolite, are frequently monitored in patients receiving primidone.

The patient had been taking the same antiepileptic medication for 9 years. Within 3 weeks of switching her to a generic primidone, there was a rise in seizure frequency and she was switched back to the original dosage form. With this change, the seizure frequency decreased to baseline. Serum drug concentrations were not measured during this period.

The patient's condition remained stable until 3 months later, when she was admitted to hospital for feeding problems. Before admission, she was taking her usual medication and serum trough levels were 10.8 mg/L for primidone and 19.1 mg/L for phenobarbital. During hospitalization, she was again switched to the primidone product that caused a problem 3 months earlier. After 6 days of receiving this product, morning trough levels were 5.1 mg/L for primidone and 15.9 mg/L for phenobarbital.

On day 6, the daily dose of primidone was increased from 500 to 625 mg, but despite this change, serum levels continued to fall and the patient had more frequent seizures. On day 10, serum primidone was less than 2.0 mg/L and serum phenobarbital was 10.4 mg/L. At this time, the patient was returned once again to the original primidone product. After 6 days of receiving this product at a dose of 500 mg/day, primidone levels were 9.0 mg/L and phenobarbital levels were 12 mg/L, and the patient's seizure frequency returned to baseline.

The evidence is clear that the two primidone products used in this patient were not bioequivalent. This observation raises concern that an initial determination of bioequivalence may change with time because of subtle changes in manufacturing or lot-to-lot variability. This problem seems to call for some stringent dissolution criteria. In any event, the investigators urged that product substitution be cautiously considered in patients who have already been titrated and maintained on an antiepileptic preparation.

Controlled-Release Medication

A basic question in developing a controlled-release product of a drug that has been used in a conventional dosage form is whether a formal clinical evaluation of the new dosage form's safety and efficacy is needed, or whether a pharmacokinetic evaluation will suffice. The FDA's position is that if there is a well-defined relationship between plasma concentration of drug and/or active metabolite and clinical response, it may be possible to rely on plasma concentration data alone as a basis for the approval of a product.

On the other hand, "where the therapeutic effect is indirect, where irreversible toxicity can occur, where there is evidence of functional (pharmacodynamic) tolerance, where peak to trough differ-ences of the immediate release form are very large, or where there is any other reasonable uncertainty concerning the relationship between plasma concentration and therapeutic and adverse effects, it will probably be necessary to carry out clinical studies."[45]

For the development of a controlled-release oral dosage form of a drug marketed in an immediate-release form for which an extensive base of pharmacodynamic-pharmacokinetic data exists, the following pharmacokinetic studies are usually required. A single dose, three-way crossover study where the immediate-release and the controlled-release products are given to fasted subjects, and the controlled-release form is also given after a high fat meal.

The fasting comparison permits an estimation of the extent of absorption from the controlled-release form relative to the immediate-release form. The food study is essentially a drug interaction assessment. If there are no differences in AUC and peak concentration following administration of the controlled-release form to fed and fasted subjects, then no further food studies are needed. If a decrease or an increase in the extent of absorption is found after a meal, it may be necessary to determine the cause of the food effect as well as the effect of time on the food-drug effect (i.e., would absorption be affected if the dosage form were given 1 or 2 hr after a meal rather than with a meal).

The FDA also requires a multiple dose, steady-state, crossover comparison of the controlled-release and immediate-release products as part of the pharmacokinetic evaluation. Ordinarily, the same daily dose is used for each regimen but the immediate-release form is given more frequently than the controlled-release form (e.g., 3 times a day versus once a day). Concentrations over at least one dosing interval should be measured in each leg of the crossover. Some investigators favor measurements over 24 hr in each leg of the study, to account for diurnal variation.

The controlled-release product should produce an AUC equivalent to the immediate release product, and the degree of fluctuation at steady-state [i.e., $(C_{max} - C_{min})/C_{av}$] for the controlled-release product should be similar to, or less than, that for the immediate release form. If appropriate, levels of major active metabolites should also be measured. For racemic drugs, consideration should be given to measurement of individual enantiomers.

Since the passage of the Drug Price Competition and Patent Restoration Act in 1984, attention has also been given to criteria needed to demonstrate the equivalence of a generic product to an approved controlled-release product. The current position of the FDA on this matter is as follows: "the new generic formulation must be comparable with respect to AUC, C_{max}, and C_{min} in a cross-over steady-state study *vs* the standard controlled-release product using the accepted Agency criteria for equivalence. In some cases, it may also be necessary to match the concentration-time profile of the approved controlled-release dosage form. The food studies described previously are also needed."[45]

SPECIFIC DRUGS

The following discussion is a summary of reports of poor bioavailability or "inequivalences" of marketed products, listed alphabetically by drug. That most of the material has been taken from previous editions of this text and that comparatively few examples of bioinequivalence have been reported in the past five years are encouraging signs, indicative of the attention given to the development of dosage forms today.

Acetazolamide

Most of the reports on differences in bioavailability of marketed products have concerned prolonged-release dosage forms. Clinical studies with acetazolamide, a carbonic anhydrase inhibitor used in treating glaucoma, provide an example.[46] Acetazolamide was only 60% available from a sustained-release capsule, Diamox Sequels, compared to that observed after an aqueous suspension. Consistent with these results, steady-state concentrations of acetazolamide for the prolonged-release capsules were about half the values observed for an immediate-release dosage form. Since Diamox Sequels is considered to be an effective product, the results suggest that lower doses of acetazolamide in rapid-release dosage forms may be useful for treating glaucoma.[47]

Aminosalicylate

Studies in Canada with various dosage forms of aminosalicylic acid (PAS), which is used, usually in combination, in the treatment of pulmonary and extrapulmonary tuberculosis, indicated large differences in drug absorption.[48] The availability of a prolonged-release product, estimated from cumulative urinary recovery of the drug in 8 subjects, was only 42% compared to that observed following

administration of a standard capsule containing drug and lactose. The relative availability of PAS from two different lots of an enteric-coated tablet and from a powder containing a polyamine resin complex of the drug was 51%, 64%, and 66%, respectively. Another investigation found no absorption of PAS in 8 subjects after administration of an enteric-coated tablet.[49]

Ampicillin

Concern for differences in bioavailability of the widely used antibiotic ampicillin was stimulated by a report from Canada demonstrating that two brands of ampicillin capsules produced lower serum concentrations than did ampicillin capsules manufactured by a third company.[50] Products B and C were only 78% and 72% as available as product A, based on the area under the serum concentration versus time curves. A second bioavailability study comparing product A with a reformulated product C indicated bioequivalence.[51] The reformulation involved a minor change in the amount of a dispersing agent. The bioavailability monograph on ampicillin published by the American Pharmaceutical Association in 1975 concluded that it is unlikely that possible differences in bioavailability among the current major United States suppliers are of clinical importance.[52] The same holds true today.

Aspirin

Poor bioavailability of aspirin has been reported only with enteric-coated products. Less than 25% of the dose was absorbed in 3 of 4 subjects after administration of a certain brand of enteric-coated aspirin tablets.[53] A clinical study with this enteric-coated product in arthritic patients showed erratic and low concentrations of salicylate, compared to those observed after regular administration of conventional aspirin tablets.[54] This problem has all but disappeared with the materials in use today to provide enteric protection.

Ascorbic Acid

This vitamin has been widely used since the claim in 1970 that daily consumption of large quantities of ascorbic acid may be beneficial for reducing the frequency and duration of the common cold. Ascorbic acid absorption was investigated in 4 subjects who received different oral dosage forms containing 1 g of vitamin C.[55] About 85% of a 1-g intravenous dose was recovered in the urine as ascorbic acid and its major metabolite. In contrast, only about 30% of the dose was recovered after an oral aqueous solution, a conventional tablet, or a chewable tablet. A still smaller fraction of the dose, about 14%, was recovered after a prolonged-release product. The incomplete availability of ascorbic acid after the solution and tablets reflects the capacity-limited absorption of the vitamin; the same daily dose given in divided doses is absorbed more efficiently. The poor results with the prolonged-release capsule may reflect the site-specific absorption of the vitamin in the proximal intestine or a poorly formulated product.

Carbamazepine

Carbamazepine is gaining wide acceptance as monotherapy for seizures and is increasingly used in children. Two formulations are marketed in the United States: 200 mg tablets and 100 mg chewable tablets. These two forms, from the same manufacturer, were compared in a single-dose randomized crossover study in fasting healthy adults with a four-week washout period between doses.[56] In each leg, a 200-mg dose of carbamazepine was given and blood was collected for 48 hr.

The area under the curve to 48 hr was about 10% larger for the chewable tablet than for the conventional tablet, but this difference was not statistically significant. A significantly higher mean C_{max} value, however, was observed with the chewable tablet (4.6 vs 3.8 mg/L). The investigators concluded that the difference in C_{max} was not clinically relevant and that carbamazepine tablets and chewable tablets could be used interchangeably. Some clinicians might take issue with this conclusion because there is evidence that adverse effects of carbamazepine are related to peak concentration.

Chloramphenicol

Although chloramphenicol is rarely the drug of choice for treating infections, it is still used in certain situations. The absorption characteristics of four different chloramphenicol products were compared in normal adults by means of blood level measurements and urinary excretion of chloramphenicol and its metabolites following single 0.5-g oral doses.[57] Mean plasma levels for groups of 10 subjects are shown in Figure 8–10. Relative bioavailabilities based on cumulative urinary excretion of total nitro compounds were 100%, 71%, 83%, and 39% for products A, B, C, and D, respectively. Similar differences in apparent bioavailability can

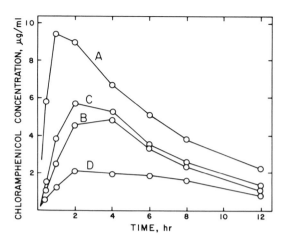

Fig. 8–10. Chloramphenicol concentrations in plasma after a single 500-mg oral dose of 4 different commercial products. (Data from Glazko, A.J., et al.[57])

be calculated from the plasma concentration data. In vitro tests indicated that products B, C, and D dissolved more slowly than did product A.

Chlorothiazide

In 1977, the FDA implemented bioequivalence requirements for tablets of chlorothiazide, a widely used diuretic, because of concern about bioavailability differences among marketed products. The availability of chlorothiazide is best determined from urinary excretion data; almost the entire dose is excreted unchanged after intravenous administration. A urinary excretion bioavailability study was conducted in 12 healthy males to evaluate three 250-mg and 500-mg chlorothiazide tablets.[58] Chlorothiazide excretion did not exceed 20% of the dose for any product, reflecting the incomplete absorption of the drug from the gastrointestinal tract. No important differences were found among the 250-mg tablets; availability ranged from 16 to 20% of the dose. Drug recovery in the urine after one of the 500-mg tablets (11% of the dose) was significantly less than that from the other two 500-mg tablets (13% and 16% of the dose).

Chlorpropamide

Chlorpropamide is an antidiabetic agent used in adult-onset diabetes. Studies in England with three marketed products showed that the rate and extent of chlorpropamide absorption were markedly impaired with one product compared to the other two.[59] The results are shown in Figure 8–11. The peak concentration of chlorpropamide after admin-

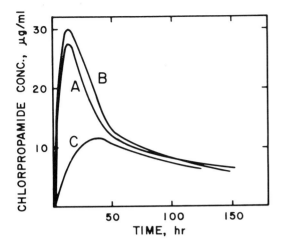

Fig. 8–11. Chlorpropamide concentrations in plasma after a single 250-mg oral dose of 3 different commercial products. (Data from Monro, A.M., and Welling, P.G.[59])

istration of product C was less than half that found after administration of the other formulations.

Diazepam

A report is available from Sweden concerning the plasma concentrations of diazepam and its major metabolite N-desmethyldiazepam after treatment with 5-mg oral doses 3 times a day.[60] A crossover study to evaluate the bioavailability of several tablet products and a marketed suspension was included in the investigation. All three tablets gave similar plasma levels but the suspension showed lower values during steady state, indicating incomplete absorption.

Differences in the rate but not the extent of absorption of marketed diazepam tablets have been reported when the drug was given after treatment with an H_2-blocker. Under these conditions, gastric pH is increased and the dissolution rate of diazepam is decreased. Some products appear to be more affected by this pH change than others. Similar differences between products might also be found in elderly patients, who tend to have elevated gastric pH. It is not likely, however, that small differences in the rate of absorption of diazepam would be of clinical interest.

Digoxin

Perhaps, more bioavailability data have been reported for digoxin than for all other drugs combined. Digoxin is poorly water-soluble and has a low therapeutic index. Relatively small differences

in bioavailability of digoxin products may be clinically significant.

The first published comparative bioavailability study for digoxin appeared in 1971.[61] The investigation was prompted by the observation that several patients in a New York City hospital required unusually large maintenance doses of digoxin but had low serum drug concentrations. Four lots of digoxin tablets from three manufacturers were evaluated in healthy subjects. The mean peak serum digoxin levels, which reflect absorption rates, varied sevenfold, with Lanoxin brand of digoxin showing the highest peak. Some of the differences observed in this investigation could have been due to low tablet potency rather than poor bioavailability.

In a later study, Lanoxin and another brand of digoxin tablets, both of which met U.S.P. specifications, were compared.[62] On the basis of areas under the serum level-time curve, the availability of the test product was only 55% of that observed with Lanoxin.

The influence of dissolution rate on the bioavailability of digoxin from commercial tablets has been appreciated since 1972. The more rapidly dissolving of two formulations marketed at different times by the same manufacturer in England resulted in higher peak serum levels.[63,64] Two digoxin products available in Sweden that differed in dissolution rate showed comparable differences in steady-state serum concentrations after chronic administration.[65] A strong correlation between dissolution rate and peak serum digoxin concentration after a single 0.5-mg dose of digoxin in tablets from 12 different lots (Fig. 8–12) and between dissolution rate and mean steady-state serum digoxin levels after 8 to 10 days of 5 different digoxin products has also been reported.[66] The U.S.P. XXI requires that not less than 65% of the labeled amount of drug from digoxin tablets dissolve in 60 min in dilute hydrochloric acid.

An unusual and potentially dangerous situation with digoxin arose in the United Kingdom.[67] The evidence indicates that three different formulations of Lanoxin tablets, the product used by more than half the British patients requiring digoxin, were marketed over a relatively short period of time. The pre-1970 and post-May 1972 tablets gave steady-state levels that were two-thirds higher than those observed after administration of tablets marketed from 1970 to 1972. The first formulation change, made in late 1969, appears to have reduced

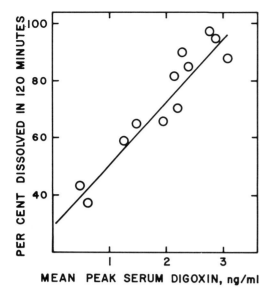

Fig. 8–12. Correlation between dissolution rate and peak serum digoxin level after a single 0.5-mg dose of different tablets. (Data from Lindenbaum, J., et al.[66])

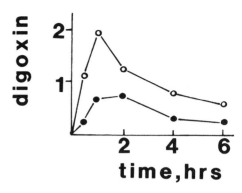

Fig. 8–13. Digoxin concentrations in plasma (ng/ml) after a single 0.5-mg oral dose in old (●) and new (○) tablets. (Data from Danon, A., et al.[71])

the bioavailability of digoxin, but this was corrected in mid-1972 by a second formulation change. From autumn 1969 to mid-1972, Lanoxin tablets were bioequivalent to most brands of digoxin marketed in England. Since mid-1972, however, there has been a significant bioavailability difference between Lanoxin tablets and the tablets of most other manufacturers.

Differences in digoxin bioavailability from different marketed tablets have also been reported in Finland[68] and Australia.[69] A useful review of digoxin bioavailability, from Sweden, was published in 1977.[70]

An interesting report from Israel, entitled "An outbreak of digoxin intoxication," has also been published.[71] Within a 2-month period between October and December 1975, 15 cases of digoxin intoxication were diagnosed on a medical ward. Almost no cases of digoxin toxicity were noted by the same physicians on the same ward during the previous year. An inquiry disclosed that the local manufacturer, without notice, had modified his formulation of digoxin to improve dissolution. Plasma levels of digoxin following single 0.5-mg doses of the old and new tablets are shown in Figure 8–13. Urinary excretion data showed more than a 2-fold difference between the two tablets in the availability of digoxin.

Furosemide

In 1979, the FDA issued a nationwide alert to patients taking the diuretic furosemide. Three manufacturers had marketed tablets of the drug without approval; these tablets were believed to be ineffective because of poor bioavailability. Patients who failed to respond to treatment with these tablets recovered when switched to an approved brand of the drug.

Martin et al.[72] compared the relative bioavailability of the brand-name tablet formulation of furosemide available in the U.S. (Lasix) and one of the generic tablets cited above. Furosemide concentrations in plasma and urine were measured after a 40-mg single dose. The bioavailability of the generic tablet was significantly less than that of the brand-name tablet. Peak furosemide levels following administration of the generic tablet were little more than 50% that observed after Lasix; total AUC was about one-third less with the generic product.

On the other hand, there was little difference with respect to 24-hr urine volume or sodium output following each product. Comparison of the effect of the two treatments is a less sensitive measure of bioequivalence and does not excuse the need for a generic product to meet expected bioavailability standards; the findings support the FDA's action against this product.

There continues to be concern about the bioavailability of furosemide tablets, fueled by differences in dissolution rate among marketed products. A recent bioavailability study compared Lasix tablets from two different lots (A, D), a generic product from two different lots (C, E), and another generic product (B), with a solution of furosemide.[73]

All of the tablets were absorbed at a slower rate (as determined by C_{max} values) and to a lesser extent (as assessed by AUC and amount excreted unchanged in the urine) than the orally administered solution of furosemide. The extent of absorption ranged from 66% for product C to 96% for product D. Variability from one lot of furosemide to another was considerable; the extent of absorption from product A was only 87% that from product D. The data suggest that products A, B, C, and E are bioequivalent but less bioavailable than product D.

Hydrochlorothiazide/Triamterene

Dyazide, a combination product containing hydrochlorothiazide 25 mg and triamterene 50 mg, is a widely prescribed potassium-sparing diuretic/antihypertensive. Since 1968, however, we have been aware that Dyazide has poor bioavailability with respect to both drugs. This was not a serious problem so long as the combination was a single source product. Matters became complicated when the period of exclusivity lapsed and other manufacturers wished to market an equivalent product. Matching precisely the incomplete bioavailability of hydrochlorothiazide and triamterene after administration of Dyazide was a difficult task and success meant the development of a poorly formulated product.

This unusual circumstance prompted the development of Maxzide, a combination product containing hydrochlorothiazide 50 mg and triamterene 75 mg. The bioavailability of both components of Maxzide is comparable to that of a liquid preparation. In fasted subjects, the absorption of both hydrochlorothiazide and triamterene from Dyazide capsules is about half that from Maxzide tablets. Maxzide was approved by the FDA on the basis of clinical studies demonstrating safety and efficacy.

A steady-state study in patients with essential hypertension concluded that the hydrochlorothiazide component of Dyazide was about two-thirds as available as that in Maxzide, while the triamterene component was less than half as bioavailable as that in Maxzide.[74] Williams et al.[75] found that the high-fat, high-calorie breakfast, recommended by the Food and Drug Administration in the evaluation of controlled-release dosage forms, had no effect on the absorption of hydrochlorothiazide or triamterene from Maxzide. On the other hand, the absorption of hydrochlorothiazide was increased by 40% and that of triamterene by 120% when Dyazide was given with the high-fat breakfast.

Levothyroxine

The bioavailability of two brands of levothyroxine, Levothroid and Synthroid, was evaluated in 34 patients who required long-term treatment with the hormone.[76] Half the patients received Levothroid for 1 month, followed by 1 month treatment with Synthroid; the other half had the opposite sequence. When patients were switched from Levothroid to Synthroid, significant decreases occurred in mean serum thyroxine levels; switching from Synthroid to Levothroid resulted in increases in thyroxine levels (Fig. 8–14). Ramos-Gabatin and co-workers concluded that marketed products of thyroxine are therapeutically inequivalent and that patients should be treated consistently with a single brand.[76] Adjustment of the dose may be necessary if the patient is switched from one brand to another.

These findings were confirmed by Sawin et al.[77] Patients with primary hypothyroidism were given oral thyroxine as Levothroid or Synthroid. Serum thyroxine was lower in all 32 patients when taking Synthroid than when taking Levothroid. Direct measurement of thyroxine in the tablets showed that Synthroid tablets contained 20 to 30% less thyroxine than label claim.

In 1984, the U.S. Pharmacopeia adopted a new method of assaying for the hormone content of levothyroxine tablets. The new assay was based on high-pressure liquid chromatography and replaced a less accurate method based on measurement of iodine content. This change required the manufacturers of Synthroid to alter their method of making the product. Synthroid tablets made before reformulation were found to contain less than 80% of labeled value, while Synthroid tablets made after the change contained 100% of the amount stated on the label.[78]

The replacement dose of the new Synthroid tablets was evaluated in 19 patients with hypothyroidism.[79] The dose was titrated monthly until thyrotropin levels become normal. The mean replacement dose was 112 μg per day, much smaller than the mean dose needed when the original product was evaluated—169 μg per day. Based on the average replacement dose, it appears that the levothyroxine content of the original tablets was approximately 70% of label claim.

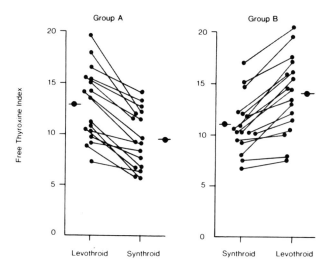

Fig. 8–14. Differences in free thyroxine index in patients switching from a regimen of Levothroid to Synthroid (group A) and in patients switching from Synthroid to Levothroid (group B). (From Ramos-Gabatin, A., Jacobson, J.M., and Young, R.L.: In vivo comparison of levothyroxine preparations. JAMA, *247*:203, 1982. Copyright 1982, American Medical Association.)

Nitrofurantoin

In single-dose bioavailability studies involving 14 different marketed products, all of which met U.S.P. specifications, significant differences between products were found in the cumulative urinary excretion of nitrofurantoin.[80] The results with two products suggested that less than 50% of the dose was absorbed. There have been several FDA recalls of nitrofurantoin tablets. Two were for failure to pass U.S.P. disintegration tests and a third was because bioavailability studies indicated poor absorption. In the latter case, urinary recovery of nitrofurantoin ranged from 2 to 14% of the dose compared to the 32% specified in the original New Drug Application.

The interest in reducing the dissolution rate of nitrofurantoin to reduce gastrointestinal upset may have led to these bioavailability problems. This situation was exacerbated by the dissolution requirement for nitrofurantoin tablets in U.S.P. XVIII, which stated that the time required for 60% of the labeled amount of nitrofurantoin to dissolve is *not less than* 1 hr. A tablet from which nitrofurantoin dissolved infinitely slowly would meet this requirement. The U.S.P. XXI requires that *not less than* 25% of the labeled amount of nitrofurantoin is dissolved in 60 min, and not less than 85% is dissolved in 120 min.

Nitrofurantoin tablets from 7 Mexican manufac-

turers as well as the innovator's tablet (Furadantin) were evaluated for disintegration, dissolution, and bioavailability.[81] The disintegration time for Furadantin was less than 1 minute; disintegration time for three lots from a single Mexican manufacturer and for one lot from another manufacturer exceeded 30 min. The percent dissolved in 60 min was less than 25% for 7 products from 3 different manufacturers. Only three products (each from a different manufacturer) dissolved sufficiently rapidly so that 85% was in solution at 120 min. Tablets from other lots made by the same manufacturers as well as the innovator's product did not meet the upper limit.

Bioavailability studies based on cumulative amount excreted after a single dose indicated that two different lots of tablets from the same manufacturer were only 30% absorbed in 1 case and 60% in the other, relative to Furadantin. For two different lots of tablets from another manufacturer, relative bioavailability was 90% for one but only 45% for the other. A statistically significant correlation ($r = 0.91$) was observed between the cumulative amount of nitrofurantoin excreted and the percent dissolved (in vitro) in 60 min for the 5 products evaluated for both dissolution and bioavailability.

Another product (Macrodantin) contains relatively large particle size nitrofurantoin, dissolves more slowly than Furadantin, and may reduce the gastrointestinal intolerance associated with rapidly dissolving products without compromising effectiveness. Mason et al.[82] evaluated the bioavailability of three macrocrystalline nitrofurantoin products, available outside the United States, relative to that of Macrodantin, the originally marketed product.

Dissolution studies indicate that at 60 min only 19% of the dose was dissolved from the Macrodantin capsule compared with 30 to 37% from the other products. The maximum rate of urinary excretion of nitrofurantoin (a parameter analogous to C_{max} and indicative of absorption rate) after a single dose of Macrodantin was 5.6 mg/hr. Maximum rates of excretion for the other products ranged from 7.5 to 8.3 mg/hr. The results indicate that some nitrofurantoin products available outside the U.S. that claim to be macrocrystalline are not bioequivalent to Macrodantin.

Oxytetracycline

In 1969, a crossover serum level study in 20 subjects was carried out on 16 lots of FDA-certified oxytetracycline hydrochloride capsules, distributed by 13 suppliers, with a single lot of Terramycin brand of oxytetracycline hydrochloride capsules as the standard in each case. The serum levels produced by capsules from 12 of these lots were significantly lower than those found with Terramycin capsules.[60]

Some time later, oxytetracycline hydrochloride capsules produced by all 11 manufacturers supplying the United States market were compared in a series of two-way crossover studies.[61] The original manufacturer's product (Terramycin) was used as the reference product. Serum concentrations of oxytetracycline after administration of 7 comparison products were more variable and markedly lower (about 50%) than those resulting from administration of the reference product.

In June 1969, the FDA stopped certification of all oxytetracycline capsules except those demonstrating acceptable bioavailability. In the next few months, some 40 million oxytetracycline capsules were recalled. Many of these products were reformulated and returned to the market in a more effective form.

Oxytetracycline bioavailability problems have also been observed in England. Significant differences in bioavailability were noted between four different marketed tablets of oxytetracycline dihydrate.[62] The results of these studies are shown in Figure 8–15. The dihydrate form of oxytetra-

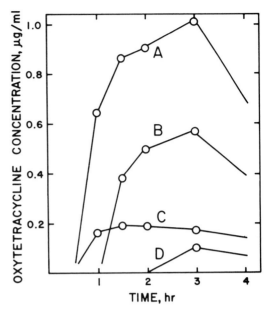

Fig. 8–15. Oxytetracycline concentrations in plasma after oral administration of different commercial tablets each containing 250 mg of oxytetracycline dihydrate. (Data from Barber, H.E., Calvey, T.N., and Muir, K.[85])

cycline is 1000 times less soluble than the hydrochloride salt and may introduce additional bioavailability problems.

Papaverine

Papaverine is used as a vasodilator and antispasmodic in the treatment of peripheral vascular disease. The bioavailability of papaverine from prolonged-release dosage forms, a conventional tablet, and an elixir was compared in healthy human subjects.[86] Plasma level data indicated equal availability of papaverine from the elixir and regular tablet; however, the AUC values for the 9 prolonged-release products ranged from 18 to 64%, relative to that resulting from the elixir. The poor performance of these marketed products may have contributed to the lack of clear-cut efficacy of the drug in various clinical trials.

Phenylbutazone

An initial report from Canada suggested significant differences in the bioavailability of phenylbutazone from different products.[87] This prompted a more comprehensive investigation of phenylbutazone blood levels after administration of 9 different tablets marketed in Canada and of an aqueous solution.[88] In comparison with the control solution, two products produced significantly lower blood levels of phenylbutazone. The absorption of phenylbutazone from one of these products was estimated to be only 60% that found from solution.

A follow-up study, in 1978, of 23 Canadian formulations of phenylbutazone found that 5 products were at least 20% less available than an oral aqueous solution of the drug.[89] Upon the advice of the Health Protection Branch Advisory Committee on Bioavailability, these products were removed from the market.

Phenytoin

The potential for variable and incomplete absorption of phenytoin from its dosage forms has been cited in many reports. Interchange of phenytoin formulations with different bioavailabilities can lead to therapeutic failure or intoxication.[90]

An unusual incidence of phenytoin intoxication in epileptic patients occurred in Australia in 1968 and 1969, following a change in the diluent of phenytoin sodium capsules from calcium sulfate to lactose. A crossover study showed that phenytoin with calcium sulfate produced lower blood levels than did phenytoin with lactose in 12 of 13 patients.[91] Presumably, the change in diluent led to greater bioavailability and a higher incidence of adverse effects with the reformulated product.

Another report, from Sweden, showed that plasma levels of phenytoin in epileptic patients were significantly higher after treatment with two preparations containing phenytoin sodium than after treatment with a third preparation containing an equivalent dose of the free acid.[92] The higher plasma levels were accompanied by better control of generalized seizures. Single-dose studies in healthy subjects showed the two preparations containing phenytoin sodium to be bioequivalent. The relative availability of phenytoin from the preparation containing the free acid was only 65%.

Substantial differences in the bioavailability of phenytoin from marketed products have also been reported in the United Kingdom[93] and in Finland.[94] The studies in the United Kingdom involved measurement of steady-state plasma phenytoin levels in 60 patients for six weeks. During the trial, the preparation of phenytoin was changed from one brand to another. A significant increase in plasma phenytoin levels was observed following the change. This was accompanied by a decrease in the number of seizures. The results of the studies in Finland are summarized in Table 8–2.

In 1978, the FDA issued new prescribing direc-

Table 8–2. Average Areas Under the Serum Phenytoin Concentration-Time Curves (AUC) in 6 Volunteers After Administration of a Single Oral Dose of 600 mg of the Drug in 4 Different Tablets and a Reference Suspension*

Dosage form	AUC (mg–hr/l)	Relative availability (%)
Tablet A	327	68
Tablet B	124	26
Tablet C	429	90
Tablet D	283	59
Suspension	480	100

*Data from Pentikäinen, P.J., Neuvonen, P.J., and Elfving, S.M.[94]

tions for phenytoin. A slow-release form, extended phenytoin sodium capsules, and a fast-release form, prompt phenytoin sodium capsules, were recognized. Only the slow-release form of the drug is approved for once-a-day dosing. On the average, the bioavailability of phenytoin is lower from the slow-release form than from the fast-release form, but considerable variability is found among patients. Patients who are maintained on one brand of phenytoin should not be switched to another brand, without considering the need for dosage adjustments.

Other reports on phenytoin bioavailability have appeared.[95,96] In 1979, Neuvonen published a review article on phenytoin bioavailability, stressing therapeutic implications.[97] For as long as phenytoin is used we must be concerned about bioavailability because this drug presents us with characteristics, including poor water solubility, low therapeutic index, and capacity-limited metabolism, that collectively are unique.

Procainamide

The bioequivalence of two prolonged-release procainamide products, Procan-SR and Pronestyl-SR, was evaluated at steady state in ten patients with cardiac arrhythmias.[98] The dose of procainamide was individualized and ranged from 2 to 3 g per day divided into 6 or 8 hourly intervals. The products were compared on a milligram-equivalent (adjusted) basis, because some patients received different daily doses of the two products.

Steady-state levels of procainamide in plasma were higher with Procan-SR than with Pronestyl-SR in 8 of 10 patients, but differences were not statistically significant. Average drug concentrations at steady state were 3.9 µg/ml for Pronestyl-SR and 4.5 µg/ml for Procan-SR. One patient, when crossed-over from Procan-SR to Pronestyl-SR, developed frequent episodes of nonsustained ventricular tachycardia. Procainamide levels in this patient were 40% less on Pronestyl-SR than on Procan-SR. These two products are probably inequivalent, but too few patients were studied to make this statement with confidence.

Quinidine

Quinidine is an old drug but still used as an antiarrhythmic agent. In a crossover study, carried out in Sweden, healthy subjects took three different formulations, each containing the same amount of quinidine base, every 12 hr for 4 days.[99] A mean steady-state serum quinidine level of 1.8 μg/ml was produced by rapidly dissolving tablets of quinidine bisulfate. One of the prolonged-release products containing quinidine bisulfate produced a mean steady-state serum level that was 23% lower than that produced by the rapidly dissolving product. A second prolonged-release preparation containing quinidine arabogalactone sulfate gave an average level that was 46% lower.

A later report from Sweden concerned the evaluation of two slow-release preparations of quinidine bisulfate (A and B).[100] The in vitro dissolution of B was unusual in that drug release was considerably faster at low pH than at neutral pH. The dissolution of quinidine from product A was essentially independent of pH. Clinical studies indicated that the availability of quinidine, as determined from AUC measurements, was about 50% greater for product A than for product B.

Bioavailability problems with prolonged-release quinidine products have also been reported in the U.S. One study compared a relatively new prolonged-release product with a widely used slow-release formulation, Quinaglute Duratabs.[101] Both products contain quinidine gluconate equivalent to 202-mg quinidine base. The extent of absorption of quinidine from the newly marketed product was only 50% that of the older product (Fig. 8–16). These findings resulted in a recall of the poorly available product by the FDA. The FDA concluded that there was a reasonable probability of serious adverse health consequences that could result from the use of this product.

Tetracycline

The first report of potential bioavailability problems with marketed dosage forms of tetracycline hydrochloride was published in 1969.[102] The ab-

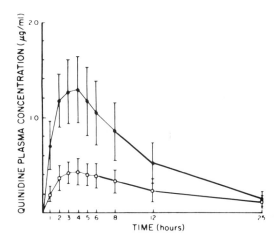

Fig. 8–16. Quinidine concentrations in plasma after single doses of quinidine gluconate tablets from 2 different manufacturers. (From Meyer, M.C., et al.[101])

sorption of tetracycline was studied after administration of four different products, including the innovator's capsule, which was used as the standard. Serum levels of tetracycline after administration of the three test products were significantly lower than those produced by the reference product.

In another study, 9 brands of tetracycline hydrochloride, marketed in Canada, were compared with an aqueous solution of the drug. Of the 9 products, 7 had relative bioavailabilities of 70 to 100%, but two products showed relative bioavailabilities of only 20 to 30%.[103] Several other reports have been summarized in a monograph.[104]

In a study reported in 1975, serum concentrations of tetracycline were compared in adults who received two different brands of tetracycline tablets.[105] Although both products passed batch certification tests of the FDA, the bioavailability of one product was only 26% that of the other.

Theophylline

The strong interest in prolonged-release theophylline for the treatment of chronic asthma has prompted several bioavailability studies that suggest clinically important differences among marketed products. One study examined several formulations in adults.[106] Absorption of theophylline from a solution or from uncoated tablets was rapid and complete. Of six prolonged-release products, three were slowly but completely and consistently absorbed. Theophylline absorption from the three other prolonged-release formulations was erratic and incomplete. One product was only 65% available relative to the solution.

Another study, comparing six prolonged-release preparations of theophylline with an elixir, found that two slow-release formulations were substantially less available than the elixir.[107] Availability of theophylline was only 48% from one slow-release product and 59% from the other.

In a recent study, 10 subjects with asthma were given the same dose of four different slow-release theophylline products twice daily for 2-week periods, to determine whether clinically important changes in serum theophylline levels occur when patients switch brands.[108] A randomized, double-blinded, crossover design was employed.

The investigators reported that on at least one occasion in every subject, switching brands was responsible for raising the serum theophylline concentrations outside the accepted therapeutic range (10 to 20 μg/ml); this was associated with adverse effects in 5 subjects. Worsening pulmonary functions were observed in 2 subjects when switching brands resulted in decreased theophylline levels. Many of the seemingly product-related changes in serum theophylline appeared to be idiosyncratic and could not be predicted by bioavailability differences between the products.

Baker et al.[108] oppose the free substitution of these formulations. They suggest that if patients are switched between different brands of slow-release theophylline, their serum theophylline concentrations need to be monitored. This is probably good advice. It is disappointing that the investigators failed to repeatedly administer a single formulation at a fixed dose for four 2-week periods to determine how frequently theophylline levels drift out of the therapeutic range when no switching occurs.

In another recent study, the relative bioavailability of two slow-release theophylline products, Slo-bid and Theo-Dur Sprinkle, was determined from saliva in preschool asthmatic children.[109] A rapidly absorbed theophylline product, Slo-Phyllin Gyrocaps was used as the bioavailability standard.

The extent of absorption was significantly less than the reference product for Theo-Dur Sprinkle but not for Slo-bid. Relative bioavailability was 66% for the Sprinkle and 109% for Slo-bid. Although Theo-Dur Sprinkle is completely absorbed in fasting subjects, under actual conditions of use a bioavailability problem is seen, probably because

food decreases the extent of absorption of theophylline from this product.

The investigators pointed out that information regarding incomplete absorption of theophylline from Theo-Dur Sprinkle is not available in the package insert. "Since substitution of more completely absorbed formulations can then inadvertently result in substantially higher serum concentrations, the availability of theophylline formulations with incomplete absorption presents a potential hazard of theophylline treatment."[109]

Tolbutamide

Tolbutamide has been identified as a drug whose clinical efficacy may be compromised by poor bioavailability. Olson et al.[110] have demonstrated that two formulations of tolbutamide, bioequivalent when newly manufactured, change differentially under certain conditions of storage.

Tablets aged by exposure to 98% relative humidity for 3 days show a decrease in dissolution rate but the effect is much greater with a generic tolbutamide product than with Orinase, the innovator's product. Before aging, 93% of the dose of Orinase was dissolved in 10 min and 100% at 30 min, compared with corresponding values of 26% and 83% for the generic tablet. Exposure of the tablets to high relative humidity decreased tolbutamide dissolution at 10 min and 30 min to 47% and 95%, respectively, for Orinase, and to 8% and 24% for the generic product.

Differences were also observed when the aged tablets were given to healthy human subjects. A single 500-mg oral dose produced a peak concentration of 52.5 μg/ml when Orinase was given, compared with a peak of 38.4 μg/ml when the generic tablet was administered. Total AUC, on the other hand, was only 10% greater after Orinase. These kinetic differences were not sufficient to significantly influence glucose concentration response.

Olson et al. also demonstrated that two tolbutamide products may be bioequivalent in fasted subjects but not when given after a meal. They administered newly-obtained tablets of Orinase and a generic tolbutamide to healthy human subjects after a standard breakfast.[110] Peak concentration was about 20% larger after Orinase; the mean time to peak concentration occurred at 2.4 hr after Orinase and 4.1 hr after the generic product. This delay in absorption resulted in a small but significant difference in glucose response at 36 min after administration, but not before or after.

The findings with tolbutamide are of interest to regulatory agencies in their effort to develop standards for demonstrating bioequivalence between products. Given the relative safety of tolbutamide, however, the changes described are of little clinical significance.

NONORAL MEDICATION

Almost all bioavailability studies reported to date have concerned oral products. This emphasis should not be construed to mean that bioavailability is not of concern with other kinds of dosage forms.

Intravenous injections, ordinarily, are free of bioavailability problems. This is not true when the injected material is a prodrug that must be hydrolyzed to parent drug. The availability of chloramphenicol after intravenous injection of chloramphenicol succinate varies considerably as a function of the patient's ability to hydrolyze the ester prodrug.

Rejection episodes in transplant patients are often treated with high doses of steroids. The aqueous solubility of prednisolone, however, is low. Intravenous injection requires the use of a soluble prodrug of prednisolone. In Switzerland, prednisolone is given intravenously as prednisolone disodium phosphate or as prednisolone sodium tetrahydrophthalate.

Patients treated for acute rejection were given on three occasions oral prednisone, iv prednisolone phosphate, and iv prednisolone phthalate, in equimolar doses.[111] Oral prednisone is biotransformed in the liver to prednisolone, the active agent. In all patients, the hydrolysis of the phosphate ester was faster than that of the phthalate ester. Mean peak concentrations of prednisolone were 18.5 µg/ml after prednisolone phosphate, 2.9 µg/ml after the phthalate, and 3.1 µg/ml after oral prednisone. Assigning a value of 100% to the AUC of prednisolone following administration of the phosphate ester, relative bioavailability was 52% for the phthalate ester and 68% for oral prednisone. The investigators concluded that "therapeutic inequivalence must be expected whenever patients are treated with equimolar doses of these three prodrugs."

Intramuscular injections of suspended material or solutions that precipitate at the injection site can also present bioavailability problems. Patients stabilized on oral phenytoin often require larger doses, at least for a period of time, when switched to the intramuscular preparation, because of the slow dissolution and absorption of crystalline phenytoin from the muscle depot.

Drug availability from rectal suppositories may be incomplete if release from the dosage form is slower than the retention time of the product. This problem has resulted in a dramatic decline in the use of theophylline suppositories.

The bioavailability of tamoxifen from rectal suppositories containing 40 mg of the drug was compared with that of oral tablets containing 20 mg in healthy male subjects.[112] Tamoxifen is widely used in the management of breast cancer. The tablets were taken with water; the suppositories were inserted after evacuation of the bowel. No defecation occurred within 6 hours after administration of a suppository.

The mean relative bioavailability from the suppositories was only 28%; the addition of a surface-active agent reduced bioavailability to 13%. The investigators concluded that rectal administration of tamoxifen leads to lower bioavailability than that found after oral administration and therefore cannot be recommended. This study, as well as others, demonstrates not only that the bioavailability of rectal tamoxifen is less than that of oral tamoxifen, but that important differences may be seen using different rectal preparations of the same drug.

Bioavailability of Topical Medication

How does one measure the bioavailability of a drug in a topical preparation? The literature concerned with this question was reviewed by Guy et al.[113] in 1986. Some investigators have applied conventional bioavailability methods and determined drug levels in plasma or urine. Usually, however, drug levels are so low that radiolabeled material is needed. Other investigators have concentrated on measuring the loss of drug from the site of application and/or the amount of drug that has penetrated the skin, using solvent washes or skin stripping with cellophane tape. Ordinarily, these methods also require labeled drug. Still others have relied on in vitro methods, measuring drug release from the ointment base into a reservoir or into or across excised animal or human skin.

For the evaluation of topical glucocorticoid preparations, most investigators have favored the so-called vasoconstrictor assay developed more than 25 years ago.[114] Application of corticosteroids to normal intact human skin results in vasoconstriction and blanching. The degree of vasoconstriction is assumed to be related to the potency of the drug; blanching is rated using a 4-point scale ranging from 0 (no vasoconstriction) to 3 (severe vasoconstriction).

Several clinical studies have generally confirmed the value of the vasoconstrictor assay, but the degree of blanching for any given product may vary widely from one person to another. The most important validation study was reported in 1985.[115] These investigators demonstrated that in 20 of 23 different comparisons the results of the vasoconstriction assay correlated with the clinical assessment of the drug.

Among the successful correlations were the following: betamethasone dipropionate 0.05% in an optimized ointment vehicle was more effective in the blanching test and in the treatment of psoriasis than was betamethasone dipropionate 0.05% in a conventional vehicle; hydrocortisone valerate cream 0.2% was more effective than hydrocortisone cream 1% in both the vasoconstrictor assay and in the clinical study; there was no difference between 1% and 2.5% hydrocortisone cream in either vasoconstriction or clinical efficacy.

For the most part, the vasoconstrictor assay has been used to predict clinical potency during the development of a new drug. More recently, it has been used to evaluate the bioequivalence of products containing the same drug, at the same strength, but differing in vehicle and/or method of preparation.[116]

The results of these comparative bioavailability studies suggest potentially important differences in clinical effects between products that are assumed to be equivalent. For example, Kenalog cream 0.1% was more potent than 5 generic creams containing triamcinolone acetonide 0.1%, Aristocort A ointment 0.1% was more potent than 2 generic ointments containing triamcinolone acetonide 0.1%, and Valisone cream 0.1% was more potent than 5 generic creams containing betamethasone valerate 0.1%. Surprisingly, no difference in the degree of blanching was noted after application of Kenalog cream 0.025%, 0.1%, or 0.5%.

These differences in marketed products that are widely assumed to be equivalent are troubling. Some will point to the failure of generic medication, but differences between generic and brand-name topical steroid products cut both ways. Some investigators have demonstrated that certain ge-

neric products produce more vasoconstriction than the "equivalent" brand-name product.[117]

An authoritative medical newsletter has observed that "different formulations of the same topical corticosteroid in the same concentration may vary in their effect on the vasoconstrictor assay and possibly in treating disease." It also notes that "some brand-name formulations appear to be more potent than their generic counterparts, but generics may also be more potent than some brand-name products. Lower concentrations of some topical corticosteroid brands may have the same effect in vasoconstrictor assays as much higher concentration of the same product."[117]

Although the results of the vasoconstrictor assay are not synonymous with clinical efficacy, there is some relationship. It is clearly imprudent to switch a patient responding to one topical corticosteroid preparation to another product. The U.S. Food and Drug Administration is working on this problem, but it is essential that the issue be resolved in a timely manner because the lack of standardization surely undermines confidence in the drug approval process.

REFERENCES

1. Shah, V.P., et al.: Comparison of plasma and urine analyses for thiazides in bioavailability/bioequivalence study. J. Pharm. Sci., 70:833, 1981.
2. Serajuddin, A.T.M., et al.: Physicochemical basis of increased bioavailability of a poorly water-soluble drug following oral administration as organic solutions. J. Pharm. Sci., 77:325, 1988.
3. Hobbs, D.C., Twomey, T.M., and Palmer, R.F.: Pharmacokinetics of prazosin in man. J. Clin. Pharmacol., 18:402, 1978.
4. Wagner, J.G., et al.: Plasma concentrations of propoxyphene in man following oral administration of the drug in solution and capsule forms. Int. J. Clin. Pharmacol., 5:371, 1972.
5. Perrier, D., and Gibaldi, M.: Influence of first-pass effect on the systemic availability of propoxyphene. J. Clin. Pharmacol., 12:449, 1972.
6. Brown, D.D., et al.: A steady-state evaluation of the effects of propantheline bromide and cholestyramine on the bioavailability of digoxin when administered as tablets or capsules. J. Clin. Pharmacol., 25:360, 1985.
7. Bjornsson, T.D., et al.: Effects of high-dose cancer chemotherapy on the absorption of digoxin in two different formulations. Clin. Pharmacol. Ther., 39:25, 1986.
8. Dickerson, J., et al.: Dose tolerance and pharmacokinetic studies of L(+) pseudoephedrine capsules in man. Eur. J. Clin. Pharmacol., 14:253, 1978.
9. Anttila, M., et al.: Comparative bioavailability of two commercial preparations of carbamazepine tablets. Eur. J. Clin. Pharmacol., 15:421, 1979.
10. Murphy, P.J., and Sullivan, H.R.: Stable isotopes in pharmacokinetic studies. Annu. Rev. Pharmacol. Toxicol., 20:609, 1980.
11. Alkalay, D., et al.: Bioavailability and kinetics of maprotiline. Clin. Pharmacol. Ther., 27:697, 1980.

12. Shinohara, Y., et al.: Stable-isotope methodology in the bioavailability study of 17-alpha-methyltestosterone using gas chromatography-mass spectrometry. J. Pharm. Sci., 75:161, 1986.
13. Heck, H., et al.: Bioavailability of imipramine tablets relative to a stable isotope-labeled internal standard: increasing the power of bioavailability tests. J. Pharmacokin. Biopharm., 7:233, 1979.
14. Gibaldi, M., and Perrier, D.: Pharmacokinetics. New York, Marcel Dekker, 1982, pp. 146–167.
15. Ronfeld, R.A., and Benet, L.Z.: Interpretation of plasma concentration-time curve after oral dosing. J. Pharm. Sci., 66:178, 1977.
16. Riegelman, S., and Collier, P.: The application of statistical moment theory to the evaluation of in vivo dissolution time and absorption time. J. Pharmacokinet. Biopharm., 8:509, 1980.
17. Hammarlund, M.M., Paalzow, L.K., Odlind, B.: Pharmacokinetics of furosemide in man after intravenous and oral administration. Application of moment analysis. Eur. J. Clin. Pharmacol., 26:197, 1984.
18. Scheline, R.R.: Metabolism of foreign compounds by gastrointestinal microorganisms. Pharmacol. Rev., 25:451, 1973.
19. Lindenbaum, J., et al.: Urinary excretion of reduced metabolites of digoxin. Am. J. Med., 71:67, 1981.
20. Lindenbaum, J., et al.: Inactivation of digoxin by the gut flora: reversal by antibiotic therapy. N. Engl. J. Med., 305:789, 1981.
21. Johnson, B.F., et al.: Effect of metoclopramide on digoxin absorption from tablets and capsules. Clin. Pharmacol. Ther., 36:724, 1984.
22. Thijssen, H.H.W., et al.: The role of the intestinal microflora in the reductive metabolism of acenocoumarol in man. Br. J. Clin. Pharmacol., 18:247, 1984.
23. Houston, J.B., Day, J., Walker, J.: Azo reduction of sulphasalazine in healthy volunteers. Br. J. Clin. Pharmacol., 14:395, 1982.
24. Rowland, M., and Tozer, T.N.: Clinical Pharmacokinetics—Concepts and Applications. 2nd Ed., Philadelphia, Lea & Febiger, 1988.
25. Shand, D.G., and Rangno, R.E.: The disposition of propranolol. I. Elimination during oral absorption in man. Pharmacology, 7:159, 1972.
26. Boyes, R.N., Scott, D.B., Jebson, P.J.: Pharmacokinetics of lidocaine in man. Clin. Pharmacol. Ther., 12:105, 1971.
27. Gram, L.F., and Christiansen, M.: First-pass metabolism of imipramine in man. Clin. Pharmacol. Ther., 17:555, 1975.
28. Garrett, E.R., et al.: Pharmacokinetics of papaverine hydrochloride and the biopharmaceutics its oral dosage forms. Int. J. Clin. Pharmacol., 16:193, 1978.
29. Ehrnebo, M., Boréus, L.O., and Lönroth, U.: Bioavailability and first-pass metabolism of oral pentazocine in man. Clin. Pharmacol. Ther., 22:888, 1977.
30. Alván, G., et al.: Importance of "first-pass elimination" for interindividual differences in steady-state concentrations of adrenergic β-receptor antagonist alprenolol. J. Pharmacokinet. Biopharm., 5:193, 1977.
31. Alván, G., et al.: First pass hydroxylation of nortriptyline: concentrations of parent drug and major metabolites in plasma. Eur. J. Clin. Pharmacol., 11:219, 1977.
32. Mistry, M., Houston, J.B.: Glucuronidation in vitro and in vivo. Comparison of intestinal and hepatic conjugation of morphine, naloxone, and buprenorphine. Drug Metabol. Dispos., 15:710, 1987.
33. Ochs, H.R., et al.: Hepatic vs gastrointestinal presystemic

34. Inaba, T., Mahon, W.A., and Stone, R.M.: Phenacetin concentrations in portal and hepatic venous blood in man. Int. J. Clin. Pharmacol., 17:371, 1979.
35. Raaflaub, J., and Dubach, U.C.: On the pharmacokinetics of phenacetin in man. Eur. J. Clin. Pharmacol., 8:261, 1975.
36. Mahon, W.A., Inaba, T., and Stone, R.M.: Metabolism of flurazepam by the small intestine. Clin. Pharmacol. Ther., 22:228, 1977.
37. Back, D.J., et al.: The gut wall metabolism of ethinylestradiol and its contribution to the pre-systemic metabolism of ethinylestradiol in humans. Br. J. Clin. Pharmacol., 13:325, 1982.
38. Back, D.J., et al.: The in vitro metabolism of ethinylestradiol, mestranol and levonorgestrel by human jejunal mucosa. Br. J. Clin. Pharmacol., 11:275, 1981.
39. Humpel, M., et al.: Investigations of pharmacokinetics of levonorgestrel to specific consideration of a first-pass effect in women. Contraception, 17:207, 1978.
40. Conolly, M.E., et al.: Metabolism of isoprenaline in dog and man. Br. J. Pharmacol., 46:458, 1972.
41. Morgan, D.J., et al.: Pharmacokinetics of intravenous and oral salbutamol and its sulphate conjugate. Br. J. Clin. Pharmacol., 22:587, 1986.
42. Leferink, J.G., et al.: Pharmacokinetics of terbutaline, a β₂-sympathomimetic, in healthy volunteers. Arzneimittelforsch., 32:159, 1982.
43. Schuirmann, D.J.: A comparison of the two one-sided tests procedure and the power approach for assessing the equivalence of average bioavailability. J. Pharmacokin. Biopharm., 15:657, 1987.
44. Wyllie, D., Pippenger, C.E., Rothner, A.D.: Increased seizure frequency with generic primidone. JAMA, 258:1216, 1987.
45. Skelly, J.P., et al.: Report of the workshop on controlled-release dosage forms: issues and controversies. Pharmac. Res., 4:75, 1987.
46. Schoenwald, R.D., and Garabedian, M.E.: Decreased bioavailability of sustained release acetazolamide dosage forms. Drug. Devel. Ind. Pharm., 4:599, 1978.
47. Friedland, B.R., Malonee, J., and Anderson, D.R.: Short-term dose response characteristics of acetazolamide in man. Arch. Ophthalmol., 95:1809, 1977.
48. Middleton, E.J., Chang, H.S., and Cook, D.: The physiologic availability and in vitro dissolution characteristics of some solid formulations of para-aminosalicylic acid and its salts. Can. J. Pharm. Sci., 3:97, 1968.
49. Wagner, J.G., et al.: Failure of U.S.P. tablet disintegration test to predict performance in man. J. Pharm. Sci., 62:859, 1973.
50. MacLeod, C., et al.: Comparative bioavailability of three brands of ampicillin. Can. Med. Assoc. J., 107:203, 1972.
51. Mayersohn, M., and Endrenyi, L.: Relative bioavailability of commercial ampicillin formulations in man. Can. Med. Assoc. J., 109:989, 1973.
52. Jusko, W.J.: Ampicillin. J. Am. Pharm. Assoc., NS 15:591, 1975.
53. Levy, G., and Hollister, L.E.: Failure of U.S.P. disintegration test to assess physiologic availability of enteric coated tablets. N.Y. State J. Med., 64:3002, 1964.
54. Clark, R.L., and Lasagna, L.: How reliable are enteric-coated aspirin preparations? Clin. Pharmacol. Ther., 6:568, 1965.
55. Yung, S., Mayersohn, M., and Robinson, J.B.: Ascorbic acid absorption in humans: a comparison among several dosage forms. J. Pharm. Sci., 71:282, 1982.

extraction of oral midazolam and flurazepam. J. Pharmacol. Exp. Ther., 243:852, 1987.

56. Maas, B., et al.: A comparative bioavailability study of carbamazepine tablets and a chewable tablet formulation. Ther. Drug Monitor, 9:28, 1987.

57. Glazko, A.J., et al.: An evaluation of the absorption characteristics of different chloramphenicol preparations in normal human subjects. Clin. Pharmacol. Ther., 9:472, 1968.

58. Staughn, A.B., Melikian, A.P., and Meyer, M.C.: Bioavailability of chlorothiazide tablets in humans. J. Pharm. Sci., 68:1099, 1979.

59. Monro, A.M., and Welling, P.G.: The bioavailability in man of marketed brands of chlorpropamide. Eur. J. Clin. Pharmacol., 7:47, 1974.

60. Berlin, A., et al.: Determination of bioavailability of diazepam in various formulations from steady-state plasma concentration data. Clin. Pharmacol. Ther., 13:733, 1972.

61. Lindenbaum, H., et al.: Variation in the biologic availability of digoxin from four preparations. N. Engl. J. Med., 285:1344, 1971.

62. Wagner, J.G., et al.: Equivalence lack in digoxin plasma levels. JAMA, 224:199, 1973.

63. Hamer, J., and Grahame-Smith, D.G.: Bioavailability of digoxin. Lancet, 2:325, 1972.

64. Whiting, B., Rodger, J.C., and Sumner, D.J.: New formulation of digoxin. Lancet, 2:922, 1972.

65. Bertler, A., et al.: Bioavailability of digoxin. Lancet, 2:708, 1972.

66. Lindenbaum, J., et al.: Correlation of digoxin tablet dissolution rate with biological availability. Lancet, 1:1215, 1973.

67. Shaw, T.R.D., Howard, M.R., and Hamer, J.: Recent changes in biological availability of digoxin. Effect of an alteration in "Lanoxin" tablets. Br. Heart J., 36:85, 1974.

68. Karjalainen, J., Ojala, K., and Reissel, P.: Nonequivalent digoxin tablets. Ann. Clin. Res., 6:132, 1974.

69. McCredie, R.M., et al.: Digoxin preparations: Variation in biological availability. Med. J. Aust., 2:922, 1973.

70. Nyberg, L.: Bioavailability of digoxin in man after oral administration of preparations with different dissolution rates. Acta Pharmacol. Toxicol., Vol. 40, Suppl. III, 1977.

71. Danon, A., et al.: An outbreak of digoxin intoxication. Clin. Pharmacol. Ther., 21:643, 1977.

72. Martin, B.K., et al.: Comparative bioavailability of two furosemide formulations in humans. J. Pharm. Sci., 73:437, 1984.

73. McNamara, P.J., et al.: Influence of tablet dissolution on furosemide bioavailability: a bioequivalence study. Pharmac. Res., 4:150, 1987.

74. Williams, R.L., et al.: Absorption and disposition of two combination formulations of hydrochlorothiazide and triamterene: influence of age and renal function. Clin. Pharmacol. Ther., 40:226, 1986.

75. Williams, R.L., et al.: Effects of formulation and food on the absorption of hydrochlorothiazide and triamterene or amiloride from combination diuretic products. Pharmac. Res., 4:348, 1987.

76. Ramos-Gabatin, A., Jacobson, J.M., and Young, R.L.: In vivo comparison of levothyroxine preparations. JAMA, 247:203, 1982.

77. Sawin, C.T., et al.: Oral thyroxine: variations in biologic action and tablet content. Ann. Intern. Med., 100:641, 1984.

78. Stoffer, S.S., Szpunar, W.E.: Potency of levothyroxine products. JAMA, 251:635, 1984.

79. Fish, L.H., et al.: Replacement dose, metabolism, and bioavailability of levothyroxine in the treatment of hypothyroidism. Role of triiodothyronine in pituitary feedback in humans. N. Engl. J. Med., 316:764, 1987.

80. Meyer, M.C., et al.: Bioavailability of 14 nitrofurantoin products. J. Pharm. Sci., 63:1693, 1974.

81. Lopez, A.A., et al.: Bioequivalence study of nitrofurantoin tablets: in vitro-in vivo correlation. Int. J. Pharmac., 28:167, 1986.

82. Mason, W.D., Conklin, J.D., Hailey, F.J.: Relative bioavailability of four macrocrystalline nitrofurantoin capsules. Int. J. Pharmac., 36:105, 1987.

83. Brice, G.W., and Hammer, H.F.: Therapeutic nonequivalence of oxytetracycline capsules. JAMA, 208:1189, 1969.

84. Blair, D.C., et al.: Biological availability of oxytetracycline HCl capsules. JAMA, 215:251, 1971.

85. Barber, H.E., Calvey, T.N., and Muir, K.: Biological availability and in vitro dissolution of oxytetracycline dihydrate tablets. Br. J. Clin. Pharmacol., 1:405, 1974.

86. Meyer, M., Gollamudi, R., and Straughn, A.B.: The influence of dosage form on papaverine bioavailability. J. Clin. Pharmacol., 19:435, 1979.

87. Searl, R.O., and Pernarowski, M.: The biopharmaceutical properties of solid dosage forms: I. An evaluation of 23 brands of phenylbutazone tablets. Can. Med. Assoc. J., 96:1513, 1967.

88. Van Petten, G.R., et al.: The physiologic availability of phenylbutazone, Part I. In vivo physiologic availability and pharmacologic considerations. J. Clin. Pharmacol., 11:177, 1971.

89. McGilveray, I.J., Mousseau, N., and Brien, R.: The bioavailability of 23 Canadian formulations of phenylbutazone. Can. J. Pharm. Sci., 13:33, 1978.

90. Feldman, S.: Phenytoin (diphenylhydantoin). J. Am. Pharm. Assoc., NS 15:647, 1975.

91. Bochner, F., et al.: Factors involved in an outbreak of phenytoin intoxication. J. Neurol. Sci., 16:481, 1972.

92. Lund, L.: Clinical significance of generic inequivalence of three different pharmaceutical preparations of phenytoin. Eur. J. Clin. Pharmacol., 7:119, 1974.

93. Stewart, M.J., et al.: Bioavailability of phenytoin. A comparison of two preparations. Eur. J. Clin. Pharmacol., 9:209, 1975.

94. Pentikäinen, P.J., Neuvonen, P.J., and Elfving, S.M.: Bioavailability of four brands of phenytoin tablets. Eur. J. Clin. Pharmacol., 9:213, 1975.

95. Neuvonen, P.J., Bardy, A., and Lehtovarra, R.: Effect of increased bioavailability of phenytoin tablets on serum phenytoin concentration in epileptic outpatients. Br. J. Clin. Pharmacol., 8:37, 1979.

96. Boréus, L.O., et al.: A comparison between microcrystalline and conventional phenytoin preparations: relative bioavailability and steady-state plasma concentrations. J. Neurol., 223:241, 1980.

97. Neuvonen, P.J.: Bioavailability of phenytoin: clinical pharmacokinetics and therapeutic implications. Clin. Pharmacokin., 4:91, 1979.

98. Hilleman, D.E., et al.: Comparative bioequivalence and efficacy of two sustained-release procainamide formulations in patients with cardiac arrhythmias. Drug Intell. Clin. Pharm., 22:554, 1988.

99. Henning, R., and Nyberg, G.: Serum quinidine levels after administration of three different quinidine preparations. Eur. J. Clin. Pharmacol., 6:239, 1975.

100. Regårdh, C.-G., et al.: Bioavailability of quinidine in slow-release form. A comparison between two preparations containing quinidine bisulphate as the active constituent. Arzneimittelforsch., 27:1716, 1977.

101. Meyer, M.C., et al.: Serious bioavailability problems with a generic prolonged-release quinidine gluconate product. J. Clin. Pharmacol., 22:131, 1982.

102. MacDonald, H., et al.: Physiologic availability of various tetracyclines. Clin. Med., 76:30, 1969.

103. Lovering, E.G., et al.: The bioavailability and dissolution behavior of nine brands of tetracycline tablets. Can. J. Pharm. Sci., 10:36, 1975.

104. Sokolski, T.D.: Tetracycline. J. Am. Pharm. Assoc., NS 15:709, 1975.

105. DeSante, K.A., et al.: Antibiotic batch certification and bioequivalence. JAMA, 232:1349, 1975.

106. Weinberger, M., Hendeles, L., and Bighley, L.: The relation of product formulation to absorption of oral theophylline. N. Engl. J. Med., 299:852, 1978.

107. Spangler, D.L., et al.: Theophylline bioavailability following oral administration of six sustained-release preparations. Ann. Allergy, 40:6, 1978.

108. Baker, J.R., Jr., et al.: Clinical relevance of the substitution of different brands of sustained-release theophylline. J. Allergy Clin. Immunol., 81:664, 1988.

109. Vaughan, L.M., et al.: Oral bioavailability of slow-release theophylline from unencapsulated beads in preschool children with chronic asthma. Ther. Drug Monitor, 10:395, 1988.

110. Olson, S.C., et al.: Effect of food and tablet age on relative bioavailability and pharmacodynamics of two tolbutamide products. J. Pharm. Sci., 74:735, 1985.

111. Frey, B.M., Seeberger, M., Frey, F.J.: Pharmacokinetics of 3 prednisolone prodrugs. Evidence of therapeutic inequivalence in renal transplant patients with rejection. Transplantation, 39:270, 1985.

112. Tukker, J.J., Blankenstein, M.A., Nortier, J.W.R.: Comparison of bioavailability in man of tamoxifen after oral and rectal administration. J. Pharm. Pharmacol., 38:888, 1986.

113. Guy, R.H., et al.: The bioavailability of dermatologic and other topically administered drugs. Pharmac. Res., 3:253, 1986.

114. McKenzie, A.W., Stoughton, R.B.: Method for comparing percutaneous absorption of steroids. Arch. Dermatol., 86:608, 1962.

115. Cornell, R.C., Stoughton, R.B.: Correlation of the vasoconstriction assay and clinical activity in psoriasis. Arch. Dermatol., 121:63, 1985.

116. Stoughton, R.B.: Are generic formulations equivalent to trade name topical glucocorticoids? Arch. Dermatol., 123:1312, 1987.

117. Generic topical corticosteroids. Med. Lett. Drugs Ther., 30:49, 1988.

9

Drug Concentration and Clinical Response

The response of an enzyme, an animal, or a human patient to a drug depends on the dose we give. There is a dose, even of the most potent chemical, that will not elicit a response. A larger dose will produce an effect that we can see or measure, and the intensity will probably increase as we increase the dose. At relatively large doses we may see new and unwanted effects added to the original effect; ultimately, we find a dose large enough to kill or destroy the test system.

The relationship between dose and response is the cornerstone of modern drug therapy. When a patient fails to respond to a dosage regimen, we consider the need for a larger, more effective dose. When a patient manifests undesirable or toxic effects in response to a dosage regimen, we consider the need for a smaller, safer dose. This method for optimization of drug therapy, based on empirical dose adjustment, sometimes succeeds, but is costly and time consuming.

The principal shortcoming of empirical dose adjustments can be found in the dose-response relationship itself. This relationship can be rigorously developed in an individual, but it will not apply to all individuals in a population. Stated another way, the same dose of a drug will produce a different intensity of effect in different individuals. Figure 9–1 shows the distribution of responses to a 0.02 mg/kg intramuscular dose of atropine. The average patient responds with an increase in heart rate of about 20 beats/min, but some patients show no change over resting heart rate, whereas others have an exaggerated response, up to 60 beats/min.[1]

There are two reasons why a single dose-response relationship does not apply to the popula-

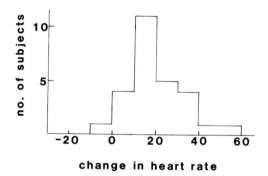

Fig. 9–1. Effect of intramuscular atropine sulfate (0.02 mg/kg) on heart rate (beats/min) in 27 subjects. (Data from Smith, S.E., and Rawlins, M.D.[1])

tion: one reason is called *pharmacodynamic variability* and the other is termed *pharmacokinetic variability*. Pharmacodynamic variability simply means that some individuals are more sensitive or more resistant to the effects of the drug than other individuals. Pharmacokinetic variability means that the same dose of a drug produces different concentrations at the sites of pharmacologic effect in different individuals because of interpatient variability in drug absorption, distribution, excretion, and metabolism.

There is now considerable evidence, from both animal and human studies, that response is better correlated with drug concentrations in blood or plasma than with the administered dose. A classical example is found in the work of Kato and co-workers.[2] The same intraperitoneal dose (110 mg/kg) of zoxazolamine, a muscle relaxant, given to 178 female rats produced a loss of righting reflex that lasted anywhere from 100 to 800 min (Fig. 9–2). Remarkably, the drug concentration in serum

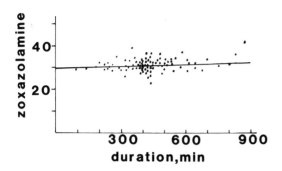

Fig. 9–2. Individual differences in zoxazolamine concentration in serum (μg/ml) on recovery from paralysis after a 110 mg/kg intraperitoneal dose to female rats. (Data from Kato, R., Takanaka, A., and Onoda, K.[2])

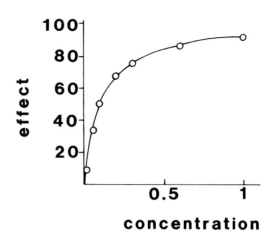

Fig. 9–3. Typical drug concentration-effect relationship resulting from the reversible interaction of drug and receptor. Effect is expressed as percent of maximum response.

at the end of paralysis was about the same in all rats irrespective of the duration of effect. Similar results were found with respect to the duration of narcosis following pentobarbital administration and the serum concentrations of pentobarbital upon recovery.[2]

Remarkable sex differences in response to drugs are well known in the rat. The same dose of hexobarbital produces 19 min of sleep in the male rat but 109 min in the female; however, the brain levels of hexobarbital upon recovery are almost identical in both male and female rats, about 53 μg/g.[3] Sex differences in the mouse are less common. Both male and female mice respond to a 100 mg/kg dose of hexobarbital with a duration of sleep of about 45 min. Despite these substantial species differences, brain levels of hexobarbital upon recovery in both male and female mice are the same as those found in rats.[3] These studies demonstrate the importance of drug concentration in determining drug effect. The relationship between drug concentration and response and the prevalence of pharmacokinetic variability form the cornerstone of clinical pharmacokinetics.

CONCENTRATION-RESPONSE RELATIONSHIPS

Quantitative relationships between drug concentration and response are based on a model for drug response. One model, which is both simple and useful, assumes that a drug interacts reversibly with a receptor in the body; the resultant effect of this interaction is proportional to the number of recep-

tors occupied. The following reaction scheme applies:

$$\text{Drug [D]} + \text{Receptor [R]} \underset{k_2}{\overset{k_1}{\rightleftharpoons}} \text{[DR]} \rightarrow \text{Effect}$$

$$(9\text{–}1)$$

This reaction sequence is analogous to the interaction of a substrate with an enzyme; it leads to the following relationship between effect and drug concentration:

$$\text{Effect} = \frac{\text{Maximum Effect [D]}}{K_D + \text{[D]}} \quad (9\text{–}2)$$

where K_D is the dissociation constant for the drug-receptor complex and [D] is drug concentration. There is no effect when [D] = 0; the effect is half-maximum when [D] = K_D (i.e., when half the receptors are occupied); as [D] increases above K_D, the maximum effect is approached asymptomatically. A more familiar form of Eq. 9–2 is:

$$E = \frac{E_{max} C}{EC_{50} + C} \quad (9\text{–}2a)$$

where EC_{50} is the concentration at which 50% of the effect is observed, E_{max} is the maximum effect, and C is drug concentration. Figure 9–3 is a plot of percent of maximum response as a function of drug concentration according to Equation 9–2. It shows a linear relationship between effect and concentration at low drug concentrations. This plot is characteristic of most concentration-response curves. It applies to in vitro experiments, which

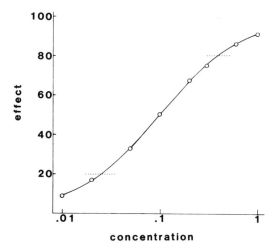

Fig. 9–4. Typical logarithmic drug concentration-effect relationship resulting from the reversible interaction of drug and receptor. Effect is expressed as percent of maximum response. The plot is approximately linear between 20% and 80% of maximum response.

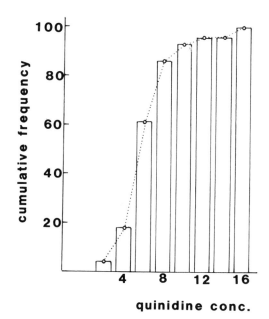

Fig. 9–5. Cumulative frequency of conversion (expressed as percent) in patients with auricular fibrillation as a function of quinidine concentration in serum (μg/ml). (Data from Sokolow, M., and Edgar, A.L.[6])

include studies of drug action on enzymes, other proteins, microorganisms, or isolated tissues or organs, to animal studies, and to clinical investigations in human patients.

A more common representation of concentration-response data is a plot of response versus the logarithm of the concentration (Fig. 9–4).[4,5] The most important feature of this transformation is the apparently linear relationship between response and drug concentration at concentrations producing effects of between 20% and 80% of the maximum effect. The logarithmic transformation of drug concentration gives rise to the following widely used, empirical relationship:

$$\text{Effect} = S \log [C] + I \qquad (9\text{–}3)$$

where S is the slope of the effect-log concentration plot and I is an empiric constant.

In some cases, the effect-concentration relationship is steeper or shallower than predicted from Eq. 9–2. A better fit may be obtained by describing the relationship as follows:

$$E = E_{max} \, C^n / (EC_{50}{}^n + C^n) \qquad (9\text{–}3a)$$

where n is a shape factor that accounts for deviations from a perfect hyperbola. If $n = 1$, Equation 9–3a is the same as Equation 9–2a and plots of effect versus drug concentration or log drug concentration will be similar to those shown in Figures 9–3 and 9–4, respectively. The larger the value of n, the steeper is the apparently linear portion of

the effect-log concentration plot. Assuming that Equation 9–3 applies, the larger the value of n, the larger is the value of S. When $n = 1$, a 16-fold increase in drug concentration around the EC_{50} is needed to increase the response from 20 to 80% of maximum; when $n = 2$, only a 4-fold increase is required.

The reversible drug-receptor interaction model adequately accounts for the *graded responses* produced by many drugs; as we increase the dose or concentration, we also increase the intensity of effect. However, there are some pharmacologic or toxic responses that cannot be measured on a continuous basis. For example, an anticonvulsant drug either prevents a seizure or does not prevent a seizure. The same is true for certain effects of antiarrhythmic drugs. The arrhythmia either is or is not suppressed. Such effects are known as *quantal* or *all-or-none* responses.

In the case of all-or-none responses, the relationship between concentration and response can be developed in terms of the frequency of an event in the patient population. Figure 9–5 shows the cumulative frequency of conversions in 28 patients with auricular fibrillation as a function of serum concentrations of quinidine.[6] This frequency histogram has roughly the same shape as the effect-concentration curve shown in Figure 9–3. The data show that serum quinidine levels of 5 to 6 μg/ml are required to get conversion in 50% of the population; serum levels of 7 to 8 μg/ml are needed for an 80% response rate.

DRUG CONCENTRATION AND THERAPEUTIC EFFECTIVENESS

Since the response to a drug increases with increasing drug concentration, it may seem reasonable to suggest that patients who do not respond to a drug should be given more drug to produce higher blood levels. This simple view of drug therapy may apply to those drugs that produce a single, specific pharmacologic effect, the so-called magic bullet, but it does not apply to most drugs. Perhaps the antibiotics come closest to this ideal. Most drugs produce multiple effects; they simultaneously affect more than one, sometimes many, organs or systems in the body. The β-blockers simultaneously affect beta-adrenergic receptors in heart and bronchi, producing desired effects on the cardiovascular system and unwanted effects, such as bronchospasm, on the pulmonary system. For this reason, a drug like propranolol should be avoided in patients with asthma or bronchitis.

The multiple effects of drugs greatly complicate the drug concentration-therapeutic effectiveness re-lationship. Figure 9–6 is a schematic representation of the desired pharmacologic effect, lack of effect, minor side effects, major side effects, and therapeutic effectiveness relationships with serum concentrations of procainamide in patients receiving this drug for the treatment of arrhythmias.[7,8] The desired pharmacologic effect is the suppression of abnormal cardiac rhythms. Side effects are classified as minor if the drug need not be withdrawn, and as serious when disturbances of cardiovascular function require discontinuation of the drug. Serious toxic effects include severe hypotension, atrioventricular and intraventricular conduction disturbances, appearance of major new ventricular arrhythmias, and cardiac arrest.

The frequency-drug concentration curves for desired pharmacologic effect, minor toxicity, and major toxicity shown in Figure 9–6 resemble portions of the concentration-effect curves shown in Figures 9–3 to 9–5. Arrhythmias will be suppressed in the majority of patients at procainamide concentrations of 4 μg/ml or more. Procainamide is a useful drug because drug concentrations associated with desired effect are lower than those associated with serious toxicity. Many patients, however, do not respond to procainamide until concentrations of 6 to 10 μg/ml are reached; some of these patients

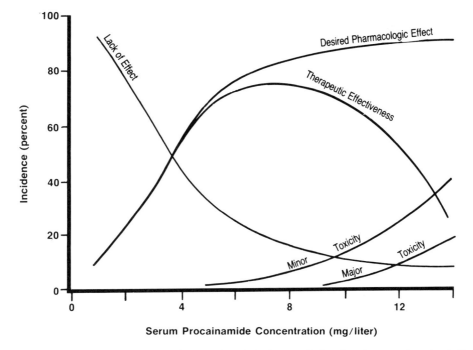

Fig. 9–6. Schematic representation of the incidence of desired pharmacologic effect (suppression of arrhythmias), lack of effect, minor and major side effects, and therapeutic effectiveness (desired pharmacologic effect minus toxicity) as a function of procainamide concentration in serum. (From Rowland, M., and Tozer, T.N.[8])

will experience minor adverse effects. Although these effects are considered minor, they may be sufficiently troubling to the patient to prompt self-discontinuation of the drug. A small number of patients do not respond to procainamide until concentrations of 10 to 14 μg/ml are achieved; many of these individuals will be plagued with minor adverse effects, and some will experience major toxicity that requires discontinuing the drug.

This description of the effects of procainamide in a patient population clearly shows that although the pharmacologic effectiveness increases with drug concentration, the therapeutic effectiveness does not. Therapeutic effectiveness may be viewed as the difference between pharmacologic effectiveness and toxicity or the benefit-to-risk ratio of a drug. Therapeutic effectiveness of procainamide increases with drug concentration to a maximum value, about 7 to 8 μg/ml, but then decreases with increasing drug concentration. These characteristics are typical of almost all drugs used today and lead us to the idea of a *therapeutic concentration range,* bounded at one end by the need to have pharmacologic effectiveness and at the other by the need to minimize toxicity.

The therapeutic concentration range of procainamide is about 4 to 10 μg/ml. Most patients do not respond to lower concentrations of the drug and some patients will experience serious adverse effects at higher concentrations. The establishment of a therapeutic concentration range for a population is hardly absolute; it requires judgment as to the importance of adverse effects. For example, if many patients elect to discontinue procainamide when faced with its minor adverse effects, it may be more realistic to define the therapeutic range as 4 to 8 μg/ml. For this reason, one may find more than one set of values cited in the literature for the therapeutic concentration range of a drug.

The therapeutic concentration range applies to an individual patient only to the extent that this patient is typical of the population. Figure 9–6 shows that some patients will benefit from serum concentrations of procainamide as low as 1 to 2 μg/ml, whereas other patients can tolerate concentrations as high as 12 to 14 μg/ml. It is helpful, therefore, to think of a therapeutic concentration range only as a guide for optimizing drug therapy.

Therapeutic concentration ranges have now been developed for perhaps 20 to 30 drugs; some are listed in Table 9–1. Experience has shown that the range for most of these drugs is narrow; the ratio

Table 9–1. Usual Therapeutic Concentration Range for Specific Drugs

Drug	Disease	Therapeutic range
Carbamazepine	Epilepsy	4–12 μg/ml
Digoxin	Congestive heart failure	0.5–2.0 ng/ml
Disopyramide	Arrhythmias	3–5 μg/ml
Gentamicin	Infection	1–10 μg/ml
Lidocaine	Arrhythmias	2–6 μg/ml
Nortriptyline	Depression	50–150 ng/ml
Phenytoin	Epilepsy	10–20 μg/ml
Procainamide	Arrhythmias	4–8 μg/ml
Salicylic acid	Rheumatoid arthritis	10–30 mg/dl
Theophylline	Asthma	10–20 μg/ml

of the upper limit to the lower limit is often only 2 or 3. The significance of the upper limit may be different for different drugs. Most often the upper limit reflects toxicity. However, in the case of nortriptyline, and perhaps other antidepressants, the upper limit reflects loss of effectiveness without signs of increasing toxicity. When toxicity is limiting it may be an extension of the pharmacologic effect of the drug (e.g., the bleeding problem associated with high concentrations of warfarin) or a different effect seemingly unrelated to the desired effect of the drug (e.g., the seizures resulting from high concentrations of theophylline). In some situations a drug may be used for more than one indication and different therapeutic ranges may apply to different conditions. The value cited in Table 9–1 for salicylic acid applies to its use as an anti-inflammatory agent in rheumatoid arthritis. Lower concentrations are adequate when the drug is used as an analgesic for simple aches and pains; but higher concentrations of salicylate may be needed for the treatment of rheumatic fever.

FACTORS COMPLICATING CONCENTRATION-RESPONSE RELATIONSHIPS

Most drugs are found in the blood in both free and bound forms. Drugs commonly bind to plasma proteins and, sometimes, to the formed elements of the blood. The degree of binding may vary widely from one patient to another. Only free drug is able to diffuse from the blood to the extravascular site of drug action. It would seem reasonable that concentration-response relationships be based on free rather than total drug concentration in blood or plasma, but usually this is not the case. All values cited in Table 9–1 refer to total drug concentrations. The determination of free drug concentration presents serious technical problems. Although progress is being made, routine measurement of free drug is still some time off.

When variability in plasma protein binding of a drug is considerable, difficulty in estimating free drug concentration is a complicating factor to establishing a concentration-response relationship for a population. The therapeutic concentration range of 10 to 20 μg/ml for phenytoin, in the treatment of epilepsy, is appropriate for patients with normal renal function, but it may be as low as 5 to 10 μg/ml for patients with uremia because plasma protein binding of phenytoin is substantially reduced in these patients.

The therapeutic range for phenytoin in terms of free drug concentration is about 1 to 2 μg/ml. On the average, phenytoin is bound to plasma proteins to the extent of about 90%. Reduced binding occurs in patients with impaired renal function, but the free drug concentration needed to produce optimal effects in most patients is still 1 to 2 μg/ml.

Some drugs have active metabolites that contribute to the pharmacologic effects and therapeutic effectiveness of the drug; examples include imipramine, propranolol, phenacetin, diazepam, procainamide, and meperidine. Concentration-response relationships based on the concentration of parent drug alone may be misleading. Efforts to establish a therapeutic concentration range for amitriptyline, an antidepressant drug, take into account the concentration of both amitriptyline and its active metabolite, nortriptyline.

Drugs that are subject to presystemic metabolism may result in higher concentrations of active metabolites after oral administration than after intravenous administration. Under these conditions, concentration-effect curves based only on the concentration of administered drug may be different for oral and intravenous doses. Figure 9–7 shows concentration-effect curves for propranolol. The drug appears to be much more active after oral than after intravenous administration. This anomalous result can be explained by the formation of significant amounts of an active metabolite, 4-hydroxypropranolol, when propranolol is given orally.[9] Presystemic formation of active metabolites also seems to explain why the change in electrocardiograph QT interval per mg/L quinidine concentration is greater after oral dosing than after intravenous administration.[10]

Many drugs are administered as racemates,

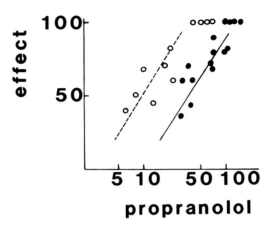

Fig. 9–7. Relationship between effect (percent block of exercise-induced tachycardia) and propranolol concentration (ng/ml) in plasma (log scale) after oral (○) and intravenous (●) administration. (Data from Coltart, D.J., and Shand, D.G.[9])

mixtures of two optically active enantiomorphs of the drug. In some cases there are considerable differences between the enantiomorphs in terms of pharmacologic activity and rates of elimination. Attempts to establish concentration-effect relationships based on total drug concentration can lead to confusing and erroneous results. Ideally, the concentration-response relationship for each enantiomorph, administered separately, should be established before attempting to resolve the effects of the racemate.

Delays in response are sometimes encountered after administering a drug. Figure 9–8 shows plasma concentrations of cocaine after rapid intravenous injection and its effect on heart rate in adult

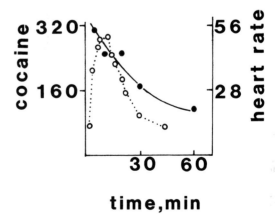

Fig. 9–8. Relationship between cocaine concentrations in plasma (●) (ng/ml) and the percent change in heart rate (○) after a 32-mg intravenous dose. (Data from Javaid, J.I., et al.[11])

cocaine users.[11] Cocaine concentrations are at a maximum almost immediately after injection, but the maximum effect of the drug is delayed 10 to 12 min. These delays usually reflect the time needed for equilibration of drug between the blood and the site of effect. They are often short, only minutes, but may be longer when the drug diffuses slowly into the site. For example, the maximum cardiac effects of digoxin are not seen for an hour or more after rapid intravenous injection of the drug.

Long delays may also be encountered when the clinical response is an indirect measure of drug effect. Warfarin and other coumarin anticoagulants directly inhibit the synthesis of certain clotting factors. The anticoagulant effect of warfarin is an indirect result of the inhibition and ultimate depletion of body stores of these clotting factors; depletion is a relatively slow process. Accordingly, the maximum effect of warfarin on blood clotting is not seen until 1 or 2 days after a rapidly absorbed oral dose of the drug. A dissociation between the direct effects of a drug and its clinical manifestations may also explain why up to 4 to 6 weeks of tricyclic antidepressant therapy may be required before maximum benefits are observed.

The effectiveness of a drug can diminish with continual use. This situation is often called an acquired tolerance to the effects of a drug. Several kinds of acquired tolerances have been described, including pharmacokinetic and pharmacodynamic tolerances. The rate of metabolism of some drugs (e.g., carbamazepine) increases with repeated administration so that a maintenance dose produces lower blood levels than those following the initial dose. This is an example of pharmacokinetic tolerance; it can usually be overcome by increasing the dose of the drug. Pharmacodynamic tolerance means that the same concentration of drug in the blood will elicit a diminished pharmacologic response after a period of drug use than after initial treatment. Animals made tolerant to barbiturates or alcohol show significantly less sedation and ataxia than do nontolerant animals at the same blood concentrations.

Tolerance to the hemodynamic effects of nitroglycerin and other organic nitrates is a serious clinical problem. The problem is most evident with transdermal nitroglycerin patches, sustained release forms of isosorbide dinitrate, and continuous intravenous infusions of nitroglycerin. In each case, relatively high and continuous plasma levels of nitrates are maintained, while the effects of the drug fade away. Intermittent application of nitroglycerin ointment or oral administration of conventional tablets or capsules of isosorbide dinitrate 2 or 3 times a day has not been found to produce tolerance, presumably because nitrate levels go up and down and there are periods when nitrate levels in plasma are negligible.

Packer et al.[12] treated patients with severe chronic heart failure with iv nitroglycerin given continuously over 48 hr. Twenty-four hr before nitroglycerin, each patient received a 40-mg oral dose of isosorbide dinitrate. A second and third dose of isosorbide dinitrate were given 2 hr and 24 hr after stopping the nitroglycerin infusion.

Within 2 hours of starting nitroglycerin, significant hemodynamic benefits were observed in all patients: an increase in stroke volume index and falls in mean arterial pressure and systolic vascular resistance. These initial responses, however, were markedly attenuated after 48 hr of uninterrupted treatment. Seventeen of the 24 patients had a complete loss of hemodynamic effects, and effects were significantly diminished in the others.

All patients responded to the first dose of isosorbide dinitrate but showed no response to the second dose, given 2 hr after the nitroglycerin infusion. Responsiveness was restored when isosorbide dinitrate was administered 24 hr after discontinuing the infusion. This study demonstrated that acute tolerance to nitroglycerin develops within hours of starting a constant rate iv infusion and that this treatment also gives rise to cross-tolerance to the effects of isosorbide dinitrate and probably other organic nitrates.

The acute tolerance to nitroglycerin has prompted prescribers to recommend that nitroglycerin patches be applied for only 12 to 16 hr a day (with a new patch applied every morning), rather than continuously as currently recommended by the manufacturers. Studies have determined that a 8 to 12 hr drug-free period is sufficient to overcome nitrate tolerance and restore responsiveness.

Cowan et al.[13] compared continuous and intermittent treatment with a nitroglycerin patch delivering 10 mg every 24 hr in patients with stable exertional angina. Patches were changed twice daily at 8 AM and 8 PM. In the continuous treatment arm of the study both patches were active; during intermittent treatment only the morning patch was active. On the eighth day, exercise testing was carried out at 8:30 AM with the previous evening's patch in place. A new (active) patch was applied at 9 AM and the patients were retested at 12:30 PM.

The first exercise test on the eighth day found no difference between those wearing an active patch (continuous group) and those wearing a placebo patch (intermittent group). Three and a half hr after application of an active patch, there was a marked improvement in exercise time for the intermittent group but no effect in the continuous group. The investigators concluded that attempts at 24-hr protection with nitrates in angina may be self-defeating.

The mechanism for the acute tolerance to organic nitrates is not completely understood. One theory suggests that nitrates increase coronary blood flow by interacting with sulfhydryl groups in vascular smooth muscle, leading to the production of S-nitrosothiols. These compounds activate guanylate cyclase and increase the intracellular concentration of cyclic guanosine monophosphate (cyclic GMP), resulting in vascular relaxation and vasodilation. Tolerance may develop if sulfhydryl availability is limited, perhaps because continuous exposure to nitrates used them up. If this hypothesis is correct, an exogenous source of sulfhydryl groups, such as N-acetylcysteine, might reverse tolerance.

To test the sulfhydryl hypothesis, Packer et al.[12] administered oral N-acetylcysteine to patients during prolonged nitroglycerin infusion. The patients were initially responsive to nitroglycerin but at the time N-acetylcysteine was given they were completely tolerant. In these patients, N-acetylcysteine produced a significant improvement in all hemodynamic variables, a response almost as strong as the initial response to nitroglycerin, but had no hemodynamic effects in patients with heart failure who were not receiving nitroglycerin.

Tolerance to the acute effects of nicotine has also been observed. When a short (10-min) intravenous infusion of nicotine is given every half hr, the increase in heart rate produced by the first infusion is greater than that produced by any of the following infusions, despite the fact that with each successive infusion higher blood levels of nicotine occur until steady state is reached.[14] Also, the increase in heart rate after iv nicotine is much smaller when the injection is given after subjects had smoked several cigarettes than after overnight abstinence from smoking.[15]

TIME COURSE OF DRUG EFFECTS

A drug that produces an all-or-none response is effective as long as its concentration remains above

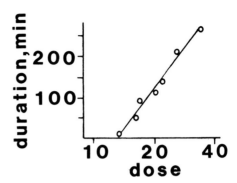

Fig. 9–9. Relationship between intravenous dose of pentobarbital (mg/kg, log scale) and duration of anesthesia in monkeys. (Data from Levy, G.[16])

some minimum concentration at the site of action. Therefore, the duration of effect is a function of dose and the rate of removal from the site of action. The larger the dose and the slower the rate of removal, the longer is the duration of action. Two factors can control the rate of removal of drug from the site of action: redistribution of drug from the site to other, less well-perfused tissues, or elimination of drug from the body. The short-lived effect of thiopental on the central nervous system is an example of redistribution-controlled removal rather than elimination-controlled removal from the site of action. In most cases, however, the rate of removal of drug from the site of action probably corresponds to its rate of removal from the body.

After a bolus intravenous dose of a drug that distributes rapidly, the amount of drug in the body (A) is given by:

$$\log A = \log Dose - kt/2.303 \qquad (9\text{–}4)$$

where k is the first-order elimination rate constant. Body levels decline until a level is reached that we shall define as the minimum effective level of drug in the body (A_{min}). At this time, $t = t_d$, the duration of effect of the drug. It follows that:

$$\log A_{min} = \log Dose - kt_d/2.303 \qquad (9\text{–}5)$$

Solving Equation 9–5 for the duration of effect (t_d) yields:

$$t_d = 2.303(\log Dose - \log A_{min})/k \qquad (9\text{–}6)$$

Equation 9–6 indicates that under these conditions a plot of duration of effect versus log dose yields a straight line with a slope equal to 2.303/k and an intercept, on the x-axis, corresponding to A_{min} (Fig. 9–9).[16] When multiple doses of a drug are administered, the duration of effect may in-

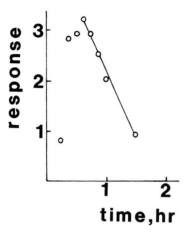

Fig. 9–10. Time course of euphoric response after an oral dose of cocaine. (Data from Mayersohn, M., and Perrier, D.[17])

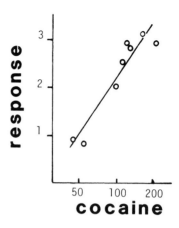

Fig. 9–11. Logarithmic cocaine concentration in plasma (ng/ml)-response relationship. (Data from Mayersohn, M., and Perrier, D.[17])

crease with each dose until steady state is reached because the initial amount of drug in the body following a dose will be higher than that of the preceding dose.

In principle, the duration of effect of a drug may be controlled by the dose. Evaluation of Equation 9–6 shows that the duration of effect increases by one half-life (0.693/k) with each doubling of the dose.[8] In practice, however, duration of effect is largely a function of the therapeutic index and half-life of the drug. The ratio of Dose to A_{min} cannot exceed the therapeutic index of the drug. If this ratio is small, on the order of two, the drug must be given no less frequently than once every half-life to avoid adverse effects.

A more useful relationship for drugs that produce graded responses is one that correlates the intensity of effect with the time after administration. We know that drug concentration declines in an exponential manner with time after administration; but to relate concentration, response, and time, we need to select a concentration-response relationship. The log concentration-effect relationship (Eq. 9–3) is a particularly useful one. Since,

$$\log C = \log C_o - kt/2.303 \qquad (9{-}7)$$

and

$$\text{Effect} = S \log C + I \qquad (9{-}8)$$

where C is drug concentration in blood or plasma, S is an effect parameter relating the change in effect to the change in log C, and I is an empirical constant, it follows that:

$$\text{Effect} = (S \log C_o + I) - Skt/2.303 \qquad (9{-}9)$$

or

$$\text{Effect} = E_o - Skt/2.303 \qquad (9{-}10)$$

Equation 9–10 indicates that the intensity of effect of a rapidly distributed drug will decline at a constant (zero-order) rate after an intravenous bolus dose. The slope of the linear plot of effect versus time is equal to $-Sk/2.303$.

Figure 9–10 shows a plot of the intensity of euphoria after an oral dose of cocaine.[17] The effect of the drug increases with time, reaches a maximum about 60 to 90 min after administration, and thereafter declines in a linear manner, in accordance with Equation 9–10. The slope of the line ($-Sk/2.303$) is equal to -0.0221 effect units/min. A plot of effect versus log concentration of cocaine, shown in Figure 9–11, is also linear; the slope (S) of this plot is equal to 3.9 effect units. From these data we may calculate that Sk = 0.051 effect units/min, k = 0.0131 min^{-1}, and $t_{1/2}$ = 53 min. This estimate of the half-life of cocaine, determined solely from effect data, agrees with the value of 57 min determined from a semilogarithmic plot of cocaine concentration versus time.

Cocchetto has applied these relationships to the constant rate intravenous infusion of short-acting drugs.[18] At steady state, the following equation applies:

$$E_{ss} = S \log K_o - (S \log Cl + I) \qquad (9{-}11)$$

where E_{ss} is the effect at steady state, k_o is the zero-order infusion rate, and Cl is the clearance of the drug. Figure 9–12 shows that the steady-state mean arterial blood pressure in a patient with malignant

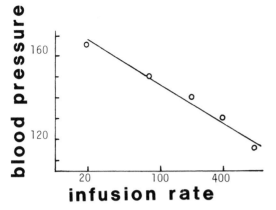

Fig. 9–12. Relationship between steady-state mean arterial blood pressure (mm Hg) and sodium nitroprusside infusion rate (μg/min, log scale). (Data from Cocchetto, D.M.[18])

hypertension is a linear function of the log of infusion rate of nitroprusside, in accordance with Equation 9–11. Based on these data and on the postinfusion rate of decline of effects, the half-life of nitroprusside was calculated to be 16 min, a value consistent with the fleeting effects of the drug when it is given as an intravenous bolus dose.

The time course of drug effects following rapid intravenous injection of a drug may be far more complicated than that suggested by Equation 9–10, because the log concentration-effect relationship applies only to a limited range of drug concentrations (i.e., those concentrations producing effects between 20% and 80% of the maximum effect). An excellent example of these complexities has been provided by Rowland and Tozer.[8]

Figure 9–13 shows the time course of effect following rapid intravenous injection of a drug. The dose is sufficiently large to yield concentrations that elicit a maximum response. The log concentration-response plot is shown in the inset. Segmenting the plots into three regions, 0 to 20% maximum response, 20 to 80% maximum, and 80 to 100% maximum, is a convenient way to describe the complex time course of effect.

The initial drug concentration produces a maximum effect. Drug concentration falls rapidly over the first hour (50% decrease) but response remains nearly constant at about 90 to 100% of maximum (region 3). Only after 2 hr, when concentration falls below 3 ng/ml and response falls below 80% maximum, does response begin to decline more

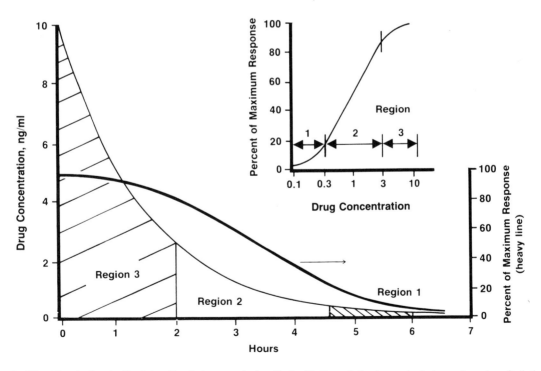

Fig. 9–13. The decline in the intensity of pharmacologic effect with time, following a single large dose, has 3 distinct parts corresponding to the regions of the concentration-response curve. There is little change in effect in region 3 despite a large change in drug concentration; effect declines linearly in region 2 and exponentially in region 1. (From Rowland, M., and Tozer, T.N.[8])

rapidly (region 2). In region 2 the drug concentration-response relationship is described by Equation 9–3, and response declines at a constant rate of about 20%/hr according to Equation 9–10. When the concentration falls below 0.3 ng/ml (region 1), the fall in response is exponential and parallels the fall in concentration.

As previously discussed, the usual response to many drugs falls in region 2; effect is lost at a constant rate. There are some reports showing an exponential loss of drug effect with time, suggesting that response to these drugs lies in region 3. The usual doses of β-blockers produce responses that appear to fall into region 1; effects on blood pressure and heart rate are relatively constant over large concentration ranges.

By focusing on drug concentration, we have learned a great deal about drug effects. In the following chapters, you will find that much is also known about the factors that influence drug concentration (pharmacokinetic variability). This information has stimulated progress in the area of individualized and optimized drug treatment. The final step, an understanding of pharmacodynamic variability, remains elusive, because it is difficult to study. Here too, however, progress is being made. We are beginning to learn that age, genetics, and diseases can alter the receptor's sensitivity to a drug. We are at the threshold of seminal advances in drug discovery, and it is vitally important that the individual patient reaps the full benefits of this windfall.

REFERENCES

1. Smith, S.E., and Rawlins, M.D.: Variability in Human Drug Response. London, Buttersworth, 1973, pp. 1–2.
2. Kato, R., Takanaka, A., and Onoda, K.: Individual difference in the effect of drugs in relation to the tissue concentration of drugs. Jpn. J. Pharmacol., *19*:260, 1969.
3. Schnell, R.C., et al.: Similarity in CNS sensitivity to hexobarbital in the rat and mouse as determined by an analytical, a pharmacokinetic, and an electroencephalographic measure. Pharmacology, *13*:20, 1975.
4. Winkle, R.A., et al.: Clinical efficacy and pharmacokinetics of a new orally effective antiarrhythmic tocainide. Circulation, *54*:884, 1976.
5. Holford, N.H.G., and Sheiner, L.B.: Understanding the dose effect relationship: clinical application of pharmacokinetic-pharmacodynamic models. Clin. Pharmacokinet., *6*:429, 1981.
6. Sokolow, M., and Edgar, A.L.: Blood quinidine concentration as a guide in the treatment of cardiac arrhythmias. Circulation, *1*:576, 1950.
7. Koch-Weser, J.: In Pharmacology and the Future: Problems in Therapy, Vol. III. Edited by G.T. Okita and G.H. Archeson, Basel, Karger, 1973, pp. 69–85.
8. Rowland, M., and Tozer, T.N.: Clinical Pharmacokinetics: Concepts and Applications. 2nd Ed. Philadelphia, Lea & Febiger, 1989.
9. Coltart, D.J., and Shand, D.G.: Plasma propranolol levels in the quantitative assessment of β-adrenergic blockade in man. Br. Med. J., *3*:731, 1970.
10. Holford, N.H.G., et al.: The effect of quinidine and its metabolites on the electrocardiogram and systolic time intervals: Concentration-effect relationships. Br. J. Clin. Pharmacol., *11*:187, 1981.
11. Javaid, J.I., et al.: Cocaine plasma concentrations: Relation to physiological and subjective effects in humans. Science, *202*:227, 1978.
12. Packer, M., et al.: Prevention and reversal of nitrate tolerance in patients with congestive heart failure. N. Engl. J. Med., *317*:799, 1987.
13. Cowan, C., et al.: Tolerance to glyceryl trinitrate patches: prevention by intermittent dosing. Br. Med. J., *294*:544, 1987.
14. Rosenberg, J., Benowitz, N.L., Wilson, M.: Disposition kinetics and effects of intravenous nicotine. Clin. Pharmacol. Ther., *28*:517, 1980.
15. Russell, M.A.H., Feyerabend, C.: Cigarette smoking. A dependence on high nicotine boli. Drug Metabolism Revs., *8*:29, 1978.
16. Levy, G.: Kinetics of pharmacologic effects. Clin. Pharmacol. Ther., *7*:362, 1966.
17. Mayersohn, M., and Perrier, D.: Kinetics of pharmacologic response to cocaine. Res. Comm. Chem. Pathol. Pharmacol., *22*:465, 1970.
18. Cocchetto, D.M.: Kinetics of pharmacological effects on constant-rate intravenous infusion. J. Pharm. Sci., *70*:578, 1981.

10

Drug Disposition—Distribution

We have known for a long time that people respond differently to drugs and now know that these differences are the result of both pharmacokinetic and pharmacodynamic variability in the patient population. Pharmacokinetic variability means that the same dose of drug results in different blood levels in different people. The association of drug concentration in blood or plasma with pharmacologic effect, described in Chapter 9, suggests that pharmacokinetic variability is an important factor in how people respond to drugs.

Pharmacokinetic variability is the result of interindividual differences in the absorption and disposition of drugs. Chapters 2 through 6 deal with various aspects of drug absorption. This chapter and the one that follows concern the basic principles of drug distribution and elimination.

The term *disposition* refers to the fate of a drug after absorption. On reaching the bloodstream, drugs are simultaneously distributed throughout the body and eliminated. Distribution usually occurs much more rapidly than elimination. The rate of distribution to the tissues of each organ is determined by the blood flow perfusing the organ and the ease with which the drug molecules cross the capillary wall and penetrate the cells of the particular tissue.

DRUG DISTRIBUTION

Distribution in Blood and Other Fluids

Drug molecules are distributed throughout the body by means of the circulation of blood. The entire blood volume (about 6 L) is pumped through the heart each minute; within minutes after a drug enters the bloodstream it is diluted into the total blood volume. A drug that is restricted to the vascular space and can freely penetrate erythrocytes has a volume of distribution of 6 L. If the drug cannot permeate the red blood cells (RBCs), the available space is reduced to about 3 L (plasma volume).

Nearly all drugs easily cross capillaries and are rapidly diluted to a much larger volume, the extracellular space. Capillaries, except those in the brain, are more like filters than lipid membranes, in terms of permeability. Drugs with molecular weights of up to 500 or 600 daltons quickly diffuse out of the vascular system and reach the interstitial fluid bathing the cells.

Certain body fluids may be relatively inaccessible to drugs in the bloodstream; these include cerebrospinal fluid (CSF), bronchial secretions, pericardial fluid, and middle ear fluid. The degree of access of antibiotics to these fluids may be a limiting factor in treating infections. Inflammation, however, often secondary to infection, increases drug penetration.

Drug concentration in body fluids also depends on the degree of drug binding in the fluid. Drug concentration in CSF and saliva, which are usually protein-free, is usually equal to free (unbound) drug concentration in plasma. Drug concentration in extracellular fluid (ECF) is frequently less than that in plasma, because the ECF has a lower albumin concentration than plasma. Drug concentration in synovial fluid varies with the degree of inflammation because albumin concentration fluctuates with the severity of the disease process.

Cellular Distribution

The penetration of drugs into cells depends on many of the factors that govern gastrointestinal absorption of drugs in solution. Small, water-soluble molecules and ions diffuse through aqueous channels or pores in the cell membrane. Lipid-soluble molecules penetrate the membrane itself. Water-soluble molecules and ions of moderate size (molecular weights of 50 daltons or more) cannot enter cells easily, except by special transport mechanisms. The penetration of weak acids or bases into cells depends on the pH of the ECF. Unlike the gastrointestinal tract, however, blood and ECF maintain a remarkably uniform pH.

Studies in dogs have shown that carbon dioxide-induced acidosis or sodium bicarbonate-induced alkalosis markedly alters the distribution of phenobarbital, a weak acid.[1] When plasma pH is lowered by carbon dioxide inhalation, there is a decrease in the plasma levels of phenobarbital. Under these conditions, a greater fraction of the drug in plasma is in the un-ionized form and a larger amount of the drug moves into the cells. Sodium bicarbonate produces an elevation of phenobarbital concentration in the plasma because of a shift of drug from the cellular space to the extracellular space. These shifts occur in all tissues, including the brain. Acidosis deepens phenobarbital anesthesia whereas alkalosis lightens it.

Sodium bicarbonate is sometimes used in the treatment of barbiturate intoxication to induce a mild systemic alkalosis to reduce the central nervous system (CNS) burden of drug. This treatment also produces urinary alkalosis, which promotes the urinary excretion of weakly acidic drugs.

Drug Penetration to Central Nervous System

The capillaries in the brain are different in their permeability characteristics from those found in the rest of the body. They possess a cellular sheath that makes them much less permeable to water-soluble substances. This sheath constitutes the so-called blood-brain barrier. The penetration rate of a drug into the brain depends on its degree of ionization in the plasma and its lipid solubility.

Highly lipid-soluble drugs, like thiopental, reach the brain almost immediately after administration. More polar compounds, like barbital, penetrate the CNS at a slower rate.

Failure of antibiotics to effectively penetrate the CNS is a long-recognized concern in the treatment of meningitis.[2] In most cases, this failure can be explained by the physicochemical properties of the drug. For example, penicillin G is a water-soluble, weak organic acid (pKa = 2.6) that is essentially ionized at the pH of plasma. The slow diffusion of penicillins into the CNS reflects the poor lipid solubility of the ionized form of the drug.

Interestingly, the permeability of the blood-brain barrier is increased in meningeal infections because of the abnormal state of the membranes. Variable but significant levels of ampicillin, penicillin G, lincomycin, and cephalothin have been found in the CSF of patients with viral, bacterial, or other meningeal inflammatory states.[3,4] Little or no detectable antibiotic activity is found in the CSF of patients with normal meninges who received these drugs. The steady-state CSF concentration of ampicillin was found to be only 2% of serum concentration in normal rabbits, but increased to 13% of serum concentration in rabbits with meningitis.[5]

Parkinsonism is associated with a depletion of dopamine in the brain. Replacement therapy is ineffective because of the inability of dopamine to cross the blood-brain barrier. On the other hand, levodopa, a precursor of dopamine, is an important drug in the treatment of this disease. Levodopa can penetrate the CNS where it is subsequently metabolized to dopamine.

A serious problem in the long-term management of parkinsonian patients treated with levodopa is the deterioration of control and the development of random fluctuations in motor performance, called the on-off phenomenon. A group of investigators in Oregon sought to determine whether the oscillating clinical response to levodopa reflected fluctuations in brain levels of the drug related to variation in gastrointestinal absorption and transport to the central nervous system.[6]

The role of absorption was evaluated by determining whether it was affected by meals and by studying the clinical response to a stable concentration of levodopa in plasma achieved by intravenous infusion. The role of transport of levodopa from plasma to brain was examined by studying the clinical response to high-protein meals and to certain amino acids given during drug infusion. The investigators hypothesized that certain amino acids might compete with levodopa for transport across the blood-brain barrier.

Patients with Parkinson's disease for at least 8 years, characterized by unpredictable and marked swings in their response to levodopa, were studied. When levodopa was given 3 times a day before meals, the typical profile of plasma levodopa concentration showed peaks about 1 hr after the dose and troughs immediately before the next dose; roughly corresponding oscillations were noted in mobility and dyskinesia. There were, however, incongruities; sometimes, a peak level was not seen after a dose, and at other times the plasma peak was not accompanied by clinical improvement even though equivalent levels at other periods of the day were effective.

When levodopa was given to patients after an overnight fast, absorption was rapid and reproducible. On the other hand, when the drug was taken after a meal, rate and extent of absorption were decreased and in some cases no peak concentration was evident. A constant rate intravenous infusion virtually eliminated fluctuations in levodopa levels in plasma and produced a stable clinical response lasting from 12 to 36 hr, except when perturbed by a meal or an amino acid challenge.

The administration of a high-protein meal during iv infusion of levodopa had no effect on drug concentration in plasma, but it did cause a deterioration of clinical response. These meals also about doubled the plasma concentration of large neutral amino acids that have been found in animal studies to affect the transport of levodopa across the blood-brain barrier.

To further characterize this loss of efficacy, patients were challenged with individual amino acids during levodopa infusion. Loss of motor control was observed when phenylalanine, leucine, and isoleucine were given but not when glycine or lysine was administered. The investigators concluded that interference with absorption of levodopa by food resulting in variable blood levels and with transport of levodopa across the blood-brain barrier by large neutral amino acids contained in the diet may be responsible, in part, for the on-off phenomenon in Parkinson's disease. The observation that constant infusion markedly decreased fluctuations offers the hope that improved methods of delivering levodopa may eliminate or at least reduce this problem.

The rapid penetration of lipid-soluble molecules in the CNS is of great importance for anticonvulsant or psychotropic drugs, which must act on the brain, but facile penetration may produce unwanted side effects with drugs intended to affect other systems, such as antiarrhythmic drugs. The CSF concentrations of lipid-soluble drugs usually reflect free drug concentrations in plasma. The CSF-plasma concentration ratio in epileptic patients undergoing temporal lobectomy was 0.12 for phenytoin and 0.46 for phenobarbital; the free to total concentration ratio in plasma was 0.15 for phen-

ytoin and 0.50 for phenobarbital.[7] The CSF-plasma concentration ratio for chlordiazepoxide in patients receiving spinal anesthesia was found to be 0.043; the free-to-total concentration ratio of the drug in plasma was 0.04.[8]

Drug levels are usually higher in brain tissue than in the CSF. Phenytoin concentrations in epileptic patients are about 6 times higher in the temporal lobe than in the CSF.[7] Propranolol concentrations are more than 250 times higher in the human brain than in the CSF.[9] This is a result of drug binding to constituents in the brain.

Adequate distribution to the central nervous system is of particular concern in the use of antineoplastic drugs. Certain parenchymal cancers are quite responsive to systemic antitumor agents, but metastases of these tumors to the CNS have been virtually unresponsive to the same chemotherapy, probably because the drugs were unable to cross the blood-brain barrier.

Several approaches are under investigation to enhance drug delivery to the CNS. Spontaneous disruption of the blood-brain barrier during the course of certain diseases (e.g., meningitis) increases the penetration of drugs to the CNS. There is now evidence that certain treatments may permit controlled transient disruption of the barrier.

For example, dimethyl sulfoxide (DMSO) seems to open the blood-brain barrier in mice to the enzyme horseradish peroxidase.[10] Uniform distribution of the enzyme was observed throughout most of the forebrain, brainstem, and cerebellum when it was given with DMSO. In the absence of this penetration enhancer, the enzyme failed to enter brain parenchyma. The effects of DMSO were no longer evident within 2 hr of administration, suggesting that disruption was transient. How DMSO opens the blood-brain barrier is unclear and whether it may be used safely in humans remains to be determined.

A more developed technique, called osmotic blood-brain barrier disruption, utilizes hyperosmolar solutions of mannitol. Osmotic disruption of the blood-brain barrier immediately before administration of methotrexate in a dog model, by infusion of 25% mannitol into the internal carotid artery, resulted in therapeutic levels of drug in the ipsilateral cerebral hemisphere but not in the contralateral hemisphere.[11] The permeability of the barrier appeared to return to normal within 1 hr after treatment.

In preliminary clinical studies, methotrexate was

administered after blood-brain barrier disruption to 6 patients with brain tumors.[12] No permanent complications were seen, and serial enhanced CT scans indicated that disruption increased drug delivery to the tumor and the surrounding brain. More recently, using this technique, Neuwelt et al.[13] documented tumor regression in patients with microglioma, medulloblastoma, and glioblastoma.

Warnke et al.[14] studied the effect of hyperosmotic blood-brain barrier disruption on transport of a water-soluble amino acid, amino-isobutyric acid, in rats with ethylnitrosourea-induced gliomas. Hyperosmotic disruption resulted in a modest, statistically insignificant, increase in tumor uptake. In contrast, a large and significant increase in the uptake of amino-isobutyric acid was found in the tumor-free brain tissue. The investigators concluded that the effects of hyperosmotic blood-barrier disruption are different in normal brain tissue and in brain tumors, and that the benefits of disruption with respect to the rate of drug delivery to brain tumors appear to be marginal. Transient disruption, however, may still be useful to increase drug delivery to brain tissue surrounding the tumor.

Boder and Farag have described a prodrug approach to enhance delivery to the CNS.[15] A biologically active compound covalently linked to a lipid-soluble dihydropyridine carrier easily penetrates the blood-brain barrier. Oxidation of the pyridine part of the drug-carrier prodrug to the ionic pyridinium salt prevents its elimination from the CNS but enhances its elimination from the general circulation. Subsequent cleavage of the prodrug in the CNS results in sustained delivery of the drug to the brain and facile elimination of the carrier.

Bodor and Farag[16] prepared the N-methyl-1,4-dihydronicotinate ester of testosterone via quaternization of testosterone nicotinate with methyl iodide followed by reduction of the quaternary salt. They postulated that the ester, by virtue of its lipid solubility, would cross the blood-brain barrier more easily than testosterone. It was also anticipated that biological oxidation to the corresponding quaternary derivative would follow, thereby capturing the corresponding ionic, hydrophilic product in the central nervous system. Oxidation in peripheral tissue not involving a permeability barrier would favor rapid clearance from the general circulation because the quaternary derivative is excreted more rapidly than the unoxidized form. Oxidation would favor both the accumulation of quaternary deriv-

ative in the brain and minimal systemic exposure outside the brain. A subsequent slow hydrolysis to free testosterone in the brain would provide a site-specific, prolonged exposure to testosterone.

After administration of the testosterone ester to female rats, no reduced material could be detected in blood or brain. However, high and persistent levels of the quaternary form of the prodrug were found in the brain, suggesting rapid oxidation. Blood levels of the charged form were initially high but fell quickly. Testosterone was found to be released from the quaternary ester very slowly giving rise to low but persistent levels in the brain ($t_{1/2}$ = 20 hours). Administration of testosterone itself results in high brain levels followed by rapid clearance ($t_{1/2}$ = 15 minutes).

Prodrugs promising brain-selective delivery have also been described for certain progestins, including ethisterone, norethindrone, and norgestrel.[17] Administration of the reduced form of a norethindrone prodrug to rats resulted in relatively high and persistent levels of the oxidized quaternary form of the prodrug in the brain. The "locked-in" quaternary salt hydrolyzed slowly to produce the pharmacologically active parent drug norethindrone. This hydrolysis produced substantially higher and more persistent levels of norethindrone in the brain than those found after the administration of norethindrone itself.

This novel prodrug approach to drug delivery and sequestration in the brain has also been applied to estradiol.[18] The maximum effect of equimolar doses of estradiol prodrug and estradiol itself in suppressing luteinizing hormone secretion in orchidectomized rats was about the same, but the effect of the prodrug persisted for a much longer time. The investigators suggested that this chemical delivery system for estradiol may be useful clinically in the treatment of vasomotor instability associated with ovariectomy or the menopause, particularly in women for whom peripheral estrogen is contraindicated. The prodrug may also be useful in the chronic reduction of gonadotropin secretion for fertility regulation or for the treatment of gonadal-steroid-dependent diseases, such as endometriosis and prostatic hypertrophy.

Placental Transfer of Drugs

Since the thalidomide tragedy, there has been keen interest in the passage of drugs across the placenta.[19–21] The membranes separating fetal capillary blood from maternal blood resemble cell

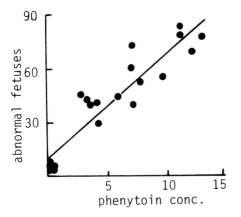

Fig. 10–1. Relationship between phenytoin concentration in maternal plasma (μg/ml) and the frequency (%) of mouse fetuses with malformations. (Data from Finnell, R.H.[24])

membranes elsewhere in the body. Many drugs of moderate to high lipid solubility, including sulfonamides, barbiturates, anticonvulsants, narcotic analgesics, antibiotics, and steroids, can be detected in appreciable concentrations in fetal blood or tissues shortly after administration to the mother.

Although its development has been greatly hampered by experimental and ethical difficulties, the theory of maternal-fetal equilibrium rates is considerable.[22,23] The shortest time possible for a drug to equilibrate between maternal blood and fetal tissue has been estimated to be about 40 min. Drugs like tubocurarine, whose passage across the placenta is impeded by low lipid solubility, large molecular size, ionization, and protein binding, probably require hours for equilibration and may not be detected in the fetus after a single dose to the mother. Fetal exposure to drugs that are rapidly eliminated by the mother is also likely to be small.

Chronic medication presents the greatest concerns. The higher the blood level of drug in pregnant patients on chronic medication, the greater is the risk to the fetus. The occurrence of malformations associated with the fetal hydantoin syndrome in the mouse are strongly correlated with maternal serum concentrations of the anticonvulsant drug phenytoin (Fig. 10–1).[24]

In man, there is some evidence that both the metabolites of phenytoin and a genetic defect in metabolic detoxification contribute to susceptibility to phenytoin-induced birth defects.[25] Lymphocytes from 24 children exposed to phenytoin throughout gestation, as well as from family members, were challenged with phenytoin metabolites generated

by isolated mouse liver. Lymphocytes from 14 children were positive, manifesting an increase in cell death on exposure to phenytoin metabolites. Each child with a positive result had at least one parent whose cells also were positive. A positive in vitro challenge was highly correlated with major birth defects, including congenital heart disease, cleft lip and/or palate, microcephaly, and major genitourinary, eye, and limb defects.

In 1982, isotretinoin, a highly effective drug for the treatment of severe chronic cystic acne, was marketed in the United States. In short order, it became the most widely criticized drug of the decade because of its potential to cause severe deformities in children born to women who had taken isotretinoin during the early weeks of pregnancy. The syndrome has been called retinoic acid embryopathy.[26]

Isotretinoin is a retinoic acid, a class of compounds related to vitamin A. Because retinoic acid as well as large doses of vitamin A were known to be teratogenic in laboratory animals, isotretinoin was labeled upon marketing as Category X, indicating that the drug was contraindicated for use during pregnancy. Despite this initial warning and subsequent stronger warnings, the use of isotretinoin during pregnancy has been associated with more than 60 documented reports of adverse reproductive outcomes since the drug went on the market. Some epidemiologists suggest that the number is actually as high as 600.

Since its marketing, the labeling of isotretinoin has become more and more restrictive. In 1984, the manufacturer added to the label a recommendation that a pregnancy test should be performed within 2 weeks of initiating treatment with isotretinoin, and that an effective form of contraception be used for at least 1 month prior to starting therapy, during therapy, and 1 month after therapy is discontinued. Furthermore, in a most unusual move, the Food and Drug Administration advised all blood banks that donations from anyone taking isotretinoin should be deferred for at least 1 month after taking the last dose. The agency, considering the potency of isotretinoin as a teratogen and the possibility that it may be present in the blood for weeks after discontinuance, suggested that there may be a risk to the developing fetus if blood from an isotretinoin-treated donor is transfused into a patient who either is or soon becomes pregnant.

Several other countries, which approved the use of isotretinoin somewhat later than the FDA, control the distribution of the drug more closely than does the United States. In the United Kingdom, only 200 dermatologists are certified to prescribe the drug. Isotretinoin is available from any licensed physician in the U.S. Sweden has elected not to approve isotretinoin for general marketing, requiring physicians to submit a special request to the government to prescribe the drug.

Since some degree of fetal exposure is likely to occur with virtually all drugs, and since the consequences of such exposure is usually unknown, many advocate that drug administration during pregnancy be severely restricted.

Some investigators are taking advantage of the ease with which drugs cross the placenta to treat the fetus by giving medication to the mother.[27] A deficiency in the enzyme 21-hydroxylase results in congenital adrenal hyperplasia, leading to masculinization of the external genitalia of affected females. This problem might be avoided if fetal adrenal gland function were suppressed.

A woman with mild 21-hydroxylase deficiency, whose previous female child was born with adrenal hyperplasia and masculinization, was given dexamethasone beginning at the tenth week of gestation of another female child. After a normal delivery at 39 weeks, the child was found to have normal external genitalia. Postnatal tests indicated that the infant, like the mother and sibling, was 21-hydroxylase-deficient. The investigators concluded that ''this study demonstrates prolonged suppression of the fetal adrenal gland with dexamethasone and suggests it might prevent abnormal masculinization in fetuses with severe congenital adrenal hyperplasia.''[27]

Blood Flow

Blood flow is the rate-limiting step in the distribution of most drugs. Accordingly, rapid equilibration of lipid-soluble drugs is observed between the blood and lungs, kidney, liver, heart, and brain, all of which are highly perfused with blood. Less rapid equilibration is found in skeletal muscle, bone, and adipose tissue, which receive a considerably smaller volume of blood per unit mass per minute. Perfusion of relatively large, solid tumors is also low. Changes in blood flow to the liver or kidneys, as a result of disease or other factors, may alter the elimination rate of a drug.

Blood flow rates may also influence drug uptake at receptor sites. Figure 10–2 shows concentrations of procainamide after a short intravenous infusion

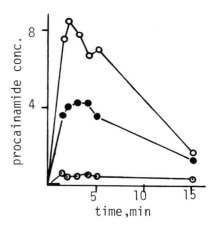

Fig. 10–2. Procainamide concentrations in the myocardium (μg/g) during and after a 1-min infusion in the dog. Key: (○) nonischemic region; (●) moderate ischemia; (◉) severe ischemia. (Data from Wenger, T.L., et al.[28])

in nonischemic and progressively ischemic regions of the dog myocardium.[28] Procainamide accumulated more slowly and peak concentrations were lower in the ischemic regions than in the nonischemic region; concentrations were lowest in the most severely ischemic region.

Redistribution of a drug into less well-perfused tissues, rather than metabolism or excretion, may limit the duration of effect of certain drugs at highly perfused sites. For example, thiopental produces anesthesia within seconds after administration because of rapid equilibration between blood and brain. The concentration of drug in the brain rapidly declines, however, and the duration of effect is short-lived despite the fact that thiopental is only slowly metabolized. The rapid decline of drug concentrations in the brain is the result of redistribution into other tissues, particularly skeletal muscle and fat. Inhibition or induction of drug-metabolizing enzymes and subsequent reduction or enhancement of the metabolism rate of thiopental is likely to have no effect on the duration of drug action because redistribution rate is the controlling factor.

Investigators in Sweden studied the distribution and elimination of the narcotic analgesic meperidine in patients recovering from surgery.[29] Five hr after the procedure, the drug was infused intravenously at a rate predicted to produce a steady-state concentration of about 500 ng/ml. Blood samples were collected simultaneously from mixed central venous blood (pulmonary artery) and peripheral arterial blood (radial artery) and assayed for meperidine.

Drug uptake by an organ is expressed as the equilibrium distribution ratio between tissue and blood (K_P). Drug clearance by an organ (CL) is expressed as the product of the organ blood flow (Q) and the extraction ratio (E).

$$CL = Q \times E \qquad (10\text{--}1)$$

The pulmonary extraction ratio (E) is calculated as follows:

$$E = (C_V - C_A)/C_V \qquad (10\text{--}1A)$$

where C_V and C_A are the venous and arterial plasma concentrations, respectively. Blood flow to the lungs is about 5,000 ml/min, the highest flow rate to any organ in the body. Accordingly (see Eq. 10–1), even a modest extraction ratio could result in a large percentage of the dose of a drug being eliminated in a single pass across the lungs.

The investigators found that the venous concentration of meperidine at steady state was 540 ng/ml, whereas the arterial concentration was 523 ng/ml. These values were not significantly different. From these results, one can calculate an extraction ratio of 0.03 which is not significantly different from zero. These findings indicate that the lungs make little or no contribution to the overall clearance of meperidine, estimated at about 800 ml/min.

On the other hand, during the infusion of meperidine before steady state, venous plasma concentrations were higher than arterial levels, suggesting an uptake of meperidine in the lungs. Equilibrium ratios of lung tissue to venous blood were estimated to be quite high, in the order of 25 to 30, suggesting that 10 to 15% of the total amount of meperidine in the body will be found in the lungs.

People exposed to nicotine develop tolerance to many of its effects. When heart rate is measured over time during and after a short constant-rate intravenous infusion of nicotine, a greater increase in heart rate is seen for a given nicotine concentration during infusion (the rising phase of concentrations) than after infusion (the declining phase). This could be the result of acute tolerance. On the other hand, similar differences in blood concentration-effect relationships in rising and falling portions of the blood concentration-time curve may be observed if drug concentrations at the effect site (brain) equilibrate more rapidly with arterial concentrations than drug levels at the (venous) blood sampling site.

To distinguish between these possibilities, rabbits were given nicotine intravenously over 1 min. Blood samples taken from the internal jugular vein (reflecting brain concentration), the femoral vein, and the femoral artery revealed that brain levels peaked before femoral venous concentrations. The results indicated that for nicotine in the rabbit, brain equilibrates with arterial blood about 3 times faster than do peripheral tissues.[30] Using typical human tissue volumes and blood flows, the investigators estimated that in humans, nicotine equilibrates with the brain about 14 times faster than with peripheral tissue.

Nicotine was also given to healthy human subjects by intravenous infusion and peripheral venous blood concentrations and cardiovascular responses were measured. Heart rate peaked before venous concentrations, suggesting more rapid distribution of drug to the heart than to venous blood. The investigators concluded that the apparent development of acute tolerance to the increase in heart rate during nicotine infusion may be due partly, if not completely, to the distribution kinetics of the drug rather than to the rapid development of functional tolerance.

Drug distribution rates are usually determined by simultaneously measuring drug concentrations in fluid or tissue (C_T) and in blood (C), as a function of time after intravenous bolus or infusion. Shortly after drug administration, the ratio of drug concentrations (C_T/C) is small. With time, the ratio increases until a constant value is achieved. This reflects equilibration of drug between the fluid or tissue and the blood.

A semilogarithmic plot of the difference between the equilibrium ratio and the ratio at a given time, as a function of time, will usually be linear, so that one may estimate a distribution half-life for a particular fluid or tissue. At least three paired samples (tissue and blood) must be obtained for this estimate. The need for multiple punctures or multiple biopsies at several times after drug administration severely limits the study of drug distribution. The alternative approach, serial sacrifice of animals at different times after administration, is limited to small species and introduces error due to interindividual variability.

A clever approach to overcome this problem and to obtain a considerable amount of information from a single sample of fluid or tissue has been described.[31] It is based on the administration of a series of different isotopes of a drug at different times before the sample is taken. The investigators suggested that this approach provides the same information about a drug's distribution to a particular site as that obtained by infusing the drug and carrying out serial collections of fluid or tissue. They applied the method to study the distribution of phenobarbital into the cerebrospinal fluid (CSF) of a dog.

Three forms of phenobarbital with different molecular weights, achieved by stable isotope labeling, were infused intravenously at different times. The heaviest form ($+5$ PB) was infused first, at -25 min. At -10 min, the next heaviest form ($+3$ PB) was given; at time 0, unlabeled phenobarbital ($+0$ PB) was infused. Blood and CSF samples were then collected at 5, 15, 30, 60, and 90 min and the concentrations of each form of phenobarbital were determined in each fluid.

Each paired sample of blood and CSF provides three data points from which a distribution half-life may be estimated. For example, the 15 min sample permits calculation of a CSF/serum ratio 15 min after drug administration ($+0$ PB), 25 min after drug administration ($+3$ PB), and 40 min after drug administration ($+5$ PB). Staggered isotope administration data from each paired sample taken at 5, 15, 30, or 60 min provided estimates of distribution half-life ranging from 22 to 24 min. These estimates were in good agreement with the distribution half-life value determined by infusing unlabeled phenobarbital and taking multiple samples of blood and CSF over time.

Distribution Volumes

There is usually a considerable difference between the apparent volume of distribution of a drug and the actual volume in which it distributes. The apparent volume of distribution is simply a proportionality constant relating the plasma concentration to the total amount of drug in the body. Depending on the degree of binding to plasma proteins and tissues, the apparent volume of distribution of a drug may vary in man from 0.04 L/kg (plasma volume) to 20 L/kg or more.

The actual distribution volume of a drug is related to body water; it can never exceed total body water (TBW), that is, about 60% of body weight or 42 L in a normal 70-kg man. Body water may be divided into 3 compartments: vascular fluid, extracellular fluid (ECF), and intracellular fluid. In man, extracellular water is about one third of the total (i.e., about 19% of body weight or 15 L). This volume includes plasma water, which is about 4% of body weight or 3 L. The whole blood (vascular) volume, including the intracellular water of

the erythrocytes, is about twice plasma volume, or about 6 L.

Certain dyes, such as Evans blue, are essentially confined to the circulating plasma and can be used to determine plasma volume (and blood volume, if the hematocrit is known). Certain substances such as chloride and bromide ions distribute rapidly throughout the ECF, but do not cross cell membranes, so they may be used to estimate extracellular water. The volume of TBW may be approximated by determining the distribution of heavy water (D_2O) or certain lipid-soluble but poorly bound substances, such as antipyrine.

The apparent volume of distribution of these tracers approximates their true volume of distribution. This, however, occurs with few substances, only those that are negligibly bound to plasma proteins and tissues. If a drug is preferentially bound to plasma proteins, the apparent volume of distribution is smaller than the real volume of distribution. On the other hand, preferential binding of drugs at extravascular sites results in an apparent volume of distribution larger than the true volume of distribution.

The following equation describes the relationship between apparent volume of distribution, drug binding, and anatomic volumes:[32]

$$V = V_B + (f_B V_T/f_T) \qquad (10\text{--}2)$$

where V is the apparent volume of distribution, V_B is blood volume, V_T is extravascular volume, and f_B and f_T are the free fractions of drug in the blood and extravascular space (tissues), respectively. If a drug is 92% bound to plasma proteins and other elements of blood, then $f_B = 0.08$. For lipid-soluble drugs, V_T is the difference between TBW and blood volume (V_B). For polar drugs, V_T is the difference between ECF volume and blood volume; this applies to most antibiotics.

Equation 10–2 indicates that the apparent volume of distribution increases with increases in anatomic volumes or tissue binding and with decreases in plasma protein or blood binding. The volume of distribution of a drug that is unbound in the body is equal to either TBW (e.g., antipyrine) or ECF volume (e.g., bromide ion), since $f_B = f_T = 1$. Disease factors and concomitant drug therapy that reduce drug binding to plasma proteins result in an increase in apparent volume of distribution.

A more physiologically correct expression for apparent volume of distribution,[33] which takes into account that plasma proteins are not limited to the blood but are distributed throughout the ECF is:

$$V = V_P (1 + R_{E/I}) + f_P V_P [(V_E/V_P)$$

$$- R_{E/I}] + V_R f_P/f_T \quad (10\text{--}3)$$

where V_P is plasma volume (3 L in a normal 70-kg man), V_E is the extracellular space minus plasma volume (15 L minus 3 L, or 12 L), V_R is the physical volume into which the drug distributes (i.e., TBW, 42 L, or extracellular space, 15 L) minus extracellular space, f_P and f_T are the free fractions of drug in plasma and tissue, and $R_{E/I}$ is the ratio of the amount of binding protein in the ECF outside the plasma to that in the plasma. Usually, 55 to 60% of the total extracellular albumin is found outside the plasma. Changes in this ratio occur with prolonged bed rest and in severe burns. Assuming that all drug binding proteins are distributed like albumin, then $R_{E/I} \simeq 1.4$.

Substituting these values into Equation 10–3 yields:

$$V = 7.2 + 7.8 f_P + V_R f_P/f_T \quad (10\text{--}4)$$

If a drug distributes only to the ECF and does not enter cells (i.e., $V_R = 0$), the apparent volume of distribution is given by:

$$V = 7.2 + 7.8 f_P \quad (10\text{--}4A)$$

When the apparent volume of distribution is large (i.e., $V >$ TBW), the first two terms in Equation 10–4 are usually negligible and the equation reduces to:

$$V = V_R f_P/f_T \quad (10\text{--}5)$$

Changes in apparent volume of distribution are found as a function of body weight, age, and disease because of differences in anatomic volumes or drug binding. The apparent volume of distribution of some drugs may differ in men and women. Studies with chlordiazepoxide show that $V = 34$ L for both sexes. When the data are normalized for differences in total body weight, a significant sex difference is found; $V = 0.58$ L/kg for women and 0.45 L/kg for men.[34]

Investigators in Japan studied factors that affected the apparent volume of distribution of cefazolin, a cephalosporin antibiotic, in newborn human infants.[35] Body weight-normalized volumes of distribution (V/BW) determined in 11 newborns ranged from 0.21 to 0.37 L/kg. The unbound fraction of cefazolin in plasma varied widely, from

about 0.2 to 0.8. A strong correlation was observed when V/kg was plotted against unbound fraction (r = 0.94). In turn, the unbound fraction was related to bilirubin levels and albumin concentrations in plasma. A statistically significant correlation (r = 0.81) between free fraction and the unconjugated bilirubin:albumin molar ratio was observed.

Cefazolin and other β-lactam antibiotics are localized in the extracellular water space and are bound to albumin in both intravascular and interstitial fluids. Predictions of the weight-adjusted apparent volume of distribution of cefazolin as a function of free fraction, based on Equation 10–3, were in good agreement with the values calculated in newborn infants.

DRUG BINDING IN BLOOD

Binding to plasma proteins affects drug distribution and elimination, as well as the pharmacologic effect of a drug. The high molecular weight of plasma proteins restricts passage across capillaries; their low lipid solubility prevents passage across cell membranes. Drug bound to plasma protein is similarly restricted. Only that fraction of the drug concentration that is freely circulating or unbound in extracellular water can penetrate cell membranes and is subject to glomerular filtration. Hepatic metabolism of most drugs is also limited by the free fraction of drug in the blood. The interaction of drugs with plasma proteins is a rapidly reversible process, however, and one may think of drug bound to plasma proteins as being in temporary storage, subject to instant recall.

Drug binding to plasma proteins may involve ionic, Van der Waals, hydrogen, and/or hydrophobic bonds. The most important contribution to drug binding in the plasma is made by albumin which comprises about one half of the total plasma proteins. In healthy individuals, albumin concentration in the plasma is about 4 g/100 ml. Lower levels are found during pregnancy (about 3.5 g/100 ml during the last trimester) and in certain diseases. Albumin binds a wide variety of drug molecules, but plays a particularly important role in the binding of weak acids and neutral drugs.

α_1-Acid glycoprotein (orosomucoid) is also an important binding protein, with an affinity for basic drugs, including imipramine, lidocaine, propranolol, and quinidine. α_1-Acid glycoprotein is a low molecular weight protein (approximately 40,000 daltons). It is an acute phase reactant, and its concentration in plasma rises in inflammation, malig-

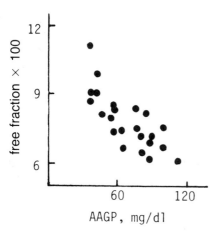

Fig. 10–3. Correlation between the levels of α_1-acid glycoprotein (AAGP) and free fraction of imipramine in healthy human subjects. (Data from Piafsky, K.M., and Borgå, O.[36])

nant disease, and stress and falls in hepatic disease and nephrotic syndrome. The average concentration of α_1-acid glycoprotein in plasma is about 40 to 100 mg/100 ml. The relationship between imipramine binding and α_1-acid glycoprotein concentration in plasma in healthy men and women is shown in Figure 10–3.[36] Other considerations concerning the plasma protein binding of basic drugs have been discussed by Routledge.[37]

The other proteins in plasma play a limited role in drug binding. There is a highly specific interaction between certain steroids, such as prednisolone, and corticosteroid-binding globulin, also known as CBG or transcortin.[38] Transcortin also binds thyroxine and vitamin B_{12}. Gamma globulins react specifically with antigens, but negligibly with most drugs.

The drug-protein interaction may be described by the law of mass action:

$$D_F + \text{Free sites} \underset{k_2}{\overset{k_1}{\rightleftharpoons}} D_B$$

where D_F and D_B are the free and bound drug, respectively, and k_1 and k_2 are the rate constants for association and dissociation, respectively. Thus,

$$K = \frac{k_1}{k_2} = \frac{[D_B]}{[D_F]\,[\text{Free sites}]}$$
$$= \frac{[D_B]}{[D_F]\,(n[P] - [D_B])} \quad (10-6)$$

where K is the equilibrium association constant, n

is the number of binding sites per mole of protein, and $[D_F]$, $[D_B]$, and $[P]$ are the molar concentrations of free and bound drug and protein, respectively.

The binding rate constants, k_1 and k_2, appear to be large since equilibrium is established almost immediately. The equilibrium constant, K, varies from about zero, where essentially no drug is bound, to about 10^6, where almost all the drug is bound to the protein.

The fraction of drug in the plasma that is free or unbound, f_P, is given by:

$$f_P = [D_F]/([D_F] + [D_B])$$
$$= [D_F]/[D_T] \quad (10-7)$$

where $[D_T]$ is the total concentration of drug in the plasma. In most cases, for a given amount of drug in the body, the greater the binding of drug to plasma proteins, the larger is the total drug concentration in plasma. Changes in binding usually affect blood levels of total drug and play a role in pharmacokinetic variability.

The fraction of drug free in the plasma depends on the magnitude of K, the total drug concentration, and the protein concentration. In principle, there are a limited number of binding sites on the protein. As the drug concentration in plasma increases, the number of free sites decreases; therefore, the fraction of free drug increases. In practice, however, the fraction of unbound drug in plasma for most drugs administered in therapeutic doses is essentially constant over the entire drug concentration range.

Concentration-dependent changes in the fraction of free drug in the plasma are most likely to occur with drugs having a high association constant (i.e., 10^5 to 10^6), and that are given in large doses (e.g., certain sulfonamides and phenylbutazone). The fraction of disopyramide unbound to plasma proteins varies from about 0.19 to 0.46 over the therapeutic range of total drug concentration in plasma (2 to 8 µg/ml).[39] A total disopyramide concentration of 2 µg/ml provides a free drug level of about 0.4 µg/ml; a 4-fold increase in total drug concentration results in a 10-fold increase in free drug concentration.

Ceftriaxone, a third generation cephalosporin, is unusual in that its plasma protein binding is concentration-dependent.[40] The percentage of free ceftriaxone in plasma increases from 4 to 17% when the total ceftriaxone concentration in plasma is increased from 0.5 µg/ml to 300 µg/ml. Concentration-dependence in plasma protein binding is also found following usual doses of valproic acid, and aspirin in the treatment of rheumatoid arthritis.

The relationship between bioavailability and area under the drug concentration-time curve (AUC) is nonlinear and absorption-rate dependent when the plasma protein binding of a drug is concentration-dependent.[41] Two products from which a drug is equally well absorbed produce different values for AUC if there is a difference in absorption rate. As a rule, AUC comparisons will overestimate the bioavailability (extent of absorption) of the more slowly absorbed product.

A large degree of intersubject variability in binding is seen with certain drugs. Studies in 26 patients who had been taking phenytoin regularly for more than 2 weeks showed that the free (unbound) phenytoin level in plasma varied from 5.8 to 12.6% of the total drug concentration.[42] A study of 31 patients with cardiovascular disease who were taking warfarin regularly has shown that the free warfarin level in plasma ranges from 0.4 to 1.9% of the total drug concentration.[43] A study concerned with the binding of benzodiazepines in human plasma found that free fraction varied 2-fold for lorazepam, 4-fold for diazepam and chlordiazepoxide, and 20-fold for oxazepam.[44] The free fraction of imipramine in plasma of depressed patients was found to vary 4-fold (5.4 to 21%). This variability may contribute to the difficulty in correlating the plasma levels of antidepressant drugs and clinical outcome.[45] Diurnal variations in plasma protein binding are responsible for variations in the total blood levels of diazepam throughout the day.[46] Normal changes in plasma lipids may account for part of the inter- and intrasubject variability in plasma protein binding found in healthy human subjects, because of potential competition between lipids and drugs for binding sites on plasma proteins.

The classic methods of studying plasma protein binding of drugs are equilibrium dialysis and ultrafiltration. Measurements are made more quickly using ultrafiltration but may not be as accurate as those based on equilibrium dialysis. The plasma protein binding of phenytoin was measured in patients with normal renal function and impaired renal function using a new, simplified ultrafiltration method as well as the traditional equilibrium dialysis method. As expected, unbound fraction was about twice as large in uremic patients as in patients with normal renal function, but in both groups of patients the values for each method were in good

agreement. The investigators concluded that the new ultrafiltration device "has a great potential for measurements of unbound concentrations of phenytoin because of its rapidity and reliability."[47]

Plasma Protein Binding and Drug Distribution

Since the protein concentration in extravascular fluid is less than in plasma, the total drug concentration in plasma is usually higher than in lymph, cerebrospinal fluid (CSF), synovial fluid, and other fluids of the extravascular space.

Normal CSF contains so little protein that it is often viewed as an ultrafiltrate of the plasma. The plasma protein binding of nortriptyline in man is about 94%. This value agrees with the finding that the steady-state concentration of nortriptyline in CSF is only 3 to 11% of the plasma level.[48] The CSF concentrations of carbamazepine and its epoxide metabolite in patients being treated for epilepsy are closely related to free drug and free metabolite concentrations in serum.[49]

Normal synovial fluid contains only 1-g albumin/100 ml; however, albumin levels may be elevated in synovial fluid from patients with arthritis or other degenerative joint diseases. The penetration of ampicillin and cloxacillin into synovial fluid has been measured after oral administration of these penicillins to patients with osteoarthritis or rheumatoid arthritis.[50] The results show that both drugs diffused rapidly into synovial fluid but that they differed appreciably with respect to total concentration relative to total concentration in plasma.

For ampicillin, which is not highly bound to plasma proteins (only 10 to 15%), the total drug levels in synovial fluid were similar to the total plasma levels. With cloxacillin, which is highly bound to plasma proteins (95%), the total levels in synovial fluid were considerably lower than those in plasma. However, the unbound levels of cloxacillin in synovial fluid and plasma were similar (Fig. 10–4).

Free and total ibuprofen levels in serum and synovial fluid were determined in patients with arthritis.[51] Albumin concentrations were found to be 3.7 g/100 ml in serum and 2.1 g/100 ml in synovial fluid. Total ibuprofen concentration in joint fluid was about 40% that in serum. The drug was bound to the extent of 99% in serum and 97.5% in synovial fluid. The ratio of total ibuprofen in synovial fluid to that in serum correlated with the albumin concentration ratio (r = 0.89). Free ibuprofen concentration in joint fluid (0.19 μg/ml) was similar

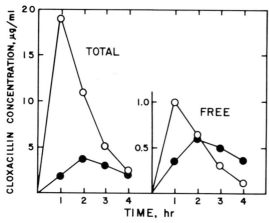

Fig. 10–4. Total and free cloxacillin concentrations in serum (○) and synovial fluid (●) after a single 500-mg oral dose to patients with arthritis. (Data from Howell, A., Sutherland, R., and Rolinson, G.N.[50])

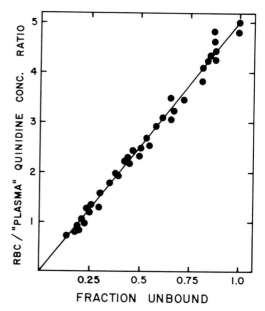

Fig. 10–5. Relationship between the red blood cell (RBC)/plasma (or diluted plasma) quinidine concentration ratio and the fraction of unbound quinidine in the plasma. (Data from Hughes, I.E., Ilett, K.F., and Jellett, L.B.[54])

to free serum levels (0.25 μg/ml), indicating that synovial fluid is easily accessible to unbound drug.

Drug Binding to Erythrocytes. Several studies have demonstrated that drug uptake by erythrocytes is a function of plasma protein binding. Linear correlations have been reported between the blood or red blood cell (RBC)/plasma concentration ratio and the percent of unbound drug in the plasma for propranolol,[52] phenytoin,[53] quinidine,[54] and haloperidol.[55] The quinidine data are shown in Figure 10–5.

Determination of the RBC-plasma concentration ratio has been suggested as a simple and rapid technique for the large-scale screening of abnormal plasma binding in routine clinical blood samples. Estimates of free rather than total drug concentration may be more useful for individualization of drug therapy.

Drugs that bind avidly to RBCs may show concentration-dependent uptake from plasma. Erythrocyte accumulation of acetazolamide appears to be a composite of two processes: a nonlinear, saturable process and a linear process (Fig. 10–6).[56] The partitioning of the diuretic, chlorthalidone between RBC and plasma is also concentration-dependent.[57] When the concentration of chlorthalidone in blood is less than 15 to 20 μg/ml, 98% of the drug is bound to the red cells. Increasing the blood concentration results in an abrupt and substantial decrease in the partition ratio, in favor of the plasma, indicating saturable binding sites of chlorthalidone on RBCs. The binding of cyclosporine, an immunosuppressant widely used to pre-

vent rejection in transplant patients, to erythrocytes is also concentration-dependent.[58] Blood/plasma ratio decreases from about 1.5 at low plasma levels of cyclosporine to 1.0 at very high levels of the drug. Whole-blood cyclosporine measurements will be difficult to interpret when hematocrit varies considerably.

Although drug binding to plasma proteins, erythrocytes, and other tissues is usually rapidly reversible, there are examples of apparently irre-

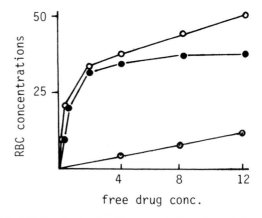

Fig. 10–6. Acetazolamide concentrations (μg/ml) in red blood cells as a function of free drug concentration in plasma. Key: (○) total concentration; (●) bound concentration; (◉) free concentration. (Data from Wallace, S.M., and Riegelman, S.[56])

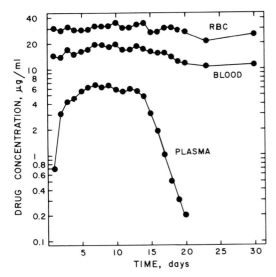

Fig. 10–7. Concentrations of an investigational carbonic anhydrase inhibitor in plasma, blood, and RBCs during and after repetitive oral dosing with 100 mg twice daily for 14 days. (Data from Lund, J., et al.[59])

versible binding. A particularly dramatic example has been reported with an investigational carbonic anhydrase inhibitor in man.[59] Drug concentrations in plasma, blood, and erythrocytes during and after repetitive dosing to human subjects are shown in Figure 10–7. The drug is found in the RBCs in measurable amounts for more than a year after the last dose.

Irreversible binding of drugs to serum albumin has also been demonstrated. Zomepirac is a nonsteroidal anti-inflammatory drug withdrawn from the market because of an unexplained high incidence of immunologic reactions. It is metabolized in humans to a reactive, unstable acyl glucuronide. Because of the similarities of zomepirac glucuronide to bilirubin glucuronide, in structure and stability, and the documented irreversible binding of bilirubin to albumin through its acyl glucuronide, Smith et al.[60] studied the reaction of zomepirac acyl glucuronide with albumin.

Irreversible binding of zomepirac to protein was demonstrated both in vitro and in vivo. Binding correlated with overall exposure to zomepirac glucuronide. When probenecid, which decreases the plasma clearance of zomepirac glucuronide and increases blood levels of the unstable metabolite, was given concurrently with zomepirac, irreversible binding was increased. The investigators concluded that the formation of irreversible protein-bound zomepirac occurs via the acyl glucuronide

and the reaction may be general for other drugs metabolized to acyl glucuronides, such as tolmetin.[61]

Plasma Protein Binding and Drug Effects

There is considerable theory but limited experimental evidence to suggest that the concentration of free drug in the plasma is the critical determinant of drug effect. To test this hypothesis, investigators studied the relationship between anticoagulant effect and the concentrations of free and total warfarin in rat plasma.[62] The concentration of total warfarin required to elicit a defined anticoagulant effect varied widely among animals (coefficient of variation of 85%), whereas the required concentration of free warfarin showed much less variation (coefficient of variation of 29%). These studies suggest that the anticoagulant effect of warfarin is more nearly a function of its free than of its total concentration in plasma.

In another study, rats were given phenytoin and its potency against maximal electroshock seizures was determined. The effect of phenylbutazone (a drug that competitively decreases the plasma protein binding of phenytoin and decreases its total plasma concentration) on the potency and on the total and unbound plasma concentrations of phenytoin was then measured. Phenylbutazone treatment increased the potency of phenytoin in terms of dose and total drug concentration (i.e., a lower plasma phenytoin concentration and a lower dose were required to protect against shock-induced seizure) but did not affect the potency of unbound phenytoin.[63] Thus, the anticonvulsant action of phenytoin appears to depend on the concentration of unbound drug in plasma rather than on the total plasma concentration or the dose.

The effects of plasma protein binding on the relationship between propranolol concentration and the antagonism of isoproterenol-induced tachycardia was investigated in healthy subjects and hypertensive patients.[64] A poor correlation was found between effect and total propranolol concentration in plasma (r = 0.46), whereas there was an excellent correlation between efficacy and free drug concentration (r = 0.89). The effect of propranolol on heart rate is a predictable function of free drug concentration in man; the contribution of individual variation in receptor sensitivity to differences in oral dosage requirement is minor compared to that of variations in systemic availability.

Plasma Protein Binding and Drug Elimination

Free rather than total drug concentration is often the driving force for drug elimination. The glomerular capillaries in the kidneys contain pores that, like those in most other capillaries, permit the passage of most drugs but restrict the passage of plasma proteins. Accordingly, in healthy individuals the glomerular filtrate is an ultrafiltrate of plasma; only free (unbound) drug is filtered. In the absence of active tubular secretion and reabsorption, drug concentration in urine is equal to free drug concentration in plasma.

If a drug or chemical is neither secreted nor reabsorbed by the tubules and is not protein bound, its renal clearance is a measure of glomerular filtration rate (GFR); inulin and creatinine have these characteristics and are often used to estimate GFR. If, on the other hand, the drug is protein bound, the renal clearance of total drug in the plasma is less than GFR but the clearance of free drug is equal to GFR. Studies have shown that the rate of renal excretion of several tetracyclines is inversely related to their extent of plasma protein binding.[65] More recently, studies in an isolated perfused rat kidney, using different amounts of serum albumin in the perfusate, showed that the renal clearance of digitoxin is linearly related to the unbound fraction of drug in perfusate.[66]

The rate of metabolism of certain drugs is also related to the degree of binding in the plasma. For example, a highly significant inverse rank-order correlation has been reported between the rate of metabolism of 11 sulfonamides in man and their degree of protein binding.[67] A strong correlation ($r = 0.95$) has been observed between total clearance of warfarin from plasma and the free fraction of drug in the serum of individual rats.[68] These data are shown in Figure 10–8. The results show that the pronounced intersubject variability (about 10-fold) in the elimination of warfarin in the rat is strongly related to intersubject differences in plasma protein binding of the drug. A statistically significant correlation between the total plasma clearance of warfarin and the free fraction of this drug in serum has also been found in patients with cardiovascular disease who were taking warfarin regularly.[43]

The plasma protein binding and metabolism of diflunisal are both capacity limited in the rat. A plot of clearance of total diflunisal from plasma vs drug concentration described a U-shaped curve. At

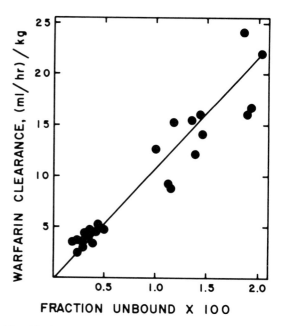

Fig. 10–8. Relationship between the clearance of warfarin from plasma and free (unbound) fraction in the serum of individual rats. (Data from Yacobi, A., and Levy, G.[68])

low diflunisal concentrations (<100 μg/ml) clearance decreased with increasing drug levels, whereas at higher concentrations (>200 μg/ml) clearance increased with increasing drug levels. On the other hand, the clearance of unbound diflunisal from plasma consistently decreased with increasing drug levels. The pattern described when the clearance of total diflunisal was plotted against drug concentration is a consequence of capacity-limited metabolism (low concentration effect) as well as capacity-limited binding (high concentration effect). The results obtained when the clearance of unbound diflunisal was studied simply reflect capacity-limited metabolism.[69]

The clearance of many drugs from the blood is directly proportional to free fraction in the plasma (f_P); the steady-state concentration of these drugs is inversely proportional to f_P. On the other hand, the clearance of some drugs is largely independent of plasma protein binding; drugs in this category include those subject to rapid and extensive hepatic metabolism, such as lidocaine or verapamil, and those undergoing extensive tubular secretion, such as the penicillins.

The effect of plasma protein binding on the half-life of a drug depends on the apparent volume of distribution (V) of the drug.[70] The half-life of drugs with a relatively small V (e.g., <0.25 L/kg) is sensitive to changes in f_P; a decrease in plasma protein binding results in a shorter half-life. Conversely, the half-life of drugs with larger values of V (e.g., >0.5 L/kg) is essentially independent of plasma protein binding.

DRUG BINDING IN TISSUES

Tissue binding plays an important part in drug distribution, at least in the sense of drug storage. In many cases, more than 90% of the drug in the body is bound in the extravascular or tissue space. Drug binding to tissues is poorly understood. Few studies have been directed to this interaction; almost all have used tissues from experimental animals.[71-73] Tissue binding has no effect on drug clearance or on average steady-state concentrations of drug in blood or plasma. Its principal influence is on the time course of drug in the body. The half-life of drugs with apparent volumes of distribution exceeding 0.5 L/kg is determined by clearance and tissue binding.[70,74] An increase in clearance or a decrease in tissue binding decreases the half-life of a drug. The role of tissue binding in the pharmacologic effects of drugs is unknown.

REFERENCES

1. Waddell, W.J., and Butler, T.C.: The distribution and excretion of phenobarbital. J. Clin. Invest., 36:1217, 1957.
2. Barling, R.W.A., and Selkon, J.B.: The penetration of antibiotics into cerebrospinal fluid and brain tissue. J. Antimicrob. Chemother., 4:203, 1978.
3. Thrupp, L.D., et al.: Ampicillin levels in the cerebrospinal fluid during treatment of bacterial meningitis. Antimicrob. Agents Chemother., Vol. 5, 1965, p. 206.
4. Lerner, P.I.: Penetration of cephalothin and lincomycin into the cerebrospinal fluid. Am. J. Med. Sci., 257:125, 1969.
5. Bodine, J.A., Strausbaugh, L.J., and Sande, M.A.: Ampicillin and an ester in experimental *Hemophilus influenzae* meningitis. Clin. Pharmacol. Ther., 20:127, 1976.
6. Nutt, J.G., et al.: The on-off phenomenon in Parkinson's disease: relation to levodopa absorption and transport. N. Engl. J. Med., 310:483, 1984.
7. Vajda, F., et al.: Human brain, cerebrospinal fluid, and plasma concentrations of diphenylhydantoin and phenobarbital. Clin. Pharmacol. Ther., 15:597, 1974.
8. Stanski, D.R., et al.: Plasma and cerebrospinal fluid concentrations of chlordiazepoxide and its metabolites in surgical patients. Clin. Pharmacol. Ther., 20:571, 1976.
9. Neil-Dwyer, G., et al.: β-Adrenoceptor blockers and the blood-brain barrier. Br. J. Clin. Pharmacol., 11:549, 1981.
10. Broadwell, R.D., Salcman, M., Kaplan, R.S.: Morphologic effect of dimethylsulfoxide on the blood-brain barrier. Science, 217:164, 1982.
11. Neuwelt, E.A., et al.: Osmotic blood-brain barrier disruption. J. Clin. Invest., 64:684, 1979.
12. Neuwelt, E.A., et al.: Monitoring of methotrexate delivery in patients with malignant brain tumors after osmotic blood-brain barrier disruption. Ann. Intern. Med., 94:449, 1981.
13. Neuwelt, E.A., Rapoport, S.I.: Modification of the blood-brain barrier in the chemotherapy of malignant brain tumors. Federation Proc., 43:214, 1984.
14. Warnke, P.C., et al.: The effect of hyperosmotic blood-brain barrier disruption on blood-to-tissue transport in ENU-induced gliomas. Ann. Neurol., 22:300, 1987.
15. Bodor, N., and Farag, H.H.: Site-specific, sustained release of drugs to the brain. Science, 214:1370, 1981.
16. Bodor, N., Farag, H.H.: Improved delivery through biological membranes XIV: brain-specific, sustained delivery of testosterone using a redox chemical delivery system. J. Pharm. Sci., 73:385, 1984.
17. Brewster, M.E., Estes, K.S., Bodor, N.: Improved delivery through biological membranes. XXIV. Synthesis, *in vitro* studies, and *in vivo* characterization of brain-specific and sustained progestin delivery systems. Pharmac. Res., 3:278, 1986.
18. Simpson, J.W., et al.: Sustained brain-specific delivery of estradiol causes long-term suppression of luteinizing hormone secretion. J. Med. Chem., 29:1809, 1986.
19. Forrest, J.M.: Drugs in pregnancy and lactation. Med. J. Aust., 2:138, 1976.
20. Green, J.P., O'Dea, R.F., and Mirkin, B.L.: Determinants of drug disposition and effect in the fetus. Ann. Rev. Pharmacol. Toxicol., 19:285, 1979.
21. Hill, R.M., and Stern, L.: Drugs in pregnancy: effects on the fetus and newborn. Drugs, 17:182, 1979.
22. Goldstein, A., Aronow, L., and Kalman, S.M.: Principles of Drug Action. John Wiley & Sons, Inc., New York, 1974, pp. 205–210.
23. Waddell, W.J., and Marlowe, C.: Transfer of drugs across the placenta. Pharmacol. Ther., 14:375, 1981.
24. Finnell, R.H.: Phenytoin-induced teratogenesis: a mouse model. Science, 211:483, 1981.
25. Strickler, S.M., et al.: Genetic predisposition to phenytoin-induced birth defects. Lancet, 2:746, 1985.
26. Lammer, E.J., et al.: Retinoic acid embryopathy. N. Engl. J. Med., 313:837, 1985.
27. Evans, M.I., et al.: Pharmacologic suppression of the fetal adrenal gland in utero. Attempted prevention of abnormal external genital masculinization in suspected congenital adrenal hyperplasia. JAMA, 253:1015, 1985.
28. Wenger, T.L., et al.: Procainamide delivery to ischemic canine myocardium following rapid intravenous administration. Circ. Res., 46:789, 1980.
29. Persson, M.P., et al.: Pulmonary disposition of pethidine in postoperative patients. Br. J. Clin. Pharmacol., 25:235, 1988.
30. Porchet, H.C., et al.: Apparent tolerance to the acute effect of nicotine results in part from distribution kinetics. J. Clin. Invest., 80:1466, 1987.
31. Evans, J.E., et al.: Staggered stable isotope administration technique for study of drug distribution. J. Clin. Pharmacol., 25:309, 1985.
32. Gibaldi, M., and McNamara, P.J.: Apparent volumes of distribution and drug binding to plasma proteins and tissues. Eur. J. Clin. Pharmacol., 13:373, 1978.
33. Øie, S., and Tozer, T.N.: Effect of altered plasma protein binding on apparent volume of distribution. J. Pharm. Sci., 68:1203, 1979.
34. Greenblatt, D.J., et al.: Kinetics of intravenous chlordiazepoxide: sex differences in drug distribution. Clin. Pharmacol. Ther., 22:893, 1977.
35. Deguchi, Y., et al.: Interindividual changes in volume of distribution of cefazolin in newborn infants and its prediction based on physiological pharmacokinetic concepts. J. Pharm. Sci., 77:674, 1988.
36. Piafsky, K.M., and Borgå, O.: Plasma protein binding of basic drugs. II. Importance of α_1-acid glycoprotein for in-

terindividual variation. Clin. Pharmacol. Ther., 22:545, 1977.

37. Routledge, P.A.: The plasma protein binding of basic drugs. Br. J. Clin. Pharmacol., 22:499, 1986.
38. Westphal, U.: Binding of steroids to proteins. J. Am. Oil Chem. Soc., 41:481, 1964.
39. Meffin, P.J., et al.: Role of concentration-dependent plasma protein binding in disopyramide disposition. J. Pharmacokinet. Biopharm., 7:29, 1979.
40. Nahata, M.C., Barson, W.J.: Ceftriaxone: a third-generation cephalosporin. Drug. Intell. Clin. Pharm., 19:900, 1985.
41. Upton, R.A., Williams, R.L.: The impact of neglecting nonlinear plasma-protein binding on disopyramide bioavailability studies. J. Pharmacokin. Biopharm., 14:365, 1986.
42. Porter, R.J., and Layzer, R.B.: Plasma albumin concentration and diphenylhydantoin binding in man. Arch. Neurol., 32:298, 1975.
43. Yacobi, A., Udall, J.A., and Levy, G.: Intrasubject variation of warfarin binding to protein in serum of patients with cardiovascular disease. Clin. Pharmacol. Ther., 20:300, 1976.
44. Johnson, R.F., et al.: Plasma binding of benzodiazepines in humans. J. Pharm. Sci., 68:1320, 1979.
45. Glassman, A.H., Hurwic, M.J., and Perel, J.M.: Plasma binding of imipramine and clinical outcome. Am. J. Psychiatry, 130:1367, 1973.
46. Naranjo, C.A., et al.: Diurnal variations in plasma diazepam concentrations associated with reciprocal changes in free fraction. Br. J. Clin. Pharmacol., 9:265, 1980.
47. Koike, Y., et al.: Ultrafiltration compared with equilibrium dialysis in the determination of unbound phenytoin in plasma. Ther. Drug Monitor, 7:461, 1985.
48. Borgå, O., et al.: Plasma protein binding of tricyclic antidepressants in man. Biochem. Pharmacol., 18:2135, 1969.
49. Johannessen, S.I., et al.: CSF concentrations and serum protein binding of carbamazepine and carbamazepine-10,11-epoxide in epileptic patients. Br. J. Clin. Pharmacol., 3:575, 1976.
50. Howell, A., Sutherland, R., and Rolinson, G.N.: Effect of protein binding on levels of ampicillin and cloxacillin in synovial fluid. Clin. Pharmacol. Ther., 13:724, 1972.
51. Whitlam, J.B., et al.: Transsynovial distribution of ibuprofen in arthritic patients. Clin. Pharmacol. Ther., 29:487, 1981.
52. Evans, G.H., Nies, A.S., and Shand, D.G.: The disposition of propranolol. III. Decreased half-life and volume of distribution as a result of plasma binding in man, monkey, dog and rat. J. Pharmacol. Exp. Ther., 186:114, 1973.
53. Kurata, D., and Wilkinson, G.T.: Erythrocyte uptake and plasma binding of diphenylhydantoin. Clin. Pharmacol. Ther., 16:355, 1974.
54. Hughes, I.E., Ilett, K.F., and Jellett, L.B.: The distribution of quinidine in human blood. Br. J. Clin. Pharmacol., 2:521, 1975.
55. Hughes, I.E., Jellett, L.B., and Ilett, K.F.: The influence of various factors on the in vitro distribution of haloperidol in human blood. Br. J. Clin. Pharmacol., 3:285, 1976.
56. Wallace, S.M., and Riegelman, S.: Uptake of acetazolamide by human erythrocytes in vitro. J. Pharm. Sci., 66:729, 1977.
57. Dieterle, W., Wagner, J., and Faigle, J.W.: Binding of chlorthalidone (Hygroton) to blood components in man. Eur. J. Clin. Pharmacol., 10:37, 1976.
58. Legg, B., Rowland, M.: Saturable binding of cyclosporin A to erythrocytes: estimation of binding parameters in renal transplant patients and implications for bioavailability assessment. Pharmac. Res., 5:80, 1988.
59. Lund, J., et al.: Early human studies of a new carbonic anhydrase inhibitor. Clin. Pharmacol. Ther., 12:902, 1971.
60. Smith, P.C., McDonagh, A.F, Benet, L.Z.: Irreversible binding of zomepirac to plasma protein in vitro and in vivo. J. Clin. Invest., 77:934, 1986.
61. Hyneck, M.L., et al.: Disposition and irreversible plasma protein binding of tolmetin in humans. Clin. Pharmacol. Ther., 44:107, 1988.
62. Yacobi, A., and Levy, G.: Effect of plasma protein binding on the anticoagulant action of warfarin in rats. Res. Comm. Chem. Pathol. Pharmacol., 12:405, 1975.
63. Shoeman, D.W., and Azarnoff, D.L.: Diphenylhydantoin potency and plasma protein binding. J. Pharmacol. Exp. Ther., 195:84, 1975.
64. McDevitt, D.G., et al.: Plasma binding and the affinity of propranolol for a beta receptor in man. Clin. Pharmacol. Ther., 20:152, 1976.
65. Kunin, C.M., Dornbush, A.C., and Finland, M.: Distribution and excretion of four tetracycline analogues in normal young men. J. Clin. Invest., 38:1950, 1959.
66. Hall, S., Rowland, M.: Relationship between renal clearance, protein binding and urine flow for digitoxin, a compound of low clearance in the isolated perfused rat kidney. J. Pharmacol. Exp. Ther., 227:174, 1983.
67. Wiseman, E.H., and Nelson, E.: Correlation of in vivo metabolism rate and physical properties of sulfonamides. J. Pharm. Sci., 53:992, 1964.
68. Yacobi, A., and Levy, G.: Comparative pharmacokinetics of coumarin anticoagulants. XIV. Relationship between protein binding, distribution, and elimination kinetics of warfarin in rats. J. Pharm. Sci., 64:1660, 1975.
69. Lin, J.H., et al.: Dose-dependent pharmacokinetics of diflunisal in rats: dual effects of protein binding and metabolism. J. Pharmacol. Exp. Ther., 235:402, 1985.
70. Faed, E.M.: Protein binding of drugs in plasma, interstitial fluid and tissues: effect on pharmacokinetics. Eur. J. Clin. Pharmacol., 21:77, 1981.
71. Ludden, T.M., Schanker, L.S., and Lanman, R.C.: Binding of organic compounds to rat liver and lung. Drug Metab. Dispos., 4:8, 1976.
72. Schneck, D.W., Pritchard, J.F., Hayes, A.H., Jr.: Studies on the uptake and binding of propranolol by rat tissues. J. Pharmacol. Exp. Ther., 203:621, 1977.
73. Fichtl, B., Bondy, B., and Kurz, H.: Binding of drugs to muscle tissue: dependence on drug concentration and lipid content of tissue. J. Pharmacol. Exp. Ther., 215:248, 1980.
74. Gibaldi, M., Levy, G., and McNamara, P.J.: Effect of plasma protein and tissue binding on the biological half-life of drugs. Clin. Pharmacol. Ther., 24:1, 1978.

11

Drug Disposition—Elimination

Drugs are eliminated from the body by *metabolism* and *excretion*. The liver is the major site of drug metabolism, but other tissues contain drug metabolizing enzymes and contribute to the biotransformation of certain drugs. The kidneys play a principal role in the excretion of drugs and/or their metabolites. Some drugs are excreted in the bile and may be eliminated in the feces. Drugs used for anesthesia are often excreted by the lungs.

This chapter concerns the basic principles of drug elimination. Emphasis is given to renal excretion of drugs and drug metabolism in the liver.

DRUG EXCRETION

Renal Excretion

The kidneys are involved in the elimination of virtually every drug or drug metabolite. Some drugs, such as gentamicin or cephalexin, are eliminated from the body almost solely by renal excretion in patients with normal renal function. Many more drugs are eliminated in part by the kidneys. Even when drug elimination from the body involves only biotransformation, the corresponding drug metabolites are usually cleared by the kidneys.

Renal Physiology. The renal excretion of a drug is a complex phenomenon involving one or more of the following processes: *glomerular filtration, active tubular secretion,* and *passive reabsorption*. These processes are depicted schematically in Figure 11–1. Depending on which one of these processes is dominant, renal clearance can be an important or negligible component of drug elimination.

The kidneys receive about 25% of cardiac output or 1.2 to 1.5 L of blood per minute. About 10% of this volume is filtered at the glomeruli. There-

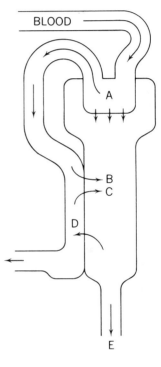

Fig. 11–1. Schematic representation of renal excretion of drugs depicting glomerular filtration of plasma water and unbound drug (A), active tubular secretion of organic acids (B) and bases (C), reabsorption of lipid-soluble drugs (D), and urinary excretion (E).

fore, about 130 ml of plasma water is filtered each minute. Although the pores of the glomerular capillaries are sufficiently large to permit the passage of most drug molecules, the glomeruli effectively restrict the passage of blood cells and plasma proteins. Accordingly, only free drug (drug that is not bound to plasma proteins) can be filtered.

Although some 180 L of protein-free filtrate pass through the glomeruli each day, only about 1.5 L is excreted as urine; the remainder is reabsorbed in the renal tubules. This often results in high urinary concentrations of certain solutes, particularly drugs that are not similarly reabsorbed. Many drugs, however, are efficiently reabsorbed from the distal portion of the nephron. In most instances, tubular reabsorption of drugs is a passive phenomenon. Nonionized, lipid-soluble drugs are rapidly and extensively reabsorbed, whereas polar compounds and ions are unable to diffuse across the renal epithelium and are excreted in the urine. For drugs that are principally eliminated by renal excretion, the more efficient the reabsorption of the drug, the longer is its biologic half-life.

The restrictive effect of plasma protein binding on glomerular filtration and the enormous capacity of the nephron to reabsorb certain solutes suggests that highly plasma protein-bound, lipid-soluble drugs would persist in the body for long periods of time after administration unless alternative elimination pathways were available. Of course, many of these drugs are subject to biotransformation in the liver or other tissues; others are subject to active tubular secretion at the proximal portion of the nephron. The fraction of drug in the blood that is not filtered may be effectively cleared by active tubular transport. The rate of tubular secretion is more closely a function of total rather than free drug concentration in blood or plasma and is independent of plasma protein binding.

Renal Clearance. The renal excretory mechanisms, filtration, reabsorption, and secretion, usually have the net effect of removing a constant fraction of the drug presented to the kidneys in renal arterial blood. The efficiency of renal excretion of a drug can be expressed in terms of a hypothetical volume of plasma that is completely *cleared* of that substance by the kidneys per unit time. This concept of *clearance* may be applied to any organ that secretes (e.g., biliary clearance) or metabolizes (e.g., hepatic clearance) a drug from the plasma. Renal clearance (Cl_R) is often a substantial fraction of the total clearance (Cl) of drug from the blood. For drugs that are essentially excreted unchanged in the urine, $Cl = Cl_R$.

Since renal clearance is a proportionality constant, relating the urinary excretion rate (dA_u/dt) of drug with its concentration (C) in blood or plasma, the following equation applies:

$$Cl_R = (dA_u/dt)/C \qquad (11–1)$$

Renal clearance is estimated by comparing the amount of drug (A_u) excreted over a short time interval (e.g., 1 hr) to the concentration of the drug in blood or plasma at the time corresponding to the midpoint of the urine collection interval.

Substances such as creatinine, the endogenous end product of creatine metabolism, or inulin, a carbohydrate, are eliminated by renal excretion but are not subject to either tubular secretion or reabsorption. Furthermore, these substances are not appreciably bound to plasma proteins. Therefore, the renal clearance of inulin or creatinine is an index of glomerular filtration rate (GFR).

In healthy individuals, the renal clearance of glucose is nearly zero because of efficient reabsorption in the renal tubules. On the other hand, certain substances are so efficiently excreted by the renal tubules that they are essentially cleared from the blood in a single pass through the kidneys. Para-aminohippuric acid (PAH) is handled in this manner. PAH is poorly lipid soluble, it does not penetrate erythrocytes, and it is not reabsorbed. Accordingly, the renal clearance of PAH is a measure of renal plasma flow rate (600 to 700 ml/min).

The renal clearance of a drug relative to GFR provides information on the mechanisms of renal excretion. Renal clearance values exceeding 130 ml/min are indicative of tubular secretion. The renal clearance of penicillin G (500 ml/min) exceeds the expected 52 ml/min calculated from the product of GFR (130 ml/min) and the fraction of drug in the plasma not bound to plasma proteins (0.4). Renal clearance values that are below 130 ml/min, even when adjusted for the degree of plasma protein binding, are indicative of tubular reabsorption. The renal clearance of phenytoin in man is about 5 ml/min. The fact that the drug is 90% bound to plasma proteins certainly contributes to this low value. Even when binding is taken into consideration, however, the renal clearance of free phenytoin (50 ml/min) is less than GFR, indicating reabsorption.

Secretion and reabsorption have opposite effects on renal clearance. When both processes are operative, presumptive evidence of either secretion or reabsorption, based on renal clearance values, does not rule out the other. Secretion may be operative even though the renal clearance of the drug is less than 130 ml/min. By the same token, reabsorption may occur with a drug having a renal clearance greater than 130 ml/min. It is also incorrect to assume that a drug with a renal clearance of about 130 ml/min is excreted simply by glomerular filtration. For example, sulfisoxazole undergoes tubular secretion and reabsorption in man but to a similar extent.[1]

Although estimates of renal clearance are informative with respect to excretion mechanisms, they give little information about the half-life of the drug. When a drug is eliminated solely by urinary excretion, the excretion rate (dA_u/dt) of the drug is given by:

$$dA_u/dt = KVC \qquad (11\text{-}2)$$

where K is the elimination rate constant of the drug, V is the apparent volume of distribution, and C is the drug concentration in blood or plasma. Accordingly, Equation 11–1 may be rewritten as follows:

$$Cl_R = \frac{KVC}{C} = KV \qquad (11\text{-}3)$$

Rearranging this expression, and recognizing that half-life ($t_{1/2}$) is equal to 0.693/K, it follows that:

$$t_{1/2} = \frac{0.693\ V}{Cl_R} \qquad (11\text{-}4)$$

Thus, the half-life of a drug is a function of both its clearance and volume of distribution. A drug may have a high clearance but still have a long half-life if V is also large.

Renal clearance also can be expressed in terms of the individual renal excretion processes, as follows:

$$Cl_R = (Cl_{RF} + Cl_{RS})(1 - FR) \qquad (11\text{-}5)$$

where Cl_{RF} is renal filtration clearance, Cl_{RS} is renal secretion clearance, and FR is the fraction of drug filtered and secreted that is reabsorbed. Renal filtration clearance (Cl_{RF}) is a function of GFR and plasma protein binding, i.e.,

$$Cl_{RF} = f_B\ GFR \qquad (11\text{-}6)$$

where f_B is the fraction of drug in the blood not bound to plasma proteins. GFR is usually estimated by determining creatinine clearance.

Drug secretion depends on the relative affinity of the drug for carrier proteins in the proximal tubule and plasma proteins, the rate of transport across the tubular membranes, and the rate of delivery of the drug to the site of secretion. These factors are included in the following equation:

$$Cl_{RS} = \frac{RBF\ f_B\ Cl_I}{RBF + f_B\ Cl_I} \qquad (11\text{-}7)$$

where RBF is renal blood flow and Cl_I is the intrinsic secretion clearance with respect to free drug.

Substituting Equations 11–6 and 11–7 for the appropriate terms in Equation 11–5, yields:

$$Cl_R = f_B\left[GFR + \frac{RBF\ Cl_I}{RBF + f_B\ Cl_I}\right](1 - FR) \qquad (11\text{-}8)$$

Equation 11–8 is a general expression for the renal clearance of drugs. An expression incorporating urine pH may be substituted for FR for those cases where tubular reabsorption is pH-dependent.

When renal excretion is not blood flow rate-limited, then $RBF \gg f_B\ Cl_I$, and Equation 11–8 reduces to:

$$Cl_R = f_B(GFR + Cl_I)(1 - FR) \qquad (11\text{-}9)$$

If tubular reabsorption is negligible or blocked by changing urine pH (i.e., FR = 0), renal clearance is given by:

$$Cl_R = f_B(GFR + Cl_I) \qquad (11\text{-}10)$$

If tubular secretion is negligible or blocked by giving a competitive inhibitor like probenecid (i.e., $Cl_I = 0$), renal clearance is given by:

$$Cl_R = f_B\ GFR\ (1 - FR) \qquad (11\text{-}11)$$

Under the conditions described by Equations 11–9 to 11–11, renal clearance is sensitive to changes in plasma protein binding.

When renal excretion is blood flow rate-limited, then $RBF \ll f_B\ Cl_I$; Equation 11–8 reduces to:

$$Cl_R = (f_B\ GFR + RBF)(1 - FR) \qquad (11\text{-}12)$$

or

$$Cl_R = RBF\ (1 - FR) \qquad (11\text{-}13)$$

because $RBF \gg f_B\ GFR$. Under these conditions, renal clearance is sensitive to changes in blood flow rate.

Equations 11–6 through 11–11 indicate that there is usually a relationship between plasma protein binding and renal clearance. When binding is capacity limited, the apparent renal clearance of a drug may show pronounced concentration dependence. This has been demonstrated with an investigational cephalosporin antibiotic in the dog.[2]

Cefixime was given by intravenous bolus injection and plasma protein binding and renal clearance were determined periodically as the drug levels in plasma declined. Renal clearance was determined by dividing the amount of drug excreted in the urine per unit time (i.e., the excretion rate) by the total drug concentration in plasma at the midpoint of the urine collection interval. Drug levels ranged from 197 μg/ml at 0.25 hours to 33 μg/ml at 11 hours after administration.

Over this 6-fold drug concentration range, free fraction in plasma (expressed as a percentage) decreased from 34% to 10% and renal clearance decreased from 1.64 to 0.33 ml/min/kg. On the other hand, the renal clearance of unbound cefixime, calculated by dividing renal clearance by free fraction, was relatively constant (mean value, 3.3 ml/min/kg). These findings indicate that the profound decrease in renal clearance was largely the result of capacity-limited binding rather than nonlinear renal excretion.

Tubular Secretion. Tubular secretion is an active transport process whereby drug diffuses against a concentration gradient from the blood capillaries across the tubular membrane to the renal tubule. This active process accounts for the fact that certain drugs, like dicloxacillin, although extensively bound to plasma protein and not subject to hepatic metabolism, are rapidly eliminated. Plasma protein binding does not affect the rate of tubular secretion because there is rapid transport of unbound drug and rapid dissociation of the drug-protein complex.

The secretion process shares many of the characteristics of the specialized transport (absorption) systems of the intestine. The process exhibits some degree of structural specificity; transport systems specific for organic acids (e.g., thiazide diuretics) and organic bases (e.g., triamterene) have been identified. Each system is characterized by a maximum rate of transport (T_m) for a specific drug. In principle, tubular secretion is saturable; in practice, however, there are few examples of nonlinear renal excretion.

The tubular excretion of several beta-lactam antibiotics has been studied in healthy human subjects.[3] Each drug was infused intravenously at different rates to achieve a wide range of concentrations in plasma. Renal clearance of each antibiotic at each steady-state concentration was calculated for the non-plasma protein bound (free) fraction of the drug. Estimation of renal clearance in terms of unbound rather than total concentration was important because the plasma protein binding of one antibiotic, cloxacillin, was capacity limited; this was not the case for benzylpenicillin or cephradine. Tubular clearance was determined from the difference between renal clearance and glomerular filtration, assumed to be equal to creatinine clearance. Tubular reabsorption was considered negligible because high urine flow rates were maintained.

In each case, a plot of tubular excretion rate *versus* free drug concentration demonstrated a saturable process. Estimates of EC_{50}, the free drug concentration at which tubular excretion rate is 50% of maximum tubular excretion rate, were 5 to 10 mg/L for cloxacillin, 50 to 100 mg/L for benzylpenicillin, and 250 to 300 mg/L for cephradine. For cloxacillin, the results indicate that capacity-limited tubular secretion is of clinical interest. An EC_{50} of 6 mg/L corresponds to a total cloxacillin concentration of 54 mg/L, a level not unusual in clinical practice.

Another similarity of tubular secretion to active intestinal absorption is competitive inhibition of one drug by another. This characteristic has been used to prolong the half-life of drugs like penicillin that are eliminated to a considerable extent by tubular secretion. Probenecid, a weak organic acid, competitively inhibits the tubular secretion of penicillin G and other penicillins, and reduces the rate of urinary excretion. Probenecid has been used clinically to increase the duration of effect of penicillins. Parenteral penicillin G or ampicillin, in high doses, with probenecid is considered to be an effective treatment for gonorrhea.[4]

Many drugs are marketed as racemic mixtures. Although enantiomers have identical physical and chemical properties, the chiral macromolecules in the body are quite specific to the spatial arrangement of drug molecules. Consequently, stereospecific or stereoselective interactions between proteins or other macromolecules and drugs are common. These interactions result in stereoselective pharmacokinetics and pharmacodynamics of drugs.

In contrast to the many studies concerning stereoselective hepatic metabolism of drugs, few studies have examined whether stereoselective renal excretion of drugs occurs. Since tubular secretion appears to be a saturable, carrier-mediated process, it is reasonable to consider the possibility of stereoselectivity. Two systems are primarily responsible for the active tubular secretion of drugs, one for organic anions and another for organic cations. Neither system has been carefully studied with respect to stereoselective tubular secretion.

Pindolol, a beta-blocker marketed as a racemic mixture, was used to study stereoselective renal clearance of organic cations.[5] Normal human subjects received an oral dose of racemic pindolol. A stereospecific assay method was used to measure the concentrations of d- and l-pindolol in plasma and urine. Renal clearance and other pharmacokinetic parameters of both enantiomers were calculated and compared.

The area under the drug concentration-time curve (AUC), half-life, and amount excreted in the urine were significantly greater for l- than for d-pindolol. Also, the renal clearance of l-pindolol was greater than that of d-pindolol in all subjects; mean values were 240 ml/min and 200 ml/min, respectively. Since binding to plasma proteins was not found to be stereoselective, differences in renal clearance between d- and l-pindolol probably reflect stereoselective renal transport.

Tubular Reabsorption. After undergoing secretion or glomerular filtration, most drugs are subject to tubular reabsorption. A large concentration gradient exists between drug in the renal tubules and free drug in the plasma, because of the efficient reabsorption of water. Tubular reabsorption of drugs is usually a passive process. The tubule membranes favor the transport of lipid-soluble drugs; compounds that are poorly lipid soluble or ionized are poorly reabsorbed. The reabsorption of drugs that are weak acids or bases depends on the pH of the tubular fluids.

Tubular Reabsorption and Urine pH. The pH of fluids in the proximal tubule approximates that of plasma (pH 7.4), whereas the pH in the distal tubule approximates that of urine, which may vary from 4.5 to 8.0; on the average, urine pH is 6.3. These extremes contrast with the narrow range of blood pH, 7.3 to 7.5. Accordingly, a large pH gradient may exist between blood and urine in the distal tubule.

Urine pH is affected by diet, drugs, and the condition of the patient. The pH of the urine also varies during the day. Respiratory and metabolic acidosis produce acid urine; respiratory and metabolic alkalosis produce alkaline urine. On the other hand, the urine is alkaline in renal tubular acidosis. Drugs like acetazolamide and sodium bi-

carbonate produce an alkaline urine; ammonium chloride and ascorbic acid produce an acid urine.

Since drug reabsorption takes place in the distal tubule, urine pH is assumed to indicate the pH at the site of reabsorption. According to the pH-partition hypothesis, acidification of the urine promotes the reabsorption of weak acids but retards the reabsorption of weak bases. The renal clearance of weak acids is increased if the urine is made alkaline because more drug is in the ionized form and cannot be reabsorbed. On the other hand, the renal clearance of weak bases is low in alkaline urine but may be increased dramatically if the urine is acidified.

The influence of pH on tubular reabsorption also depends on the pKa of the drug. Relatively strong acids or bases are virtually completely ionized over the entire range of urine pH and undergo little reabsorption. The critical range of pKa values for pH-dependent excretion is about 3.0 to 7.5 for acids and 7.5 to 10.5 for bases.[3]

The extent to which changes in urine pH alter the rate of drug elimination depends on the contribution of renal clearance to total clearance. Although weak acids like tolbutamide and warfarin are susceptible to pH-dependent changes in reabsorption, such changes have little effect on their elimination, which depends essentially on hepatic metabolism.

Studies to determine pH-dependent urinary excretion often maintain urine pH at the acid or alkaline extreme by continually administering either ammonium chloride or sodium bicarbonate during the course of the study. These studies are also useful for detecting renal mechanisms that are not evident under normal urine pH conditions. For example, in women subjects, a change in urine pH from 5.3 to 7.4 increases the renal clearance (corrected for protein binding) of sulfisoxazole from 92 ml/min to 187 ml/min.[1] Although sulfisoxazole renal clearance at the average value of urine pH is consistent with glomerular filtration, the data at the extremes of urine pH indicate that both tubular secretion and reabsorption contribute to the renal excretion of this sulfonamide.

The influence of urine pH on the elimination of sulfonamides has been studied by many investigators; often, the effects are considerable. Changes in urine pH from 5 to 8 have been shown to decrease the half-life of sulfaethidole in man from 11.4 to 4.2 hr.[7] The rate of elimination of sulfalene and sulfasymazine in healthy subjects was doubled

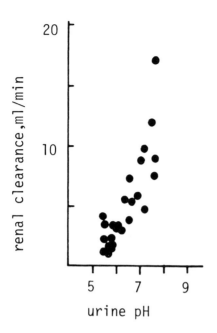

Fig. 11–2. Effect of urine pH on the renal clearance of sulfamethoxazole. (Data from Vree, T.B., et al.[9])

by administration of sodium bicarbonate, which increased urine pH from about 6 to 8.[8] Half-lives were decreased from 72 to 14 hr for sulfalene and from 32 to 7 hr for sulfasymazine. The effect of urine pH on the renal clearance of sulfamethoxazole is shown in Figure 11–2.[9]

Blood levels of salicylate commonly found in patients on high-dose aspirin therapy for rheumatoid arthritis fluctuate considerably with changes in urine pH. Patients concomitantly receiving antacids that alkalinize the urine may require higher doses of aspirin to maintain adequate blood levels of salicylate.

The renal clearance of methotrexate varies from 48 to 300 ml/min over a urine pH range of 5.5 to 8.3 in patients with various malignancies but normal renal function.[10] Preliminary data indicate that the increase in renal clearance, resulting from urinary alkalinization in these patients, is reflected by a shorter half-life of methotrexate.

pH-dependent renal excretion has also been demonstrated for many weak bases, including amphetamine, ephedrine, methadone, and fenfluramine. In some cases, the change in renal clearance also results in a change in the half-life of the drug. For example, the average half-life of pseudoephedrine in human subjects decreased from 13.4 to 4.7 hr when urine pH was reduced from 8 to 5.[11] Unanticipated toxicity after ordinary doses of

pseudoephedrine in a patient with renal tubular acidosis was associated with high blood levels and low renal clearance, as a result of persistently alkaline urine.[12]

Large differences in elimination rate, as a function of urine pH, are found with amphetamine.[13] On the average, about a sevenfold difference in the total clearance of amphetamine from the plasma is evident when data from subjects with controlled acid urine are compared with data from the same subjects with uncontrolled urine pH.[14]

Urine pH also influences the fraction of drug excreted unchanged. For example, about 57% of a dose of amphetamine is excreted unchanged in subjects with acid urine (pH 4.5 to 5.6) compared to about 7% in subjects with alkaline urine (pH 7.1 to 8.0).[13] Renal excretion of unchanged drug accounts for about 90% of an oral dose of ephedrine in subjects with acid urine but only about 25% in subjects with alkaline urine.[15] Administration of amphetamine or related drugs with sodium bicarbonate not only enhances pharmacologic effects but also makes it much more difficult to detect unchanged drug in the urine of athletes who illicitly ingest stimulants to enhance performance.

The influence of urine pH on the pharmacokinetics of flecainide, an antiarrhythmic agent, has also been studied.[16] The cumulative urinary excretion following a 300 mg oral dose was 134 mg (45% of the dose) under acid conditions but only 22 mg (7% of the dose) under alkaline conditions. Renal clearance of flecainide in individual subjects ranged from 2 to 172 ml/min under alkaline conditions and from 98 to 968 ml/min under acid conditions.

Important differences in half-life and AUC were also observed. The mean half-life of flecainide was 33 hours under alkaline conditions and about 8 hours under acid conditions. The mean value for total AUC was more than 3 times greater under alkaline than under acid conditions. From a clinical toxicology point of view, efforts to acidify urine might be a useful therapeutic measure in patients with dangerously high serum levels of flecainide.

The occurrence of diurnal variation in urine pH, possibly related to decreased sensitivity of the respiratory center during sleep, is well known. Urine pH in most individuals is relatively low during sleep but increases after awakening. Accordingly, a corresponding diurnal cycle may occur in the rate of elimination of certain drugs. Clinical studies show that the mean half-life of sulfasymazine (pKa

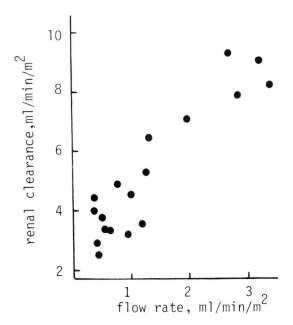

Fig. 11–3. Effect of urine flow rate on the renal clearance of theophylline. (Data from Levy, G., and Koysooko, R.[18])

= 5.5) during the night (35 hr) is about three times higher than during the day (13.5 hr).[17]

Tubular Reabsorption and Urine Flow Rate. Diuresis increases the renal clearance of drugs that are extensively reabsorbed, because it decreases the concentration gradient between the tubular fluid and the blood. The relationship between the renal clearance of theophylline and urine flow rate is shown in Figure 11–3.[18] Fluctuations in the excretion rate of chlorpheniramine[19] and pseudoephedrine[12] coincide with fluctuations in urine flow rate. Suppression of tubular reabsorption by altering urine pH and flow rate is the basis for the use of forced alkaline diuresis in the treatment of certain drug intoxications.

Active Tubular Reabsorption. Although the tubular reabsorption of most drugs is a passive process, there are some important exceptions. Lithium and fluoride appear to undergo active tubular reabsorption. Uric acid is thought to be reabsorbed by an active transport system that is inhibited by uricosuric drugs. The renal clearance of riboflavin in man increases with increasing vitamin concentrations in the plasma, suggesting capacity-limited tubular reabsorption.[20]

Crystalluria. In principle, a drug may be so concentrated in the renal tubules after water reabsorption that precipitation and kidney damage may occur. This phenomenon is termed *crystallu-*

ria. It is of concern with drugs that are given in high doses and are excreted unchanged or converted to a metabolite with limited solubility in the urine. The use of certain sulfonamides has been associated with the formation of crystalline deposits of unchanged and/or acetylated drug in the kidney.[21] Crystalluria has also been observed in patients treated with large doses of ampicillin.[22] Precipitation can be avoided by assuring an adequate rate of urine flow. The minimum rate of urine flow may be calculated by dividing the excretion rate of drug or metabolite by its solubility in urine at a given pH.[23] A minimum urine flow rate of 190 ml/hr is required to prevent precipitation of sulfisoxazole in acidic urine (pH = 5); a flow of only 5 ml/hr is required if urine pH is 7. Hydration and alkalinization of urine during and after large doses of methotrexate are recommended procedures to prevent crystalluria.[10]

Biliary Excretion

A drug may be secreted by the liver cells into the bile and pass into the intestine. Some or most of the secreted drug may be reabsorbed in the small intestine and undergo *enterohepatic cycling;* the rest is excreted in the feces. This cycle may be repeated many times, until biotransformation, renal excretion, and fecal excretion ultimately eliminate the drug from the body. In this way, enterohepatic cycling may increase the persistence of drug in the body.

Often, biotransformation of a drug occurs in the liver, and a glucuronide or some other conjugate is secreted in the bile. In some instances, the polar metabolite cannot be reabsorbed, and fecal excretion occurs. In other cases, deconjugation takes place in the intestine, and the liberated parent drug may be absorbed.

Biliary excretion and renal tubular secretion share certain characteristics. Both are active, capacity-limited processes, subject to competitive inhibition. Concentrations of drug or metabolites in bile are often much higher than in plasma, consistent with an active transport mechanism. Many examples of competitive inhibition of biliary secretion have been reported.[24] Probenecid inhibits the biliary secretion of methotrexate in the rat; this inhibition is associated with increased toxicity.[25] A 25 mg/kg dose of methotrexate produces no mortality. The same dose given with a nontoxic dose of probenecid results in an 80% mortality rate.

In man, bile flow rate ranges from 0.5 to 0.8

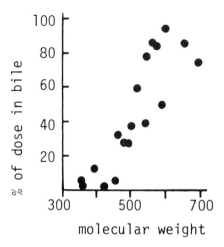

Fig. 11–4. The influence of molecular weight on the biliary excretion of various cephalosporins in the rat. (Data from Wright, W.E., and Line, V.D.[28])

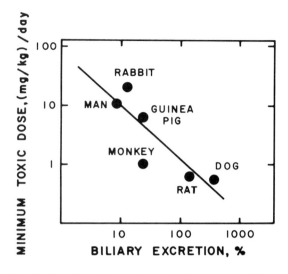

Fig. 11–5. Correlation between total (cumulative) biliary excretion (expressed as percent of dose) and the sensitivity to intestinal lesions in different species. (Data from Duggan, D.E., et al.[31])

ml/min. Factors affecting hepatic bile formation have been reviewed by Javitt.[26] Since the bile to plasma drug concentration ratio can approach 1000, biliary clearances of 500 ml/min or higher may be achieved. In most animal species, including man, drug excreted in the bile enters the intestine after storage in the gallbladder; the rat is unusual in that it has no gallbladder.

Seemingly, the most important factor influencing the excretion of a drug in bile is the molecular weight of the form of the compound excreted. Studies in the rat indicate that compounds having a molecular weight of less than about 300 tend to be excreted in urine, whereas compounds of molecular weight exceeding 300 are found in the bile in appreciable quantities.[27] Figure 11–4 shows the relationship between molecular weight and the biliary excretion of 18 cephalosporins in rats.[28] The molecular weight threshold for appreciable biliary excretion (i.e., > 5 to 10% of the dose) in man appears to be on the order of 400 to 500.[27]

Biliary excretion of drugs seems to be a more important elimination process in laboratory animals, including the rat and dog, than in man.[24] Its actual importance in man, however, is not clear, because information on the biliary excretion of drugs and metabolites in man is limited. Appreciable amounts of indocyanine green, digitoxin, cromolyn, erythromycin, and rifampin are excreted unchanged in the bile in man. Indomethacin, sulfobromophthalein, morphine, carbenoxolone, and estradiol also undergo biliary excretion in man, but largely in the form of conjugates.[29]

Biliary excretion is important in the elimination of rifampin. The half-life of the drug is about twice as long in patients with biliary obstruction as in patients without obstruction (5.7 hr vs 2.6 hr).[30] Unusually pronounced accumulation with repeated doses is found in patients with obstructive jaundice.

Biliary excretion of indomethacin and its conjugates appears to be an important if not a causative factor for intestinal lesions following indomethacin administration in many species.[31] The correlation between the cumulative biliary excretion of indomethacin and its conjugates and the sensitivity to intestinal lesions in different species is shown in Figure 11–5. Note that enterohepatic cycling in the dog and rat is so extensive that the intestine is exposed to more than 100% of the dose. Biliary excretion is also a factor in the elimination of sulindac, another nonsteroidal anti-inflammatory, in man.[32]

Recent investigations have been directed toward detecting enterohepatic cycling in man by interrupting the cycle in the intestine. For example, oral administration of cholestyramine, a nonabsorbable ion-exchange resin that strongly binds acid and neutral drugs, decreases the half-life of digitoxin from 6.0 to 4.5 days and reduces the effects of the drug on ECG values.[33] These results suggest that a significant fraction of the dose of digitoxin undergoes enterohepatic cycling; cholestyramine interrupts the cycle and promotes fecal excretion.

Cholestyramine has also been reported to decrease the half-life and anticoagulant effect and increase the clearance of warfarin in healthy human subjects.[34]

Oral administration of charcoal, a nonspecific adsorbent, is expected to produce results similar to those of cholestyramine. Charcoal administration decreases the half-life of the antileprotic drug dapsone from 20.5 to 10.8 hr.[35] Charcoal also enhances the elimination of phenobarbital, carbamazepine, and phenylbutazone in man.[36] Repeated doses of activated charcoal from 6 hr on after oral administration of a single dose of amitriptyline resulted in a significant decrease in half-life and total AUC of parent drug as well as of nortriptyline, its active metabolite.[37]

The results with nonabsorbable adsorbents are surprising, because they suggest that a far wider variety of drugs is cycled between the gut and systemic circulation in man than we suspected, based on our understanding of biliary excretion. An alternative explanation is that some drugs are secreted into the gut lumen by a nonbiliary mechanism and that this secretion is promoted by intestinal adsorbents. Studies with the toxic organochlorine pesticide chlordecone (Kepone) support this alternative mechanism.

Cholestyramine is useful in the treatment of chlordecone intoxication, because it increases the excretion of the pesticide in the stools.[38] These findings suggest that enterohepatic cycling of chlordecone is significant. Fecal excretion of chlordecone, however, is observed in man and rat even when bile is totally diverted from the small intestine.[39] Therefore, chlordecone must enter the human and rat small intestine by a nonbiliary mechanism as well as through bile. This alternative entry mechanism probably involves direct secretion or partitioning from the bloodstream to the lumen across the gut wall. This mechanism may apply to other drugs and chemicals.

Salivary Excretion

Transfer of drugs from blood to saliva depends on lipid solubility, pKa, and plasma protein binding. The concentration of a lipid-soluble nonionized drug in saliva approximates the free (unbound) drug concentration in plasma. Since the average pH of saliva (6.5) is lower than the pH of plasma (7.4), saliva/plasma free drug concentration ratios are less than unity for weak acids, and exceed unity for weak bases. Some drugs may be actively transported from blood to saliva. For example, the concentration of lithium in saliva of healthy subjects is reported to be 2 to 3 times higher than in plasma.[40] Metoprolol concentrations in saliva have been reported to be much higher than can be predicted from the pKa of the drug.[41]

Salivary excretion is of little quantitative importance in drug disposition; however, the salivary excretion of certain drugs may be of therapeutic interest. For example, the effectiveness of rifampin against meningococci harbored in the nasopharynx is thought to be related to the fact that salivary concentrations in patients receiving the drug exceed the minimum inhibitory concentration of rifampin for the carrier strains.[42] Salivary excretion of antibiotics may be a cause of lingua nigra or black hairy tongue in patients receiving these drugs.[43] Gingival hyperplasia in epileptics may be related to salivary excretion of phenytoin.

The relatively constant saliva/plasma drug concentration ratio for certain drugs has created interest in the use of drug concentration in saliva as an indicator of total or free drug concentration in plasma. Good to excellent correlations between drug concentrations in saliva and plasma or serum have been reported for antipyrine, theophylline, lithium, salicylate, phenytoin, phenacetin, carbamazepine, sulfapyridine, caffeine, ethanol, diazepam, phenobarbital, primidone, quinidine, acetaminophen, tolbutamide, and digoxin.

Although many reports suggest little variability in saliva-plasma concentration ratios among subjects, other reports are less encouraging. Large differences among relatively sick patients and within individual patients in saliva/plasma procainamide concentration ratios have been reported;[44] ratios ranged from 0.3 to 8.8. One patient had a ratio of 7.2 on one occasion and 2.8 on another. In general, the variability in ratios was related to variability in saliva pH, which ranged from 6.2 to 8.0. Patients with relatively low saliva pH values had relatively high saliva/plasma procainamide concentration ratios. These findings are consistent with the fact that procainamide is a weak base, with a pKa of 9.4.

The relationship between saliva/plasma drug concentration ratio, pKa, pH, and binding is expressed in the following equations:

$$\frac{C_s}{C_p} = \frac{1 + 10^{(pH_s - pKa)}}{1 + 10^{(pH_p - pKa)}} \times \frac{f_p}{f_s} \quad (11\text{--}14)$$

which applies to weak acids, and

$$\frac{C_s}{C_p} = \frac{1 + 10^{(pKa - pH_s)}}{1 + 10^{(pKa - pH_p)}} \times \frac{f_p}{f_s} \quad (11\text{--}15)$$

which applies to weak bases. The terms C_s and C_p refer to drug concentrations, pH_s and pH_p refer to pH, and f_p and f_s refer to free fractions in saliva and plasma. No drug binding has been reported in saliva; therefore, $f_s = 1$. The saliva to plasma concentration ratio of tolbutamide, a weak acid, has been calculated to be 0.012, based on the following values: $pKa = 5.4$, $pH_s = 6.5$, $pH_p = 7.4$, $f_p = 0.09$, and $f_s = 1.0$. This estimate agrees with experimental observations.[45] The difference in pH between saliva and plasma results in a saliva level that is much smaller than free tolbutamide concentration in plasma. The saliva/plasma concentration ratios of tolbutamide and chlorpropamide (weak acids), and procainamide and meperidine (weak bases) are sensitive to saliva pH over a wide range of values, from 6.0 to 8.0.[46] The saliva/plasma concentration ratio of phenobarbital is relatively independent of saliva pH up to pH 7.

Secretion of Drugs into Milk

The excretion of drugs in breast milk has received considerable attention.[47–49,50] Drugs ingested by a lactating mother must be expected to appear in her milk and be ingested by a breast-feeding infant.

Distribution into milk has been studied in some detail in goats and cows. These studies suggest that drug transfer between milk and plasma occurs by passive diffusion, consistent with pH-partition theory. Milk is generally more acidic than plasma, so weak bases tend to concentrate there, whereas weak acids tend to have milk-to-plasma (M/P) concentration ratios less than one.

Milk is a complex fluid with high fat and protein levels, but composition varies widely among species. This has hampered the development of animal models. A useful approach, which takes into account milk and plasma pH, milk and plasma protein binding, and milk fat partitioning, has been proposed for predicting M/P ratios in breast-feeding women.[51] The model was developed by assuming that only the unbound, un-ionized form of a drug located in the aqueous phases of blood and milk can diffuse across mammary membranes and that no carrier-mediated transfer occurs. Under these condition, at steady state, un-ionized free drug concentration in plasma equals un-ionized free drug

concentration in skim milk, the aqueous phase of milk.

Drug concentration in skim milk (C_{SM}) is related to concentration in whole milk (C_M) as follows:

$$C_{SM} = (S/M)\, C_M \quad (11\text{--}16)$$

where S/M refers to the skim-to-whole milk drug concentration ratio.

Only that fraction of the drug in the aqueous phase not bound to milk proteins (f_{SM}) and un-ionized ($f_{SM\,un}$) is available for diffusion. Therefore,

C_{SM}, unbound, un-ionized

$$= (f_{SM})(f_{SM\,un})(S/M)\, C_M \quad (11\text{--}17)$$

A similar expression can be written for the un-ionized, free drug concentration in plasma, i.e.,

C_P, unbound, un-ionized

$$= (f_P)(f_{P\,un})\, C_P \quad (11\text{--}18)$$

Therefore, at steady state,

$$(f_{SM})(f_{SM\,un})(S/M)\, C_M = (f_P)(f_{P\,un})\, C_P \quad (11\text{--}19)$$

and the milk-to-plasma drug concentration ratio is given by:

$$M/P = C_M/C_p$$

$$= (f_P)(f_{P\,un})/\,(f_{SM})(f_{SM\,un})(S/M) \quad (11\text{--}20)$$

Fleishaker et al.[51] used this approach, adding drugs to milk and plasma in vitro, to predict the distribution of diazepam, phenytoin, and propranolol in breast milk from lactating women. Single milk and serum samples were collected in the morning from each woman participating in the study. Milk was obtained by completely emptying the breast using an electric pump. After collection, pH and fat content were determined. Skim milk was prepared by centrifuging whole milk. Serum and skim milk protein binding was determined by equilibrium dialysis. S/M ratios were estimated after incubation of whole milk with drug for 1 hr.

The test drugs were bound to a smaller extent in skim milk than in serum. For example, at phenytoin concentrations ordinarily found in plasma during treatment with the drug, binding was 86% in serum but only 42% in milk. The S/M ratio was less than one for each drug indicating significant partitioning into milk fat. Diazepam showed the highest affinity with an S/M ratio of only 0.22.

The values of S/M, free fraction in skim milk

and plasma, and fraction of drug un-ionized in skim milk and plasma (estimated by assuming a plasma pH of 7.4 and a milk pH of 7.1) for each drug were used to calculate M/P ratios, according to Equation 11–20. Estimates were 0.16 for diazepam, 0.50 for propranolol, and 0.30 for phenytoin, in good agreement with published in vivo values found in nursing mothers.

The lowest M/P ratio was found with diazepam because it is the most extensively bound to plasma proteins (99.7%). If plasma protein binding were ignored, the M/P ratio would be about 1.0 rather than 0.16. Binding to milk proteins and partitioning into milk fat are also important. If these factors were ignored, the M/P ratio would be 0.013. Only when all factors are taken into account are reasonable predictions obtained.

Using the M/P ratio and the measured or calculated average steady-state drug concentration in maternal plasma (C_{ss}), one can predict the average drug concentration in milk and the amount of drug that will be ingested by the infant. Steady-state levels in the mother may be calculated as follows:

$$C_{ss} = DR \times F/Cl \qquad (11–21)$$

where DR is the dosing rate (i.e., the daily dose divided by 24 hours), F is the bioavailability of the drug, and Cl is drug clearance in the mother.

Average drug concentration in milk is the product of C_{ss} and M/P. The dose of drug ingested by the infant is the product of average drug concentration in milk and the volume of milk consumed. However, more drug will be ingested if breast feeding coincides with peak drug concentration in the mother, and less drug will be ingested if nursing takes place immediately before the mother's next dose. An average infant consumes about 150 ml of milk per kg of body weight per day. The ingested dose can then be compared, on a mg/kg basis, to the usual adult dose to assess the level of risk.

One commentary on breast feeding concluded that most drugs taken by a nursing mother will be excreted in her milk, but in amounts that are unlikely to harm the infant. Theophylline is a likely example. An average steady-state theophylline concentration of 15 μg/ml in the plasma of a nursing mother gives rise to an average level of about 12 μg/ml in breast milk.[52] If the infant nursed 1 liter of milk per day, about 12 mg of theophylline would be ingested or 2 mg/kg/day for a 6-kg infant. This amount of theophylline is relatively small

compared with the usual initial adult dose of 4 mg/kg every 8 to 12 hr and is unlikely to cause harm.

A direct comparison of the infant dose with the usual adult dose may be misleading. Drug elimination in the infant may be comparatively poor because of immature renal function and incomplete development of hepatic microsomal enzymes. One report suggests that an adjustment factor accounting for the likely impairment of drug clearance in the infant is needed to assess the relative risk of drug ingestion in the breast-feeding infant.[50] These investigators suggest that a 3-day old term infant ingesting one-half the maternal dose in breast milk, on a mg/kg or mg/M^2 basis, must be assumed to have 50% greater exposure to the drug because of reduced clearance.

A review dealing specifically with psychotropic drugs in breast milk states:[53]

With our present inadequate knowledge, it is difficult to prepare a list of drugs that are safe or are harmful to the breast-fed infant. However, we do know that drugs such as diazepam, lithium, bromides, reserpine and opium alkaloids are to be avoided and that barbiturates, haloperidol, and penfluridol should be administered (to the mother) with caution.

The Medical Letter on Drugs and Therapeutics updated information on drugs in breast milk in 1979.[54] It concluded as follows:

Wherever possible, nursing mothers should not take drugs. Mothers who must take antithyroid drugs (especially radioactive iodine), lithium, chloramphenicol and probably most anticancer drugs should not nurse. The safety of many other drugs for use during nursing is not known.

A committee on drugs[54a] concluded in 1983 that the following agents are contraindicated during breast feeding: amethopterin, cyclophosphamide, and perhaps other cytotoxic agents because of possible immune suppression, association with carcinogenesis, and unknown effects on growth, bromocriptine because it suppresses lactation, and methimazole and thiouracil because of potential effects on the infant's thyroid function. Cimetidine, clemastine, ergotamine, gold salts, and phenindione were also cited as contraindicated. Metronidazole and various radiopharmaceuticals were listed as drugs that require temporary cessation of breast feeding for 1 to 14 days to allow elimination of the dose.

DRUG METABOLISM

Drug metabolism or biotransformation refers to the biochemical (enzymatic) conversion of a drug to another chemical form. Many tissues in the body are capable of metabolizing drugs, but most drugs are mainly metabolized in the liver by enzymes localized in hepatic microsomes, a cellular fraction derived from the endoplasmic reticulum.

Drug-metabolizing enzymes oxidize, reduce, hydrolyze, or conjugate compounds. Reduction, oxidation, and hydrolytic reactions (Phase I pathways) result in metabolites with functional groups (e.g., hydroxyl, amine, or carboxyl) that can be conjugated (Phase II pathways). In man the most common conjugations of drugs or metabolites occur with acetate, sulfate, glycine, or glucuronic acid. Examples of the more important drug metabolism pathways in man are given in Table 11-1.

Most oxidative processes take place in liver microsomes. They require reduced nicotinamide phosphate (NADPH), molecular oxygen, and a complex of enzymes in the endoplasmic reticulum; the terminal oxidizing enzyme is cytochrome P-450, a hemeprotein. Many drugs, as well as steroid hormones, are oxidized by this microsomal system. Oxidation of certain drugs, such as alcohols and xanthines, may be catalyzed by nonmicrosomal enzymes; ethanol, mercaptopurine, and azothioprine are examples.

Reduction is a relatively uncommon pathway of drug metabolism. Azo dyes, used as food coloring, are reduced to form amines, both in the liver and by intestinal flora. Sulfasalazine is also cleaved by intestinal bacteria to form aminosalicylate, the active component, and sulfapyridine. Prednisone and cortisone are also reduced to active metabolites, prednisolone and hydrocortisone.

Digoxin is metabolized by anaerobic intestinal bacteria in the lower gastrointestinal tract to cardioinactive compounds called *digoxin reduction products*.[55] Digoxin inactivation by this pathway affects the bioavailability of the cardiac glycoside and results in increased dosage requirements for some patients. Factors found to increase inactivation include rapid gastric emptying and hypermotility as well as the administration of slowly dissolving dosage forms of digoxin. In such cases, a significant fraction of the dose reaches the lower bowel and is subject to reduction and inactivation.

Other investigators observed that although the oral anticoagulant acenocoumarol is efficiently metabolized by intestinal flora to its inactive amino metabolite, this is not a clinical problem because the drug is rapidly absorbed from the upper gastrointestinal tract after oral administration of commercial tablets and never reaches sites in the gut with a high density of microflora. On the other hand, appreciable amounts of reduced metabolites are recovered in the urine when acenocoumarol is given in a slowly-dissolving dosage form.[56]

Hydrolysis of esters and amides is a common pathway of drug metabolism. The liver microsomes contain nonspecific esterases, as do other tissues and plasma.

Glucuronide formation is the most common conjugation process of drug metabolism. It involves the reaction between uridine diphosphate glucuronic acid (UDPG) and drugs containing hydroxyl, carboxyl, or amine groups. The reaction is mediated by the microsomal enzyme glucuronyltransferase. Glucuronides are water soluble acids that are easily excreted in urine and bile. Some ester glucuronides are labile and can be hydrolyzed in urine or plasma to parent drug. High blood levels of clofibrate in patients with renal disease are the result of accumulation and hydrolysis of the glucuronide conjugate in the plasma.[57]

Aromatic acids are sometimes converted to glycine conjugates. The acids are activated by combining with ATP to form coenzyme A derivatives before conjugation with glycine. The conversion of benzoic acid to hippuric acid and salicylic acid to salicyluric acid are examples of this metabolic pathway.

Many amine compounds, including sulfonamides, isoniazid, dapsone, hydralazine, and procainamide, are metabolized to their acetyl derivative by acetylcoenzyme A and acetyltransferase.

Conjugation with sulfate is a common pathway of metabolism of hydroxy compounds, particularly steroids. The sulfate donor is 3'-phosphoadenosine-5'-phosphosulfate (PAPS). Sulfate conjugates, like glucuronides, have a high renal clearance.

Drugs subject to biotransformation usually produce several metabolites. In some instances, dozens of metabolites originate from the administration of a single drug (e.g., chlorpromazine). Metabolites can arise from parallel or consecutive pathways. For example, meperidine is simultaneously metabolized to normeperidine (N-dealkylation) and meperidinic acid (ester hydrolysis); salicylate is simultaneously conjugated with glycine and glucuronic acid. On the other hand, phenytoin is largely metabolized to 5-phenyl-5-hydroxyphenylhydantoin (aromatic hydroxylation), which in turn is conjugated with glucuronic acid; phenacetin is oxi-

Table 11–1. Metabolic Pathways for Drugs in Man

Type of reaction	Example
1. Oxidation	

1. Oxidation
   a. Aromatic hydroxylation

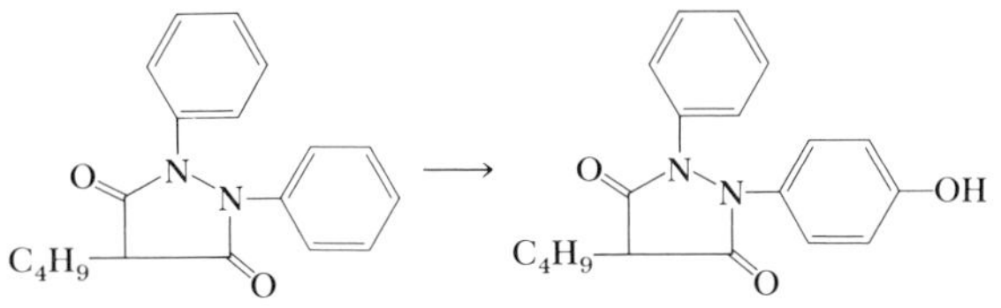

Phenylbutazone

   b. Aliphatic hydroxylation

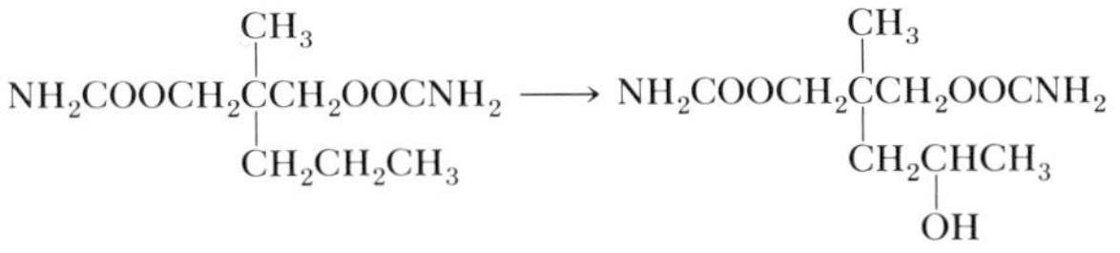

$$NH_2COOCH_2CCH_2OOCNH_2 \longrightarrow NH_2COOCH_2CCH_2OOCNH_2$$

Meprobamate

   c. Oxidative N-dealkylation

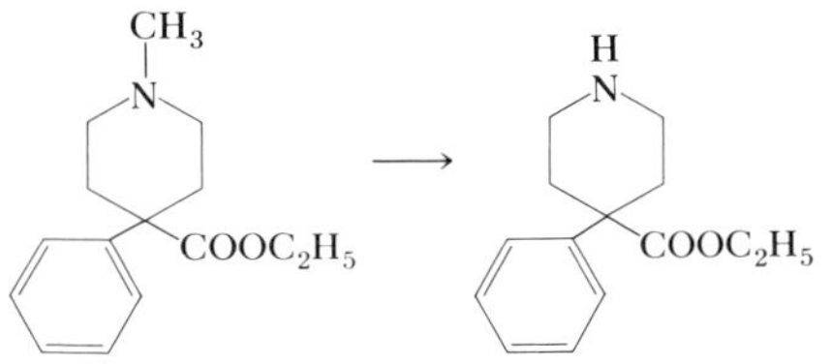

Meperidine

   d. Oxidative O-dealkylation

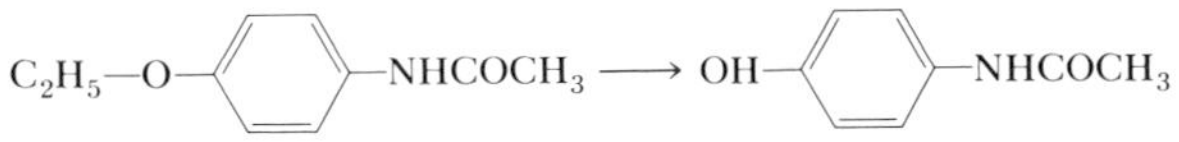

$$C_2H_5{-}O{-}{-}NHCOCH_3 \longrightarrow OH{-}{-}NHCOCH_3$$

Phenacetin   Acetaminophen

   e. S-oxidation

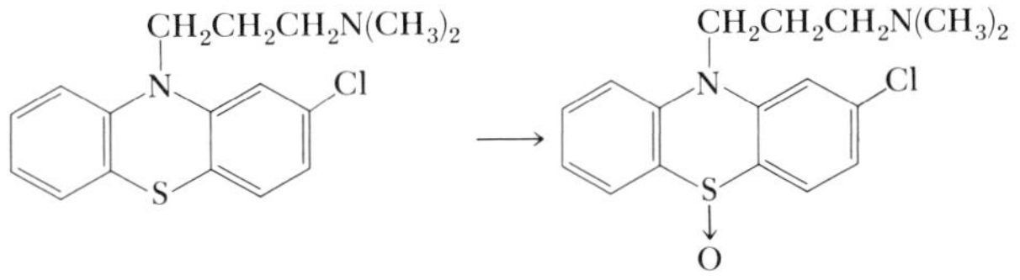

Chlorpromazine

2. Reduction

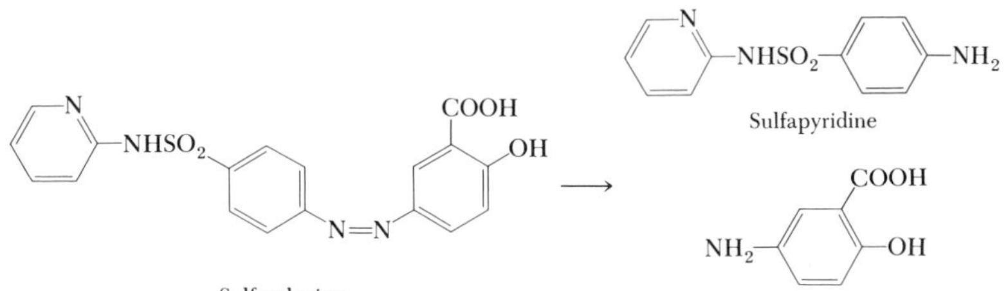

Sulfapyridine

Sulfasalazine

5-Aminosalicylate

3. Hydrolysis

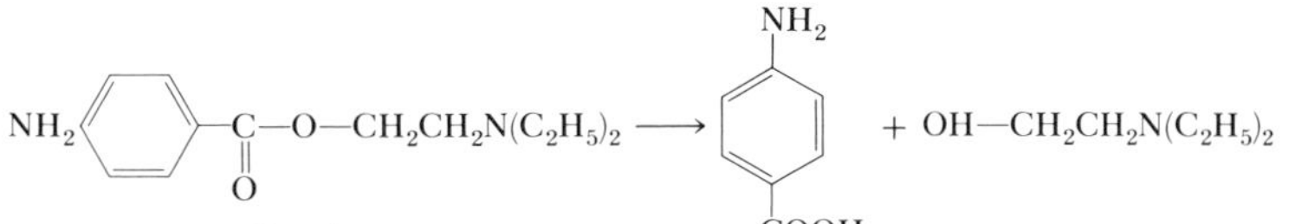

$$NH_2{-}{-}C{-}O{-}CH_2CH_2N(C_2H_5)_2 \longrightarrow + OH{-}CH_2CH_2N(C_2H_5)_2$$

Procaine

Table 11–1. (Cont.)

Type of reaction	Example

4. Conjugation
    a. Glycine

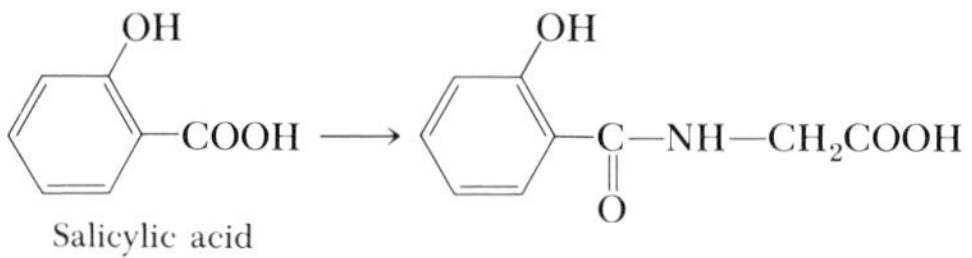

Salicylic acid

    b. Glucuronic acid

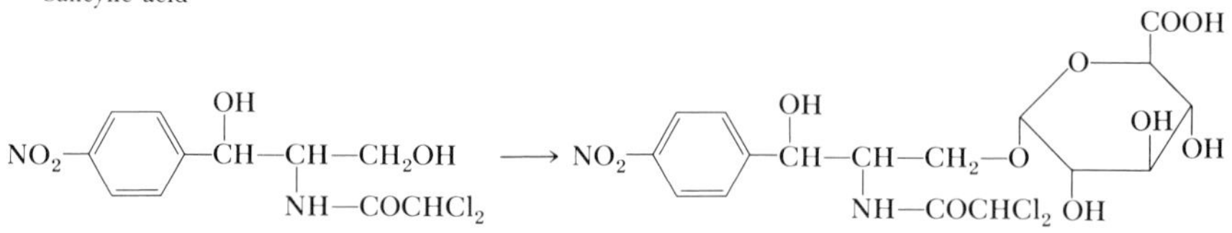

Chloramphenicol

    c. Sulfate

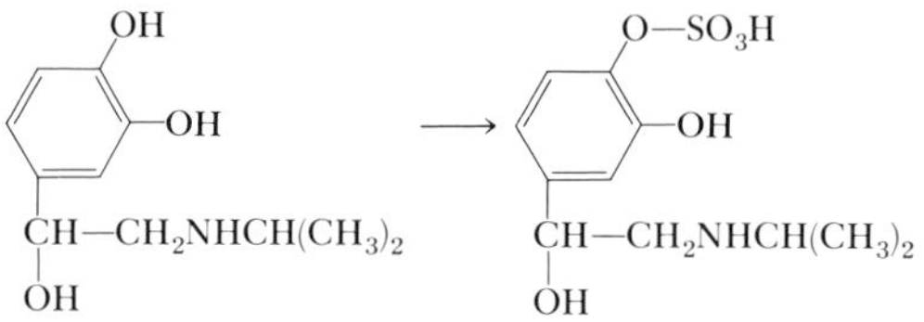

Isoproterenol

    d. Acetylation

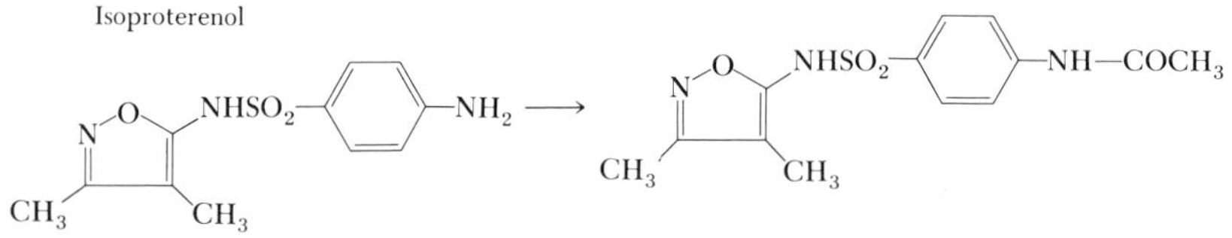

Sulfisoxazole

dized (dealkylation) to acetaminophen, which in turn is sulfated and glucuronidated.

Induction and Inhibition of Drug Metabolizing Enzymes

Microsomal drug metabolism can be stimulated by a large number of drugs and chemicals by a process known as enzyme induction.[58] Microsomal enzyme induction is a complex process associated with an increase in liver weight, proliferation of the endoplasmic reticulum, and increases in microsomal protein and cytochrome P-450. Elevated levels of cytochrome P-450 are the result of increased synthesis.

At least two kinds of inducers have been found, exemplified by phenobarbital and polycyclic aromatic hydrocarbons. Differences between these kinds of inducers have been discussed by Conney.[58] Phenobarbital-type inducers stimulate a wide range of metabolic pathways in liver microsomes, including oxidation, reduction, and glucuronide formation. Polycyclic aromatic hydrocarbons, such as 3-methylcholanthrene or cigarette smoke, stimulate a more limited group of metabolic reactions. Phenobarbital enhances the metabolism of meper-

idine to normeperidine but polycyclic hydrocarbons do not. Cigarette smoke stimulates the metabolism of theophylline but phenobarbital does not.

The effect of smoking on estrogen metabolism was studied in postmenopausal women treated for 1 year with different doses of oral estradiol. Estrogen levels were lower in smokers than nonsmokers, particularly so in subjects receiving high-dose estradiol (4 mg). In this group, serum levels of estrone and estradiol in smokers were only 50% of those in nonsmokers. Moreover, a significant inverse correlation was found between the number of cigarettes smoked daily and the changes in the levels of serum estrone and estradiol. This report suggests that increased hepatic metabolism results in lower estrogen levels among postmenopausal smokers, which may contribute to the reported increased risk of osteoporosis among smokers.[59]

Some drugs induce microsomal enzymes that play a role in their own metabolism. This phenomenon has been called self-induction or autoinduction. Carbamazepine, a widely used anticonvulsant, is a well-known example. The metabolic clearance of carbamazepine increases on continuous administration until the microsomal enzymes are fully induced.

Rapid development of enhanced clearance after high-dose cyclophosphamide, possibly indicative of autoinduction, has also been reported.[60] The mean clearance of cyclophosphamide was observed to increase from 93 ml/min on the first day of treatment to 178 ml/min on the second day. This was associated with an increase in the mean clearance of coadministered dexamethasone from 369 ml/min to 526 ml/min. An increased rate of formation of phosphoramide mustard, an active metabolite of cyclophosphamide, with higher peak concentrations was also seen. These results suggest that high-dose cyclophosphamide causes an increase in its own clearance through an apparent induction of hepatic-metabolizing enzymes, detectable 24 hours after initial exposure to cyclophosphamide.

Today, far more drug metabolism and interaction studies are concerned with inhibition of microsomal enzymes rather than induction. Certain drugs, including monoamine oxidase inhibitors, such as isocarboxazid, phenelzine, and tranylcypromine, and xanthine oxidase inhibitors, such as allopurinol, are used clinically to inhibit specific enzyme systems. Usually, these drugs are not as specific as we wish, and more than one enzyme system is inhibited. This lack of specificity applies to many drugs. The antiulcer drug cimetidine is recognized as one of the most potent and comprehensive inhibitors of microsomal drug metabolism used in clinical medicine.

The mechanisms by which drugs produce enzyme inhibition are poorly understood. Possibilities include:[61] (1) substrate competition (two drugs competing for the same enzyme); (2) competitive or noncompetitive inhibition (a substance, which is not necessarily a substrate, reduces the affinity of the enzyme for its substrate); (3) product inhibition (the product of the enzyme reaction, the metabolite, competes with the substrate); and (4) repression (the amount of enzyme is reduced, either by decreased formation or increased destruction).

Ordinarily, the administration of a drug with an inhibitor of drug-metabolizing enzymes signals a potentially undesirable drug interaction, occasionally requiring a reduction in the dose of the drug to avoid dangerously high blood levels. Sometimes, inhibition may be used to advantage to improve the delivery or extend the persistence of a drug.

A well recognized example is the combination of levodopa and carbidopa. This combination is considered the treatment of choice by most neurologists when symptoms of Parkinson's disease significantly interfere with normal daily activities. Carbidopa is a dopa decarboxylase inhibitor that does not cross the blood-brain barrier and, therefore, does not prevent the conversion of levodopa to dopamine in the central nervous system. By preventing the extracerebral metabolism of levodopa, carbidopa increases the amount available in the brain for decarboxylation to dopamine. This serves to enhance the therapeutic response and reduce adverse events caused by peripheral effects of dopamine and other catecholamines. This combination increases the plasma concentration of levodopa, reduces dosage requirements by about 75%, and significantly decreases the incidence of nausea and vomiting.

Cytarabine (Ara-C) must be given by intravenous infusion for the treatment of lymphatic cancers because absorption from the gastrointestinal tract is poor. Rectal administration results in a bioavailability of only 6%. Poor bioavailability may be related in part to inactivation of cytarabine to Ara-U by deaminase enzymes in the lower bowel and/or in the liver. With this in mind, investigators administered rectal cytarabine with 3,4,5,6-tetrahydrouridine (THU), which inhibits deamination. This combination resulted in nearly a 4-fold increase in the blood levels of cytarabine. The investigators concluded that a suppository containing cytarabine and THU may be a useful alternative to slow iv infusion of the drug.[62]

Imipenem is the first of a new class of beta-lactam antibiotics called carbapenems. These compounds have broader activity against bacteria than even the third-generation cephalosporins. Studies early in the development of imipenem indicated that the beta-lactam ring was hydrolyzed by a renal dehydropeptidase enzyme in the brush border of the kidney. Seemingly associated with this process was the occurrence of nephrotoxicity in several animal species. The simultaneous administration of cilastatin, a dehydropeptidase inhibitor with no antibacterial activity, eliminated the nephrotoxicity potential. The commercial dosage form contains imipenem and cilastatin in a 1:1 ratio. Cilastatin has no effect on the pharmacokinetics of imipenem but does increase the fraction of the dose excreted unchanged in the urine.[63]

Active Metabolites

Metabolites usually differ considerably from the parent drug with respect to pharmacologic effects and disposition. Most are rapidly eliminated and have little pharmacologic activity, but some play an important role in the effects of the drug.

Oxyphenbutazone (from phenylbutazone), acetaminophen (from phenacetin), nortriptyline (from amitriptyline), morphine (from codeine), prednisolone (from prednisone), mesoridazine (from thioridazine), and desipramine (from imipramine) are examples of metabolites that have been used as drugs in their own right. Primidone, an anticonvulsant, is appreciably metabolized to phenobarbital, which undoubtedly contributes to the efficacy of this drug in the treatment of seizures. Several of the metabolites of diazepam, including nordiazepam and oxazepam, are active, as is the acetyl metabolite of procainamide.

The activity of some drugs may reside wholly in one or more metabolites. Drugs that require bioactivation to be useful are sometimes called prodrugs. Cyclophosphamide is an example. It was developed with the intention of slowly releasing phosphoramide mustard, one of several active metabolites, in order to prolong the cytotoxic effects of the mustard. Levodopa is an inactive precursor of dopamine. It is used because, unlike dopamine, levodopa can cross the blood-brain barrier and then undergo decarboxylation to form the active drug.

Prednisone and clorazepate are also prodrugs but not very useful ones. Prednisone is not active per se but is the precursor of prednisolone. Prednisolone, however, is formed so rapidly after the administration of prednisone that there is no difference in clinical use in giving prednisolone or prednisone. Clorazepate is a precursor of N-desmethyl diazepam (nordiazepam). Ordinarily, rapid and complete conversion of clorazepate to nordiazepam occurs in gastric acid after oral administration. However, since the elimination half-life of nordiazepam is several days, it is difficult to understand why clorazepate should be used instead of nordiazepam, other than to avoid patent infringement.

Some active metabolites exert the same kind of pharmacologic effect as the parent compound. N-acetylprocainamide is an antiarrhythmic agent, acetaminophen like phenacetin is an analgesic, and nortriptyline and desipramine are antidepressants

as well as metabolites of amitriptyline and imipramine, respectively.

The major pathway for the biotransformation of morphine is hepatic glucuronidation to morphine-3-glucuronide and to a lesser extent to morphine-6-glucuronide (M6G). The results of recent studies point to the potential significance of M6G in the clinical effects of morphine. Persistent narcotic effects in the presence of M6G accumulation in patients with renal failure provide circumstantial evidence for the metabolite's clinical activity. More directly, significant analgesic activity has been found after iv administration of M6G to cancer patients.[64] No morphine or morphine-3-glucuronide was detected in plasma at any time after administration.

While encainide is an effective antiarrhythmic agent, there is considerable evidence to suggest that active metabolites mediate most of the effects seen during long-term treatment. In most patients concentrations of the active metabolites O-desmethyl encainide (ODE) and 3-methoxy-O-desmethyl encainide (MODE) are higher than those of encainide. Moreover, the correlations between antiarrhythmic activity and either ODE or MODE plasma levels are much stronger than with plasma levels of encainide itself.

In perhaps 5 to 10% of patients, however, who appear to be genetically poor metabolizers of encainide and certain other drugs, mean plasma encainide concentrations are unusually high while low or negligible levels of ODE and MODE are seen. In these patients, the long-term effects of encainide may be mediated largely by the parent drug.[65]

In some cases, active metabolites appear to have a mechanism of action different from the parent drug. For example, normeperidine is much less potent as an analgesic but more potent as a central nervous system stimulant and convulsant than meperidine, the parent drug. Normeperidine is thought to be largely responsible for the adverse effects of meperidine.

Some investigators hold that the cardiotoxicity of doxorubicin is more closely related to its major metabolite doxorubicinol than to the parent drug itself.[66] The reduced metabolite was markedly more potent than parent drug at compromising both systolic and diastolic cardiac function in isolated dog tissue. On the other hand, the cytotoxicity of doxorubicinol in tumor cell lines was far less than doxorubicin. The investigators suggested that inhibition of aldoketo reductases that catalyze the reduction of doxorubicin to doxorubicinol would result in more drug to kill cancer cells but less metabolite to compromise cardiac function.

A clue as to the source of drug toxicity—metabolite or parent—may be obtained in some instances by administering the parent with an inhibitor of drug metabolism. A more favorable safety profile implicates one or more metabolites. Cyproheptadine, a drug with both antihistaminic and antiserotonergic activity, damages the insulin-secreting cells of the pancreas to produce a diabetic state. Administration of an inhibitor of drug metabolism effectively protects against the insulin loss induced by cyproheptadine.[67] These findings suggest that a metabolite may be involved in the pancreatic beta-cell toxicity of cyproheptadine.

Sometimes, the formation of relatively small amounts of a reactive metabolite is singularly responsible for toxic effects of the drug.[68] Large doses of acetaminophen are hepatotoxic because of the reaction of a minor metabolite with liver proteins. Metabolites of halothane are also reactive, combining with phospholipids and proteins of the endoplasmic reticulum in the liver. Methoxyflurane and, to a lesser extent, enflurane produce renal toxicity because of the liberation of inorganic fluoride.

In a small number of patients, perhaps as few as 1 in 10,000, treatment with anticonvulsant medication results in a hypersensitivity syndrome usually requiring discontinuance of therapy. Typically, the reaction is delayed in onset after initiation of drug therapy and can cause severe morbidity or even result in death.

The low incidence of anticonvulsant hypersensitivity suggests that this risk may be secondary to a genetic defect in drug metabolism. With this in mind, investigators have studied aromatic anticonvulsants to help understand the pathogenesis of idiosyncratic reactions.[69]

Phenytoin, phenobarbital, and carbamazepine are metabolized to hydroxylated aromatic compounds. Reactive aromatic epoxides called arene oxides are intermediates in this process. Arene oxides may bind to cellular macromolecules, interfering with cell function and initiating immunologic response. Epoxide hydrolases are cellular enzymes critical for the detoxification of arene oxides. Studies have suggested that genetically-deficient detoxification of arene oxides might predispose patients to toxicity.

Lymphocytes from patients with suspected hypersensitivity to anticonvulsants were incubated in vitro with metabolites of phenytoin, phenobarbital, or carbamazepine, generated by hepatic microsomes from enzyme-induced mice. Healthy human subjects never exposed to anticonvulsant drugs and patients with seizure disorders chronically treated with anticonvulsants without immunologically-based adverse effects provided the control lymphocytes.

Defining cytotoxicity as the percentage of dead cells above baseline, the investigators determined that the toxic effects of drug metabolites on lymphocytes from control subjects were < 1% for phenytoin and phenobarbital and 3.6% for carbamazepine. Toxicity of the drug metabolites to cells from patients with suspected hypersensitivity differed significantly from controls: 13.5% for phenytoin, 13.3% for phenobarbital, and 20.6% for carbamazepine.

The correlation of clinical response to treatment with anticonvulsants with in vitro lymphocyte results was impressive. All 34 patients who had hypersensitivity reactions to phenytoin, also had positive in vitro results (i.e., true positives). One patient treated with phenytoin with no adverse effects, had a negative in vitro test (true negative). Results were similar for carbamazepine: 25 true positives and 2 true negatives. For patients treated with phenobarbital, there were 21 true positives and 3 true negatives, but two false positives and one false negative were also obtained.

The investigators concluded that ''the in vitro lymphocyte toxicity assay provides a model for the investigation of some hypersensitivity reactions. Our work suggests that it may aid in diagnosis and in the prediction of adverse reactions.''[69]

The offspring of women with epilepsy treated during pregnancy have a higher incidence of congenital malformations than do those born to women with untreated epilepsy or women without epilepsy. A major risk factor for this high incidence of malformation is the administration of valproic acid in combination with other anticonvulsants, particularly phenytoin and carbamazepine.[70] Recent evidence suggests that valproic acid inhibits epoxide hydrolase, the microsomal enzyme required to detoxify unstable, reactive arene oxide metabolites, including those formed in the oxidative metabolism of phenytoin and carbamazepine.[71] These findings support the recommendation that combination drug therapy with valproic acid should be avoided during pregnancy.

Disposition of Metabolites

Although important exceptions exist, most biotransformations result in metabolites that are considerably less pharmacologically active than the parent compounds. Most metabolites are also more polar than their precursors. Distribution of certain metabolites, such as glucuronide and sulfate conjugates, tends to be limited to the extracellular space. The apparent volume of distribution of a metabolite is usually less than that of the parent drug. Metabolites are excreted in the urine more readily than their precursors because often they are not subject to tubular reabsorption.

Renal excretion plays a major role in the elimination of metabolites. Considerable accumulation of drug metabolites is found in patients with renal impairment. Steady-state levels of propranolol glucuronide, 4-hydroxypropranol glucuronide, and naphthoxylactic acid, the principal metabolites of propranolol in plasma, in uremic patients are 20 to 30 times as high as in patients with normal renal function.[72] Some active metabolites may also accumulate in patients with renal failure.[73] Examples include the metabolites of allopurinol, procainamide, and clofibrate.

Metabolite Kinetics

The amount of a metabolite in the body at any time after administration of parent drug is a function of its formation rate and its elimination rate. Either step in this process may be rate limiting. When the elimination rate constant of the drug is smaller than that of the metabolite, metabolite levels decline in parallel with levels of parent drug (i.e., the half-life of both the drug and metabolite appear to be the same). When administered as such, the real elimination half-life of the metabolite may be found to be much shorter than that of the parent drug, but when it is formed from parent drug, the apparent half-life of the metabolite is never less than that of the parent.

When the second step in the process is rate limiting (i.e., the elimination rate constant of the metabolite is smaller than that of the drug), levels of drug and metabolite do not decline in parallel. The half-life of the metabolite is always greater than that of the drug and is the same whether administered or formed.

When metabolite levels are formation rate-lim-ited, the metabolite is cleared so quickly that the amount in the body is kept quite low, always lower than the amount of parent drug. When metabolite levels are elimination rate-limited, it is likely that metabolite will accumulate on repetitive dosing of the parent drug and steady-state levels will be higher than those of the parent.

Sometimes, a pharmacokinetic study will find that the apparent half-life of a metabolite is equal to that of the parent drug, suggesting formation-rate limited elimination, but metabolite concentrations in plasma are higher than those of parent drug. This appears to be contradictory because formation-rate limited means that only small amounts of metabolite are in the body at any time. However, if the metabolite has a much smaller volume of distribution than the parent drug, this small amount of metabolite may result in a higher blood level than will a larger amount of parent drug.

After administration of drug, the total area under the plasma level-time curve (AUC) can be calculated for both metabolite and drug. The ratio of these AUC values is as follows:

$$AUC(m)/AUC = Cl_f/Cl(m) \quad (11\text{--}22)$$

where AUC(m) is the area for the metabolite, AUC is the area for the drug, Cl_f is the formation clearance for converting the drug to the particular metabolite, and Cl(m) is the elimination clearance of the metabolite.

Substituting fm (Cl) for Cl_f, where fm is fraction of the dose of drug converted to the metabolite and Cl is drug clearance, yields

$$\frac{AUC(m)}{AUC} = \frac{fm \text{ Clearance of drug}}{\text{Clearance of metabolite}} \quad (11\text{--}23)$$

After a single dose of parent drug, AUC, AUC(m), and drug clearance can be calculated. Sometimes, fm may also be estimated, from urinary excretion data. When this is possible, the clearance of the metabolite may be calculated by means of Equation 11–23.

When the entire dose of a drug, or nearly so, can be accounted for by drug-related compounds in the urine, then fm is the amount of the particular metabolite excreted in the urine divided by the dose. Often, urinary recovery is far less than the administered dose. This may result from alternative excretion pathways (e.g., bile) or the formation and excretion of unrecognized metabolites. Some investigators have estimated fm from these data by comparing the amount of the particular metabolite excreted in the urine to the total amount of drug-related material in the urine. Error may be introduced by this approach. For example, if a metabolite were eliminated by both biliary and urinary excretion, the amount recovered in the urine would be less than the amount formed and both fm and metabolite clearance would be miscalculated.

The mean residence time of a metabolite can usually be calculated after intravenous or oral administration of parent drug. After iv drug, the apparent mean residence time of metabolite ($MRT_{M/P}$) is given by

$$MRT_{M/P} = MRT + MRT_M \qquad (11-24)$$

where MRT is the mean residence time of the drug and MRT_M is the mean residence time of the metabolite. On rearrangement,

$$MRT_M = MRT_{M/P} - MRT \qquad (11-25)$$

After oral administration,

$$MRT_M = MRT_{M/P(ORAL)} - MRT_{(ORAL)} \qquad (11-26)$$

where $MRT_{M/P(ORAL)}$ is the apparent mean residence time of metabolite after oral administration of parent drug and $MRT_{(ORAL)}$ is apparent mean residence time of drug after oral administration.

If a drug distributes rapidly, so that a one-compartment model applies, the half-life of a metabolite can be estimated from mean residence time. Under these conditions, the following applies to parent drug and metabolite, respectively.

$$MRT = 1.44 \ t_{1/2}(drug) \qquad (11-27)$$

and

$$MRT_{M/P} = 1.44 \ [t_{1/2}(drug) + t_{1/2}(M)] \qquad (11-28)$$

The mean residence time for a metabolite is always larger than the mean residence time of its precursor; the difference between them is an estimate of the true half-life of the metabolite, i.e.,

$$t_{1/2}(M) = [MRT_{M/P} - MRT]/\ 1.44 \qquad (11-29)$$

Species Differences

Drug metabolism studies in laboratory animals are often useful in suggesting likely drug metabolites to be found in man. Some species may be more useful than others. A survey of drug metabolism studies in laboratory animals and man, covering 32 compounds, among which were amphetamines, arylacetic acids, and sulfonamides, concluded that the rhesus monkey resembles man most closely in terms of urinary metabolite patterns; patterns in the dog and rat were much less useful for predicting results in man.[74] For example, sulfadimethoxine is mainly acetylated in the rat, but in man the major urinary metabolite is a glucuronide. Scores of similar examples can be found.

Species differences in the activity of microsomal enzyme systems are usually so great as to render the results of studies in laboratory animals meaningless as a guide for assessing the duration of drug activity in man. Table 11–2 shows the duration of effect of the skeletal muscle relaxant, carisoprodol, in different laboratory animals.[75] A range of 0.2 to 21.5 hr was observed in response to the same mg/kg dose. Interestingly, brain or serum concentrations of carisoprodol at the end of paralysis were similar in all species.

Many drugs are metabolized much more rapidly in the rat or dog than in man. A certain dose of a drug may have fleeting activity in a test animal but elicit an adequate response in man. These differences are of concern to those involved in the development of new drugs, because present methods of drug screening may overlook potentially useful drugs. These considerations are also important for the toxicologic evaluation of drugs in laboratory animals.

Stereoselective Drug Metabolism

Chemical synthesis of a drug with an asymmetric or chiral center usually results in two enantiomers,

Table 11–2. Species Differences in the Hepatic Oxidation (μmoles/g liver per 30 min) and Half-Life (hr), Duration of Paralysis (hr), and Brain and Serum Concentrations (μg/g or μg/ml) at the End of Paralysis of Carisoprodol After a 200 mg/kg Single Intraperitoneal Dose*

Species	Hepatic oxidation	Half-life	Paralysis	Concentration	
				Brain	Serum
Mouse	0.60	0.3	0.2	112	130
Guinea pig	0.44	0.8	0.5	105	129
Rat (male)	0.42	0.8	0.5	90	105
(female)	0.16	2.4	1.6	108	128
Rabbit	0.07	7.5	5.4	93	112
Cat	0.02	36	21.5	113	135

*Data from Kato, R.[75]

mirror images that cannot be superimposed on one another. This 50:50 mixture is called a racemate. In contrast, enzymes and receptor sites are stereoselective. Therefore, stereoisomers often exhibit pronounced differences in pharmacologic and toxicologic properties. Furthermore, various aspects of drug disposition (e.g., binding, metabolism, renal excretion) also exhibit stereoselectivity.

Despite the important differences in both pharmacologic and pharmacokinetic properties that may exist between two enantiomers, less than 20% of all racemic drugs are marketed as preparations containing only one isomer. In most cases, stereospecific synthesis is difficult and separation of the enantiomers is a major challenge. Often, a racemate will contain an "active" and "inactive" enantiomer. The "inactive" enantiomer, however, may not be an inactive compound. It may contribute partially to overall drug effect, be an antagonist, or have actions at other receptors resulting in undesirable side effects.

Warfarin is used as a racemic mixture of R- and S-warfarin. The S-enantiomer is about 5 times more potent than the R-enantiomer and is eliminated more rapidly. The metabolism of warfarin is highly stereoselective. The major metabolic route of S-warfarin is oxidation through ring hydroxylation of the coumarin nucleus to form primarily 7-hydroxy-S-warfarin. R-warfarin is primarily metabolized by oxidation to 6-hydroxy-R-warfarin and by reduction to R,S-warfarin alcohols.[76]

Studies in young adults have shown that l-hexobarbital is eliminated more rapidly than d-hexobarbital.[77] More recently, the pharmacokinetics of the hexobarbital enantiomers were compared in young (mean 23 years) and elderly adults (mean 68 years).[78] In each group, the apparent clearance of l-hexobarbital was considerably larger than that of d-hexobarbital. In the younger subjects, a mean value of 16.9 ml/min per kg was determined for l-hexobarbital compared with a mean value of 1.9 ml/min per kg for d-hexobarbital.

The apparent clearance of d-hexobarbital was nearly the same in young and elderly subjects. In contrast, the apparent clearance of l-hexobarbital was about twice as high in young subjects as in elderly subjects (16.9 versus 8.2 ml/min per kg). This is the first demonstration of age-related preferential decline in metabolism of one enantiomer over another for any racemic drug in animals or humans.

The (+)-isomer of amphetamine is metabolized more rapidly than the (−)-isomer.[79] When urine pH is maintained above 7, the half-life of the (+)-isomer is about 16 hr, whereas that of the (−)-isomer is about 26 hr. When the urine is acidified by administration of ammonium chloride, so that metabolism plays a smaller role in the overall elimination of amphetamine, half-life differences between the isomers almost disappear.

Differences in rates of metabolism have also been observed with the enantiomers of propranolol[80,81] and ibuprofen.[82] Propranolol is used clinically as an equal mixture of S- and R-enantiomers. S-Propranolol is about 100 times more potent as a beta-blocker than the R-enantiomer and is believed to be largely responsible for the clinical effects of the racemic drug. Repeated dosing of the racemate resulted in higher steady-state levels of S-propranolol than of R-propranolol, suggesting that propranolol undergoes stereoselective metabolism.[81]

For most 2-arylpropionic acid nonsteroidal antiinflammatory drugs (NSAIDs), the S-enantiomer is the active species. Only one of these drugs, naproxen, is available as the S-enantiomer; all the others are racemic mixtures. Interest in their stereochemistry was aroused by observations that the differences in potency between the two enantiomers in in vitro tests of antiinflammatory activity were much greater than in in vivo tests. For example, S-ibuprofen is 160 times more potent than R-ibuprofen in the inhibition of prostaglandin synthetase but has only about 50% greater potency than the R-enantiomer in an acetylcholine writhing test in mice or a pain threshold test in rats.[83]

This inquiry led to the discovery of a novel stereospecific pathway for the metabolism of the inactive R-enantiomers. These enantiomers undergo a stereospecific metabolic inversion, which progressively transforms the inactive enantiomers to the pharmacologically active S-enantiomers. This inversion has been shown for ibuprofen and benoxaprofen and may occur with ketoprofen and fenoprofen.[84] No inversion has been observed with indoprofen; preliminary studies suggest that carprofen may also exhibit little, if any, inversion.[83] Quantitatively, a 50% inversion of R- to S-benoxaprofen has been observed in human subjects, and nearly two thirds of R-ibuprofen has been found to be stereospecifically inverted to S-ibuprofen.

Lam[84] points out that even when the rate of inversion is rapid and the extent of inversion is considerable, the inactive R-enantiomer serves no therapeutic purpose and is, at best, merely a prodrug for the active S-enantiomer. Differences in the rate and extent of inversion in patients is a potential source of variability in therapeutic response to NSAIDs and allows for variable amounts of possibly toxic metabolites to be formed from the inactive R-enantiomer. Administration of the S-enantiomer would remove such variability and increase the therapeutic ratio.

In another study, boys with attention-deficit disorder were given single doses of dl-methylphenidate.[85] Drug levels in plasma were determined with an enantioselective assay method. In all 6 children, plasma levels of d-methylphenidate were at least 5-fold greater than those of the l-enantiomer. Mean AUC values were 24.5 ng-hr/ml for the d-form and 3.8 ng-hr/ml for the l-form. The plasma level-time curve for total methylphenidate $(d + l)$ is almost superimposed on that of the d-enantiomer because the contribution of the l-enantiomer to the total level is very small.

Nicoumalone, like warfarin, is a racemic, coumarin-type oral anticoagulant, available in the UK and other countries but not in the U.S. It is the second most commonly prescribed oral anticoagulant in the United Kingdom and is the most widely used oral anticoagulant in continental Europe. Preliminary studies indicated important differences in both pharmacokinetics and pharmacodynamics when each enantiomer of nicoumalone was given separately. More recently, a stereospecific assay for nicoumalone has been developed, permitting more detailed study. The kinetics of the individual enantiomers were determined after a single oral dose of the racemic mixture to 3 healthy human subjects.[86]

Dramatic differences were observed: mean apparent clearance was 21 ml/min for the R-enantiomer and 292 ml/min for the S-enantiomer; mean half-life was about 7 hr for the R-form and about 1 hr for the S-form. The protein binding of the enantiomers of nicoumalone was also found to be different. Percent unbound was 1.0 for the S-enantiomer and 0.7 for the R-form. Further evaluation of the data suggest that about 30% of an oral dose of S-nicoumalone would be lost to first-pass metabolism, whereas only 3% of an oral dose of R-nicoumalone would be similarly affected.

Verapamil, a widely used calcium channel blocker, is also subject to stereoselective first-pass metabolism.[87] Suspicions of an extensive first-pass effect were raised when clinicians realized that an iv dose of 5 to 10 mg was effective in terminating various supraventricular tachyarrhythmias, whereas an oral dose of 80 to 160 mg was needed to elicit an effect comparable to that seen after iv administration. The reason for this, at least in part, is that despite its almost complete absorption, the bioavailability of verapamil is only 20 to 30% because of extensive presystemic hepatic elimination. Based on a bioavailability of 20 to 30%, however, an oral dose of 25 to 50 mg should be sufficient to elicit a response equivalent to a 5 to 10 mg iv dose.

Analysis of the concentration-effect relationship revealed the reason for this seeming discrepancy. The same concentration of verapamil (i.e., dl-verapamil) is more effective after intravenous than after oral administration. On average, verapamil plasma levels 3 times higher were needed after oral administration to produce the same prolongation on the ECG as after iv administration. This is contrary to all precepts of pharmacokinetics.

The standard analytical method for assaying verapamil measures both the d- and l-forms. l-Verapamil, however, is about 8–10 times more potent than d-verapamil. Therefore, the most plausible explanation for this anomaly is that the more active l-isomer is preferentially metabolized during hepatic first-pass metabolism. It follows that a given plasma level after iv administration will be richer in the more potent l-verapamil than after oral administration and thus produce a greater pharmacologic effect.

It has been demonstrated that after oral administration, the d-enantiomer has a bioavailability of 50%, about 2.5 times greater than that of l-verapamil. The d- to l- isomer ratio of plasma verapamil after iv administration is about 2, whereas after oral administration the ratio is about 5. These differences in the d- to l-enantiomer ratio of plasma verapamil in relation to route of administration explain the observed differences in the concentration-effect relationships.

Labetalol is sometimes claimed to provide alpha- and beta-blocking activity in a single drug and is indicated for the treatment of high blood pressure. In fact, labetalol has two asymmetric centers and is therefore a mixture of four diastereomers. The alpha- and beta-blocking activities are not distributed uniformly among the four isomers. The RR-isomer of labetalol, also called dilevalol, is primarily responsible for the beta-adrenergic receptor blocking activity, but has only weak alpha-activity.

The SR-isomer produces most of the alpha-blocking activity. Of the four diastereomers, only dilevalol has an antihypertensive effect in spontaneously hypertensive rats comparable to that of labetalol. Although the two inactive isomers are without toxicity, some clinicians believe it would be preferable to use only the active RR-isomer to lessen the potential for interactions among the isomers or with other drugs.[84]

Ariens[88] caustically observed that "too often, and without it being noticed, data in the scientific literature on mixtures of stereoisomers, racemates, are presented as if only one compound were involved. This neglect of stereochemical aspects of drug action, including metabolism, excretion, etc. notwithstanding, computerized curve fitting, generation of extensive tables with pharmacokinetic constants, and postulation of complex multicompartment systems, degrades many pharmacokinetic studies to expensive 'highly sophisticated pseudoscientific nonsense.' "

A report from Australia[89] described a theoretical analysis to illustrate the potential which exists for misinterpretation of drug disposition and plasma drug concentration-effect data generated for a racemic drug using a nonstereoselective assay. The investigators demonstrated convincingly that the use of a nonselective analytical method can lead to the collection of data which may be both quantitatively and qualitatively inaccurate with respect to the individual enantiomers. For example, the clearance of the unresolved drug (i.e., the sum of the R- and S-enantiomers) may indicate nonlinear pharmacokinetics, even though the kinetics of the enantiomers are concentration- and time-independent. We would never think of carrying out a pharmacokinetic analysis on levels of radioactivity in plasma after administration of a labeled drug. The same caution should be applied to the pharmacokinetic analysis of data obtained after administration of a racemate.

Capacity-Limited Metabolism

The rate of an enzymatic process, like biotransformation, can usually be described by the Michaelis-Menten equation:

$$\text{Rate of metabolism} = \frac{V_{max}C}{K_m + C} \quad (11\text{--}30)$$

where C is the drug concentration in the plasma, V_{max} is the maximum production rate of metabolite, and K_m is the Michaelis constant. The constant V_{max}

is a function of the total amount of metabolizing enzyme; $1/K_m$ reflects the affinity between drug (substrate) and enzyme. Operationally, K_m is the drug concentration at which the rate of metabolism is one half of the maximum.

Experience suggests that the usual dose of most drugs results in plasma concentrations that are much smaller than the K_m values associated with their metabolism. Since $C \ll K_m$, it follows from Equation 11–30 that:

$$\text{Rate of metabolism} = \frac{V_{max}}{K_m} C = k_m C \quad (11\text{--}31)$$

where k_m is the apparent first-order metabolic rate constant. Accordingly, the elimination of most drugs that are eliminated totally or in part by biotransformation can be described by first-order kinetics.

Some drugs, including ethanol, salicylate, and phenytoin, have one or more K_m values that are comparable to or less than their usual concentrations in the plasma following therapeutic doses. One study suggests that the apparent K_m for phenytoin in patients is as low as 4 μg/ml.[90] The usual desired concentration range for phenytoin in treating seizures is 10 to 20 μg/ml. Calculations based on studies in normal adults suggest that the K_m values (expressed in terms of amount of drug in the body) for the glycine conjugation and for the acyl glucuronidation of salicylate are about 340 and 640 mg, respectively.[91] Considerably larger amounts of salicylate are found in patients taking aspirin or other salicylate preparations for rheumatoid arthritis or rheumatic fever.

The elimination of drugs like phenytoin or salicylate cannot be described by first-order kinetics; their pharmacokinetics are said to be *nonlinear*. The relative rate of elimination is slower at higher concentrations than at lower concentrations of drug in the plasma. In other words, it takes longer to decrease a high drug concentration by 50% than to decrease a low concentration by the same percentage. Because the apparent half-life (actually, the time required to decrease the peak concentration of drug in blood or plasma by 50%) of these drugs increases with increasing dose, their elimination is said to be *dose-dependent*. Strictly speaking, however, Michaelis-Menten elimination is *concentration-dependent* rather than dose-dependent.

Drugs manifesting dose-dependent elimination present unusual challenges in therapeutic manage-

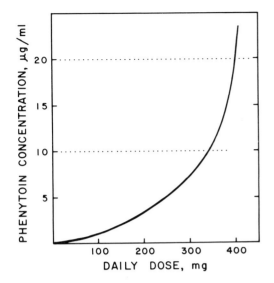

Fig. 11–6. Relationship between steady-state serum concentration of phenytoin and daily dose. (Data from Mawer, G.E., et al.[90])

ment, because steady-state concentrations change disproportionately with changes in dose. For example, a 50% increase in the daily dose of aspirin produces about a 300% increase in the concentration of salicylate in the plasma.[92] The nonlinear relationship between steady-state concentration and dose also explains why a relatively small (20%) increase in the daily dose of aspirin can produce a pronounced therapeutic response in patients with rheumatic fever or acute arthritis who have not responded to the lower dose.[93]

The unusual pharmacokinetics of salicylate elimination presents a dilemma in the design of rational dosage regimens. The problem is particularly serious in patients with rheumatoid arthritis, because effective salicylate therapy requires the use of doses that result in near-toxic levels. Small changes in dose can produce a change in blood concentrations from ineffective levels to levels causing serious adverse effects. It is significant that the most severe instances of aspirin intoxication result from therapeutic overdosage,[94] and that more children die of therapeutic than of accidental aspirin poisoning.[95]

Serious problems may occur when ethotoin or phenytoin is used in the treatment of seizures. Increasing the daily dose of ethotoin 2-fold (from 30 to 60 mg/kg) produced, on the average, a 3-fold change in steady-state plasma concentrations in epileptic patients.[96] In one patient, this dosage change produced a 7-fold increase in steady-state levels.

The theoretical curve relating steady-state serum concentrations to daily dose of phenytoin, derived from studies in 15 epileptic patients, is shown in Figure 11–6.[90] The curve rises steeply when the daily dose exceeds 340 mg. The steepness of the curve is illustrated by a case report of a female patient with grand mal epilepsy.[90] Serum concentrations of 7.6 and 4.6 μg/ml were observed on 2 consecutive visits while she was taking 300 mg of phenytoin daily. These levels are subtherapeutic in many adult patients. Between the visits she had a major convulsion. The maintenance dose was increased to 350 mg daily. About 5 weeks later she returned to the clinic complaining of ataxia, a common sign of phenytoin intoxication. Her serum phenytoin concentration had risen to 27 μg/ml, a level at which adverse effects of the drug are frequent. In this patient, a modest (17%) increase in the daily dose of phenytoin produced about a 5-fold change in steady-state serum concentration of the drug.

Dosage adjustments for theophylline therapy have traditionally been based on a linear pharmacokinetic model, whereby a change in dose at steady state would result in a proportional change in the serum concentration of theophylline. Increasingly, however, investigators have suggested that the pharmacokinetics of theophylline following therapeutic doses may not be linear in certain patients. Children treated aggressively with serum theophylline levels close to 20 μg/ml, for example, have been found to become toxic during a bout of influenza, which only modestly decreased the clearance of theophylline.

In view of these reports, investigators in Japan[97] determined the incidence and implications of capacity-limited elimination in pediatric and adult patients with chronic asthma receiving a sustained-release form of theophylline as principal therapy. Patients in whom at least two steady-state concentration measurements were obtained at two or more different doses were selected. Nonlinearity was defined as a percent change in plasma levels exceeding the change in dose by at least 50%.

Nonlinear elimination was observed in 40% of the children and 42% of the adults. In these patients, the mean maximum elimination rate (V_{max}) was significantly greater in children than in adults, 32 *versus* 22 mg/kg per day, indicating that the metabolic capacity for theophylline is greater in children than in adults. Also, V_{max} values were significantly correlated with age. Mean values for

K_m, on the other hand, were similar in the two groups, 13.0 and 12.9 μg/ml, respectively, and individual K_m values were independent of age. These values for K_m are well within the therapeutic concentration range of theophylline (usually considered to be 10 to 20 μg/ml).

Nonlinear pharmacokinetic characteristics have also been reported for propranolol. Steady-state levels were higher when a daily dose of 80 mg was given as 40 mg twice daily than when given as 20 mg 4 times daily.[98] The 24-hour steady-state AUC values were 340 ng-hr/ml after dosing 4 times a day and 446 ng-hr/ml after dosing twice a day, a difference in apparent bioavailability of 30%. These findings suggest nonlinear first-pass metabolism of propranolol. In general, the bioavailability of first-pass drugs that obey Michaelis-Menten kinetics will be sensitive to rate of drug input.[99] This helps us to understand why the relative bioavailability of slow-release dosage forms of propranolol is only about 50% compared with conventional tablets given 3 times a day.

Propafenone is an investigational antiarrhythmic agent that markedly slows conduction. It is eliminated almost entirely by hepatic metabolism. Propafenone is very well absorbed but bioavailability is incomplete, because of first-pass metabolism, and dose-dependence.[100] When the oral dose was increased from 150 to 450 mg, peak concentration of propafenone in serum increased by a factor of six. In other subjects, a 3-fold increase in dose from 300 to 900 mg/day produced a 10-fold increase in steady-state propafenone serum concentrations.

Nicardipine, a potent, orally active vasodilator, related to nifedipine, is under investigation for use in hypertension, angina, and cerebrovascular disease. In one study, oral doses of nicardipine ranging from 10 to 40 mg every 8 hours were given to healthy subjects. The steady-state bioavailability of nicardipine was found to be dose-dependent and averaged 19% at 10 mg, 22% at 20 mg, 28% at 30 mg, and 38% at 40 mg. The investigator cautioned that if one wished to increase the oral dose higher than 40 mg every 8 hours, such increases should be very conservative and plasma concentrations should be monitored.[101]

Other Examples of Nonlinear Metabolism

Certain drugs display nonlinear pharmacokinetics that are not consistent with Michaelis-Menten kinetics. These drugs display dose-dependent or time-dependent pharmacokinetics rather than concentration-dependent pharmacokinetics.

Concentration-dependent or Michaelis-Menten kinetics means that clearance decreases with increasing drug concentration; however, drug clearance at a given drug concentration is the same whether a high or low dose is given.

Dose-dependent kinetics implies that clearance changes with dose rather than concentration. For example, clearance of acetaminophen from the blood at any concentration is lower following a toxic dose than after a therapeutic dose. This occurs because high doses of acetaminophen cause hepatotoxicity, which reduces the liver's ability to metabolize the drug.

Dose-dependent kinetics have also been found in laboratory animals with doses of acetaminophen that do not cause hepatotoxicity.[102] The underlying mechanism involves depletion of the sulfate pool in the body, which is only slowly restored. Sulfate conjugation plays a principal role in the elimination of acetaminophen; a reduction in the rate of acetaminophen sulfate formation reduces the overall rate of elimination of the drug.

Product inhibition of drug metabolism can also produce dose-dependent kinetics.[103] Studies in laboratory animals with phenytoin and phenylbutazone indicate that certain hydroxylated metabolites can inhibit the metabolism of their precursors. In man, however, evidence of product inhibition is scant, possibly because safety considerations limit the administration of drug metabolites. Diazepam, however, provides an opportunity for investigation because several of its metabolites are used as drugs in their own right. It has been found that nordiazepam inhibits the metabolism of diazepam.[104]

Unusual, nonlinear pharmacokinetic characteristics have also been observed with nitroglycerin.[105] As nitroglycerin iv infusion rates were increased from 10 to 40 μg/min, the steady-state concentration in plasma increased disproportionately, from 0.4 to 4.2 ng/ml. However, when the infusion rate was then decreased to 10 μg/min, steady-state concentrations of nitroglycerin were always higher during the second 10 μg/min infusion than during the first 10 μg/min infusion. On average, steady-state levels were 1.0 ng/ml during the second low-dose infusion compared with 0.4 ng/ml during the first.

The investigators pointed out that high concentrations of the dinitrate metabolites accumulate after administration of nitroglycerin. These high metabolite levels may inhibit the clearance of the parent drug (end-product inhibition). Alternatively, capacity-limited binding of nitroglycerin to blood vessels at or near the infusion site would also explain the unusual results.[105]

Time-dependent kinetics means that the clearance of the drug changes with continuous administration of the same dose, whether or not there is significant accumulation of the drug on multiple dosing. For example, the elimination of diazepam is slower after multiple dosing than following a single dose.[106] This change in clearance appears to be a consequence of the considerable accumulation of nordiazepam on multiple dosing of diazepam and of nordiazepam's ability to inhibit the metabolism of diazepam.[104]

Time-dependent pharmacokinetics is also observed with drugs that stimulate their own metabolism. The steady-state concentration of drugs with linear pharmacokinetics can be predicted from data obtained after a single dose because clearance is assumed to remain constant throughout treatment. If a drug is subject to autoinduction, however, clearance is higher after multiple doses than following a single dose. Studies with the anticonvulsant carbamazepine illustrate this point.[107]

Carbamazepine was given to patients as a single oral dose; 1 week later the patients received the drug 3 times a day for 2 to 3 weeks. The half-life of carbamazepine was shorter in all patients after multiple doses (21 hr, on the average) than after the initial single dose (36 hr, on the average). The average steady-state concentration predicted from the single dose data was higher (17 μg/ml) than the steady-state levels observed during treatment (8 μg/ml). The results are consistent with self-induction of microsomal enzymes; the clearance of carbamazepine doubles on repeated dosing. Similar results have been observed in the rhesus monkey during constant rate intravenous infusion of carbamazepine (Fig. 11–7).[108]

There is also evidence that salicylate metabolism is autoinduced.[109] Healthy subjects receiving 3.9 g aspirin per day show maximum salicylate concentrations in plasma after about 4 days; thereafter, salicylate levels decline by about 25 to 30% despite a constant daily dose. The results may be a consequence of self-induction of a metabolic pathway (e.g., salicylurate formation).[110]

Another kind of time-dependent pharmacokinetics, as yet unexplained, has been observed with certain drugs having no obvious similarities in chemical structure but sharing the common characteristic of a high hepatic clearance; each of these drugs shows a large first-pass effect after oral administration because of presystemic hepatic metabolism. Propranolol accumulates during continued oral administration to a greater extent than predicted from its half-life and area under the curve (AUC) after a single oral dose.[111] Presystemic extraction decreases from 78% after a single dose to 66% at steady state following 80 mg given every 8 hr. In other words, the systemic availability of propranolol increases from 22 to 34% during multiple dosing; steady-state levels are about 50% greater than expected.

During chronic oral treatment of hypertensive patients with labetalol, an α,β-adrenoceptor block-

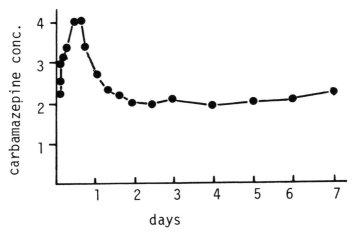

Fig. 11–7. Carbamazepine concentrations in serum (μg/ml) in a monkey during constant rate intravenous infusion of the drug. (Data from Pitlick, W.H., and Levy, R.H.[108])

ing drug, observed mean steady-state levels in patients were almost twice those predicted from a single oral dose.[112] Unexpected accumulation at steady state has also been observed with the analgesic propoxyphene.[113]

In patients with atrial fibrillation, oral and intravenous single dose studies with verapamil, a calcium channel blocker, indicate that only 35% of the oral dose is available; about two thirds of the dose is subject to first-pass hepatic metabolism. The first-pass metabolism of oral verapamil decreases considerably on multiple dosing; mean verapamil concentration in plasma at steady state was nearly twice the value predicted from the single-dose studies.[114,115]

Nonlinear accumulation of verapamil does not occur on intravenous administration. Steady-state concentrations of verapamil following constant-rate intravenous infusion were similar to those predicted from single-dose intravenous studies.[114] On the other hand, the antiarrhythmic drug lidocaine, which is also subject to a large first-pass effect on oral administration, does show clinically significant, nonlinear accumulation during continuous constant-rate intravenous infusion.[116,117]

Some believe that the decline in lidocaine clearance during continuous intravenous infusion may be related to inhibition by monoethylglycinexylidide (MEGX), a metabolite of lidocaine. In support of this hypothesis, investigators in Scotland found that the clearance of lidocaine when given with MEGX decreased from 970 ml/min to 800 ml/min.[118]

The nonlinear pharmacokinetics of drugs subject to first-pass hepatic metabolism presents a confusing picture at this time. Not all drugs display this characteristic. For example, the antidepressant nortriptyline, which is subject to significant presystemic hepatic metabolism, accumulates in a highly predictable manner on multiple oral dosing.[119] Some drugs (e.g., verapamil) show nonlinearity on oral dosing but not on intravenous dosing. Lidocaine shows nonlinear accumulation on intravenous dosing, but has not been studied on oral dosing. Saturation of a high affinity, low capacity enzyme system or binding site in the liver may explain some of the results, but more than one mechanism is likely.

Extrahepatic Metabolism

Many tissues other than the liver contain microsomal and soluble drug metabolizing enzymes, but for the most part their role in drug disposition is poorly understood.

The liver seems to be the only consistently important organ for drug metabolism, as it relates to the elimination of drugs from the body. The drug metabolizing activity of certain organs, including the skin, the gut, and the lungs, is of general interest, however, because their anatomic position permits them to exert a kind of first-pass effect that limits drug availability to sites of pharmacologic effect.

The epidermis can carry out several metabolic reactions including glucuronide conjugation. There is evidence for the cutaneous metabolism of adrenal steroids, hydrocortisone, and fluorouracil. Recent in vitro studies indicate that the antiviral drug vidarabine is extensively metabolized in skin.[120] Drug metabolism in skin could decrease the potency and duration of effects of topically applied drugs intended to act locally, or produce a first-pass effect for drugs intended for systemic effects.

The most important extrahepatic site of drug metabolism is the gastrointestinal tract. Certain drugs may be extensively conjugated after oral administration by enzymes in the intestinal epithelium. The consequence of this presystemic metabolism is incomplete bioavailability.

Intestinal metabolism explains why isoproterenol is 1000 times less active after oral than after intravenous administration, despite the fact that there is little difference in the total urinary recovery of drug-related material after equal intravenous and oral doses of radiolabeled drug. Oral administration of isoproterenol in man produces a pattern of metabolism that differs markedly from that seen after intravenous dosing.[121] After intravenous dosing, unchanged isoproterenol accounts for more than 60% of the urinary radioactivity; the remainder is present as free or conjugated 3-0-methyl isoproterenol. In contrast, the major metabolite in plasma and urine after oral administration is a sulfate conjugate of isoproterenol that is formed in the intestinal wall.

Similar differences in metabolic pattern in man, as a function of route of administration, have been reported for terbutaline.[122] After intravenous administration, unchanged terbutaline accounts for 70 to 90% of the urinary radioactivity. The remainder is present as a sulfate conjugate of terbutaline. On the other hand, the sulfate conjugate accounts for about 70% of drug-related material in the urine after oral administration. Sulfate conjugation in the gut wall during absorption of terbutaline is a likely explanation for this difference.

Drug metabolism studies in man suggest that at least two other bronchodilator drugs are metabolized in the intestine after oral administration. A sulfate conjugate accounts for about 50% of the total urinary radioactivity after oral administration of rimiterol but for only 2% after intravenous administration.[123] A similar difference with respect to the extent of formation of sulfate conjugate after oral and intravenous administration has been found with isoetharine.[124]

Albuterol (salbutamol), the most widely used beta-agonist in the world, is also subject to gut metabolism after oral administration.[125] After iv administration of albuterol, urinary excretion of unchanged drug accounts for 64% of the dose and the sulfate conjugate accounts for 12%. With oral administration, bioavailability was 50% and urinary excretion of unchanged drug and sulfate conjugate accounted for 32% and 48% of the dose, respectively. The incomplete bioavailability suggests that oral albuterol is subject to presystemic metabolism. The markedly different composition of drug-related material after iv and oral albuterol suggests that presystemic metabolism occurs in the gastrointestinal mucosa.

The low plasma morphine levels observed in man after oral administration compared to those that result from parenteral administration are probably due to the rapid conjugation of the drug with glucuronic acid in the cells of the intestinal mucosa during absorption.[126]

The relatively high activity of β-glucuronidase in the intestine may contribute to the duration of effect of drugs that undergo biliary secretion in the form of glucuronide conjugates. The conjugates may be hydrolyzed, thereby promoting reabsorption and enterohepatic cycling of parent drug.

Esterases in the intestine appear to contribute to the less than complete bioavailability of aspirin after oral administration.[127] These enzymes may also be important for the bioactivation of drugs that are given in the form of ester prodrugs.

The intestinal flora in the distal small intestine and colon metabolize certain poorly absorbed drugs or drugs that are subject to biliary excretion. Intestinal bacteria play an important role in the metabolism of sulfasalazine in man.[128] The drug consists of 5-aminosalicylate in azo linkage with sulfapyridine (see Table 11–1). On oral administration, sulfasalazine is partially absorbed during

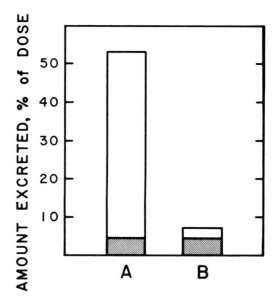

Fig. 11–8. Urinary excretion of sulfasalazine (shaded area) and its metabolite sulfapyridine (open area) in a patient before (A) and after (B) colectomy. (Data from Schroder, H., Lewkonia, R.M., and Price Evans, D.A.[129])

its transit through the small intestine and is excreted unchanged in the urine. The unabsorbed portion of the dose enters the cecum and colon where the molecule is cleaved at the azo linkage by bacteria. Most of the sulfapyridine thus formed is absorbed and subsequently metabolized. The fate of the 5-aminosalicylate moiety is probably similar. The cleavage is believed to be essential for the therapeutic effects of the drug, to liberate 5-aminosalicylate.

The importance of microflora metabolism in the intestine to the disposition of sulfasalazine is evident from the results of studies in a patient before and after total colectomy (Fig. 11–8). The excretion of unchanged sulfasalazine in urine was unaffected by the surgery. The effect on sulfapyridine, however, was dramatic; its excretion in urine decreased from about 50 to 3% of the dose.[129] It is also likely that far less 5-aminosalicylate was formed in this patient.

Sulindac is a nonsteroidal antiinflammatory drug that undergoes conversion to a sulfide compound, which is 5 times more potent than sulindac, and an inactive sulfone. Studies in patients with surgical ileostomies suggest that gut microflora are important for the reduction of sulindac to sulfide.[130] It appears that about 50% of the active sulfide metabolite found in normal subjects given sulindac is formed by gut bacteria mostly from sulindac excreted in the bile.

Of late, there has been considerable interest in the metabolism of drugs by the lungs. Since the lungs are perfused by the entire blood supply, even a relatively low degree of drug metabolism activity could make an important contribution to the overall disposition of a drug. The unique anatomic location of the lungs means that drug metabolizing activity could result in a first-pass effect for drugs given intravenously, with respect to the arterial circulation and sites of pharmacologic effect. In other words, the area under the drug concentration in arterial blood versus time curve may be greater after intra-arterial administration of drugs subject to lung metabolism than after intravenous administration. Direct administration of drugs to the lungs may avoid this first-pass effect. Drug metabolism by the lungs has been reviewed by Brown,[131] and more recently by Roth and Wiersma.[132] The contribution of lung metabolism to the clearance of drugs from the blood has been clearly presented by Collins and Dedrick and associates.[133,134]

REFERENCES

1. Cohen, M., and Pocelinko, R.: Renal transport mechanisms for the excretion of sulfisoxazole. J. Pharmacol. Exp. Ther., 185:703, 1973.
2. Tonelli, A.P., Bialer, M., Yacobi, A.: Relationship between protein binding and renal clearance of a new oral cephalosporin in the dog. J. Pharm. Sci., 74:1242, 1985.
3. Bins, J.W., Mattie, H.: Saturation of the tubular excretion of beta-lactam antibiotics. Br. J. Clin. Pharmacol., 25:41, 1988.
4. Treatment of syphilis and gonorrhea. Med. Lett. Drugs Ther., 18:29, 1976.
5. Hsyu, P.-H., Giacomini, K.M.: Stereoselective renal clearance of pindolol in humans. J. Clin. Invest., 76:1720, 1985.
6. Milne, M.D.: Influence of acid-base balance on efficacy and toxicity of drugs. Proc. R. Soc. Med., 58:961, 1965.
7. Kostenbauder, H.B., Portnoff, J.B., and Swintosky, J.V.: Control of urine pH and its effect on sulfaethidole excretion in humans. J. Pharm. Sci., 51:1084, 1962.
8. Dettli, L., Spring, P., and Raeber, I.: The influence of alkali administration on the biological half-life of two sulfonamides in human blood serum. Int. J. Clin. Pharmacol., 2:130, 1967.
9. Vree, T.B., et al.: Pharmacokinetics of sulfamethoxazole in man: effects of urinary pH and urine flow on metabolism and renal excretion of sulfamethoxazole and its metabolite N₄-acetylsulfamethoxazole. Clin. Pharmacokin., 3:319, 1978.
10. Sand, T.E., and Jacobsen, S.: Effects of urine pH and flow on renal clearance of methotrexate. Eur. J. Clin. Pharmacol., 19:453, 1981.
11. Kuntzman, R.G., et al.: The influence of urinary pH on the plasma half-life of pseudoephedrine in man and dog and a sensitive assay for its determination in human plasma. Clin. Pharmacol. Ther., 12:62, 1971.
12. Brater, D.C., et al.: Renal excretion of pseudoephedrine. Clin. Pharmacol. Ther., 28:690, 1980.
13. Rowland, M., and Beckett, A.H.: The amphetamines: Clinical and pharmacokinetic implications of recent studies of an assay procedure and urinary excretion in man. Arzneimittelforsch., 16:1369, 1966.
14. Beckett, A.H., Salmon, J.A., and Mitchard, M.: The relation between blood levels and urinary excretion of amphetamine under controlled acidic and under fluctuating urinary pH values using (¹⁴C) amphetamine. J. Pharm. Pharmacol., 21:251, 1969.
15. Wilkinson, G.R., and Beckett, A.H.: Absorption, metabolism and excretion of the ephedrines in man. I. The influence of urinary pH and urine volume output. J. Pharmacol. Exp. Ther., 102:139, 1968.
16. Muhiddin, K.A., Johnston, A., Turner, P.: The influence of urinary pH on flecainide excretion and its serum pharmacokinetics. Br. J. Clin. Pharmacol., 17:447, 1984.
17. Dettli, L., and Spring, P.: Diurnal variations in the elimination rate of a sulfonamide in man. Helv. Med. Acta, 33:291, 1966.
18. Levy, G., and Koysooko, R.: Renal clearance of theophylline in man. J. Clin. Pharmacol., 16:329, 1976.
19. Beckett, A.H., and Wilkinson, G.R.: Influence of urine pH and flow rate on the renal excretion of chlorpheniramine in man. J. Pharm. Pharmacol., 17:257, 1965.
20. Jusko, W.J., and Levy, G.: Pharmacokinetic evidence for saturable renal tubular reabsorption of riboflavin. J. Pharm. Sci., 59:765, 1970.
21. Nelson, E.: Kinetics of the excretion of sulfonamides during therapeutic dosage regimens. J. Theor. Biol., 2:193, 1962.
22. Potter, J.L., Weinberg, A.G., West, R.: Ampicillinuria and ampicillin crystalluria. Pediatrics, 48:636, 1971.
23. Nelson, E.: Minimum rate of flow in therapy with sulphonamides. Nature, 189:928, 1961.
24. Levine, W.G.: Biliary excretion of drugs and other xenobiotics. Annu. Rev. Pharmacol. Toxicol., 18:81, 1978.
25. Kates, R.E., Tozer, T.N., and Sorby, D.L.: Increased methotrexate toxicity due to concurrent probenecid administration. Biochem. Pharmacol., 25:1485, 1976.
26. Javitt, N.B.: Hepatic bile formation. N. Engl. J. Med., 295:1464, 1976.
27. Hirom, P.C., Millburn, P., and Smith, R.L.: Some physiological factors influencing the concentration of drugs at body sites. J. Mond. Pharm., 1:15, 1972.
28. Wright, W.E., and Line, V.D.: Biliary excretion of cephalosporins in rats: influence of molecular weight. Antimicrob. Agents Chemother., 17:842, 1980.
29. Rollins, D.E., and Klaassen, C.D.: Biliary excretion of drugs in man. Clin. Pharmacokinet., 4:368, 1974.
30. Spring, P.: The pharmacokinetics of Rimactane in patients with impaired liver and kidney function. Ciba Found. Symp., 1968, pp. 32–34.
31. Duggan, D.E., et al.: Enterohepatic circulation of indomethacin and its role in intestinal irritation. Biochem. Pharmacol., 25:1749, 1975.
32. Duggan, D.E., and Kwan, K.C.: Enterohepatic recirculation of drugs as a determinant of therapeutic ratio. Drug Metab. Rev., 9:21, 1979.
33. Caldwell, J.H., Bush, C.A., and Greenberger, N.J.: Interruption of the enterohepatic circulation of digitoxin by cholestyramine. II. Effect on metabolic disposition of tritium-labeled digitoxin and cardiac systolic intervals in man. J. Clin. Invest., 50:2638, 1971.
34. Jähnchen, E., et al.: Enhanced elimination of warfarin during treatment with cholestyramine. Br. J. Clin. Pharmacol., 5:437, 1978.
35. Neuvonen, P.J., Elonen, E., and Matilla, M.J.: Oral ac-

tivated charcoal and dapsone elimination. Clin. Pharmacol. Ther., 27:823, 1980.

36. Neuvonen, P.J., and Elonen, E.: Effect of activated charcoal on absorption and elimination of phenobarbitone, carbamazepine and phenylbutazone. Eur. J. Clin. Pharmacol., 17:51, 1980.

37. Karkkainen, S., Neuvonen, P.J.: Pharmacokinetics of amitriptyline influenced by oral charcoal and urine pH. Int. J. Clin. Pharmacol., 24:326, 1986.

38. Cohn, W.J., et al.: Treatment of chlordecone (Kepone) toxicity with cholestyramine. N. Engl. J. Med., 298:243, 1978.

39. Boylan, J.J., et al. : Excretion of chlordecone by the gastrointestinal tract: evidence for a nonbiliary mechanism. Clin. Pharmacol. Ther., 25:579, 1979.

40. Groth, U., Prellwitz, W., and Jähnchen, E.: Estimation of pharmacokinetic parameters of lithium from saliva. Clin. Pharmacol. Ther., 16:490, 1974.

41. Dawes, C.P., and Kendall, M.J.: Comparison of plasma and saliva levels of metoprolol and oxprenolol. Br. J. Clin. Pharmacol., 5:217, 1978.

42. Devine, L.F., et al.: Rifampin: Effect of two-day treatment on the meningococcal carrier state and the relationship to the levels of drug in sera and saliva. Am. J. Med. Sci., 261:79, 1971.

43. Ellinger, P., and Shattock, F.M.: Black tongue and oral penicillin. Br. Med. J., 2:208, 1946.

44. Koup, J., Jusko, W.J., and Goldfarb, A.L.: pH-dependent secretion of procainamide into saliva. J. Pharm. Sci., 64:2008, 1975.

45. Matin, S.B., Wan, S.H., and Karam, J.H.: Pharmacokinetics of tolbutamide: prediction of concentration in saliva. Clin. Pharmacol. Ther., 16:1052, 1974.

46. Mucklow, J.C., et al.: Drug concentration in saliva. Clin. Pharmacol. Ther., 24:563, 1978.

47. Anderson, P.O.: Drugs and breast feeding—a review. Drug Intell. Clin. Pharm., 11:208, 1977.

48. Welch, R.M., and Findlay, J.W.A.: Excretion of drugs in human breast milk. Drug Metab. Rev., 12:261, 1981.

49. Forrest, J.M.: Drugs in pregnancy and lactation. Med. J. Aust., 2:138, 1976.

50. Atkinson, H.C., Begg, E.J., Darlow, B.A.: Drugs in human milk: clinical pharmacokinetic considerations. Clin. Pharmacokin., 14:217, 1988.

51. Fleishaker, J.C., Desai, N., McNamara, P.J.: Factors affecting the milk-to-plasma drug concentration ratio in lactating women: physical interactions with protein and fat. J. Pharm. Sci., 76:189, 1987.

52. Yurchak, A.M., and Jusko, W.J.: Theophylline secretion into breast milk. Pediatrics, 57:518, 1976.

53. Ananth, J.: Side effects in the neonate from psychotropic agents excreted through breast feeding. Am. J. Psychiatry, 135:801, 1978.

54. Anon.: Update: Drugs in breast milk. Med. Lett. Drugs Ther., 21:21, 1979.

54a. Committee on Drugs: The transfer of drugs and other chemicals into human breast milk. Pediatrics, 72:375, 1983.

55. Lindenbaum, J., et al.: Urinary excretion of reduced metabolites of digoxin. Am. J. Med., 71:67, 1981.

56. Thijssen, H.H.W., et al.: The role of the intestinal microflora in the reductive metabolism of acenocoumarol in man. Br. J. Clin. Pharmacol., 18:247, 1984.

57. Faed, E.M., and McQueen, E.G.: Plasma half-life of clofibric acid in renal failure. Br. J. Clin. Pharmacol., 7:407, 1979.

58. Conney, A.H.: Pharmacological implications of microsomal enzyme induction. Pharmacol. Rev., 19:317, 1967.

59. Jensen, J., Christiansen, C., Rodbro, P.: Cigarette smoking, serum estrogens, and bone loss during hormone-replacement therapy early after menopause. N. Engl. J. Med., 313:973, 1985.

60. Moore, M.J., et al.: Rapid development of enhanced clearance after high-dose cyclophosphamide. Clin. Pharmacol. Ther., 44:622, 1988.

61. Smith, S.E., and Rawlin, M.D.: Variability in Human Drug Response. London, Butterworths, 1973, pp. 94–98.

62. Liversidge, G.G., et al.: Enhanced serum concentrations of Ara-C using suppositories containing tetrahydrouridine as a deamination inhibitor of Ara-C. J. Pharm. Pharmacol., 38:223, 1986.

63. Lyon, J.A.: Imipenem/cilastatin: the first carbapenem antibiotic. Drug. Intell. Clin. Pharm., 19:894, 1985.

64. Osborne, R., et al.: Analgesic activity of morphine-6-glucuronide. Lancet, 1:828, 1988.

65. Brabey, J.T., et al.: Antiarrhythmic activity, electrocardiographic effects and pharmacokinetics of the encainide metabolites O-desmethyl encainide and 3-methoxy-O-desmethyl encainide in man. Circulation, 77:380, 1988.

66. Olson, R.D., et al.: Doxorubicin cardiotoxicity may be caused by its metabolite, doxorubicinol. Proc. Natl. Acad. Sci., 85:3585, 1988.

67. Chow, S.A., Rickert, D.E., Fischer, L.J.: Evidence that drug metabolites are involved in cyproheptadine-induced loss of pancreatic insulin. J. Pharmacol. Exp. Ther., 246:143, 1988.

68. Nelson, S.D.: Metabolic activation and drug toxicity. J. Med. Chem., 25:753, 1982.

69. Shear, N.H., Spielberg, S.P.: Anticonvulsant hypersensitivity syndrome. In vitro assessment of risk. J. Clin. Invest., 82:1826, 1988.

70. Kaneko, S., et al.: Teratogenicity of antiepileptic drugs: analysis of possible risk factors. Epilepsia, 29:459, 1988.

71. Kerr, B.M., Levy, R.H.: Inhibition of epoxide hydrolase by anticonvulsants and risk of teratogenicity. Lancet, 1:610, 1989.

72. Stone, W.J., and Walle, T.J.: Massive propranolol metabolite retention during maintenance hemodialysis. Clin. Pharmacol. Ther., 28:449, 1980.

73. Drayer, D.E.: Pharmacologically active drug metabolites: therapeutic and toxic activities, plasma and urine data in man, accumulation in renal failure. Clin. Pharmacokinet., 1:426, 1976.

74. Caldwell, J.: The current status of attempts to predict species differences in drug metabolism. Drug Metab. Rev., 12:222, 1981.

75. Kato, R.: Characteristics and differences in the hepatic mixed function oxidases of different species. Pharmacol. Ther., 6:41, 1979.

76. Hewick, D.S., and McEwen, J.: Plasma half-lives, plasma metabolites and anticoagulant efficacies of the enantiomers of warfarin in man. J. Pharm. Pharmacol., 25:458, 1973.

77. Breimer, D.D., and vanRossum, J.M.: Pharmacokinetics of (+)-, (−)- and (±)-hexobarbitone in man after oral administration. J. Pharm. Pharmacol., 25:762, 1973.

78. Chandler, M.H.H., Scott, S.R., Blouin, R.A.: Age-associated stereoselective alterations in hexobarbital metabolism. Clin. Pharmacol. Ther., 43:436, 1988.

79. Wan, S.H., Matin, S.B., and Azarnoff, D.L.: Kinetics, salivary excretion of amphetamine isomers, and effect of urinary pH. Clin. Pharmacol. Ther., 23:585, 1978.

80. George, C.F., et al.: Pharmacokinetics of dextro-, laevo-, and racemic propranolol in man. Eur. J. Clin. Pharmacol., 4:74, 1972.

81. Silber, B., Holford, N.H.G., and Riegelman, S.: Stereoselective disposition and glucuronidation of propranolol in humans. J. Pharm. Sci., 71:699, 1982.

82. Vangiessen, G.J., and Kaiser, D.G.: GLC determination of ibuprofen [dl-2-(p-isobutylphenyl) propionic acid] enantiomers in biological specimens. J. Pharm. Sci., *64*:798, 1975.

83. Williams, K., Lee, E.: Importance of drug enantiomers in clinical pharmacology. Drugs, *30*:333, 1985.

84. Lam, Y.W.F.: Stereoselectivity: an issue of significant importance in clinical pharmacology. Pharmacother., *8*:147, 1988.

85. Srinivas, N.R., et al.: Stereoselective disposition of methylphenidate in children with attention-deficit disorder. J. Pharmacol. Exp. Ther., *241*:300, 1987.

86. Gill, T.S., Hopkins, K.J., Rowland, M.: Stereospecific assay of nicoumalone: application to pharmacokinetic studies in man. Br. J. Clin. Pharmacol., *25*:591, 1988.

87. Eichelbaum, M.: Pharmacokinetic and pharmacodynamic consequences of stereoselective drug metabolism in man. Biochem. Pharmacol., *37*:93, 1988.

88. Ariens, E.J.: Stereochemistry, a basis for sophisticated nonsense in pharmacokinetics and clinical pharmacology. Eur. J. Clin. Pharmacol., *26*:663, 1984.

89. Evans, A.M., et al.: Stereoselective drug disposition: potential for misinterpretation of drug disposition data. Br. J. Clin. Pharmacol., *26*:771, 1988.

90. Mawer, G.E., et al.: Phenytoin dose adjustment in epileptic patients. Br. J. Clin. Pharmacol., *1*:163, 1974.

91. Levy, G., and Tsuchiya, T.: Salicylate accumulation in man. N. Engl. J. Med., *287*:430, 1972.

92. Paulus, H.E., et al.: Variation of serum concentrations and half-life of salicylate in patients with rheumatoid arthritis. Arthritis Rheum., *14*:527, 1971.

93. Calabro, J.J., and Marchesano, J.M.: Fever associated with juvenile rheumatoid arthritis. N. Engl. J. Med., *276*:11, 1967.

94. Done, A.K.: Salicylate poisoning. JAMA, *192*:770, 1965.

95. Craig, J.O., Ferguson, I.C., and Syme, J.: Infants, toddlers and aspirin. Br. Med. J., *1*:757, 1966.

96. Sjö, O., et al.: Dose-dependent kinetics of ethotoin in man. Clin. Exp. Pharmacol. Physiol., *2*:185, 1975.

97. Ishizaki, T., Kubo, M.: Incidence of apparent Michaelis-Menten kinetic behavior of theophylline and its parameters (V_{max} and K_m) among asthmatic children and adults. Ther. Drug Monitor., *9*:11, 1987.

98. Dvornik, D., et al.: Propranolol concentrations in healthy men given 80 mg daily in divided doses: effect of food and circadian variation. Curr. Ther. Res., *32*:214, 1982.

99. Wagner, J.G.: Propranolol: pooled Michaelis-Menten parameters and the effect of input rate on bioavailability. Clin. Pharmacol. Ther., *37*:481, 1985.

100. Parker, R.B., McCollam, P.L., Bauman, J.L.: Propafenone: a novel type 1c antiarrhythmic agent. Drug. Intell. Clin. Pharm., *23*:196, 1989.

101. Wagner, J.G.: Single intravenous dose and steady-state oral dose pharmacokinetics of nicardipine in healthy subjects. Biopharm. Drug Disposition, *8*:133, 1987.

102. Galinsky, R.E., and Levy, G.: Dose- and time-dependent elimination of acetaminophen in rats: Pharmacokinetic implications of cosubstrate depletion. J. Pharmacol. Exp. Ther., *219*:14, 1981.

103. Perrier, D., Ashley, J.J., and Levy, G.: Effect of product inhibition in kinetics of drug elimination. J. Pharmacokinet., Biopharm., *1*:231, 1973.

104. Klotz, U., and Reimann, I.: Clearance of diazepam can be impaired by its major metabolite desmethyldiazepam. Eur. J. Clin. Pharmacol., *21*:161, 1981.

105. Noonan, P.K., Williams, R.L., Benet, L.Z.: Dose dependent pharmacokinetics of nitroglycerin after multiple intravenous infusions in healthy volunteers. J. Pharmacokin. Biopharm., *13*:143, 1985.

106. Klotz, U., Antonin, K.H., and Bieck, P.R.: Comparison of the pharmacokinetics of diazepam after single and subchronic doses. Eur. J. Clin. Pharmacol., *10*:121, 1976.

107. Eichelbaum, M., et al.: Plasma kinetics of carbamazepine and its epoxide metabolite in man after single and multiple doses. Eur. J. Clin. Pharmacol., *8*:337, 1975.

108. Pitlick, W.H., and Levy, R.H.: Time dependent kinetics. I. Exponential autoinduction of carbamazepine in monkeys. J. Pharm. Sci., *66*:647, 1977.

109. Rumble, R.H., Brooks, P.M., and Roberts, M.S.: Metabolism of salicylate during chronic aspirin therapy. Br. J. Clin. Pharmacol., *9*:41, 1980.

110. Furst, D.E., Gupta, N., and Paulus, H.E.: Salicylate metabolism in twins: Evidence suggesting a genetic influence and induction of salicylurate formation. J. Clin. Invest., *60*:32, 1977.

111. Routledge, P.A., and Shand, D.G.: Clinical pharmacokinetics of propranolol. Clin. Pharmacokinet., *4*:73, 1979.

112. McNeil, J.J., et al.: Labetalol steady-state pharmacokinetics in hypertensive patients. Br. J. Clin. Pharmacol., *13*:755, 1982.

113. Inturrisi, C.E., et al.: Propoxyphene and norpropoxyphene kinetics after single and repeated doses of propoxyphene. Clin. Pharmacol. Ther., *31*:157, 1982.

114. Kates, R.E., et al.: Verapamil disposition kinetics in chronic atrial fibrillation. Clin. Pharmacol. Ther., *30*:44, 1981.

115. Schwartz, J.B., et al.: An investigation of the cause of accumulation of verapamil during regular dosing in patients. Br. J. Clin. Pharmacol., *19*:512, 1985.

116. Prescott, L.F., et al.: Impaired lignocaine metabolism in patients with myocardial infarction and cardiac failure. Br. Med. J., *1*:939, 1976.

117. Bauer, L.A., et al.: Influence of long-term infusions on lidocaine kinetics. Clin. Pharmacol. Ther., *31*:433, 1982.

118. Thomson, A.H., et al.: The pharmacokinetics and pharmacodynamics of lignocaine and MEGX in healthy subjects. J. Pharmacokin. Biopharm., *15*:101, 1987.

119. Alexanderson, B.: Prediction of steady state plasma levels of nortriptyline from single oral dose kinetics: A study in twins. Eur. J. Clin. Pharmacol., *6*:44, 1973.

120. Ando, H.Y., Ho, N.F., and Higuchi, W.I.: *In vitro* estimates of topical bioavailability. J. Pharm. Sci., *66*:755, 1977.

121. Conolly, M.E., et al.: Metabolism of isoprenaline in dog and man. Br. J. Pharmacol., *46*:458, 1972.

122. Davies, D.S., et al.: Metabolism of terbutaline in man and dog. Br. J. Clin. Pharmacol., *1*:129, 1974.

123. Evans, M.E., et al.: The pharmacokinetics of rimiterol in man. Xenobiotica, *4*:681, 1974.

124. Williams, F.M., et al.: The influence of the route of administration on urinary metabolites of isoetharine. Xenobiotica, *4*:345, 1974.

125. Morgan, D.J., et al.: Pharmacokinetics of intravenous and oral salbutamol and its sulphate conjugate. Br. J. Clin. Pharmacol., *22*:587, 1986.

126. Brunk, S.F., and Delle, M.: Morphine metabolism in man. Clin. Pharmacol. Ther., *16*:51, 1974.

127. Levy, G., and Angelino, N.J.: Hydrolysis of aspirin by rat small intestine. J. Pharm. Sci., *57*:1449, 1968.

128. Goldman, P.: Therapeutic implications of the intestinal microflora. N. Engl. J. Med., *289*:623, 1973.

129. Schroder, H., Lewkonia, R.M., and Price Evans, D.A.: Metabolism of salicylazosulfapyridine in healthy subjects and in patients with ulcerative colitis. Effects of colectomy

and of phenobarbital. Clin. Pharmacol. Ther., *14*:802, 1973.

130. Strong, H.A., et al.: Sulindac metabolism: the importance of an intact colon. Clin. Pharmacol. Ther., *38*:387, 1985.

131. Brown, E.B.B.: The localization, metabolism and effects of drugs and toxicants in lung. Drug Metab. Rev., *3*:33, 1974.

132. Roth, R.A., and Wiersma, D.A.: Role of the lung in total body clearance of circulating drugs. Clin. Pharmacokinet., *4*:355, 1979.

133. Collins, J.M., et al.: Nonlinear pharmacokinetic models for 5-fluorouracil in man: Intravenous and intraperitoneal routes. Clin. Pharmacol. Ther., *28*:235, 1980.

134. Collins, J.M., and Dedrick, R.L.: Contribution of lungs to total body clearance: linear and nonlinear effects. J. Pharm. Sci., *71*:66, 1982.

12

Pharmacokinetic Variability—
Body Weight, Age, Sex, and
Genetic Factors

When individuals are given identical doses of a drug, large differences in pharmacologic response may be seen. For example, the sleeping times of 72 rats after intraperitoneal administration of pentobarbital sodium (30 mg/kg) ranged from about 30 to 190 min; the duration of paralysis in 96 rats after intraperitoneal administration of zoxazolamine (110 mg/kg) varied from 100 to 850 min.[1]

The decrease in blood glucose (expressed as percent of control level) 30 min after a 1 g intravenous dose of tolbutamide in 97 human subjects ranged from 10% to more than 50%.[2] The variable effect of 1 drop of an ophthalmic solution containing 30 mg/ml phenylephrine hydrochloride instilled into the conjunctival sac on pupil diameter in 39 subjects is shown in Figure 12–1.[3]

The dose required to produce a certain response may vary widely from individual to individual. For example, the dose of warfarin required to increase prothrombin time to the range of 18 to 21.5 sec in 15 patients with cardiovascular disease varied from 0.04 to 0.20 mg/kg per day.[4] The daily dose of phenindione required to achieve an adequate degree of anticoagulation ranges from 25 to 200 mg.[5]

Two sources of variability are differences in drug levels at the site of action (as inferred by drug concentration in the plasma), and differences in effect produced by a given drug concentration. Although both sources contribute to the variability in response, there is increasing evidence for many drugs that the principal variation is the drug concentration resulting from a given dose. This is called pharmacokinetic variability.

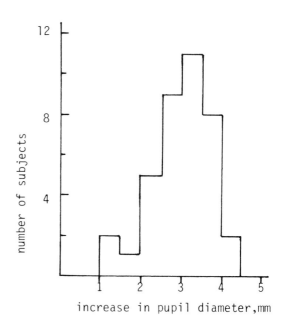

Fig. 12–1. Variable effect of 1 drop of an ophthalmic solution containing 30 mg/ml phenylephrine hydrochloride instilled into the conjunctival sac on pupil diameter in 39 subjects. (Data from Bertler, Å., and Smith, S.E.[3])

The typically large variability in blood levels of drugs is seen in the results of a study in 24 patients with meningitis treated with continuous intravenous infusion of ampicillin, 150 mg/kg per day.[6] On day 5 of treatment, serum levels of ampicillin ranged from 9 to 92 µg/ml. Differences in renal function among the patients partly explain the large range of serum concentrations.

A great deal of variability, both pharmacokinetic and pharmacodynamic, has been seen with midazolam, an intravenous benzodiazepine widely used for sedation before and during surgery. Investigators in The Netherlands studied the pharmacokinetics of midazolam in 17 patients on mechanical ventilation in a general intensive care unit who were receiving a continuous iv infusion of the drug, adjusted according to the level of sedation.[7] The half-life of midazolam was less than 2 hours in 1 patient, ranged from 3.5 to 6 hr in 10 patients, and was greater than 10 hr in 6 patients.

The investigators noted that a "wide range of midazolam serum levels was associated with adequate sedation, and similarly the midazolam levels at the moment of awakening were highly variable." Apparently, it is very difficult to establish a relationship between level of consciousness and midazolam concentration in patients in intensive care because of the variety of drugs that are used and the state of the patient.

Not only is a high degree of variability routinely found between subjects, a wide range of blood levels may also be seen when the same subject takes a drug on different occasions. It is widely believed, however, that intersubject variability is much greater than intrasubject variability. Wagner[8] determined the inter- and intrasubject variation of digoxin renal clearance in normal adult males, using data from 5 different studies. He found that intrasubject coefficients of variation averaged 24% (with a range of 15 to 29%). Depending on the method used to calculate variance, intersubject coefficients of variation averaged 30% (with a range of 18 to 42%) or 42% (with a range of 19 to 50%). Consistent with the prevailing wisdom, intersubject variability in the renal clearance of digoxin was greater than intrasubject variability, but clearly, intrasubject variability is not trivial.

The greatest difference between maximum and minimum renal clearances of digoxin in the five studies averaged 115 ml/min within subjects and 183 ml/min between subjects. The ratio of intra- to intersubject variability ranged from 0.47 to 0.71 with a mean value of 0.64. Physical activity is one factor contributing to intrasubject variability. The renal clearance of digoxin is significantly higher during a period of normal physical activity than during a period of immobilization.

Some drugs show greater variability than others. It is particularly difficult to prescribe the appropriate dose for drugs with nonlinear pharmacoki-

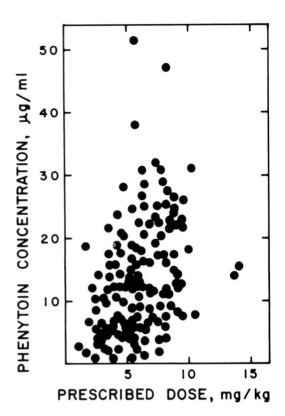

Fig. 12–2. Relationship between the steady-state plasma concentration of phenytoin in epileptic patients and the prescribed daily dose. (Data from Lund, L.[9])

netics because of interpatient variability in blood levels. The relationship between the concentration of phenytoin in the plasma and the prescribed daily dose is shown in Figure 12–2. More than a 20-fold difference was found in the apparent steady-state phenytoin concentrations in plasma among patients who had been prescribed the same daily dose.[9] The steady-state plasma chlorthalidone concentrations in 10 patients during treatment with a standard dose of 50 mg/day varied 5-fold between individuals, ranging from 211 to 1138 ng/ml.[10]

Particularly pronounced pharmacokinetic variability is consistently observed with drugs subject to a high hepatic clearance and substantial presystemic metabolism. An example is shown for the tricyclic antidepressant desipramine in Figure 12–3. The upper and lower curves show the extreme results in 2 patients. The middle curve shows mean values for 9 other patients. All 11 patients were treated with 25 mg of desipramine orally 3 times a day. Plasma levels differed by 30-fold.[11] Steady-state levels of nortriptyline in patients with psychiatric illness receiving 75 mg/day varied from

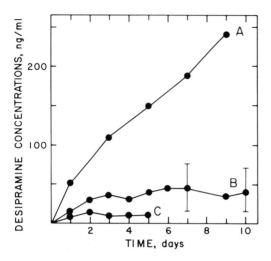

Fig. 12–3. Desipramine concentrations in plasma in patients during repetitive dosing with 25 mg 3 times a day. Curves A and C indicate the levels in 2 patients who showed the highest and lowest degree of drug accumulation, respectively. Curve B reflects the average of 9 other patients. The vertical bars at days 7 and 10 on curve B indicate the range of desipramine concentrations in the individual patients. (Data from Hammer, W., Idestrom, C.M., and Sjöqvist, F.[11])

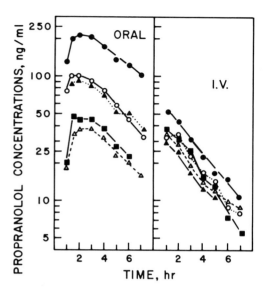

Fig. 12–4. Propranolol concentrations in plasma after a single 80-mg oral or 10-mg intravenous (iv) dose to 5 healthy adults. Less variability is observed after iv administration. (Data from Shand, D.G., Nuckolls, E.M., and Oates, J.A.[14])

about 10 to 260 ng/ml.[12] Steady-state plasma concentrations of alprenolol, a beta-blocking drug, in 30 patients treated for a prolonged period varied 25-fold between individuals receiving identical oral doses.[13]

Theory suggests that a drug subject to substantial presystemic metabolism should show less pharmacokinetic variability after parenteral administration than after oral administration. Figure 12–4 indicates that this is the case after oral and intravenous administration of propranolol.[14]

Many factors contribute to the variability in the relationship between the amount of drug administered or prescribed and the resulting drug concentration in the body. This relationship is influenced by the bioavailability of the drug from the dosage form, a subject discussed in earlier chapters, as well as other factors that may affect the completeness of absorption. It is also influenced by a host of factors that affect drug disposition. Drug absorption, distribution, metabolism, and excretion processes are subject to individual variation from age-related phenomena, genetic and environmental factors, the consequences of disease, and concomitant administration of other drugs. An additional and possibly important source of variability

is that certain patients frequently fail to follow directions about taking medicine.

This chapter and the two that follow are concerned with factors that contribute to intersubject differences in drug concentrations in blood and tissues.

BODY WEIGHT AND SIZE

The apparent volume of distribution of a drug is determined by the anatomic space into which it distributes and its relative degree of vascular and extravascular binding. Because the volume of both total body water (TBW) and extracellular fluid (ECF) in adults with normal lean-to-fat ratios is directly proportional to body weight, there is a relationship between apparent volume of distribution and body weight. This relationship is particularly evident for drugs that are poorly bound in the body.

Initial blood levels following a single dose or a loading dose of a drug that is rapidly absorbed are largely dependent on apparent volume of distribution; the larger is the volume of distribution, the lower is the blood level. Whenever peak blood levels are of concern during drug therapy, body weight should be considered in determining the appropriate dose.

Organ size, function, and blood flow are also

related to body weight, but the relationship between drug clearance and body weight is not clear. The correlation between drug clearance and body weight in normal young adults is poor; studies that also include infants, children, and the elderly are confounded by well known age effects on drug clearance. Therefore, there are no general guidelines to relate maintenance doses of drugs to body weight.

Because of pharmacokinetic variability in drug absorption, binding, and elimination and because of pharmacodynamic variability in response, weight adjustments are generally thought unnecessary unless the weight of an individual differs by more than 50% from the average adult weight (70 kg). In practice, adjustments for weight are made only for children and for unusually small, emaciated, or obese adult patients.[15]

Obesity

Obesity, defined as that condition when a patient's total body weight is more than 25% above desirable weight, occurs in almost 20% of the population of the United States and is more prevalent in women than men. Ideal body weight (IBW) is usually defined as follows:

IBW (men) = 50 kg ± 1 kg/2.5 cm above or below 150 cm in height   (12–1)

IBW (women) = 45 kg ± 1 kg/2.5 cm above or below 150 cm in height   (12–2)

Drug distribution may change as a result of the changes in body composition in the obese patient. The percentage of fat and lean body mass in an individual may be estimated by measuring height (in inches), weight (in kilograms), and girth (in inches, using the umbilical level at exhalation), and using these data in the following equations:[16]

Percent fat

$$= 90 - 2 \text{ (Height} - \text{Girth)} \quad (12\text{–}3)$$

Lean body mass

$$= (100 - \text{Percent fat}) \times \text{Weight} \quad (12\text{–}4)$$

The smaller ratio of body water and muscle mass to total body weight, and the greater proportion of body fat in the obese could lead to changes in drug partitioning into the various body compartments. Fat contains less extracellular fluid than other tissues. Therefore, the distribution space for polar drugs, like antibiotics, is relatively less in obese

patients and may be a reason for reducing the daily dose, calculated on a mg/kg total body weight basis. On the other hand, the relative distribution space for lipid-soluble drugs may be the same or even larger in obese patients; this may call for the same or even larger daily doses, calculated on a mg/kg total body weight basis. Furthermore, in principle, drug binding, metabolism, and excretion may be affected by obesity. For these reasons, the selection of appropriate dosing regimens for the severely obese patient is a formidable challenge.

Intuitively, one expects an obese patient to need a larger dose than a normal-weight patient. Dosing regimens based on milligrams of drug per kg of total body weight or per square meter of body surface area will indeed deliver a larger dose to the obese patient. But, studies comparing pharmacokinetics in obese and normal-weight subjects suggest that this approach is frequently wrong and may result in drug toxicity.

A dosing regimen that is safe and effective in the average patient may require modification if the apparent volume of distribution, clearance, or half-life of the drug in the patient under consideration is sufficiently different from the average value. The volume of distribution of most drugs is greater, sometimes dramatically greater, in obese subjects than in normal-weight subjects. Largely for this reason, one may find much longer half-lives in obese subjects. On the other hand, differences in drug clearance between significantly overweight and normal-weight patients are often small; in many cases, there is no need to change the total daily dose of a drug when it is given to an obese patient.

Changes in dosing regimen for obese patients might be anticipated if a drug is largely excreted unchanged or eliminated through formation of sulfate or glucuronide conjugates. Creatinine clearance is increased in obese patients and the renal clearance of a drug may be increased to a similar or greater extent. Renal excretion of a drug may be greater in obese patients because of changes in renal blood flow and glomerular filtration rate secondary to increased blood volume and cardiac output. Metabolic clearance reflecting conjugation with sulfate or glucuronic acid also seems to increase as a function of body weight. Oxidative metabolism, on the other hand, does not appear to be affected by weight changes.

If a drug distributes poorly or not at all into the excess body space found in the obese patient, one would expect the same plasma drug concentrations after administration of the same absolute amount of drug to a patient with normal body weight or to an obese patient, provided their lean body masses were comparable. This is illustrated by the results of studies with digoxin.[17] A single intravenous dose of 0.5 mg of digoxin was given to 5 obese patients before and after an average weight loss of 46 kg. There were no significant differences in the blood concentrations before and after weight reduction.

In another study, the pharmacokinetics of digoxin were determined in 13 obese subjects (average total body weight 100 kg, 162% of IBW) and 16 control subjects (average total body weight 65 kg, 98% of IBW). No important differences were found in absolute volume of distribution (approximately 950 L), clearance (approximately 300 ml/min), or half-life (approximately 35 to 40 hr).[18]

The results of these studies indicate that the obese patient should receive the same average loading and maintenance doses of digoxin as the normal-weight patient. If the drug is dosed on a body weight basis, the obese patient should receive the same mg/kg of IBW dose as the normal-weight patient but a smaller mg/kg total body weight dose of digoxin. Digoxin dosage may be dangerously high if calculated on the basis of total body weight in obese patients.

Several studies have examined the pharmacokinetics of aminoglycoside antibiotics in obese subjects. Schwartz and associates[19] administered 1 mg/kg gentamicin to 6 obese subjects (average body weight 104 kg) and 6 normal-weight subjects (average body weight 55 kg). The apparent volume of distribution was significantly larger in the obese subjects than in the normal-weight subjects (19 L vs 13 L). On the other hand, the apparent volume of distribution corrected for *total* body weight was significantly smaller in the obese subjects than in the normal-weight subjects (0.185 L/kg vs 0.244 L/kg).

These results indicate that gentamicin distributes into the excess body space of obese patients but not as efficiently as it distributes into lean body mass. Korsager confirmed these results and calculated that the uptake of gentamicin into the excess body space in the obese subjects was about 40% of the uptake into lean body mass.[20] Similar findings have been reported for tobramycin[19,21] and amikacin.[22] Dosing these antibiotics on a mg/kg IBW basis produces lower peak blood levels in an obese patient than in a normal-weight patient; dosing on a mg/kg total body weight basis results in higher peak blood levels in obese patients than in patients of normal weight.

Bauer and associates recommend that the loading dose of amikacin in the severely obese patient be based on an apparent volume of distribution (V) calculated as follows:[22]

$$V = 0.26 [IBW + 0.38 (FW)] \quad (12–5)$$

where IBW is ideal body weight, FW is fat weight (total body weight minus IBW), 0.26 L/kg is the apparent volume of distribution in normal-weight individuals, and 0.38 is a factor accounting for the more limited distribution of amikacin in excess body space than in lean body mass.

A patient weighing 150 kg (IBW = 70 kg) is predicted to have an apparent volume of distribution of 26.1 L; a normal-weight patient will have an apparent volume of distribution of 18.2 L. The loading dose of amikacin (in mg or mg/kg IBW) should be about 40% higher for the obese patient than for the normal-weight patient.

Some drugs (e.g., caffeine, lidocaine, lorazepam, and theophylline) distribute about equally between lean body mass and excess body mass (largely adipose tissue). In this case, apparent volume of distribution is larger in obese patients but distribution volume per kg of total body weight is about the same in obese and normal-weight individuals. Other drugs (e.g., phenytoin, thiopental, and diazepam), because they are lipid soluble, distribute disproportionately into excess body weight and volume per kg total body weight is larger in obese subjects. The distribution volume of thiopental per kg total body weight is 1400 ml in normal-weight subjects and 4720 ml in obese subjects. Plots of apparent volume of distribution per kg total body weight vs total body weight tend to be linear, with a negative slope for drugs such as gentamicin, a slope approximating zero for drugs such as caffeine, and a positive slope for drugs such as thiopental.

Blouin and co-workers have studied the pharmacokinetics of vancomycin in obese subjects.[23] The apparent volume of distribution of vancomycin was considerably larger in obese subjects than in normal-weight subjects (50 L vs 33 L). Like the aminoglycosides, however, the apparent volume of distribution of vancomycin normalized for total body weight was smaller in the obese subjects than in the normal-weight subjects, indicating limited distribution into the excess body space. Loading doses of vancomycin (in mg or mg/kg IBW) should be higher for obese patients than for normal-weight patients.

Another important finding of the vancomycin studies is that the clearance of vancomycin was more than twice as large in obese subjects than in normal-weight subjects (188 ml/min vs 81 ml/min). This result was consistent with the larger creatinine clearance in the obese subjects compared to that observed in normal-weight subjects (180 ml/min vs 138 ml/min). The same mg/kg total body weight daily dose in obese and normal-weight subjects yields comparable average vancomycin concentrations at steady state.[21] Higher drug clearance in obese subjects than in normal-weight subjects has also been reported with aminoglycoside antibiotics.[19-22]

Bauer et al.[24] studied the clearance of cimetidine in normal-weight (62 kg) and obese (140 kg) subjects. In subjects with normal total body weight and renal function, about one-half of an iv dose of cimetidine is excreted unchanged in the urine. The investigators observed that the clearance of cimetidine from serum was much greater in obese subjects than normal-weight subjects (1147 vs 637 ml/min). This difference was almost entirely the result of a substantially higher renal clearance of cimetidine in obese than in control subjects (808 vs 318 ml/min).

Studies with theophylline in obese subjects are of interest because, unlike the aminoglycosides, theophylline is almost completely metabolized via oxidative pathways. The large increase in absolute volume of distribution of theophylline in obese subjects, compared to that observed in normal-weight subjects, indicates that theophylline readily distributes into fat. Loading doses of theophylline should be calculated on the basis of total body weight; however, the absolute clearance of theophylline (in ml/min) is remarkably similar in obese and normal-weight patients.[25] Therefore, maintenance dose calculations for theophylline should be based on IBW; total daily dose (in mg or mg/kg IBW) should be similar in obese and normal weight patients. The clearance of nordiazepam (desmethyldiazepam), the active metabolite of clorazepate, is also similar in obese and normal-weight subjects.[26]

The effects of obesity on the kinetics of three other drugs subject to oxidative metabolism (viz, propranolol, trazodone, and verapamil) have also been reported. Bowman et al.[27] compared the pharmacokinetics of propranolol in obese and control subjects. Clearance, determined after iv dosing, was nearly identical in the two groups. A trend toward decreased first-pass metabolism in the obese group after oral administration was not statistically significant. The half-life of propranolol was longer in the obese group because of a nearly 2-fold change in volume of distribution.

Similar results were observed with trazodone.[28] Clearance was about the same in obese and control subjects but the large difference in apparent volume of distribution (162 vs 67 L) resulted in a prolonged half-life in obese subjects (13 vs 6 hr). The investigators concluded that the dose of trazodone should be based on ideal rather than total body weight; average daily dose should be about the same in normal-weight and obese patients.

Abernethy and Schwartz[29] gave iv verapamil to obese and normal-weight patients with hypertension and found that elimination half-life was prolonged in obese patients (10 vs 4 hr) because of a marked increase in volume of distribution (713 vs 301 L) with no significant change in total verapamil clearance [1340 (obese) vs 1250 ml/min].

Ibuprofen, a widely used NSAID, appears to be an exception to the general rule that obesity has a minimal effect on the clearance of drugs eliminated by oxidative metabolism.[30] A 600 mg oral dose of ibuprofen resulted in a significantly lower peak concentration in obese subjects than in controls (37 vs 48 mg/L) consistent with a larger volume of distribution. Surprisingly, the total area under the ibuprofen concentration in plasma vs time curve was also lower in obese subjects. This difference could be explained by decreased absorption or increased clearance in obese subjects; plasma protein binding was nearly the same in each group.

Ibuprofen undergoes aliphatic hydroxylation and carboxylation rather than ring hydroxylation or oxidative N-demethylation, the more common oxidative pathways. Perhaps the cytochrome P-450(s) concerned with aliphatic hydroxylation and carboxylation is increased selectively in obese subjects. The results suggest that larger doses of ibuprofen are required for obese patients to attain plasma levels similar to those in normal-weight patients.

Relatively few drugs are eliminated by nitroreduction but this pathway applies to one of the most widely used benzodiazepines in Europe: nitrazepam. Investigators have determined that the half-life of nitrazepam is markedly greater in obese subjects than in controls (33.5 vs 24 hr) due to increased distribution volume (290 vs 137 L), calculated by assuming complete absorption after oral administration.[31]

Plasma levels of nitrazepam after a single dose were appreciably lower in obese subjects, suggesting an increased clearance. Mean oral clearance was 101 ml/min in the obese group compared with a value of 67 ml/min in the control group. A correlation analysis involving all subjects indicated a statistically significant relationship between apparent nitrazepam clearance and percent of ideal body weight.

These investigators observed that "benzodiazepines which undergo hydroxylation or oxidative N-demethylation, including diazepam, desmethyldiazepam, alprazolam, and midazolam have minimal if any change in clearance in obese subjects . . . In contrast, the benzodiazepines lorazepam and oxazepam, which are biotransformed in man by glucuronide conjugation, have increases in clearance in obese man which are well correlated with degree of obesity. The increased clearance of nitrazepam in obese subjects suggests that the nitroreduction pathway for biotransformation of xenobiotics may also be increased in obese individuals."

In addition to the elimination of lorazepam and oxazepam, drugs subject to glucuronide conjugation, the elimination of acetaminophen, which is subject largely to sulfate conjugation, is also enhanced in obese subjects.[32] Another example of the effects of obesity on conjugative metabolism is seen with salicylate.[33] The major elimination pathways for salicylate are glycine and glucuronide conjugation. The clearance of salicylate after administration of aspirin was about 20% greater in obese subjects (113 kg TBW) than in normal-weight subjects (67 kg TBW).

As a rule, an increase in distribution volume results in an increase in half-life, whereas an increase in clearance produces a decrease in half-life. Most drugs have a longer half-life in obese than in normal-weight subjects, reflecting changes in volume of distribution. A most dramatic example of the effect of obesity on half-life has been reported with theophylline in a study involving a patient who weighed 523 kg.[34] Although theophylline clearance in this patient was similar to values observed in normal-weight subjects, a half-life of about 34 hr was determined, about 4 times longer

than expected for normal-weight individuals with average clearances.

Neonates, Infants, and Children

Dosing guidelines for children are more complicated than those for adults. Evidence indicates that children require and tolerate larger mg/kg doses of many drugs than do adults. For example, the usual doses of digoxin are 15 to 20 μg/kg per day for children 4 weeks to 2 years of age, 10 to 15 μg/kg per day for children 2 to 12 years of age and 4 to 5 μg/kg per day for adults.[35] These doses result in average digoxin concentrations in plasma of about 1 to 1.5 ng/ml when given to patients of the appropriate age.[36]

Estimates of the dose required for infants and children are often obtained on the basis of the surface area of the young patient relative to the surface area of an adult. Body surface area (SA) can be calculated using the following height-weight formula:[37]

$$SA\ (m^2)\ =\ weight\ (kg)^{0.5378}$$

$$\times\ height\ (cm)^{0.3964}\ \times\ 0.024265\quad(12\text{--}6)$$

A less accurate but still useful estimate of surface area in children can be calculated from the following equation:[38]

$$SA\ (m^2)\ =\ weight\ (kg)^{0.728}\quad(12\text{--}7)$$

The body surface area of the average adult is assumed to be 1.73 m².

A still simpler equation to calculate body surface area, one that is easily solved using a calculator with a square root function, has also been proposed.[39] In this relationship, surface area (in m²) is equal to the square root of the product of height (in cm) and weight (in kg), divided by 60. That is,

$$SA\ =\ (height\ \times\ weight)^{1/2}\ /60\quad(12\text{--}8)$$

Validation of this equation was based on measurements in adolescent and adult subjects. A 185-cm tall, 80-kg patient is predicted to have a body surface area of 2.03 cm². Other investigators tested the accuracy of this simplified equation when applied to children.[40] The body surface area of 168 children between the ages of 1 and 14 years was calculated. The resulting values were then compared to the classic equation of DuBois and DuBois.[41] That is,

$$SA = 0.007184 \times height^{0.725}$$
$$\times weight^{0.425} \quad (12-9)$$

The investigators found a correlation coefficient between the two methods of calculation of greater than 0.99, suggesting that this simplified approach to the estimation of body surface area is reliable in both adults and children.

Calculations based on body surface area indicate that, in general, the average 3-month-old child weighing 6 kg should receive twice the mg/kg dose given to an average adult, whereas the average 5-yr-old child weighing 20 kg should receive 1.5 times the mg/kg dose given to adults.[38] Because of age-related differences in drug metabolism, however, still larger doses are sometimes required.

One study examined the variability in peak serum concentration of gentamicin in patients from different age groups, ranging from 6 months to 42 years of age, who received parenteral doses standardized for body weight (1 mg/kg) or body surface (30 mg/m²).[42] Age-related variability was less after administration of a dose calculated on surface area than after a dose calculated on weight. Children under 10 years of age require a larger mg/kg dose than older patients to achieve comparable serum gentamicin concentrations. The same mg/m² dose of gentamicin results in roughly comparable serum levels in all age groups.

The requirement for larger mg/kg doses in children than in adults is related in part to the fact that TBW and ECF make up a larger percentage of the total body weight in children than in adults. Total body water decreases with age, from 78% of the newborn's body weight to 60% of the adult's weight.[43] Differences in extracellular water (ECW) are even greater. Extracellular water represents about 45% of the body weight in the newborn but only 20% of the adult's body weight.[44] This means that the same mg/kg dose of a drug that is not bound and is distributed only in the ECW produces less than half the blood level in the newborn as in the adult, and about 70% of the blood level in a 2-year-old child as in an adult.[45]

In general, age-related changes in drug distribution tend to decrease the volume of distribution in adults compared with neonates for most water-soluble drugs. Drugs that are lipid soluble may have a lower volume of distribution in neonates

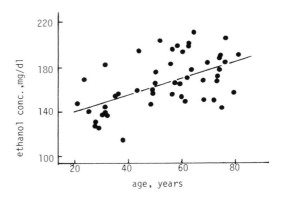

Fig. 12–5. Ethanol concentrations in blood at the end of a constant rate intravenous infusion as a function of age. (Data from Vestal, R.E., et al.[47])

because of age-related differences in adipose tissue.

Fisher and his colleagues[46] have studied the pharmacokinetics of vecuronium, a polar nondepolarizing muscle relaxant, in 5 infants (3 to 11 months old) and 5 children (1 to 5 years old). The muscle relaxant was given by iv infusion after anesthesia during elective surgery. The apparent volume of distribution of vecuronium was larger (357 vs 204 ml/kg) and the mean residence time was longer (66 vs 34 min) in infants than in children.

The investigators pointed out that they expected changes in the distribution volume because of several factors. "First, the distribution of muscle relaxants such as vecuronium is limited to extracellular fluid (ECF). ECF volume decreases markedly during the first year of life, starting at approximately 44% of body weight at birth and approaching the adult value of 22% at 1 year of age." Previous studies by these investigators found that the volume of distribution for d-tubocurarine, a related drug, was 514 ml/kg for infants, 405 ml/kg for children, and 309 ml/kg for adults, values that shadow the age-related changes in ECF.

No significant difference was observed in clearance between infants and children. Values of 5.6 and 5.9 ml/kg/min, respectively, were calculated. Therefore, the longer mean residence time of vecuronium in infants is almost strictly related to the larger volume of distribution in these patients.

Elderly Patients

Age-related changes in body composition at the other end of life may also affect drug distribution. On the average, lean body mass decreases and body fat increases in relation to total body weight in the

242 **Biopharmaceutics and Clinical Pharmacokinetics**

aging individual. The percentage of total body weight composed of adipose tissue is on the order of 36% in elderly men and 48% in elderly women, much higher than that found in young adults, 18% in men and 33% in women. It follows that the apparent volume of distribution of a relatively water-soluble drug such as antipyrine may remain the same or decrease slightly with age, whereas that of lipid-soluble drugs such as diazepam may be much larger in elderly patients than in younger ones.

Vestal and co-workers have observed a decrease in the lean body mass per unit surface area as a function of age, over an age range of 21 to 81 years, in healthy human subjects.[47] The apparent volume of distribution of ethanol, which is largely unbound and distributed in TBW, also decreased with age. The smaller volume of body water and the decreased lean body mass in elderly subjects probably account for the higher peak ethanol levels in blood after administration of a constant dose of ethanol as compared with young subjects (Fig. 12–5).

AGE

Age itself, rather than body size and composition, also affects the distribution and elimination of many drugs. Drug binding, metabolism, and excretion may change as a function of age. A study that documents changes in pharmacokinetic parameters from newborns to elderly particularly well is that of Sereni et al., who examined the pharmacokinetics of sulfamethoxypyridazine in subjects of different ages.[48] The study panel was divided into 5 groups: newborns (2 to 3 days), infants (1 to 12 months), children (4 to 9 years), adults (16 to 37 years), and elderly subjects (>70 years). The half-lives and apparent volumes of distribution of the sulfonamide in each age group are summarized in Table 12–1.

The half-life of sulfamethoxypyridazine was

Table 12–1. Half-Lives (t₁/₂) and Apparent Volumes of Distribution (V) of Sulfamethoxypyridazine in Human Subjects of Different Ages*

Age groups	t½ (hr)	V (L/kg)
Newborns	136	0.47
Infants	54	0.36
Children	51	0.20
Adults	63	0.22
Elderly subjects	98	0.26

*Data from Sereni, F., et al.[48]

Table 12–2. Elimination Half-Lives (hr) of Various Drugs in Neonates and Adults*

Drug	Neonates	Adults
Amobarbital	17 to 60	12 to 27
Carbamazepine	8 to 28	21 to 36
Diazepam	25 to 100	15 to 25
Indomethacin	14 to 20	2 to 11
Meperidine	22	3 to 4
Nortriptyline	56	18 to 22
Phenylbutazone	21 to 34	12 to 30
Phenytoin	21	11 to 29
Theophylline	24 to 36	3 to 9
Tolbutamide	10 to 40	4 to 9

*Data from Rane, A., and Tomson, G.[51]

considerably longer in newborns and elderly subjects than in young adult subjects. On the other hand, infants and children eliminated the drug more rapidly than did adults. The apparent volume of distribution was larger in newborns and infants than in adults, suggesting differences in binding and/or in the relative size of body compartments.

Another comprehensive examination of the effect of age on drug elimination has been reported for ceftriaxone.[49] Clearance increased from 0.9 to 2.5 ml/min when comparing patients 1 to 8 days old with patients 9 to 30 days old. The mean clearance of ceftriaxone in children ranging in age from 1 to 12 months and from 1 to 6 years was 6.2 ml/min and 9.1 ml/min, respectively. The 18 to 49 year old age group had the highest clearance of ceftriaxone, 17 ml/min. Older groups of patients had progressively lower values of clearance. Very elderly patients, 75 to 92 years of age, had an average clearance of about 8 ml/min.

These findings are generally consistent with results from other studies that compare the pharmacokinetics of drugs in a more limited number of age groups. For example, the clearance of cyclosporine, normalized for either total body weight or surface area, is greatest in bone marrow transplant recipients less than 10 years old (82 ml/min/kg), lowest in patients older than 40 years (20 ml/min/kg), and intermediary in patients ranging in age from 11 to 40 years (43 ml/min/kg).[50]

In general, drug elimination is impaired in newborns, particularly premature newborns; it improves with age and tends to be more efficient in older infants and children. Thereafter, drug elimination declines with age.

Drug Metabolism in Newborns

The most dramatic age-related differences in drug elimination often occur between the newborn and the adult. Most of the enzymatic microsomal systems required for drug metabolism are present at birth, but their titers are usually lower than adult levels. In general, drugs subject to biotransformation are eliminated more slowly in newborns than in adults (Table 12–2).[51]

Apparent exceptions to this generalization include the anticonvulsant drugs phenytoin and carbamazepine. The similarity of plasma half-lives of these drugs in newborns and adults is in contrast to the other drugs listed in Table 12–2. These data, however, were obtained in newborns who acquired the drug in utero from the mother who was receiving anticonvulsant treatment during pregnancy. Chronic exposure of the fetus to antiepileptic drugs throughout gestation may lead to induction of drug-metabolizing enzymes.

Although drug oxidation in the neonate seems to be almost uniformly impaired, drug conjugation in the newborn presents a mixed picture. Sulfate conjugation seems to be as efficient in newborns as in adults, but conjugation with glucuronic acid is considerably reduced, reaching adult levels only after 3 years of age. This deficiency is responsible for the serious adverse effects observed in newborns after administration of chloramphenicol, a drug that is ordinarily conjugated with glucuronic acid. Blood levels of chloramphenicol are higher and persist considerably longer in 1- and 2-day-old infants than in 4- to 5-year-old children.[52]

Reports of the variable effectiveness of indomethacin in the closure of significant patent ductus arteriosus in preterm infants have prompted an examination of the relationship between gestational age and indomethacin elimination in the newborn. One investigator found that the half-life of indomethacin decreased with gestational age.[35] Improved indomethacin elimination during development may be associated with treatment failures. Infants who did not respond to indomethacin eliminated the drug more rapidly and had lower plasma levels than those infants who did respond to the drug.[54]

Investigators in Seattle studied the pharmacokinetics of morphine in infants less than 10 weeks of age.[55] The clearance of morphine in newborns (1 to 4 days old) was less than half that found in older infants (6 vs 24 ml/min/kg). Differences in volume of distribution between the two groups modulated the effect of clearance on half-life but the half-life of morphine was longer in the newborns (7 vs 4 hr). The investigators suggested that

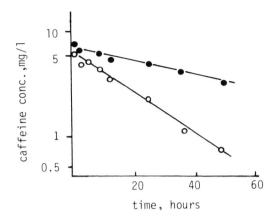

Fig. 12–6. Semilogarithmic plot of caffeine concentrations after a single iv dose to the same infant at ages 1.5 mo (●) and 2.5 mo (○). Half-life decreased from 41 to 16 hr from one administration to the next. (Data from Aranda, J.V., et al.[58])

the combination of lower clearance and longer elimination half-life in newborns may explain a prolonged duration of action for morphine in very young infants.

Theophylline is used frequently in newborns for treatment of apnea associated with immaturity, weaning from mechanical ventilation, and as a bronchodilator in infants with bronchopulmonary dysplasia. Compared with an adult, the preterm infant has a low clearance for theophylline. The amount of unchanged theophylline in urine in premature infants decreases with postnatal age, whereas the excretion of metabolites increases with age. One study found a strong correlation between theophylline half-life and postnatal age in premature infants 12 to 191 days old; half-life decreased from about 50 hr to 5 hr over this age range.[56]

Differences in the elimination of caffeine in newborns and adults are among the most remarkable reported for any drug.[57,58] The half-life of caffeine in the newborn is about 4 days; in adults, it is about 4 hr. Adults eliminate less than 2% of a dose of caffeine unchanged in the urine; the rest of the dose is metabolized to demethylated xanthines and urates. In the newborn, however, unmetabolized caffeine accounts for more than 85% of the urinary excretion products.[57] Caffeine remains the predominant urinary component for the first 3 months of life, but its percentage decreases gradually to the adult level of less than 2% by the age of 7 to 9 months. Figure 12–6 shows plasma levels of caffeine in the same infant at ages 1.5 months and

2.5 months. The long half-life of caffeine in the neonate is the result of slow urinary excretion of unchanged drug, which is the primary route of elimination in the infant because there is little or no metabolism.

Some drugs are metabolized in the gastrointestinal tract by intestinal bacteria in the large bowel. Cardioinactive digoxin reduction products can be detected by radioimmunoassay in the urine of about one-third of adults during treatment, signalling inactivation of digoxin by reduction of the lactone ring, mediated by anaerobic intestinal bacteria. About 10% of adult patients excrete large amounts of reduced metabolites. In these patients, more than 40% of total urinary digoxin and its derivatives is in the form of digoxin reduction products.

Investigators in New York carried out a study to determine whether infants and children metabolize digoxin in this way.[59] Eighty-nine patients on chronic digoxin therapy, younger than 21 years of age, were evaluated. None of the 36 digitalized infants 8 months of age or less excreted reduced digoxin metabolites in the urine; about 12 patients would have been expected in this category if the adult pattern prevailed. Among the 45 children older than 16 months, digoxin reduction products were found in the urine of 20. However, large quantities of digoxin reduction products in the urine, such as are found in 10% of adults, were not found in children less than 9 years of age.

Even though reduced metabolites were not found early in life, stool cultures of 20 of 73 infants younger than 8 months of age contained high concentrations of bacteria that reduced and inactivated digoxin in vitro, in some cases as early as the second week of life. In summary, children were found to be colonized with intestinal bacteria early in life but the capacity to inactivate digoxin developed only gradually. The investigators concluded that "the discrepancy between the time digoxin reduction product-forming organisms appear in the stool and production is detectable in vivo dictate caution in characterizing gut flora metabolic processes based only on in vitro observations."

Plasma Protein Binding in Newborns

Differences in plasma protein binding and tissue binding of drugs have also been reported between newborns and adults. Table 12–3 shows binding data and apparent volumes of distribution for several drugs in neonates and adults.[60] In each case, binding to plasma proteins is less in the newborns than in the adults. Generally consistent with the decrease in plasma protein binding is an increase in apparent volume of distribution in the newborn. Diazepam, despite the fact that the fraction unbound to plasma proteins is 4 times larger in neonates than in adults, is an exception. Apparently, the extravascular (tissue) binding of diazepam is even more impaired in the newborn than is plasma protein binding.

The relatively low plasma protein binding in neonates is often associated with elevated levels of bilirubin, which is avidly bound to albumin and may compete with drug for binding sites. At one time it was thought that competition between drugs and bilirubin for binding sites on albumin could result in displacement of bilirubin leading to its deposition in the central nervous system and kernicterus. Current thinking is that displacement of bilirubin by a drug is unlikely because the affinity of bilirubin for albumin is greater than that of any drug studied to date. Other mechanisms are probably involved in the development of CNS toxicity in neonates with elevated bilirubin and jaundice.

Decreased plasma protein binding of drugs and differences in body composition with respect to TBW and ECW largely explain why larger mg/kg doses are required to produce peak blood levels in neonates comparable to those in adults.

Table 12–3. Plasma Protein Binding (Fraction Free in Plasma), and Apparent Volume of Distribution in Neonates and Adults

Drug	Free fraction		Volume (L/kg)	
	Neonates	Adults	Neonates	Adults
Diazepam	0.16	0.04	1.6	2.4
Digoxin	0.8	0.7	5 to 10	7
Phenobarbital	0.68	0.53	1.0	0.55
Phenytoin	0.2	0.1	1.3	0.63
Sulfamethoxypyrazine	0.43	0.38	0.47	0.24
Sulfisoxazole	0.32	0.16	0.38	0.16

*Data from Morselli, P.L.[60]

Renal Excretion in Newborns

Although the ratio of kidney weight to total body weight in the newborn is twice that in the adult, the organ is anatomically and functionally immature; all aspects of renal function are reduced. Neonatal renal plasma flow and glomerular filtration rates normalized for body surface are still only 30 to 40% those of the adult, as indicated by aminohippurate and inulin studies.[61,62] One would anticipate that drugs subject to renal excretion would be eliminated more slowly in the newborn than in the adult patient.

The different processes of renal excretion mature at different rates. Average glomerular filtration rate is 38.5 ml/min/1.73 sq m and maximal tubular secretory capacity for para-aminohippurate (PAH) is 16 mg/min/1.73 sq m in full-term neonates, compared with adult values of 127 and 80, respectively. At 6 months of age, glomerular filtration rate is nearly 90% that found in the average adult, whereas maximal tubular secretory capacity for PAH is only about 60% of the adult value.[63] Immature renal function affects the elimination of aminoglycosides, indomethacin, digoxin, penicillins, sulfonamides, and many other drugs. The risk of adverse drug effects in newborns is high unless close attention is paid to the size of the dose.

Studies with digoxin are illustrative. Repetitive administration of 12 to 13 µg/kg per day of digoxin to full-term neonates (3 to 30 days), infants (1 to 12 mo), and children (1 to 10 years) results in mean steady-state plasma digoxin levels of 2.1, 1.2, and 1.4 ng/ml, respectively.[64] The elevated digoxin levels in the neonates are related to the low renal clearance of digoxin, which is, on the average, less than half that found in children and adults with normal renal function.

Drug Metabolism in Children

Although drug metabolism is impaired in neonates compared to adults, older infants and children actually metabolize certain drugs more rapidly than adults. Rates of drug metabolism for many drugs reach a maximum somewhere between 6 months and 12 years of age and thereafter decline with age. Accordingly, children often require higher mg/kg doses than do adults.

Drugs showing faster elimination in children than in adults include antipyrine, clindamycin, diazoxide, phenobarbital, carbamazepine, valproic acid, ethosuximide, and theophylline. Theophylline has been the most carefully documented.

In one study the pharmacokinetics of theophylline were determined in asthmatic children (6 to 17 years of age) and in normal adults, after a 4 mg/kg intravenous dose of aminophylline.[65] The average total clearance of theophylline was 87 ml/hr per kg in the children and 57 ml/hr per kg in the adults. The average half-life of theophylline was 3.7 hr in the children and 5.5 hr in the adults.

Wyatt and co-workers determined that the average daily dose of theophylline required to maintain serum levels in the therapeutic range of 10 to 20 µg/ml was 24 mg/kg for children up to 9 years of age, 18 mg/kg for children aged 12 to 16 years, and 13 mg/kg for patients older than 16 years.[66] Administration of the adult dose to the younger children seldom produces therapeutic levels; administration of the dose required for children to adults results in blood levels usually associated with adverse effects.

Body surface area has been found to be a better correlate of dosing requirements in children than body weight, perhaps because it is a better correlate of cardiac output, of hepatic and renal blood flow, and of glomerular filtration rate in children and adults. According to one approach based on body surface area, a child's maintenance dose is calculated as follows:

$$\text{Child's dose} = \frac{\text{SA of child (m}^2)}{1.73 \text{ m}^2}$$

$$\times \text{ Adult dose (mg/day)}$$

$$(12-10)$$

where 1.73 m² is the surface area (SA) of the average 70-kg adult. The SA of the child may be estimated from Equations 12–6 or 12–7. Equation 12–10 leads to higher mg/kg doses for a child than for the adult. The larger mg/kg dose resulting from the use of Equation 12–8, however, is still inadequate to meet the requirements for theophylline in children.

Clinical experience in pediatric patients has suggested that children often require large doses of procainamide for suppression of arrhythmias. In adults, the half-life of procainamide ranges from 2.5 to 5 hr, with rapid acetylators grouped at the lower end of the range; plasma clearance averages about 8 to 9 ml/min/kg. A study in 5 children 7 to 12 years of age found an average half-life of 1.7 hr and a clearance of nearly 20 ml/min/kg.[67] Quinidine is also metabolized more rapidly in children than adults.[68]

Drug Elimination in the Aged

The probability of experiencing adverse effects from a drug in adults appears to increase with age. This is related in part to the decline in organ function that occurs as a result of advancing age. For example, cardiac output decreases by 30 to 40% between the ages of 25 and 65 years.[69] Glomerular filtration rate (GFR) declines progressively with age after the age of 20 yr.[70] Differences in the pharmacokinetics of certain drugs between young and old adults are anticipated, and, indeed, some important differences have been observed.[71,72]

Glomerular filtration falls at a rate of about 1 ml/min per 1.73 m² per year between the ages of 20 and 90 years.[70] Parallel declines in tubular secretion and active tubular reabsorption have also been observed. The total clearance of drugs largely eliminated by renal excretion declines approximately in proportion to the reduced GFR. The 50% decline in renal function in the elderly patient relative to the young patient is often of little clinical importance, but must be considered in determining the appropriate dose of certain drugs in the elderly; these drugs include digoxin, cimetidine, lithium, and the aminoglycoside antibiotics.[71,72]

The same amount (0.5 mg) of digoxin administered intravenously to elderly men (73 to 81 years) and young men (20 to 33 years) resulted in higher blood concentrations and longer half-lives in the elderly.[73] This is principally due to diminished urinary excretion of digoxin in the elderly. Renal clearance of digoxin averaged 53 ml/min per 1.73 m² in the old and 83 ml/min per 1.73 m² in the young men. Although serum creatinine levels in the old and young subjects were not different, creatinine clearance averaged 56 ml/min per 1.73 m² in the elderly and 122 ml/min per 1.73 m² in the young subjects.

A report from Europe showed that the total plasma clearance of cimetidine decreased by half between the ages of 30 and 65 years, largely as a result of a profound decrease in the renal clearance of cimetidine with age.[74] The clearance of ranitidine was also found to be significantly lower in an elderly group compared with a group of young adults, consistent with the difference in creatinine clearance between the two groups.[75] These investigators predicted that ranitidine levels in plasma would be about 60% higher in the elderly compared with young adults, but suggested that dose reduc-

tion may not be necessary because ranitidine is substantially free of dose-related adverse effects.

Other investigators found marked differences in the disposition of the angiotensin-converting enzyme inhibitor enalapril and its active metabolite, enalaprilat, between healthy young and elderly subjects.[76] The apparent clearance of enalapril after oral administration and the clearance of enalaprilat after iv administration were about 30% lower in the elderly subjects. The clearance of each was significantly correlated with creatinine clearance, which averaged 92 ml/min in the younger group and 66 ml/min in the older group.

The decreased clearance and higher blood levels of enalaprilat may explain in part the greater hypotensive effect and prolonged converting enzyme inhibition observed in elderly subjects. Some dosage adjustments based on creatinine clearance may be necessary.

During the development of a new diuretic/antihypertensive combination product of triamterene (T) and hydrochlorothiazide (HCT) (Maxzide), with bioavailability characteristics superior to the original combination product (Dyazide), Williams et al.[77] compared the two formulations in patients with mild to moderate hypertension. For each product, they found higher blood levels of HCT than they had observed in earlier studies with healthy subjects. The clearance of HCT appeared to be lower in the patients than in healthy subjects.

An important difference between the two groups was age. The mean age was 50 years for the patients and 24 years for the healthy subjects. Age in the patient population ranged from 22 to 69 years. Those patients less than 60 years of age had a peak HCT concentration in plasma of 455 ng/ml, whereas those greater than 60 years of age had a mean peak level of 600 ng/ml. Similar differences were noted with regard to the plasma levels of the principal metabolite of T, hydroxytriamterene sulfate (HTS), which like HCT is eliminated by renal excretion. Relatively small differences in levels of T were observed.

Analysis of the data suggested that age is an important factor in determining the elimination of HCT and HTS. The investigators observed that ''because increasing age is associated with reduced renal function, decreasing renal function might also have contributed to the alteration in drug disposition seen in our data.'' In fact, highly significant correlations were observed between the renal clearance values of HCT, T, and its active metabolite,

HTS, and both age and measured creatinine clearance when the data from both the patients and the healthy subjects were combined.

Hydrochlorothiazide is eliminated primarily by renal excretion. Between the ages of 25 and 50 years, the renal clearance of HCT declined by about one-third. In subjects older than 60 years, the clearance of HCT may be reduced 50% or more. Therefore, a given dose of HCT will result in higher blood levels in elderly individuals than in young adults. Because of the important role of metabolism in the elimination of triamterene, little accumulation occurs in the presence of renal impairment. On the other hand, renal excretion is the major route of elimination of HTS, and considerable accumulation occurs in older patients.

In evaluating renal function in the elderly patient one must bear in mind the decline of muscle mass and lean body mass relative to total body weight that occurs with old age. Since serum creatinine concentration depends on creatinine turnover, which is a function of muscle mass, as well as renal creatinine clearance, the decline in renal function may not be accompanied by an elevation in serum creatinine. Estimates of creatinine clearance from serum creatinine levels must take the patient's age into account.

Changes in drug metabolism with age are not nearly as predictable as changes in the renal excretion of drugs. There is a growing list of drugs subject to oxidative metabolism that are cleared less efficiently in the elderly, but this is not the case for all such drugs. Drug conjugation reactions, on the other hand, seem to be largely independent of age.

Hepatic blood flow declines with age, partly because of reduced cardiac output. Accordingly, the clearance of drugs with liver blood flow-dependent elimination may decrease in the elderly. Important age-related changes have also been reported for drugs showing marked first-pass metabolism.

The prototypical drug for studying metabolic oxidation in humans has been antipyrine. Swift et al.[78] measured liver volume and antipyrine kinetics in two groups of healthy individuals aged 20 to 29 years and 75 to 89 years. Liver volume and antipyrine clearance were reduced in the elderly group. On the average, clearance was 42 ml/min in the young subjects and 24 ml/min in the elderly subjects. The investigators concluded that "hepatic drug oxidation as measured by antipyrine clearance declines in man with aging and this is partly due

to a decrease in liver size and partly to reduction in microsomal enzyme activity."

Most studies examining the effect of age on human liver size in vivo have used ultrasound. Swift et al.[78] found a reduction in estimated liver volume from a mean of 1300 ml in subjects 30 to 39 years of age to 990 ml in subjects aged 75 to 86 years. Bach et al.[79] reported a 17% decrease in liver volume over a similar age range. In a review of age-related changes in liver size and blood flow, and the implications for drug metabolism in the elderly, Woodhouse and Wynne[80] noted that the largest study of this kind found a significant negative correlation between estimated liver volume and age. A 28% fall in liver volume was noted in those over 65 years of age compared with those under 40.

Other investigators measured the plasma clearance of antipyrine after intravenous injection in normal male subjects aged 22 to 72 years.[81] They found that antipyrine clearance declined with age in the group as a whole, but that the change was much greater in smokers than nonsmokers. Antipyrine clearance was higher in smokers than nonsmokers among subjects less than 40 years of age but there was little difference between them among subjects older than 40. These findings suggest that the enzyme-inducing effects of smoking diminish with age.

The effects of aging on the pharmacokinetics of anticonvulsants is also of interest. Investigators determined the pharmacokinetics of phenytoin after an intravenous injection of 100 mg to a group of young healthy adults with a mean age of 29 years and to a group of elderly patients with a mean age of 83 years.[79] The clearance of phenytoin appeared to be similar in each group, about 50 ml/min, but plasma protein binding was considerably decreased in the elderly. Therefore, the clearance of unbound (free) phenytoin was significantly lower in the older patients (309 vs 569 ml/min), suggesting a need for lower doses of phenytoin in such patients.

The pharmacokinetics of valproic acid were compared in healthy young and elderly subjects during repeated dosing with oral valproate, 250 mg every 12 hr.[82] Steady-state concentrations of valproic acid were practically identical in both groups, about 40 to 45 mg/L. Free fraction in plasma, however, was significantly larger in the elderly than in the young subjects (0.11 vs 0.06). Calculation of unbound valproic acid concentrations indicated that

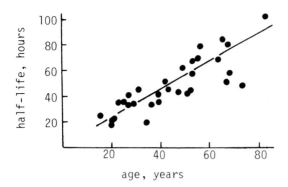

Fig. 12–7. Relationship between the half-life of diazepam and age in a group of healthy subjects. (Data from Klotz, U., et al.[83])

free drug levels at steady state are almost twice as high in the elderly as in the young subjects.

Changes in plasma protein and tissue binding on aging complicate the evaluation of the effects of age on drug metabolism. For example, Klotz and associates found a striking increase in the half-life of diazepam as a function of age in a panel of subjects ranging in age from 15 to 82 years; half-life increased from 20 to 90 hr (Fig. 12–7).[83] The clearance of diazepam, however, was independent of age. The entire change in half-life can be accounted for by an age-dependent increase in the apparent volume of distribution of diazepam secondary to changes in tissue binding of the drug. A similar situation has been reported for nitrazepam.[84]

An even more striking increase in the half-life of chlordiazepoxide with age has been reported. Unlike the situation with diazepam, this age-related increase in half-life is the result of both an increase in apparent volume of distribution and a decrease in the metabolic clearance of chlordiazepoxide.[85]

The effects of aging on the elimination of two short-acting benzodiazepines, triazolam and midazolam, have also been studied. The elimination of both drugs principally involves hepatic metabolism to hydroxylated metabolites.

Plasma triazolam concentrations were measured in male and female subjects, ranging in age from 21 to 87 years after a single 0.5-mg oral dose.[86] The apparent oral clearance of triazolam in male and female elderly subjects (>61 years) was only about half that observed in the younger subjects (<34 years). The initial hypnotic dose of triazolam in elderly patients with insomnia should be about

half that recommended for a young adult of similar weight.

Similar but less pronounced effects have been observed with midazolam.[87] Elderly are not only less efficient in their ability to metabolize midazolam, they are also much more sensitive to the effects of the drug.[88]

Several benzodiazepines, including oxazepam, lorazepam, and temazepam, are not subject to oxidative metabolism but are eliminated by conjugation with glucuronic acid. Several studies have shown little or no effect of age on drug clearance. In regard to these drugs, Greenblatt and his colleagues have observed in a widely-cited literature review[89] that "total clearance tends to decline with age, but the amount of variability attributable to age is small, making age-related changes in clearance either insignificant or of border-line significance."

Early population pharmacokinetic studies suggested a need to lower theophylline doses in elderly patients because of reduced clearance. Subsequent studies, however, indicated that these preliminary observations may have been confounded by not controlling for disease state and smoking habits. These later reports suggested that theophylline clearance was independent of age in both smokers and nonsmokers and that cigarette smoking increased the clearance of theophylline in both young and elderly subjects.[90,91]

A carefully controlled investigation of the effect of age on theophylline metabolism in young and old cigarette smokers, using stable isotope methodology, may have resolved this controversy.[92] These investigators found that the plasma clearance of theophylline in old nonsmokers was about one-third less than in young nonsmokers. Theophylline clearance was also lower in older smokers than in young smokers but the difference, in the order of 20%, was less than that observed in nonsmokers. It appears the metabolism of theophylline is slightly impaired in the elderly but the change is difficult to detect because the variability in theophylline kinetics is large.

Age-related changes in hepatic blood flow and in the effects of smoking on microsomal drug metabolizing enzyme activity can also complicate the evaluation of the effects of age on drug metabolism. Vestal and co-workers determined in a group of 27 healthy subjects, consisting of smokers and nonsmokers and ranging in age from 21 to 73 years, that the systemic clearance of propranolol, deter-

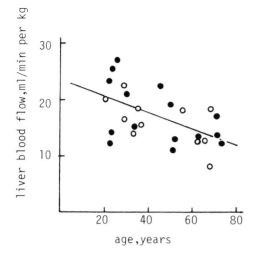

Fig. 12–8. Relationship between liver blood flow and age in smokers (●) and nonsmokers (○), r = 0.55. (Data from Vestal, R.E., et al.[93])

mined after intravenous administration, decreased as a function of age.[93] Propranolol has a high metabolic (hepatic) clearance that depends on both hepatic blood flow rate and the intrinsic ability of the hepatic enzymes to metabolize the drug (intrinsic clearance). The decline in the systemic clearance of propranolol as a function of age is largely the result of an age-dependent decrease in liver blood flow (Fig. 12–8). A similar age-related decline in the systemic clearance of indocyanine green has also been reported.[94]

Vestal and co-workers also found that the intrinsic hepatic metabolism of propranolol (determined after oral administration) decreased with age in smokers but not in nonsmokers.[93] Cigarette smoke induces hepatic microsomal enzymes involved in the metabolism of propranolol. Young smokers metabolize propranolol more efficiently than young nonsmokers; however, there is little difference in the intrinsic metabolic clearance of propranolol in elderly smokers and nonsmokers. The results are consistent with a decreased induction of drug-metabolizing enzymes with aging. This age-related effect on enzyme induction has also been found with antipyrine.[94]

The effects of aging on the kinetics of other beta-blockers have also been investigated. The bioavailability of metoprolol, which like propranolol undergoes substantial first-pass metabolism after oral administration, was studied in healthy young and elderly subjects.[95] Large intersubject differences were observed in both groups, but no sig-

nificant difference in area under the drug concentration in plasma versus time curve (AUC), peak concentration, or half-life was found between the groups.

The pharmacokinetics of labetalol, a mixed alpha- and beta-blocker has also been studied after oral and iv administration to a small group of patients with hypertension, ranging in age from 28 to 75 years.[96] Labetalol bioavailability, incomplete because of first-pass metabolism, varied from 9 to 68% but was significantly correlated with age. The regression equation predicts a bioavailability of 15 to 20% in a 20-year-old patient and 55 to 60% in a 70-year-old patient.

These preliminary findings were confirmed by Abernethy et al.[97] On comparing the pharmacologic effects and pharmacokinetics of labetalol in young and elderly patients with systemic hypertension, they concluded that ''the combination of increased antihypertensive effect and decreased clearance suggests that smaller labetalol doses may be required in elderly hypertensive persons to achieve antihypertensive effects comparable to those in young hypertensive patients.''

In another study,[98] a prolonged-release tablet containing oxprenolol, a beta-blocker used outside the United States, was given once daily for 8 days to normal young adult subjects and elderly hypertensive patients. The elderly patients had a significantly higher AUC and peak drug concentration after the first and last dose of oxprenolol, presumably related to decreased clearance. Although it is not possible to sort out the effects of disease from those of age per se on the kinetics of oxprenolol, it is clear that the results of pharmacokinetic studies in young healthy subjects do not apply to an older population with hypertension.

This important distinction of age and disease may apply to other beta-blockers. Rigby et al.[99] measured steady-state blood levels in elderly patients with hypertension and in young healthy adults after repeated oral dosing of atenolol, metoprolol, oxprenolol, and propranolol. In each case, drug levels were considerably higher in the elderly patients than in the young healthy subjects. The ratios of steady-state concentrations (elderly: young) were 2.0 for atenolol, 1.6 for metoprolol, 1.5 for oxprenolol, and 2.1 for propranolol.

Calcium channel blockers produce a greater hypotensive effect in elderly patients than in younger ones. Studies with verapamil, nifedipine, and felodipine indicate age-related changes in drug disposition contribute to the enhanced effects.

Abernethy et al.[100] studied the pharmacodynamics and pharmacokinetics of verapamil in young (23 to 36 years), elderly (61 to 74 years), and very elderly (75 to 102 years) male patients with hypertension. After a single 10-mg dose of iv verapamil, mean arterial blood pressure decreased more in elderly and very elderly patients than in young patients. The plasma clearance of verapamil was lower in the elderly and very elderly patients, resulting in prolonged elimination half-lives in these patients.

It is worth noting that few studies have included subjects beyond 75 years of age. Although statistically significant differences between the elderly and very elderly patients were not seen in this study, the investigators point out "there was a trend toward even greater changes in the very elderly compared with the young hypertensive patients in both pharmacodynamic and pharmacokinetic data." Age-related changes appear to continue with advancing age into the eighth and ninth decades of life.

Robertson et al.[101] studied the kinetics of nifedipine in healthy normotensive subjects aged 22 to 35 years and 73 to 83 years. Following a small iv dose, the clearance of nifedipine was 348 ml/min in the elderly compared with 519 ml/min in the young but volume of distribution was similar in each group. Mean peak concentration and AUC after oral administration were also much higher in the elderly than in the young subjects.

No hemodynamic effects were observed in the group of young subjects after oral nifedipine. In contrast, nifedipine had a significant acute hypotensive effect in the elderly. The investigators concluded that the results are consistent with an age-related decrease in the hepatic clearance and first-pass metabolism of nifedipine, as well as impaired baroreceptor function, all of which contribute to its increased hypotensive effect in elderly patients.

Other dihydropyridine calcium channel blockers will probably be found to show age-related changes in pharmacokinetics similar to nifedipine. For example, Landahl et al.[102] found blood levels of felodipine, an investigational dihydropyridine, to be 3 times higher in elderly than in young subjects. Moreover, the effect on blood pressure correlated with plasma concentration of felodipine.

Anesthesiologists have long been concerned about dosing requirements for anesthetics in elderly patients undergoing surgery. There is considerable evidence to show that the dose of thiopental required to induce or maintain a light level of anesthesia decreases with age. Many have assumed that this is because elderly patients are more sensitive to the effects of thiopental than younger patients. In fact, there is a general clinical impression that the aged brain is pharmacodynamically more sensitive to sedative, hypnotic, and anesthetic drugs.

Homer and Stanski[103] reexamined the question of dosing requirements of thiopental in the elderly and confirmed earlier findings. The dose of thiopental needed to achieve a measured degree of suppression of brain activity, as determined by the electroencephalogram (EEG) decreased linearly with age. The regression equation predicted a dosage requirement of 10.4 mg/kg for a 20-year-old patient but one of only 4.4 mg/kg for an 80-year-old patient. For each 10-year increment in age, the dose of thiopental decreased about 1 mg/kg.

The decreased dosage requirement for thiopental could result from either age-related changes in brain response or pharmacokinetics. These investigators, however, were unable to find a relationship between age and serum concentration of either total or unbound thiopental needed to reach half-maximum EEG suppression. This means that the need for smaller doses of thiopental in older patients must be due to age-related changes in pharmacokinetics. This aspect was investigated further in patients ranging in age from 24 to 88 years, who were given a bolus or very short iv infusion of thiopental. Blood samples were taken frequently after administration.

After a bolus dose of thiopental or after terminating a short infusion, there is pronounced multiexponential decline of drug levels in serum with time. Although no age-related changes were found with respect to clearance, unbound clearance, volume of distribution, or half-life, marked differences in the initial distribution kinetics of thiopental were found. The apparent volume of the so-called central compartment changed markedly with age, ranging from about 25 L in young adults (20 to 30 years of age) to 5 L or less in patients more than 60 years old. This smaller initial distribution volume in the elderly results in much higher serum levels (and presumably brain levels) immediately after dosing.

The investigators concluded that "this pharmacokinetic difference explains the clinical impression of 'increased sensitivity' of the elderly to thiopental. Having a smaller central compartment, the elderly develop high serum levels of thiopental quickly and require less drug to show an effect. Thus, the dose of thiopental required to reach a surgical level of anesthesia significantly decreased with increasing age.''

Considerable attention has also been given to the disposition of antidepressant drugs in the elderly. These drugs are widely used in older patients; some estimate that clinically important depression is present at any given time in at least 10% of the elderly population.

In 1977, Nies et al.[104] reported that older depressed patients treated with imipramine developed higher steady-state plasma levels of imipramine and desipramine, its active metabolite, than younger patients. The age-related differences in imipramine and desipramine levels occurred despite the fact that all of the younger patients, less than 65 years, were receiving 150 mg imipramine per day, but the dosage for the older group ranged from 50 to 150 mg/day with a mean value of 92 mg daily. Despite the lower dose, higher drug levels were generated.

More recently, Abernethy et al.[105] studied the disposition of imipramine and desipramine directly in healthy subjects older than 65 years or younger than 40 years. Each subject was given iv and oral doses of imipramine and an oral dose of desipramine. After iv administration, imipramine half-life was considerably prolonged in elderly subjects compared with younger subjects (30 vs 17 hours). This change was almost entirely due to reduced clearance.

Still greater differences were noted after oral administration of imipramine because of a decreased first-pass effect in the elderly. Peak levels of imipramine in elderly men were about twice those found in younger men; a 4-fold difference was seen in women as a function of age. In contrast, small age-related differences were observed after oral desipramine.

These findings suggest that the metabolism of imipramine, a tertiary amine predominantly subject to demethylation, may be more sensitive to effects of age than the metabolism of desipramine, which largely involves hydroxylation. The investigators are cautious in offering dosage recommendations, pointing out that ''total pharmacologic activity for both imipramine and desipramine may be related to the quantity of parent drug, demethylated metabolites, and hydroxylated metabolites present.''

Unfortunately, the findings with imipramine and desipramine cannot be generalized to other tricyclic antidepressants. This is clearly illustrated by the findings of Schulz et al.[106] who studied the effects of age on the kinetics of amitriptyline after iv and oral administration. Although the half-life of amitriptyline was marginally longer in the elderly group (22 vs 16 hours), there was no change in clearance with age. Furthermore, drug levels were similar in both groups after oral administration; first-pass metabolism eliminated 52% of the dose in the young adult subjects and 57% in the older subjects. These findings indicate that amitriptyline kinetics in healthy subjects, unlike those of imipramine, are relatively insensitive to age.

On the other hand, the elimination of nortriptyline, the demethylated active metabolite of amitriptyline, is much lower in the elderly, at least in those who are hospitalized and depressed, than in young healthy subjects. According to Dawling et al.,[107] the apparent clearance of nortriptyline in young healthy subjects following an oral dose ranged from 16 to 115 L/hour, with a mean of 54 L/hour; the mean apparent clearance in elderly patients was only 20 L/hour, with a range of 8 to 38 L/hour.

These age-related differences in the pharmacokinetics of tricyclic antidepressants provide, at least in part, an explanation for the increased susceptibility of older patients to side effects, including postural hypotension, urinary retention, tachycardia, and mental confusion. They also provide a rationale for using lower doses in the elderly.

Reports of serious adverse reactions with benoxaprofen, a nonsteroidal anti-inflammatory drug (NSAID) subsequently recalled from the market because of toxicity, heralded the current era of heightened concern as to drug dosage in the elderly. No other drug class has undergone greater scrutiny in this regard. Some of the more important studies with NSAIDs are reviewed below.

Upton et al.[108] studied naproxen pharmacokinetics in healthy elderly and young men. They found a substantial decrease in plasma protein binding of naproxen in the elderly panel of subjects. Consequently, although serum levels of total naproxen were similar in each group, steady-state concentrations of unbound naproxen were about twice as great in the elderly individuals than in the younger subjects. These findings support the view of some clinicians who recommend that geriatric patients be treated, at least initially, with only one-half the usual dose of naproxen.

The elimination of ketoprofen, one of the more recently introduced NSAIDs, also appears to be impaired in the elderly. On oral dosing, plasma concentrations of ketoprofen were consistently higher in elderly patients than in young adult subjects.[109] The mean apparent clearance of ketoprofen was 89 ml/min for the panel of young adults but only 37 ml/min in the elderly panel. Ketoprofen, like naproxen, is highly bound to plasma proteins, and even greater differences may exist in the unbound clearance of ketoprofen between young and elderly subjects but the investigators did not report binding data.

Conjugation with glucuronic acid, resulting in an ester glucuronide, is the major route of ketoprofen elimination. About two-thirds of an oral dose is recovered in urine as ketoprofen glucuronide; a negligible amount of unchanged ketoprofen is excreted in urine. The investigators concluded that the decreased elimination of ketoprofen in the elderly is due to decreased conjugation with glucuronic acid.

An alternative explanation, based on the susceptibility of ester glucuronides to hydrolysis in biological fluids, has been advanced.[110] "Since the elderly have reduced renal function, old age should also result in a decreased excretion of ketoprofen glucuronide. The resulting accumulation of this ester glucuronide may lead to increased systemic deconjugation (regeneration of the parent compound)."

In 1987, a leading representative of the Food and Drug Administration discussed guidelines for the clinical investigation of drugs for use by the elderly.[111] The underlying principle of these guidelines is that age-related differences in response to drugs can arise from either pharmacokinetic or pharmacodynamic changes, but studies to evaluate possible differences in the elderly should focus initial attention on assessment of pharmacokinetic differences between age groups.

The critical features of a proper evaluation of a new drug with respect to the elderly are the following: "1. Include the elderly in clinical trials if they will be exposed to the new drug after it is marketed . . . Although it is reasonable and necessary to exclude patients too infirm to participate in clinical trials, patients unable to provide meaningful informed consent, and patients with too much complicating illness, rigid age cutoffs and routine exclusion of all patients with concomitant illness and medication is unnecessary and counter productive. It tends merely to delay discovery of important problems and interactions: it cannot prevent them . . . 2. Analyze the influence of age on adverse events and effectiveness . . . In the past, it was uncommon to examine trial experience to see whether age affected response . . . Any attempt to relate benefit or adverse effect to factors such as age will be greatly improved by good pharmacokinetic data . . . 3. Seek and transmit via labeling better information on all of the factors that affect pharmacokinetics of the drug, including age."

We are still a long way off from understanding why some drugs show important age-related changes in clearance while others do not. Many factors have been examined but one factor that has not been considered is the possibility of age-related stereoselective changes in elimination. About 10 to 15% of all drugs are marketed as racemic mixtures. Racemic drugs whose enantiomers use different oxidative metabolic pathways could exhibit selective age-related changes in drug metabolism.

In pursuit of this idea, investigators in Kentucky studied the disposition of hexobarbital enantiomers in young and elderly healthy male subjects.[112] The well-recognized and striking difference in the elimination of d- and l-hexobarbital was clearly seen in the panel of young subjects. Oral clearance was 16.9 ml/min/kg for the l-form but only 1.9 ml/min/kg for the d-form.

Interestingly, the difference between the hexobarbital enantiomers was considerably less in the elderly subjects. The reason for this was that although the oral clearance of d-hexobarbital was about the same in elderly and young subjects (1.7 vs 1.9 ml/min/kg), the mean oral clearance of l-hexobarbital in the elderly panel was less than half that found in the young panel (8.2 vs 16.9 ml/min/kg). A substantial age-related fall in the clearance of the l-form of hexobarbital but not of the d-form was observed. The investigators pointed out that age-related preferential decline in metabolism of one enantiomer over another has never been reported for any racemic drug in animals or humans.

Gender

Large sex-related differences in the capacity of rats to metabolize drugs are widely recognized.[113]

These differences are routinely considered in designing toxicology studies for new drugs. An example may be found in a recent report by Trenk et al.,[114] who studied the pharmacokinetics of phenprocoumon, an oral anticoagulant, in female and male inbred Lewis-Wistar rats. The clearance of phenprocoumon was significantly lower in females than males (7.9 vs 24.5 ml/min/kg) and its apparent volume of distribution was also much smaller in females than males (288 vs 617 ml/kg).

The low clearance of phenprocoumon in female rats is consistent with a slower metabolism found for many drugs metabolized by P-450 enzymes in rats and appears to be related to differences in sex hormones. In this species, androgens strongly stimulate the activity of microsomal mixed function oxidases. The smaller distribution volume of phenprocoumon in females relates, at least in part, to a higher degree of plasma protein binding. Percent unbound was 0.96% in females and 1.24% in males.

Important gender-related differences in metabolism are not generally observed in the mouse, guinea pig, dog, rabbit, or human. A review of the literature in 1977 concluded that although sex-related differences in drug metabolism did exist in human subjects, the differences were small and did not warrant modification of dosage as a function of gender. This conclusion still applies, but today we recognize that if sex-related differences are to be found, other variables including age, smoking habits, and the use of oral contraceptives need to be controlled.

The kinetics of a large number of benzodiazepines have been studied with respect to sex-related differences. Findings with compounds that are largely eliminated by oxidative metabolism are inconclusive. More consistent results have been observed with benzodiazepines eliminated by metabolic conjugation. The clearance or apparent clearance of temazepam,[115] oxazepam,[116] and lorazepam[117] is significantly less in human female subjects than in males. These differences parallel those found in rats but are far smaller.

Two studies in human subjects with acetaminophen indicate that clearance is about 40% greater in males than in females. Based on the data provided by Miners et al.,[118] we can calculate that most of the difference is due to increased activity of the glucuronidation pathway in males; the formation clearance of acetaminophen glucuronide was 252 ml/min in males and 173 ml/min in females. The formation clearances for acetaminophen sulfate (105 vs 80 ml/min) and for acetaminophen oxidation products (38 vs 28 ml/min) were also higher in men than in women. The major elimination pathway for temazepam, oxazepam, and lorazepam also involves conjugation with glucuronic acid.

In another study by Miners and his associates,[119] salicylic acid clearance was found to be about 60% higher in male than in female subjects, an effect due largely to enhanced activity of the glycine conjugation pathway (salicyluric acid formation) in males. Still lower clearance values were found in women using oral contraceptives.

It is clearly established that combination oral contraceptives, consisting of a synthetic estrogen and a progestin, inhibit the oxidative metabolism of many drugs. Studies comparing users with non-users have found that oral contraceptives decrease the clearance of antipyrine, chlordiazepoxide, diazepam, prednisolone, imipramine, and metoprolol, among other drugs. In one study, in women using the same oral contraceptive for 6 months to 4 years, antipyrine clearance was 28 ml/min during use but increased to 37 ml/min 4 weeks after stopping medication.[124]

Pregnancy

The possible effects of pregnancy on plasma drug concentrations have been reviewed by Eadie and co-workers.[121] Late pregnancy is associated with delayed gastric emptying and decreased motility of the gastrointestinal tract. These changes may reduce the rate of drug absorption.

The volume available for drug distribution increases during pregnancy, with the growth of the uterus, placenta, and fetus. Maternal plasma volume and ECF volume also increase. The concentration of plasma proteins tends to fall gradually during pregnancy, and drug binding may be reduced.

Perucca and Crema[122] reviewed the literature dealing with plasma protein binding of drugs in pregnancy. They noted that "experimental studies conducted mostly in vitro have shown that the plasma protein binding of many (but not all) drugs is decreased during pregnancy, particularly during the last trimester. Notable examples . . . include diazepam, valproic acid, phenytoin, phenobarbitone, salicylic acid, pethidine, lignocaine, dexamethasone, sulphafurazole and propranolol."

Chen et al.[123] studied the serum protein binding

of phenytoin and phenobarbital in vitro in healthy pregnant and nonpregnant women and in vivo in pregnant and nonpregnant women with epilepsy who were under treatment with phenytoin, phenobarbital, or combinations of either or both with other anticonvulsants. They found for both phenytoin and phenobarbital that binding to plasma proteins was reduced during pregnancy in both healthy women and women with epilepsy.

There was a clear trend toward decreased drug binding during the course of the pregnancy. Compared with the mean value found in nonpregnant women with epilepsy, the free fraction of phenytoin was 13% higher in the first trimester and 24% higher in the third trimester. The same applied to phenobarbital. The degree of impaired binding during pregnancy paralleled the decrease in serum albumin over this period. In the absence of changes in drug excretion or metabolism, impaired plasma protein binding alone during pregnancy should present few problems. One would expect to see a decrease in total drug concentration in plasma but no change in free drug concentration. Under these conditions, there is no need to change the dose. A decision to increase the dose because total drug concentration is below some preconceived therapeutic level may result in drug toxicity.

Plasma protein binding decreases in pregnancy but glomerular filtration increases. One study in pregnant women showed that creatinine clearance fell from 136 ml/min per 1.73 m^2 during the third trimester to 98 ml/min per 1.73 m^2 6 to 12 weeks postpartum.[124] In some cases, notably for drugs largely eliminated by renal excretion, this change may result in unusually rapid elimination and undermedication in pregnant patients.

For example, the plasma clearance of ampicillin is about 50% greater in pregnant women than in nonpregnant controls.[125] Consistent with this finding, ampicillin levels in plasma following treatment with pivampicillin, a prodrug, are much lower in pregnant women.[126] Controlled studies with ampicillin, cephradine, and cefuroxime have found 30 to 50% lower plasma levels and substantially shorter half-lives during pregnancy than after delivery.[127] Other investigators reported that the mean plasma clearance of cephradine was nearly 60% greater during pregnancy than afterwards.[128] Higher mg/kg doses of ampicillin and other antibiotics may be required in pregnant patients to avoid the risk of treatment failure.[129]

In parallel with the changes in glomerular filtra-

tion rate, the clearance of digoxin is also increased during pregnancy.[124] One study determined that renal clearance of digoxin fell from 103 ml/min per 1.73 m^2 during the third trimester to 86 ml/min per 1.73 m^2 postpartum and that digoxin renal clearance and creatinine clearance were significantly correlated. Consistent with these findings, the 24-hour urinary excretion of digoxin in patients treated with 0.375 mg/day oral digoxin fell from 186 μg during the third trimester to 134 μg postpartum.

These results suggest the possibility of inadequate serum levels of digoxin in pregnant patients treated with ordinarily adequate doses. Surprisingly, the opposite has been found.[124] Twelve of 15 patients evaluated had higher serum digoxin concentrations during pregnancy than after delivery. On the average, serum digoxin was 1.28 ng/ml in the third trimester and 1.0 ng/ml postpartum.

Several reasons come to mind to explain the elevated serum digoxin level during pregnancy in the face of increased renal clearance: a decrease in nonrenal clearance, an increase in the bioavailability of digoxin, or a combination of the two. Although it is usually assumed that digoxin is largely excreted unchanged, the nonrenal component is considerable, accounting for about 40% of digoxin clearance.

A substantial decrease in the nonrenal clearance of digoxin during pregnancy, on the order of 50%, could account for the higher serum levels of digoxin despite the enhanced renal excretion of the drug. Alternatively, an increase from about 60% (pre- or post-pregnancy) to about 85% (during pregnancy) in the bioavailability of digoxin would also produce the elevated serum levels that were observed. This explanation appears to be more likely, although one cannot rule out some decrease in the nonrenal clearance of digoxin during pregnancy.

In the later stages of pregnancy, bowel motility decreases as a result of high progesterone levels, leading to increased transit time in the small bowel and increased absorption of certain drugs. Studies have shown that decreased gastric emptying and intestinal transit time significantly increase the bioavailability of digoxin, particularly from slowly dissolving preparations.

Considerable attention has been given to the effects of pregnancy on the pharmacokinetics of anticonvulsants.[130] The major concerns in the pregnant epileptic patient are loss of seizure control and the teratogenic effects of anticonvulsant drugs on the fetus. One investigator found that seizure frequency increased during pregnancy in 45% of the women treated for idiopathic epilepsy.[131]

Epileptic patients must be carefully monitored when they become pregnant. At least part of the reason for the seeming deterioration in seizure control during pregnancy is a decline in the plasma levels of anticonvulsant drugs even though the dose is maintained and compliance appears to be unaffected. This problem is well documented[132,133] and may be related to accelerated metabolism of anticonvulsants during pregnancy, but the interpretation is complicated by concomitant changes in drug binding to plasma proteins.

Phenytoin, phenobarbital, and valproic acid binding to serum proteins is significantly decreased in pregnant women, consistent with the mild hypoalbuminemia that occurs during pregnancy. As a result, there is a decrease in total drug concentration at steady state during pregnancy. However, Chen et al.[123] found that the fall in phenytoin and phenobarbital serum levels during pregnancy was greater than could be accounted for by changes in protein binding and free drug levels were lower in pregnant women than in nonpregnant women. The mean free concentration of phenytoin at steady state was 0.51 μg/ml in pregnant subjects and 0.75 μg/ml in nonpregnant controls; for phenobarbital, the respective values were 8.6 and 10.1 μg/ml.

These findings suggest either accelerated metabolism or reduced absorption of anticonvulsants during pregnancy. In view of the physiologic changes in gastrointestinal motility that occur during pregnancy, reduced absorption appears to be an unlikely explanation. Most investigators favor a mechanism involving decreased plasma protein binding and accelerated metabolism to explain the declining serum levels of anticonvulsant drugs during pregnancy. This hypothesis, however, remains to be proven.

Induction of hepatic drug metabolizing enzymes by circulating progesterone may be a factor contributing to the suspected increased clearance of anticonvulsants during pregnancy. One study found the apparent clearance of methimazole, the active metabolite of carbimazole, to be significantly higher in pregnant hyperthyroid patients than in nonpregnant hyperthyroid patients.[134] In one patient, the clearance of methimazole increased about 40% from the first trimester to the third trimester of pregnancy.

Further evidence for the accelerated metabolism hypothesis is found in studies with metoprolol, the cardioselective beta-blocker widely used in the treatment of hypertension during pregnancy. In one report, single 100-mg oral doses were given to pregnant women during the last trimester of pregnancy and again 3 to 5 months after delivery.[135]

Individual peak plasma levels in the last trimester were only 20 to 40% of those found postpartum. The apparent oral clearance ranged from 251 to 502 ml/min/kg with a mean value of 362 ml/min/kg./ In contrast, apparent clearance values determined after delivery ranged from 53 to 108 ml/min/kg with a mean of 82 ml/min/kg. These results suggest that pregnancy profoundly affects the intrinsic hepatic metabolism of metoprolol. The binding of metoprolol to plasma proteins is low, on the order of 10%, and changes in binding cannot explain the differences observed during and after pregnancy.

In another study, investigators examined the effects of pregnancy on the pharmacokinetics of metoprolol after both oral and intravenous administration.[136] Women who developed hypertension during pregnancy received in the third trimester a single 10-mg intravenous dose of metoprolol; 3 days later each patient received a single 100-mg oral dose of the drug. The procedure was repeated 3 to 6 months after delivery.

Again, the metabolism of metoprolol appeared to be markedly accelerated during pregnancy. The clearance of iv metoprolol decreased from 1.38 L/min during pregnancy to 0.65 L/min after delivery, and the apparent oral clearance fell from 9.56 to 1.71 L/min. The bioavailability of oral metoprolol, which reflects only first-pass metabolism because metoprolol is probably completely absorbed, was 21% in the third trimester and 42% postpartum.

These results convincingly demonstrate that the increased clearance of metoprolol during pregnancy is a result of increased hepatic metabolism and a substantially greater first-pass effect after oral administration. The investigators note that the recommended doses of metoprolol for hypertension do not differ from different patient categories and urge that dose-effect and plasma concentration-effect relationships be studied in pregnant women to determine if larger than average doses of metoprolol are needed.

GENETIC FACTORS

A major cause of intersubject differences in drug concentrations in the blood or plasma is variability in drug metabolism. In any large population, one finds individuals who metabolize a drug much more slowly or much more rapidly than the average person. It is now evident that genetic factors contribute substantially to the large differences among people in metabolic clearance of drugs. The study of these differences is called *pharmacogenetics*.

Studies in Twins

The genetic component of individual variation in drug metabolism can be estimated by comparing the pharmacokinetics of a drug in identical and fraternal twins. If the differences among individuals are largely related to genetic factors, the variability in rates of drug metabolism will be much smaller in monozygotic (identical) twin pairs than in dizygotic (fraternal) twin pairs.

Estimation of the half-lives of antipyrine, dicumarol, and phenylbutazone, all of which are eliminated by oxidative metabolism, in identical and fraternal twins indicates that differences are appreciably greater in fraternal twins.[137] These data are summarized in Table 12–4. Similar findings have been reported for the metabolism of ethanol,[138] halothane,[139] salicylate,[140] and nortriptyline[141] in human twin pairs. For nortriptyline, plasma protein binding as well as metabolic clearance appears to be principally under genetic control.[142]

Polymorphic Acetylation

Isoniazid. The metabolism of most drugs in man seems to be under multifactorial or polygenetic control. This judgment prevails because frequency distribution plots of metabolic parameters usually yield continuous unimodal curves similar to a normal distribution curve. Metabolism data for some drugs, however, show a bimodal distribution.

Figure 12–9 is a frequency distribution histogram for isoniazid concentrations in the plasma 6

Table 12–4. Antipyrine, Dicumarol, and Phenylbutazone Half-Lives in Identical and Fraternal Twins*

			Half-life		
Twin	Age	Sex	Antipyrine (hr)	Dicumarol (hr)	Phenylbutazone (days)
Identical Twins					
H.M.	48	M	11.3	25.0	1.9
H.M.	48	M	11.3	25.0	2.1
D.T.	43	F	10.3	55.5	2.8
V.W.	43	F	9.6	55.5	2.9
J.G.	22	M	11.5	36.0	2.8
P.G.	22	M	11.5	34.0	2.8
J.T.	44	M	14.9	74.0	4.0
J.T.	44	M	14.9	72.0	4.0
C.J.	55	F	6.9	41.0	3.2
F.J.	55	F	7.1	42.5	2.9
G.L.	45	M	12.3	72.0	3.9
G.L.	45	M	12.8	69.0	4.1
D.H.	26	F	11.0	46.0	2.6
D.W.	26	F	11.0	44.0	2.6
Fraternal Twins					
A.M.	21	F	15.1	45.0	7.3
S.M.	21	M	6.3	22.0	3.6
D.L.	36	F	7.2	46.5	2.3
D.S.	36	F	15.0	51.0	3.3
S.A.	33	F	5.1	34.5	2.1
S.M.	33	F	12.5	27.5	1.2
J.H.	24	F	12.0	7.0	2.6
J.H.	24	F	6.0	19.0	2.3
F.D.	48	M	14.7	24.5	2.8
P.D.	48	M	9.3	38.0	3.5
L.D.	21	F	8.2	67.0	2.9
L.W.	21	F	6.9	72.0	3.0
E.K.	31	F	7.7	40.5	1.9
R.K.	31	M	7.3	35.0	2.1

*Data from Vesell, E.S.[137]

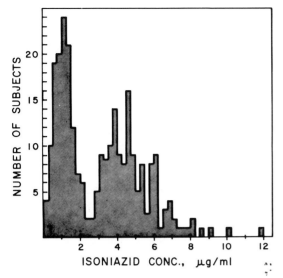

Fig. 12–9. Distribution of isoniazid concentrations in plasma 6 hr after an oral dose to 267 human subjects. (Data from Evans, D.A.P., Manley, K.A., and McKusick, V.C.[143])

hr after administration of a 10 mg/kg oral dose to 267 subjects.[143] A bimodality is evident with a mean of about 1 µg/ml for one subpopulation and a mean of about 4 to 5 µg/ml for the other. The subpopulations are designated rapid inactivators and slow inactivators of isoniazid; they are assumed to represent two distinct phenotypes. The main route of elimination of isoniazid in man is conjugation with acetylcoenzyme A to form acetylisoniazid. Slow inactivators of isoniazid have less N-acetyltransferase in their liver than do rapid inactivators.

The half-life of isoniazid depends on how rapidly the drug is acetylated. In rapid inactivators the half-life of the drug ranges from 45 to 80 min; in slow inactivators the half-life of isoniazid is about 140 to 200 min.[144] At a given dosing rate, the steady-state plasma isoniazid level is lower in rapid inactivators than in slow inactivators. Rapid acetylators excrete small amounts of the drug unchanged in the urine (about 3% of the dose), whereas slow acetylators may excrete up to 30% of dose as unmetabolized isoniazid.

Widely different geographic and racial distributions of the acetylator phenotypes have been reported.[145] The upper extremes are the Eskimos and most populations of an Oriental origin; about 80 to 100% of these populations are rapid acetylators. The lower extremes investigated are Egyptians and certain groups of European origin; these popula-

tions consist of about 20 to 40% rapid acetylators. About one half of the United States population is classified as rapid acetylators.

Slow acetylators treated with isoniazid are more prone to develop peripheral neuropathy, are more prone to the adverse effects of phenytoin when simultaneously treated with isoniazid, and show greater tendency to develop antinuclear antibodies (ANA) and clinical signs of a systemic lupus erythematosus-like syndrome (SLE).[145] Rapid acetylators respond less favorably to treatment for pulmonary tuberculosis with a once-weekly isoniazid dosage regimen and may be more prone to develop isoniazid-related hepatitis.[145]

Polyneuritis is a well known adverse effect of isoniazid; it occurs more frequently in slow acetylators than in rapid acetylators. In one study, polyneuritis occurred during isoniazid therapy in 4 of 5 slow inactivators but in only 2 of 10 rapid inactivators.[146] Another study found peripheral neuropathy in 20% of slow inactivators compared with an incidence of 3% in rapid inactivators of isoniazid.[147]

As a consequence of the inhibitory effect of isoniazid on phenytoin metabolism, slow acetylators are more prone to the side effects of phenytoin than are rapid acetylators when both drugs are given together.[148] The dose of phenytoin should be reduced in such situations to avoid this complication.

Under certain conditions, slow acetylators show a higher cure rate than rapid acetylators. A study in 775 patients with pulmonary tuberculosis on standard isoniazid regimens showed that sputum conversion generally occurred earlier in slow than in rapid inactivators.[149] After 6 months, however, no clinically detectable differences were observed between rapid and slow phenotypes. If isoniazid is administered only once a week, then responses are better in slow than in rapid inactivator patients with tuberculosis.[150] A more recent report indicated that when patients were treated once a week for 12 months with isoniazid plus rifampin, 5% of the rapid acetylators had an unsatisfactory response; the treatment was completely successful in slow acetylators.[151]

Isoniazid is metabolized to acetylisoniazid and subsequently to acetylhydrazine, which can be converted to a potent acylating agent that produces liver necrosis. This metabolic sequence is the basis for the hypothesis that fast acetylators, who form more acetylisoniazid, are more susceptible to isoniazid-associated liver injury than slow acetylators.

Clinical evidence for this, however, is conflicting.[152] One reason that acetylator phenotype may not be a major determinant of isoniazid-induced hepatitis is that acetylhydrazine is inactivated by acetylation to form diacetylhydrazine, a nontoxic metabolite; this acetylation is subject to the same phenotype as the conversion of isoniazid to acetylisoniazid.[153]

There is a strong correlation of acetylator phenotype between isoniazid and many other drugs, including sulfadiazine, sulfamethazine (sulfadimidine), dapsone, procainamide, hydralazine, and nitrazepam.[145] Sulfanilamide, aminosalicylate, and aminobenzoate are also acetylated but show no correlation with phenotype, suggesting that the enzyme system or rate-limiting step for acetylation of these drugs is different than that of isoniazid. A recent investigation found no correlation between acetylator status and the formation of the acetyl metabolite of acebutolol, a β-blocker.[154] Unlike isoniazid and related drugs, where the acetyl metabolite is formed directly from the parent drug, acebutolol is probably first hydrolyzed to an amine which is then N-acetylated. This hydrolysis step is not genetically controlled and may be rate limiting.

Sulfonamides. Sulfadiazine, sulfamethazine, and sulfapyridine are subject to polymorphic acetylation. Sulfamethazine (sulfadimidine) is widely used to determine acetylator phenotype.[155] Urine is collected for 8 hr after oral administration of sulfamethazine (45 mg/kg) and assayed for unmetabolized sulfamethazine and "total" sulfamethazine. Acetylsulfamethazine is assumed to represent the difference between "total" and unmetabolized sulfamethazine. People who excrete more than 64% of the dose as acetyl metabolite are classified as rapid acetylators; those who excrete less are classified as slow acetylators. Phenotype can also be determined from the concentration ratio of acetylsulfamethazine to sulfamethazine in plasma at certain times after administration of a test dose.

The adverse effects of sulfasalazine are related to acetylator phenotype because it is metabolized by intestinal bacteria to sulfapyridine. Most of the toxic symptoms ascribed to the drug can be related to high serum concentrations of sulfapyridine. One study found that the mean serum concentration of sulfapyridine at steady state in patients with ulcerative colitis treated with sulfasalazine was 54 μg/ml for slow acetylators and 31 μg/ml for fast acetylators.[156] In another study, 24 of 28 patients with ulcerative colitis or Crohn's disease who experienced side effects during sulfasalazine therapy were phenotyped as slow acetylators.[157] Adverse effects to sulfasalazine regularly occur when serum concentrations of sulfapyridine exceed 50 μg/ml.[158]

Dapsone. Dapsone is used in the treatment of leprosy and dermatitis herpetiformis. Acetylation is an important elimination pathway of the drug. Slow acetylators treated with dapsone may be more prone to hematologic side effects; rapid acetylators may require higher doses for effective treatment.[145]

Dapsone has also been used for determining acetylator phenotype by calculating the concentration ratio of monoacetyldapsone (MAD) to dapsone (DDS) in plasma 3 hr after a single 100-mg dose of dapsone. A study of acetylator phenotype in 50 healthy Caucasians found 50% to be rapid acetylators (MAD/DDS ratio of 0.14 to 0.28), 44% to be slow acetylators (MAD/DDS ratio of 0.42 to 1.06), and 6% to be of indeterminate phenotype (MAD/DDS ratio of 0.32 to 0.34).[159]

Procainamide. Procainamide (PA) is an orally effective drug for the treatment of ventricular arrhythmias. In patients with normal renal function, more than half the dose is excreted unchanged; from 20 to 40% of the dose is acetylated to give N-acetylprocainamide (NAPA). The amount of NAPA formed depends on the acetylator phenotype of the patient. The steady-state serum concentration ratio of NAPA to PA is about 1.3 in fast acetylators and about 0.5 in slow acetylators.[160] This ratio increases with decreasing renal function because urinary excretion is more important to the elimination of NAPA than to that of PA. For a given dosage regimen, steady-state blood levels of PA will be about 30% higher in slow acetylators than in fast acetylators. Accordingly, fast acetylators may require higher daily doses of PA than slow acetylators, to achieve comparable blood levels.[161]

The long-term use of PA is limited by the development of a systemic lupus erythematosus (SLE)-like syndrome, almost invariably preceded by high titers of antinuclear antibodies (ANA). Early reports estimated the incidence of ANA in PA therapy to be 50%, but with longer duration of therapy it rises to almost 100%. The incidence of clinical lupus has been estimated to be 30% but may be higher with a longer duration of PA treatment.[162]

It is widely held that NAPA is far less likely to induce SLE than is PA. Therefore, the acetylator phenotype of the patient may affect the onset or incidence of PA-related ANA or SLE.

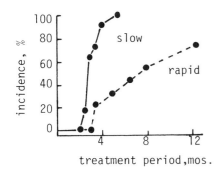

Fig. 12–10. Incidence (expressed as percent of patient population) of development of antinuclear antibodies (ANA) during treatment with procainamide (PA) in slow and rapid acetylators. (Data from Woosley, R.L., et al.[163])

Woosley and co-workers determined the rate of development of ANA in 20 patients, 11 slow acetylators and 9 fast acetylators, receiving chronic PA therapy.[163] As shown in Figure 12–10, the duration of therapy required to induce antibodies in 50% of slow and rapid acetylators was about 3 months and 7 months, respectively. After 5.5 months, ANA had developed in all the slow acetylators, but in only 36% of the rapid acetylators. After 1 year of treatment, antibodies had developed in all but two patients.

These investigators also evaluated the effect of acetylator phenotype on the rate of development of the lupus syndrome in 7 patients, 4 slow acetylators and 3 fast acetylators.[163] The mean duration of therapy before development of lupus was 12 months for the slow acetylators and 54 months for the rapid acetylators. These findings suggest that acetylation of the arylamine group of PA serves as a protective pathway of biotransformation, reducing the amount of drug or reactive metabolite available for initiating the immunopathology associated with drug-induced lupus.

Hydralazine. The metabolism of the antihypertensive drug hydralazine is complicated, but acetylation plays an important role. Plasma concentrations of hydralazine after a standard oral dose vary by as much as 15-fold among individuals, but are lower in rapid acetylators than in slow acetylators.[164] Current dosing guidelines for hydralazine specify a maximum of 200 mg/day for patients with unknown acetylator status and a maximum dose of 300 mg/day for fast acetylators.

Hydralazine, like PA, induces ANA and an SLE-like syndrome. In a study of 57 patients treated with hydralazine for hypertension, a 54% incidence of ANA was found; the incidence was 38% for rapid acetylators and 67% for slow acetylators.[165] More recently, 27 hypertensive patients were treated with hydralazine and followed for evidence of autoimmunity.[166] Acetylation phenotype profoundly affected this response; slow acetylators had a much higher incidence and larger amounts of autoantibodies than rapid acetylators.

Other investigators have studied the role of acetylator phenotype in determining the response to hydralazine in patients with hypertension.[167] Hydralazine was added to diuretic and beta-blocker at doses not exceeding 200 mg daily, consistent with current dosing recommendations for patients with unknown acetylator status. Phenotype was determined with sulfamethazine. About 37% of the 57 patients were classified as rapid acetylators and the rest were considered to be slow acetylators.

The addition of hydralazine satisfactorily lowered blood pressure in only 47% of the patient population. Most rapid acetylators reached the maximum dosage of hydralazine (200 mg/day), but only 27% of these patients were controlled at the end of the 6-month trial. In contrast, satisfactory control of blood pressure was achieved in 65% of the slow acetylators at daily doses of 50 or 100 mg.

The investigators recommended that patients who do not respond to hydralazine at daily doses of 200 mg and for whom continued use of hydralazine at higher dosage is deemed preferable to the use of another drug be phenotyped for acetylator status. They further suggested that about 70% of those evaluated will be rapid acetylators for whom the daily dose of hydralazine may be safely increased to 300 mg or even 400 mg.

Other Drugs. Amrinone is a positive inotropic agent with vasodilatory properties used to a limited extent in the treatment of congestive heart failure. In both animals and man, amrinone has been shown to be converted to its N-acetyl metabolites. Hamilton et al.[168] studied the influence of acetylator phenotype on the pharmacokinetics of amrinone in healthy human subjects. After being phenotyped, the subjects received iv amrinone 75 mg over 10 minutes.

The clearance of amrinone was significantly lower in slow acetylators than in fast acetylators (277 vs 620 ml/min). There was more than a 4-fold difference between the highest clearance in the fast acetylators and the lowest clearance in the slow acetylators. As expected, the ratio of N-acetylamrinone to amrinone in urine was much higher in fast acetylators.

Both isoniazid and sulfamethazine have been used to determine acetylator status but these agents may produce adverse effects in certain patients. The search for a safer phenotyping agent has focused on caffeine. The urinary ratios of two caffeine metabolites, 5-acetylamino-6-formylamino-3-methyluracil (AFMU) and 1-methylxanthine (MX) are closely related to acetylation phenotypes determined with the use of sulfamethazine.

Evans et al.[169] administered caffeine, in the form of a cola beverage, to children and adolescents and measured the ratio of metabolites in urine collected over the first 4 hours. Subjects with a molar ratio (AFMU:MX) less than 0.3 were defined as slow acetylators; those with ratios greater than 0.4 were classified as rapid acetylators. Fifteen children were ranked as rapid acetylators, nine were classified as slow acetylators, and two had intermediate metabolic ratios. It is likely that caffeine will become the probe of choice to determine acetylator phenotype.

Polymorphic Oxidation—Debrisoquin Type

The hydroxylation of debrisoquin, an adrenergic-blocker used in the treatment of hypertension is expressed as two phenotypes, designated extensive metabolizer (EM) and poor metabolizer (PM).[170] The ratio of debrisoquin to 4-hydroxy-debrisoquin in urine collected for 8 hr after a 10-mg oral test dose of debrisoquin ranged from 0.6 to 1.5 in EM subjects and from 19.3 to 22.9 in PM subjects. The frequency of 4-hydroxylation defect (PM phenotype) was about 3% (3 of 94 subjects).

The metabolism of guanoxan, an antihypertensive drug chemically related to debrisoquin and guanethidine, and phenacetin was studied in healthy subjects previously phenotyped for their ability to hydroxylate debrisoquin.[171] From 31 to 60% of the guanoxan dose was excreted unchanged in the urine in PM subjects, whereas only 1.2 to 1.9% was excreted unchanged in EM subjects. The rate of formation of acetaminophen, an active metabolite of phenacetin, was considerably slower in the PM group than in the EM group. Therefore, the hydroxylation defect shown for debrisoquin also applies to the oxidative metabolism of phenacetin and guanoxan.

More recent studies suggest a correlation of oxidation phenotype between debrisoquin and nor-

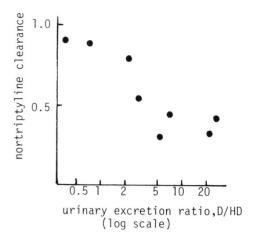

Fig. 12–11. Relationship between nortriptyline clearance (hr per kg) and the urinary excretion ratio of debrisoquin (D) to 4-hydroxydebrisoquin (HD). (Data from Bertilsson, L., et al.[172])

triptyline,[172] phenytoin,[173] metoprolol,[174] phenformin,[175] and perhexiline,[176] but not antipyrine.[172] A correlation was also observed between the plasma clearance of nortriptyline and the debrisoquin to 4-hydroxydebrisoquin urinary excretion ratio in the same individual (Fig. 12–11).[172]

The clinical consequences of polymorphic oxidation continue to be examined. The small percentage of the population who are poor metabolizers may be at risk of adverse effects from the usual doses of many drugs.

Shah and co-workers have suggested a relationship between the incidence of neuropathy in patients with ischemic heart disease treated with perhexiline and the oxidative metabolism status of the patient.[176] The average debrisoquin/4-hydroxydebrisoquin ratio was 14.4 in patients with neuropathy but only 0.65 in patients with no signs of neuropathy.

Debrisoquin and sparteine have been used most frequently to study genetic polymorphism in oxidative metabolism of the debrisoquin type. The impaired metabolism of debrisoquin and sparteine in PMs has been shown to follow Mendelian inheritance. PM subjects are homozygous for an autosomal recessive gene.

The molecular mechanism of impaired drug oxidation is under study in laboratories throughout the world. The findings to date suggest impaired metabolism is the result of the absence of or altered catalytic properties of the P-450 cytochrome involved in the oxidative metabolism of debrisoquin and other drugs.

To better understand polymorphic oxidation, investigators from Germany and Switzerland studied sparteine metabolism in human liver microsomes prepared from liver samples obtained from patients undergoing cholecystectomy.[177] The patients had been phenotyped with sparteine before laparotomy. The ratio of sparteine to the sum of 2- and 5-dehydrosparteine in urine, termed the metabolic ratio (MR), was the basis for phenotyping. The study panel consisted of 6 patients with MR <1 (EMs), 4 patients with MR >20 (PMs), and 3 patients classified as intermediates with MR values ranging from 3 to 18.

In hepatic microsomes from PMs, the Michaelis-Menten constant (K_M) for the formation of 2-dehydrosparteine was 30 times larger than in microsomes from EMs (1880 vs 58 μmol/L). Intermediary metabolizers had an average K_m of 658 μmol/L. The K_m values for 2-dehydrosparteine formation correlated strongly ($r = 0.98$) with urinary MR values. There were no significant differences in V_{max} values between EM and PM subjects. 5-Dehydrosparteine was detected only in microsomal preparations from EMs. The investigators concluded that "the data obtained in this study indicate that the basis of the differences in oxidative capacity between PMs and EMs is more likely to be the result of a variant isozyme with defective catalytic properties rather than a decreased amount of enzyme."

Difficulty in obtaining debrisoquin as well as its potential for adverse effects have prompted investigators to evaluate other probes for phenotyping. Dextromethorphan (DM) is quickly becoming the agent of choice. There is a strong relationship between dextromethorphan O-demethylation and debrisoquin 4-hydroxylation.

Investigators in Sweden[178] determined serum concentrations of DM and its metabolites in healthy subjects given DM orally. The same subjects were phenotyped using the urinary ratio of debrisoquin and 4-hydroxydebrisoquin; 4 of 29 subjects were classified as PMs.

PMs had very low serum levels of the O-demethylated metabolite of DM, dextromethorphan (D), whereas the serum levels of DM were highest in these subjects. The opposite was seen in EMs. The two groups were characterized by a large difference in DM/D ratio and were easily identified after a single dose of DM. The ratios in PMs were 3.6 or more compared with ratios of 0.11 or less in EMs.

Evans et al.[169] reported the use of dextromethorphan to phenotype children and adolescents. These investigators also found that analysis of urine collected for 4 hours after coadministration of DM and caffeine permits the simultaneous determination of both oxidation (debrisoquin type) and acetylation phenotypes in an individual subject.

Gene frequencies for the loci involved in impaired metabolism may vary among racial and ethnic groups, resulting in differences in polymorphic distribution. A well-established difference between Caucasians and Orientals is the responsiveness to ethanol, involving differences in both alcohol and aldehyde dehydrogenases. More recently, interethnic differences in debrisoquin hydroxylation were studied in healthy white subjects living in the U.S. ($n = 183$) and Japanese subjects living in Japan ($n = 100$), using the 8-hour urinary metabolic ratio of debrisoquin to identify EMs and PMs.[179]

In white subjects, the frequency of PMs for debrisoquin was 8.7%. In contrast, no PMs of debrisoquin were found among the Japanese subjects. These findings are important because differences in polymorphic distribution of oxidative drug metabolizing ability have implications for interethnic efficacy and toxicity of drugs and other chemicals metabolized by the involved cytochrome P-450. "Given the international nature of drug development and use and the multiracial nature of the populations of many countries, it appears that the potential for genetically determined interethnic differences in drug responsiveness caused by drug dispositional factors should be given increased recognition."[179]

The relative importance of genetic and environmental factors in determining differences among individuals in debrisoquin hydroxylation was studied in 52 families in Sweden.[180] The major influence on interindividual variation was genetic heritability, accounting for 79% of the variance. Only a minor part of family resemblance was actually due to common culture and environment. The investigators concluded that "the debrisoquin metabolic phenotype seems to be extensively controlled by a monogenic system and not significantly influenced by environmental factors or age."

Genetic polymorphism in oxidative metabolism raises an intriguing question. What other tendencies cosegregate with the metabolism phenotype? There is some evidence that lung cancer is more frequent in EMs than in PMs, suggesting that metabolic activation of environmental carcinogens by the involved hydroxylase has a part in the disease.[181,182] More recently, differences in personality between EMs and PMs have been reported.[183]

Fifty-one PMs and 102 EMs, matched for age and sex, were evaluated using standardized tests. Significant differences in personality were measured. Scores for PMs implied high vitality, alertness, efficiency, and ease of decision making. Consistent with lack of hesitation in making a decision was the significantly higher frequency of extreme responses in the PMs. The investigators speculated that "the relation between debrisoquin hydroxylation phenotype and personality may indicate that debrisoquin hydroxylase is also involved in the metabolism of endogenous substances important for central nervous system function."

Beta-Blockers. The metabolism of several beta-adrenoceptor blocking drugs (e.g., metoprolol, alprenolol, timolol) appears to be linked to debrisoquin oxidative polymorphism. Poor metabolizers of debrisoquin may have relatively high plasma concentrations of these drugs when treated with usual doses and may be susceptible to adverse effects.

Lewis et al.[184] studied timolol and atenolol in 6 EMs and 4 PMs of debrisoquin. Timolol is extensively metabolized in humans, largely by oxidative pathways. Atenolol undergoes little metabolism and is largely excreted unchanged.

Mean plasma concentration of timolol were more than twice as high in poor metabolizers of debrisoquin than in extensive metabolizers. Beta-blockade, determined by bicycle ergometry, following a 20-mg oral dose of timolol was also greater in PMs than in EMs. At 24 hours after the dose, the mean degree of blockade was 16% in the PMs and 6% in the EMs. Statistically significant correlations were found between the debrisoquin/4-hydroxy-debrisoquin ratio in urine after a test dose and the AUC of timolol ($r = 0.75$) as well as between the urinary ratio and the degree of beta-blockade at 24 hours ($r = 0.66$). There was no relation between oxidation phenotype and plasma atenolol levels or the degree of beta-blockade following a single 100 mg dose of atenolol.

Other investigators studied propranolol in EMs and PMs of debrisoquin.[185] Dramatic differences were observed between the two groups with respect to the formation of 4-hydroxypropranolol (4-HP). Total AUC for unconjugated 4-HP following a single 160 mg oral dose of propranolol averaged 21 ng-hr/ml in PMs and 94 ng-hr/ml in EMs. The AUC for total 4-HP, determined after hydrolysis, was also more than 4 times greater in PMs than in EMs. Similar differences in plasma concentrations of unconjugated and total 4-HP were found after multiple oral doses of propranolol. At steady-state, 4-HP accounted for about 20–25% of drug-related material in urine in PMs but for less than 5% in EMs.

Despite the differences in 4-HP plasma levels and urinary recoveries, plasma concentrations of propranolol were about the same in EMs and PMs. Furthermore, although propranolol and 4-HP are equipotent, no difference in beta-blockade was found between the two groups. These findings suggest that formation of 4-HP is a minor pathway in the overall metabolism of propranolol and that 4-HP does not contribute significantly to beta-blockade during treatment with propranolol.

Encainide. Encainide is a class I antiarrhythmic agent recently approved for use in the United States. Disturbing findings suggesting excess deaths in patients treated with encainide, reported shortly after the drug's approval, foreshadow that the use of encainide will be limited in the United States. Nevertheless, its metabolism, pharmacokinetics, and pharmacodynamics are sufficiently interesting to merit discussion.

Encainide is extensively metabolized to form O- and N-desmethylencainide (ODE and NDE); ODE is further metabolized to 3-methoxy-O-desmethylencainide (MODE). Studies in laboratory animals suggest that all three metabolites are active, potency decreasing as follows: ODE > MODE = encainide > NDE.

Early clinical trials with encainide turned up a nonresponder who, paradoxically, had much higher plasma levels of encainide than patients responding to the drug. Further probing indicated that this patient was also a poor metabolizer of debrisoquin. These results prompted Wang et al.[186] to study encainide in EMs and PMs of debrisoquin.

Dramatic differences in the pharmacokinetics of encainide were observed. Total clearance, determined after intravenous administration, was 1.8 L/min in EMs but only 0.22 L/min in PMs. After an oral dose, bioavailability was 26% in EMs and 88% in PMs, reflecting large differences in first-pass metabolism. Plasma levels of ODE after a single oral dose of encainide were more than 10 times higher in EMs than PMs. Substantial plasma concentrations of MODE were also found in EMs but this metabolite could not be detected in slow metabolizers.

Important differences were also found in the pharmacologic effects of encainide in EMs and PMs. Measurement of ECG changes after 3 days of oral encainide showed a significant delay in intraventricular conduction in EMs but not in PMs. Although poor metabolizers have substantially higher and more persistent levels of encainide than extensive metabolizers, PMs appear to be less responsive to the effects of the drug than EMs. These findings suggest an important role for ODE and MODE in the clinical effects of encainide.

These investigators also studied encainide in 8 patients with ventricular arrhythmias, 2 of whom were phenotyped as PMs of debrisoquin.[187] Encainide suppressed ventricular ectopic beats by greater than 90% in all patients. QRS interval on the ECG was prolonged by 31 to 62% in the 6 EMs and by 22% and 29% in the 2 PMs. At steady-state, encainide concentrations in plasma were about 5 times higher in the 2 PMs than in the EMs. On the other hand, unlike the PMs, the EMs had appreciable levels of both ODE and MODE.

In both PMs, arrhythmia suppression and prolongation of the QRS interval were significantly correlated with encainide levels in plasma. This was not the case in the EMs. Arrhythmia suppression and effects on the ECG in EMs were strongly correlated with concentrations of ODE and MODE.

These findings support the hypothesis that among EMs, who probably constitute more than 90% of the U.S. population, metabolites of encainide are primarily responsible for the clinical effects of the drug. On the other hand, encainide seems to be an effective antiarrhythmic agent in its own right, at least at the high concentrations found in poor metabolizers of debrisoquin.

"In both phenotypic groups, there is an active compound in plasma with a relatively long half-life: ODE in EMs ($t_{1/2}$ = >6 hours) and encainide in PMs (>8 hours)."[187] Frequency of dosing of encainide should reflect these half-lives rather the relatively short half-life of encainide itself, about 3 hours, found in EMs.

More recently, Barbey et al.[188] studied the pharmacokinetics and antiarrhythmic effects of ODE and MODE directly in 9 patients with ventricular arrhythmias, 2 of whom were PMs. Intravenous infusion of both ODE and MODE suppressed chronic ventricular arrhythmias. The clearance of ODE was also a function of debrisoquin phenotype.

Mean clearance in EMs was 914 ml/min, with a range from 554 to 1314 ml/min. ODE clearance was 434 ml/min in one poor metabolizer and 298 ml/min in the other. MODE was detected during ODE infusion in all 7 EMs but in neither poor metabolizer. The clearance of MODE in EMs ranged from 180 to 410 ml/min. MODE clearance in one PM was well within this range but was only 78 ml/min in the other. Whether MODE clearance is a function of metabolic phenotype requires a larger panel of subjects to answer.

Propafenone. Propafenone is a new antiarrhythmic agent undergoing clinical testing in the U.S. At least one active metabolite of propafenone is recognized, 5-hydroxypropafenone, with antiarrhythmic properties similar to the parent drug. Large variability in blood levels has been observed during the early clinical trials with propafenone. Some patients, for no obvious reason, exhibit unusually long half-lives and high plasma levels.

The occurrence of high blood levels and slow elimination in a small fraction of the patients taking propafenone prompted Siddoway and his colleagues[189] to consider the possibility of polymorphic metabolism. These investigators studied the pharmacokinetics and pharmacodynamics of propafenone in symptomatic patients with more than 30 ventricular ectopic depolarizations (VEDs) per hour, who had been phenotyped with debrisoquin.

The half-life of propafenone was 5.5 hr in EMs and 17.2 hr in PMs. The apparent clearance after oral administration was about 4 times greater in EMs than in PMs, 1115 vs 264 ml/min. The concordance between debrisoquin and propafenone metabolism suggest a low capacity for hydroxylation of propafenone in PMs. Consistent with this hypothesis, the ratio of propafenone to the 5-hydroxy metabolite is much smaller in EMs than in PMs.

Surprisingly, the relationship between propafenone dose and concentration in plasma was also different in EMs and PMs. A total of 17 patients (13 EMs and 4 PMs) received doses of 600 mg/day and 900 mg/day. This 50% increase in dose, as expected, resulted in a mean increase of about 50% in steady-state trough levels in PMs, from 1340 to 2030 ng/ml. In EMs, however, this modest increase in dose resulted in more than a 200% increase in drug levels. These results suggest that the pharmacokinetics of propafenone are markedly nonlinear in EMs, whereas, over the dosage range studied, the kinetics of propafenone appear to be linear in PMs.

The nonlinear kinetics of propafenone have been confirmed by Zoble et al.[190] These investigators followed 169 patients of unknown phenotype with chronic ventricular arrhythmia during treatment with various doses of propafenone. They found that for a doubling of the daily dose from 450 to 900 mg/day, mean steady-state trough propafenone concentrations increased 4.3-fold.

Siddoway et al.[189] also reported that the trough plasma concentrations of propafenone at which more than 70% suppression of VEDs was realized ranged from 40 to 1800 ng/ml. This range could be divided into two groups, based on metabolic phenotype: 42–1356 ng/ml for EMs and 1408–1801 ng/ml for PMs. Although higher levels of propafenone are found in PMs, this group appears to be less sensitive to the antiarrhythmic effects of the drug. Consequently, there were no significant differences in the mean effective dose of propafenone for EMs and PMs, 828 mg/day vs 800 mg/day, respectively.

In another study, examining the effects of food on the bioavailability of propafenone, Axelson et al.[191] found that food had no effect in poor metabolizers of propafenone, but resulted in a marked increase in bioavailability in extensive metabolizers. Bioavailability was increased by 250%, on the average. There was a strong correlation between the food-related increase in AUC and the fasting AUC. Those subjects showing the largest change in propafenone AUC due to food had the lowest AUC after oral administration of propafenone in the fasting state.

Other Drugs. Imipramine is eliminated by demethylation to the active metabolite desipramine and both imipramine and desipramine are subject to 2-hydroxylation. The demethylation of imipramine and the 2-hydroxylation of both drugs are carried out by at least two different isozymes of cytochrome P-450. The 2-hydroxylation expresses the activity of the isozyme also known to oxidize debrisoquin, sparteine, and other drugs.

Brosen and Gram[192] administered imipramine and desipramine intravenously and orally to extensive and poor metabolizers of sparteine. They assumed that the absorption of both drugs was complete and calculated the extent of first-pass metabolism in each subject. Consistent with theory, the mean degree of first-pass metabolism of imipramine was about 60% in EMs but only 30%

in PMs. In other words, about 40% of a 50-mg oral dose of imipramine was systemically available in EMs compared with 70% of the dose in PMs.

Desipramine showed similar results but a closer relationship was found between the extent of first-pass metabolism and metabolic ratio (MR), determined from the ratio of sparteine to dehydrosparteine in a 12-hour urine sample. Mean first-pass metabolism was 44% in EMs with an MR of 0.31 or less, 27% in EMs with MR values ranging from 0.72–0.98, and 14% in PMs with MR values ranging from 62–140.

There is also evidence that the metabolism of flecainide, an orally effective antiarrhythmic agent, is under monogenic control. Interestingly, flecainide like encainide has been found to produce excess deaths in patients treated for arrhythmias. Flecainide is both metabolized and excreted unchanged. Urinary excretion is pH-dependent.

Mikus et al.[193] administered oral flecainide to extensive and poor metabolizers of the debrisoquin type. Urine pH was controlled, on the acid side, with oral ammonium chloride given before and after flecainide. This measure decreased variability but also maximized the urinary excretion of unchanged drug.

The average clearance of flecainide, assuming complete absorption and no first-pass effect, was 1,041 ml/min in EMs and 600 ml/min in PMs. Renal clearance, measured directly, was 315 ml/min in EMs and 308 ml/min in PMs. Renal excretion accounted for about 30% of the overall elimination of flecainide in EMs and for about 50% in PMs.

Mikus and his colleagues have shown that the total clearance of flecainide is dependent on debrisoquin phenotype whereas its renal clearance is not. The difference between total clearance and renal clearance is called the nonrenal clearance and in some cases may faithfully reflect metabolic clearance. Nonrenal clearance of flecainide was calculated to be 726 ml/min in EMs and 292 ml/min in PMs.

The investigators concluded that "under conditions of uncontrolled urinary . . . pH, renal excretion of flecainide will be reduced and the difference in disposition will be greater. In PMs with renal impairment, accumulation of flecainide to very high levels may be anticipated, and this may result in proarrhythmic effects." In patients with renal impairment, flecainide levels will be elevated in both PMs and EMs unless dosage is adjusted.

In patients with no renal function, one may calculate from the nonrenal clearance values reported in this study that flecainide levels will be 2.5 times greater in PMs than in EMs.

Polymorphic Oxidation—Mephenytoin Type

Poor hydroxylators of phenytoin have been recognized for about 25 years. These individuals are at risk of severe adverse effects because hydroxylation is the principal elimination pathway for phenytoin. Many investigators believe that this problem is an inherited one, but evidence for concordance with the debrisoquin phenotype has not been forthcoming.

The hydroxylation of mephenytoin, a closely related drug, also demonstrates polymorphism. In one study,[194] the urinary excretion of hydroxymephenytoin was determined after a single oral dose of mephenytoin in 118 Caucasians and 70 Asians. The urinary excretion of the metabolite was bimodal in these populations; 13% of the Asians and 4% of the Caucasians were classified as poor metabolizers. Hydroxymephenytoin accounted for about 40 to 45% of the dose of mephenytoin in EMs but for only 1 to 3% for the dose in PMs. Family studies have suggested that deficient hydroxylation of mephenytoin is genetically determined.

Mephenytoin is a racemate and its metabolism is stereoselective; hydroxylation strongly favors the S-enantiomer. It follows that the ratio of S- to R-mephenytoin in urine will be very small in EMs but nearly 1.0 in PMs. Wedlund et al.[195] tested this hypothesis by determining the urinary recovery of hydroxyphenytoin and the urinary S:R enantiomeric ratio of mephenytoin after a single 100-mg dose of mephenytoin.

On the basis of urinary excretion data, 4 of the 156 Caucasians studied were classified as PMs of mephenytoin. These individuals excreted negligible quantities of the hydroxy metabolite, whereas the rest of the panel excreted about 40% of the dose as hydroxymephenytoin. The mean S:R ratio of mephenytoin was 0.99 in the 4 PMs but only 0.16 in the EMs. This difference is consistent with the stereoselective metabolism of mephenytoin in EMs but not in PMs.

The panel was also phenotyped with debrisoquin. Using this probe, 11 subjects (7%) were classified as PMs. All 4 poor metabolizers of mephenytoin were classified as extensive metabolizers of debrisoquin and all 11 poor metabolizers of debri-

soquin were found to be extensive metabolizers of mephenytoin. On the basis of these results, the investigators concluded that "4-hydroxylation of mephenytoin is a new polymorphism independent of that for debrisoquin."

More recently, Wedlund et al.[196] determined the plasma levels of the enantiomers of both mephenytoin and its pharmacologically active N-demethylated metabolite, phenylethylhydantoin (PEH), after a single oral dose of mephenytoin in subjects who had been phenotyped. In extensive metabolizers of mephenytoin, substantial plasma levels of both R-mephenytoin and R-PEH were measured, whereas very low levels of the S-form of mephenytoin and its metabolite were seen. A 100- to 200-fold difference in the oral clearance of S- and R-mephenytoin was calculated. Average values were 4700 ml/min for the S-enantiomer and 27 ml/min for the R-enantiomer. Mean half-lives were 2 hours for S- and 76 hours for R-mephenytoin.

In these same extensive metabolizers, R-PEH concentrations accumulated over several days after a single dose of mephenytoin and then declined with a half-life of about 200 hours. Plasma levels of S-PEH were negligible.

A different picture emerged in poor metabolizers of mephenytoin. The stereoselective elimination of mephenytoin essentially disappeared. Average oral clearance values in PMs were 29 ml/min for S-mephenytoin and 20 ml/min for R-mephenytoin. Almost comparable plasma levels of S- and R-PEH were also found. The investigators suggested that such large differences between EMs and PMs would be expected to have clinical consequences for both desired and untoward effects of mephenytoin when it is used as an anticonvulsant.

The rate of 4-hydroxylation of S- and R-mephenytoin has also been studied in human liver microsomes from 13 extensive metabolizers of mephenytoin and 2 poor metabolizers.[197] Microsomal metabolism of S-mephenytoin in the two subjects classified as PMs was characterized by a larger K_m (150 and 180 μmol/L versus a mean value of 38 μmol/L in EMs), a smaller V_{max} (0.8 and 0.7 nmol/mg protein per hour versus a mean value of 4.8 nmol/mg protein per hour in EMs), and loss of stereoselectivity. On the other hand, the formation of 4-hydroxymephenytoin from R-mephenytoin was not dependent on mephenytoin phenotype. The investigators concluded that "these results support our hypothesis that the mephenytoin polymorphism is caused by a partial or complete absence or inactivity of a cytochrome P-450 isozyme with high affinity for S-mephenytoin.''

Not surprisingly, reports are now being published suggesting that the metabolism of many drugs may be influenced by the mephenytoin phenotype. For example, Kupfer and Branch[198] found that the metabolism of mephobarbital cosegregates with mephenytoin hydroxylation. They measured the 8-hour urinary recovery of 4-hydroxymephobarbital (4-HP) after a single oral dose of racemic mephobarbital in 17 EMs and 6 PMs of mephenytoin.

The recovery of 4-HP in EMs ranged from 2.5 to 48%, with a mean value of about 10%. No metabolite was detected in the urine of poor metabolizers of mephenytoin. One extensive metabolizer received similar doses of R- and S-mephobarbital on separate occasions. Urinary recovery of the 4-hydroxy metabolite was 33% of the dose when R-mephobarbital was given but less than 1% of the dose when S-mephobarbital was administered. Studies as to absolute configuration have shown that S-mephenytoin is the analog of R-mephobarbital. Based on their findings, Kupfer and Branch suggested that ''mephobarbital is stereoselectively hydroxylated by the same drug metabolizing enzyme that is responsible for the stereoselective aromatic hydroxylation of mephenytoin.''

Investigators in Sweden studied the importance of genetic factors in the metabolism of diazepam.[199] They administered single oral doses of diazepam and its metabolite, desmethyldiazepam (DMD), on separate occasions to 4 poor metabolizers of debrisoquin, 3 poor metabolizers of mephenytoin, and 9 extensive metabolizers of both drugs.

Among the 16 subjects, a statistically significant correlation ($r = 0.83$) was found between the total plasma clearance of diazepam and that of DMD. There was no relationship between diazepam or DMD disposition and debrisoquin status. Diazepam clearance was 22 ml/min in EMs and 26 ml/min in PMs of debrisoquin. However, poor metabolizers of mephenytoin had less than half the plasma clearance of both diazepam and DMD than extensive metabolizers. Mean diazepam clearance was 26 ml/min in EMs and 12 ml/min for PMs of mephenytoin. Corresponding values for DMD were 11 ml/min and 5 ml/min. Mean half-life of diazepam was 88 hours in PMs and 41 hours in EMs. ''This study shows that the metabolism of diazepam (mainly demethylation) and desmethyl-

diazepam (mainly hydroxylation) is related to the mephenytoin but not to the debrisoquin hydroxylation phenotype.''[199]

Ward et al.[200] examined the relative contributions of the debrisoquin and mephenytoin isozymes to the stereoselective metabolism of oral propranolol in a panel of healthy subjects who had been phenotyped. Six subjects were extensive metabolizers of both drugs (EM), 4 were poor metabolizers of debrisoquin (PM_D), 5 subjects were poor metabolizers of mephenytoin (PM_M), and 1 subject was a poor metabolizer of both drugs ($PM_{D/M}$).

The total oral clearance of R-propranolol was significantly greater than that of the S-form in the EM, PM_D, and PM_M groups. The highest mean clearance of R-propranolol was seen in the EM group (2666 ml/min) and the lowest values occurred in the one individual who was deficient for both drugs (918 ml/min). Oral clearance values in the other two groups were similar and intermediary, 1860 ml/min for the PM_D group and 2012 ml/min for the PM_M group. The same pattern emerged for S-propranolol.

The partial metabolic clearance of each propranolol enantiomer to 4-hydroxypropranolol in the PM_D group was only about 25% that found in the EM and PM_M groups, suggesting a major contribution of the debrisoquin isozyme to this route of metabolism. The partial metabolic clearance to naphthoxylactic acid (NLA) in the PM_M group was about half that found in the EM and PM_D groups, suggesting that the mephenytoin isozyme contributes to the metabolic conversion of propranolol to NLA.

It appears that the 4-hydroxylation of propranolol cosegregates with the debrisoquin polymorph but the side-chain oxidation of propranolol to NLA is catalyzed in part by the mephenytoin isozyme. Propranolol is the first drug identified where two independent isozymes of cytochrome P-450, identified as being responsible for debrisoquin and mephenytoin hydroxylation, contribute to the two separate oxidative pathways. A deficiency in both routes will probably result in impaired total clearance of propranolol.

REFERENCES

1. Kato, R., Takanaka, A., and Onoda, K.: Individual difference in the effect of drugs in relation to the tissue concentration of drugs. Jpn. J. Pharmacol., 19:260, 1969.
2. Swerdloff, R.S., et al.: Influence of age on the intravenous tolbutamide response test. Diabetes, 10:161, 1967.
3. Bertler, Å., and Smith, S.E.: Genetic influences in drug

responses of the eye and the heart. Clin. Sci., *40*:403, 1971.

4. Yacobi, A., Udall, J.A., and Levy, G.: Serum protein binding as a determinant of warfarin body clearance and anticoagulant effect in patients. Clin. Pharmacol. Ther., *19*:552, 1976.

5. Nichols, E.S., et al.: Long term anticoagulant therapy in coronary atherosclerosis. Am. Heart J., *55*:142, 1958.

6. Bouvet, E., et al.: Differences in serum ampicillin concentrations among patients under constant-rate infusion. Br. Med. J., *139*:1164, 1980.

7. Odenhof, H., et al.: Clinical pharmacokinetics of midazolam in intensive care patients, a wide interpatient variability? Clin. Pharmacol. Ther., *43*:263, 1988.

8. Wagner, J.G.: Inter- and intrasubject variation of digoxin renal clearance in normal adult males. Drug Intell. Clin. Pharm., *22*:562, 1988.

9. Lund, L.: Effects of phenytoin in patients with epilepsy in relation to its concentration in plasma. *In* Biological Effects of Drugs in Relation to Their Plasma Concentrations. Edited by D.S. Davies and B.N.C. Prichard. New York, Macmillan, 1973, pp. 227–238.

10. Collste, P., et al.: Interindividual differences in chlorthalidone concentrations in plasma and red cells of man after single and multiple doses. Eur. J. Clin. Pharmacol., *9*:319, 1976.

11. Hammer, W., Idestrom, C.M., and Sjöqvist, F.: Chemical control of antidepressant drug therapy. *In* Proceedings of the First International Symposium on Antidepressant Drugs. Edited by S. Garrattini and M.N.G. Dukes. Amsterdam, Excerpta Medica, 1967, pp. 301–310.

12. Sjoqvist, F., et al.: Plasma level of monomethylated tricyclic antidepressants and side-effects in man. Excerpta Medica International Congress Series, *145*:246, 1968.

13. Rawlins, M.D., et al.: Steady-state plasma concentrations of alprenolol in man. Eur. J. Clin. Pharmacol., *7*:353, 1974.

14. Shand, D.G., Nuckolls, E.M., and Oates, J.A.: Plasma propranolol levels in adults with observations in four children. Clin. Pharmacol. Ther., *11*:112, 1970.

15. Rowland, M., and Tozer, T.N.: Clinical Pharmacokinetics. Concepts and Applications. Philadelphia, Lea & Febiger, 1980, pp. 218–229.

16. Weisberg, H.F.: Electrolytes and Acid-Base Balance. 2nd Ed. Baltimore, Williams & Wilkins, 1962.

17. Ewy, G.A., et al.: Digoxin metabolism in obesity. Circulation, *44*:810, 1971.

18. Abernethy, D.R., Greenblatt, D.J., and Smith, T.W.: Digoxin disposition in obesity. Clinical pharmacokinetic investigation. Am. Heart J., *102*:740, 1981.

19. Schwartz, S.N., et al.: A controlled investigation of the pharmacokinetics of gentamicin and tobramycin in obese subjects. J. Infect. Dis., *138*:499, 1978.

20. Korsager, S.: Administration of gentamicin to obese subjects. Int. J. Clin. Pharmacol. Ther. Toxicol., *18*:549, 1980.

21. Blouin, R.A., et al.: Tobramycin pharmacokinetics in morbidly obese patients. Clin. Pharmacol. Ther., *26*:508, 1979.

22. Bauer, L.A., et al.: Amikacin pharmacokinetics in morbidly obese patients. Am. J. Hosp. Pharm., *37*:519, 1980.

23. Blouin, R.A., et al.: Vancomycin pharmacokinetics in normal and morbidly obese subjects. Antimicrob. Agents Chemother., *21*:575, 1982.

24. Bauer, L.A., et al.: Cimetidine clearance in the obese. Clin. Pharmacol. Ther., *37*:425, 1985.

25. Gal, P., et al.: Theophylline disposition in obesity. Clin. Pharmacol. Ther., *23*:438, 1978.

26. Abernethy, D.R., et al.: Prolongation of drug half-life

due to obesity: studies of desmethyldiazepam (clorazepate). J. Pharm. Sci., *71*:942, 1982.

27. Bowman, S.L., et al.: A comparison of the pharmacokinetics of propranolol in obese and normal volunteers. Br. J. Clin. Pharmacol., *21*:529, 1986.

28. Greenblatt, D.J., et al.: Trazodone kinetics: effect of age, gender, and obesity. Clin. Pharmacol. Ther., *42*:193, 1987.

29. Abernethy, D.R., Schwartz, J.B.: Verapamil pharmacodynamics and disposition in obese hypertensive patients. J. Cardiovasc. Pharmacol., *11*:209, 1988.

30. Abernethy, D.R., Greenblatt, D.J.: Ibuprofen disposition in obese individuals. Arthritis Rheum., *28*:1117, 1985.

31. Abernethy, D.R., et al.: Obesity effects on nitrazepam disposition. J. Clin. Pharmacol., *22*:551, 1986.

32. Abernethy, D.R., et al.: Obesity, sex, and acetaminophen disposition. Clin. Pharmacol. Ther., *31*:783, 1982.

33. Greenblatt, D.J., et al.: Influence of age, gender, and obesity on salicylate kinetics following single doses of aspirin. Arthritis Rheum., *29*:1117, 1985.

34. Koup, J.R., Vawter, T.K.: Theophylline pharmacokinetics in an extremely obese patient. Clin. Pharm., *2*:181, 1983.

35. Soyka, L.: Clinical pharmacology of digoxin. Pediatr. Clin. North Am., *19*:241, 1972.

36. Cree, J.E., Coltart, D.J., and Howard, M.R.: Plasma digoxin concentration in children with heart failure. Br. Med. J., *1*:443, 1973.

37. Haycock, G.B., Schwartz, G.J., and Wisotsky, D.H.: Geometric method for measuring body surface area: a height-weight formula validated in infants, children, and adults. J. Pediatr., *93*:62, 1978.

38. Wagner, J.G.: Biopharmaceutics and Relevant Pharmacokinetics. Washington, DC, Drug Intelligence Publications, 1971, pp. 18–25.

39. Mosteller, R.D.: Simplified calculation of body-surface area. N. Engl. J. Med., *317*:1098, 1987.

40. Lam, T.-K., Leung, D.T.Y.: More on simplified calculation of body-surface area. N. Engl. J. Med., *318*:1130, 1988.

41. DuBois, D., DuBois, E.F.: A formula to estimate the approximate surface area if height and weight be known. Arch. Intern. Med., *17*:863, 1916.

42. Echeverria, P., et al.: Age dependent dose response to gentamicin. J. Pediatr., *87*:805, 1975.

43. Diem, K., and Letner, C. (eds.): Documenta Geigy—Scientific Tables. 7th Ed. Basel, Ciba-Geigy Ltd., 1970.

44. Friis-Hansen, B.: Body water compartments in children: changes during growth and related changes in body composition. Pediatrics, *28*:169, 1961.

45. Gill, M.A., and Ueda, C.T.: Novel method for the determination of pediatric dosages. Am. J. Hosp. Pharm., *33*:389, 1976.

46. Fisher, D.M., Castagnoli, K., Miller, R.D.: Vecuronium kinetics and dynamics in anesthetized infants and children. Clin. Pharmacol. Ther., *37*:402, 1985.

47. Vestal, R.E., et al.: Aging and ethanol metabolism. Clin. Pharmacol. Ther., *21*:343, 1977.

48. Sereni, F., et al.: Pharmacokinetic studies with a long-acting sulfonamide in subjects of different ages. Pediatr. Res., *2*:29, 1968.

49. Hayton, W.L., Stoeckel, K.: Age-associated changes in ceftriaxone pharmacokinetics. Clin. Pharmacokin., *11*:76, 1986.

50. Yee, G.C., et al.: Age-dependent cyclosporine: pharmacokinetics in marrow transplant recipients. Clin. Pharmacol. Ther., *40*:438, 1986.

51. Rane, A., and Tomson, G.: Prenatal and neonatal drug metabolism in man. Eur. J. Clin. Pharmacol., *18*:9, 1980.

52. Weiss, C.F., Glazko, A.J., and Weston, J.K.: Chloramphenicol in newborn infant: Physiologic explanation of its toxicity when given in excessive doses. N. Engl. J. Med., 262:787, 1960.

53. Evans, M.A., et al.: Gestational age and indomethacin elimination. Clin. Pharmacol. Ther., 26:746, 1979.

54. Brash, A.R., et al.: Pharmacokinetics of indomethacin in the neonate. Relation of plasma indomethacin levels to response of the ductus arteriosus. N. Engl. J. Med., 305:67, 1981.

55. Lynn, A.M., Slattery, J.T.: Morphine pharmacokinetics in early infancy. Anesthesiol., 66:136, 1987.

56. Dothey, C.I., et al.: Maturational changes of theophylline pharmacokinetics in preterm infants. Clin. Pharmacol., Ther., 45:461, 1989.

57. Aldridge, A., Aranda, J.V., and Neims, A.H.: Caffeine metabolism in newborns. Clin. Pharmacol. Ther., 25:447, 1979.

58. Aranda, J.V., et al.: Maturation of caffeine elimination in infancy. Arch. Dis. Child., 54:946, 1979.

59. Lindsay, L., et al.: Digoxin inactivation by the gut flora in infancy and childhood. Pediatrics, 79:544, 1987.

60. Morselli, P.L.: Clinical pharmacokinetics in neonates. Clin. Pharmacokinet., 1:81, 1976.

61. McCance, R.A.: Renal function in early life. Physiol. Rev., 28:331, 1948.

62. Rubin, M.I., Bruck, E., and Rapoport, M.: Maturation of renal function in childhood. J. Clin. Invest., 28:1144, 1949.

63. Stewart, C.F., Hampton, E.M.: Effect of maturation on drug disposition in pediatric patients. Clin. Pharm., 6:548, 1987.

64. Wettrell, G., et al.: Concentrations of digoxin in plasma and urine in neonates, infants, and children with heart disease. Acta Paediatr. Scand., 63:705, 1974.

65. Ellis, E.G., Koysooko, R., and Levy, G.: Pharmacokinetics of theophylline in children with asthma. Pediatrics, 58:542, 1976.

66. Wyatt, R., Weinberger, M., and Hendeles, L.: Oral theophylline dosage for the management of chronic asthma. J. Pediatr., 92:125, 1978.

67. Singh, S., et al.: Procainamide elimination kinetics in pediatric patients. Clin. Pharmacol. Ther., 32:607, 1982.

68. Szefler, S.J., et al.: Rapid elimination of quinidine in pediatric patients. Pediatrics, 70:370, 1982.

69. Brondfonbreaur, M., Landowne, M., and Shock, N.W.: Changes in cardiac output with age. Circulation, 12:557, 1955.

70. Davies, D.F., and Shock, N.W.: Age changes in glomerular filtration rate, effective renal plasma flow, and the tubular excretory capacity in adult males. J. Clin. Invest., 29:496, 1950.

71. Crooks, J., O'Malley, K., and Stevenson, I.H.: Pharmacokinetics in the elderly. Clin. Pharmacokinet., 1:280, 1976.

72. Greenblatt, D.J., Sellers, E.M., and Shader, R.I.: Drug disposition in old age. N. Engl. J. Med., 306:1081, 1982.

73. Ewy, G.A., et al.: Digoxin metabolism in the elderly. Circulation, 39:449, 1969.

74. Somogyi, A., Rohner, H.-G., Gugler, R.: Pharmacokinetics and bioavailability of cimetidine in gastric and duodenal ulcer patients. Clin. Pharmacokin., 5:84, 1980.

75. Young, C.J., Daneshmend, T.K., Roberts, C.J.C.: Effects of cirrhosis and aging on the elimination and bioavailability of ranitidine. Gut, 23:819, 1982.

76. Hockings, N., Ajayi, A.A., Reid, J.L.: Age and the pharmacokinetics of angiotensin converting enzyme inhibitors enalapril and enalaprilat. Br. J. Clin. Pharmacol., 21:341, 1986.

77. Williams, R.L., et al.: Absorption and disposition of two combination formulations of hydrochlorothiazide and triamterene: influence of age and renal function. Clin. Pharmacol. Ther., 40:226, 1986.

78. Swift, C.G., et al.: Antipyrine disposition and liver size in the elderly. Eur. J. Clin. Pharmacol., 14:149, 1978.

79. Bach, B., et al.: Disposition of antipyrine and phenytoin correlated with age and liver volume in man. Clin. Pharmacokinet., 6:389, 1981.

80. Woodhouse, K.W., Wynne, H.A.: Age-related changes in liver size and hepatic blood flow. The influence on drug metabolism in the elderly. Clin. Pharmacokin., 15:287, 1988.

81. Wood, A.J.J., et al.: Effect of aging and cigarette smoking on antipyrine and indocyanine green elimination. Clin. Pharmacol. Ther., 26:16, 1979.

82. Bauer, L.A., et al.: Valproic acid clearance: unbound fraction and diurnal variation in young and elderly adults. Clin. Pharmacol. Ther., 37:697, 1985.

83. Klotz, U., et al.: The effects of age and liver disease on the disposition and elimination of diazepam in man. J. Clin. Invest., 55:347, 1975.

84. Kangas, L., et al.: Human pharmacokinetics of nitrazepam: Effect of age and disease. Eur. J. Clin. Pharmacol., 15:163, 1979.

85. Roberts, R.K., et al.: Effect of age and parenchymal liver disease on the disposition and elimination of chlordiazepoxide. Gastroenterology, 75 :479, 1978.

86. Greenblatt, D.J., et al.: Reduced clearance of triazolam in old age: relation to antipyrine oxidizing capacity. Br. J. Clin. Pharmacol., 15:303, 1983.

87. Greenblatt, D.J., et al.: Effect of age, gender, and obesity on midazolam kinetics. Anesthesiol., 61:27, 1984.

88. Bell, G.D., et al.: Intravenous midazolam for upper gastrointestinal endoscopy: A study of 800 consecutive cases relating dose to age and sex of patient. Br. J. Clin. Pharmacol., 23:241, 1987.

89. Greenblatt, D.J., et al.: Benzodiazepine kinetics: implications for therapeutics and pharmacogeriatrics. Drug. Metabol. Revs., 14:251, 1983.

90. Bauer, L.A., and Blouin, R.A.: Influence of age on theophylline clearance in patients with chronic obstructive pulmonary disease. Clin. Pharmacokinet., 6:469, 1981.

91. Cusack, B., et al.: Theophylline kinetics in relation to age: the importance of smoking. Br. J. Clin. Pharmacol., 10:109, 1980.

92. Vestal, R.E., et al.: Aging and drug interactions. I. Effect of cimetidine and smoking on the oxidation of theophylline and cortisol in healthy men. J. Pharmacol. Exp. Ther., 241:488, 1987.

93. Vestal, R.E., et al.: Effects of age and cigarette smoking on propranolol disposition. Clin. Pharmacol. Ther., 26:8, 1979.

94. Wood, A.J.J., et al.: Effect of aging and cigarette smoking on antipyrine and indocyanine green elimination. Clin. Pharmacol. Ther., 26:16, 1979.

95. Briant, R.H., et al.: Bioavailability of metoprolol in young adults and the elderly, with additional studies on the effects of metoclopramide and propantheline. Eur. J. Clin. Pharmacol., 25:353, 1983.

96. Kelly, J.G., et al.: Bioavailability of labetolol increases with age. Br. J. Clin. Pharmacol., 14:303, 1982.

97. Abernethy, D.R., et al.: Comparison in young and elderly patients of pharmacodynamics and disposition of labetolol in systemic hypertension. Am. J. Cardiol., 60:697, 1987.

98. Bradbook, D., et al.: Comparison of pharmacokinetic profiles of single and multiple doses of a slow release Oros oxprenolol delivery system in young normotensive and

elderly hypertensive subjects. Br. J. Clin. Pharmacol., *21*:371, 1986.

99. Rigby, J.W., et al.: A comparison of the pharmacokinetics of atenolol, metoprolol, oxprenolol, and propranolol in elderly hypertensive and young healthy subjects. Br. J. Clin. Pharmacol., *20*:327, 1985.

100. Abernethy, D.R.: Verapamil pharmacodynamics and disposition in young and elderly hypertensive patients. Ann. Intern. Med., *105*:329, 1986.

101. Roberston, D.R.C., et al.: Age-related changes in the pharmacokinetics and pharmacodynamics of nifedipine. Br. J. Clin. Pharmacol., *25*:297, 1988.

102. Landahl, S., et al.: Pharmacokinetics and blood pressure effects of felodipine in elderly hypertensive patients. A comparison with young healthy subjects. Clin. Pharmacokin., *14*:374, 1988.

103. Homer, T.D., Stanski, D.R.: The effect of increasing age on thiopental disposition and anesthetic requirement. Anesthesiol., *62*:714, 1985.

104. Nies, A., et al.: Relationship between age and tricyclic antidepressant plasma levels. Am. J. Psychiatry, *134*:790, 1977.

105. Abernethy, D.R., Greenblatt, D.J., Shader, R.I.: Imipramine and desipramine disposition in the elderly. J. Pharmacol. Exp. Ther., *232*:183, 1985.

106. Schulz, P., et al.: Amitriptyline disposition in the elderly. J. Pharmacol. Exp. Ther., *232*:183, 1985.

107. Dawling, S., Crome, P., and Braithwaite, R.: Pharmacokinetics of single oral doses of nortriptyline in depressed elderly hospital patients and young healthy volunteers. Clin. Pharmacokinet., *5*:394, 1980.

108. Upton, R.A., et al.: Naproxen pharmacokinetics in the elderly. Br. J. Clin. Pharmacol., *18*:207, 1984.

109. Advenier, C., et al.: Pharmacokinetics of ketoprofen in the elderly. Br. J. Clin. Pharmacol., *16*:65, 1983.

110. Verbeeck, R.K., Wallace, S.M., Loewen, G.R.: Reduced elimination of ketoprofen in the elderly is not necessarily due to impaired glucuronidation. Br. J. Clin. Pharmacol., *17*:783, 1984.

111. Temple, R.: The clinical investigation of drugs for use by the elderly: Food and Drug guidelines. Clin. Pharmacol. Ther., *42*:681, 1987.

112. Chandler, M.H.H., Scott, S.R., Blouin, R.A.: Age-associated stereoselective alterations in hexobarbital metabolism. Clin. Pharmacol. Ther., *43*:436, 1988.

113. Kato, R.: Sex-related differences in drug metabolism. Drug Metab. Rev., *3*:1, 1974.

114. Trenk, D., Jahnchen, E., Oie, S.: Sex-related differences in disposition and response to phenprocoumon in rats. J. Pharm. Pharmacol., *40*:403, 1988.

115. Divoll, M., et al.: Effect of age and gender on disposition of temazepam. J. Pharm. Sci., *70*:1104, 1981.

116. Greenblatt, D.J., et al.: Oxazepam kinetics: effects of age and sex. J. Pharmacol. Exp. Ther., *215*:86, 1980.

117. Greenblatt, D.J., et al.: Lorazepam kinetics in the elderly. Clin. Pharmacol. Ther., *26*:103, 1979.

118. Miners, J.O., Attwood, J., Birkett, D.J.: Influence of sex and oral contraceptive steroids on paracetamol metabolism. Br. J. Clin. Pharmacol., *16*:503, 1983.

119. Miners, J.O., et al.: Influence of gender and oral contraceptive steroids on the metabolism of salicylic acid and acetylsalicylic acid. Br. J. Clin. Pharmacol., *22*:135, 1986.

120. Homeida, M., Halliwell, M., Branch, R.A.: Effects of an oral contraceptive on hepatic size and antipyrine metabolism in premenopausal women. Clin. Pharmacol. Ther., *24*:228, 1978.

121. Eadie, M.J., Lander, C.M., and Tyrer, J.H.: Plasma drug level monitoring in pregnancy. Clin. Pharmacokinet., *2*:427, 1977.

122. Perucca, E., Crema, A.: Plasma protein binding of drugs in pregnancy. Clin. Pharmacokin., *7*:336, 1982.

123. Chen, S.-S., et al.: Serum protein binding and free concentration of phenytoin and phenobarbitone in pregnancy. Br. J. Clin. Pharmacol., *13*:547, 1982.

124. Luxford, A.M.E., Kellaway, G.S.M.: Pharmacokinetics of digoxin in pregnancy. Eur. J. Clin. Pharmacol., *25*:117, 1983.

125. Philipson, A.: Pharmacokinetics of ampicillin during pregnancy. J. Infect. Dis., *136*:370, 1977.

126. Philipson, A.: Plasma levels of ampicillin in pregnant women following administration of ampicillin and pivampicillin. Am. J. Obstet. Gynecol., *130*:674, 1978.

127. Philipson, A.: The use of antibiotics in pregnancy. J. Antimicrob. Chemother., *12*:101, 1983.

128. Philipson, A., Stiernstedt, G., Ehrnebo, M.: Comparison of the pharmacokinetics of cephradine and cefazolin in pregnancy and nonpregnant women. Clin. Pharmacokin., *12*:136, 1987.

129. Assael, B.M., et al.: Ampicillin kinetics in pregnancy. Br. J. Clin. Pharmacol., *8*:286, 1979.

130. Montouris, G.D., Fenichel, G.M., and McLain, W.M.: The pregnant epileptic. A review and recommendations. Arch. Neurol., *36*:601, 1979.

131. Knight, A.H., and Rhind, E.G.: Epilepsy and pregnancy: A study of 153 pregnancies in 59 patients. Epilepsia, *16*:99, 1975.

132. Dalessio, D.J.: Seizure disorders and pregnancy. N. Engl. J. Med., *312*:559, 1985.

133. Levy, R.H., Yerby, M.S.: Effects of pregnancy on antiepileptic drug utilization. Epilepsia 26(Suppl 1):S52, 1985.

134. Skellern, G.G., et al.: The pharmacokinetics of methimazole in pregnant patients after oral administration of carbimazole. Br. J. Clin. Pharmacol., *9*:145, 1980.

135. Hogstedt, S., Lindberg, B., Rane, A.: Increased oral clearance of metoprolol in pregnancy. Eur. J. Clin. Pharmacol., *24*:217, 1983.

136. Hogstedt, S., et al.: Pregnancy-induced increase in metoprolol metabolism. Clin. Pharmacol. Ther., *37*:688, 1985.

137. Vesell, E.S.: Advance in pharmacogenetics. Prog. Med. Genet., *9*:291, 1973.

138. Vesell, E.S., Page, J.G., and Passananti, G.T.: Genetic and environmental factors affecting ethanol metabolism in man. Clin. Pharmacol. Ther., *12*:192, 1971.

139. Cascorbi, H.F., et al.: Genetic and environmental influence on halothane metabolism in twins. Clin. Pharmacol. Ther., *12*:50, 1971.

140. Furst, D.E., Gupta, N., and Paulus, H.E.: Salicylate metabolism in twins. Evidence suggesting a genetic influence and induction of salicylurate formation. J. Clin. Invest., *60*:32, 1977.

141. Alexanderson, B.: Prediction of steady-state plasma levels of nortriptyline from single oral dose kinetics: A study in twins. Eur. J. Clin. Pharmacol., *6*:44, 1973.

142. Alexanderson, B., and Borga, O.: Interindividual differences in plasma protein binding of nortriptyline in man. A twin study. Eur. J. Clin. Pharmacol., *4*:196, 1972.

143. Evans, D.A.P., Manley, K.A., and McKusick, V.C.: Genetic control of isoniazid metabolism in man. Br. Med. J., *2*:485, 1960.

144. Kalow, W.: Pharmacogenetics: Heredity and the Response to Drugs. Philadelphia, W.B. Saunders, 1962.

145. Lunde, P.K.M., Frislid, K., and Hansteen, V.: Disease and acetylation polymorph. Clin. Pharmacokinet., *2*:182, 1977.

146. Hughes, H.B., et al.: Metabolism of isoniazid in man as related to the occurrence of peripheral neuritis. Am. Rev. Tuberc., 70:266, 1954.

147. Devadatta, S., et al.: Peripheral neuritis due to isoniazid. Bull. WHO, 23:587, 1960.

148. Kutt, H., et al.: Diphenylhydantoin intoxication. A complication of isoniazid therapy. Am. Rev. Resp. Dis., 101:377, 1970.

149. Harris, H.W.: High-dose isoniazid compared with standard dose isoniazid with PAS in the treatment of previously untreated cavity pulmonary tuberculosis. In Transactions of the 20th Conference on Chemotherapy of Tuberculosis, 1961, p. 39.

150. Evans, D.A.P.: Genetic variations in the acetylation of isoniazid and other drugs. Ann. NY Acad. Sci., 151:723, 1968.

151. Ellard, G.A., and Gammon, P.T.: Acetylator phenotyping of tuberculosis patients using matrix isoniazid or sulphadimidine and its prognostic significance for treatment with several intermittent isoniazid-containing regimens. Br. J. Clin. Pharmacol., 4:5, 1977.

152. Bernstein, R.E.: Isoniazid hepatotoxicity and acetylation during tuberculosis chemoprophylaxis. Am. Rev. Resp. Dis., 121:429, 1980.

153. Lauterburg, B.H., et al.: Pharmacokinetics of the toxic hydrazine metabolites formed from isoniazid in humans. J. Pharmacol. Exp. Ther., 235:566, 1985.

154. Gulaid, A., et al.: Lack of correlation between acetylator status and the production of the acetyl metabolite of acebutolol in man. Br. J. Clin. Pharmacol., 5:261, 1978.

155. White, T.A., and Evans, D.A.P.: The acetylation of sulfamethazine and sulfamethoxypyridazine by human subjects. Clin. Pharmacol. Ther., 9:80, 1968.

156. Das, K.M., et al.: The metabolism of salicylazosulphapyridine in ulcerative colitis. The relationship between metabolites and the response to treatment in patients. Gut, 14:631, 1973.

157. Das, K.M., et al.: Adverse reactions during salicylazosulfapyridine therapy and the relation with drug metabolism and acetylator phenotype. N. Engl. J. Med., 289:491, 1973.

158. Das, K.M., and Dubin, R.: Clinical pharmacokinetics of sulphasalazine. Clin. Pharmacokinet., 1:406, 1976.

159. Carr, K., et al.: Simultaneous analysis of dapsone and monoacetyldapsone employing high performance liquid chromatography: a rapid method for determination of acetylator phenotype. Br. J. Clin. Pharmacol., 6:421, 1978.

160. Lima, J.J., and Jusko, W.J.: Determination of procainamide acetylator status. Clin. Pharmacol. Ther., 23:25, 1978.

161. Campbell, W., et al.: Acetylator phenotype and the clinical pharmacology of slow-release procainamide. Br. J. Clin. Pharmacol., 3:1023, 1976.

162. Uetrecht, J.P., and Woosley, R.L.: Acetylator phenotype and lupus erythematosus. Clin. Pharmacokinet., 6:118, 1981.

163. Woosley, R.L., et al.: Effect of acetylator phenotype on the rate at which procainamide induces antinuclear antibodies and the lupus syndrome. N. Engl. J. Med., 298:1157, 1978.

164. Shepherd, A.M.M., et al.: Plasma concentration and acetylator phenotype determine response to oral hydralazine. Hypertension, 3:580, 1981.

165. Perry, H.M., Jr., et al.: Relationship of acetyltransferase activity to antinuclear antibodies and toxic symptoms in hypertensive patients treated with hydralazine. J. Lab. Clin. Med., 76:114, 1970.

166. Litwin, A., et al.: Prospective study of immunological effects of hydralazine in hypertensive patients. Clin. Pharmacol. Ther., 29:477, 1981.

167. Ramsay, L.E., et al.: Should the acetylator phenotype be determined when prescribing hydralazine for hypertension? Eur. J. Clin. Pharmacol., 26:39, 1984.

168. Hamilton, R.A., et al.: Effect of acetylator phenotype on amrinone pharmacokinetics. Clin. Pharmacol. Ther., 40:615, 1986.

169. Evans, W.E., et al.: Dextromethorphan and caffeine as probes for simultaneous determination of debrisoquin-oxidation and N-acetylation phenotypes in children. Clin. Pharmacol. Ther., 45:568, 1989.

170. Mahgoub, A., et al.: Polymorphic hydroxylation of debrisoquine in man. Lancet, 2:584, 1977.

171. Sloan, T.P., et al.: Polymorphism of carbon oxidation of drugs and clinical implications. Br. Med. J., 2:655, 1978.

172. Bertilsson, L., et al.: Nortriptyline and antipyrine clearance in relation to debrisoquine hydroxylation in man. Life Sci., 27:1673, 1980.

173. Sloan, T.P., Idle, J.R., and Smith, R.L.: Influence of D^H/D^L alleles regulating debrisoquine oxidation on phenytoin hydroxylation. Clin. Pharmacol. Ther., 29:493, 1981.

174. Lennard, M.S., et al.: Defective metabolism of metoprolol in poor hydroxylators of debrisoquine. Br. J. Clin. Pharmacol., 14:301, 1982.

175. Oates, N.S., et al.: Genetic polymorphism of phenformin 4-hydroxylation. Clin. Pharmacol. Ther., 32:81, 1982.

176. Shah, R.R., et al.: Impaired oxidation of debrisoquine in patients with perhexiline neuropathy. Brit. Med. J., 284:295, 1982.

177. Osikownska-Evers, B., et al.: Evidence for altered catalytic properties of the cytochrome P-450 involved in sparteine oxidation in poor metabolizers. Clin. Pharmacol. Ther., 41:320, 1987.

178. Mortimer, O., et al.: Dextromethorphan: polymorphic serum pattern of the O-demethylated and didemethylated metabolites in man. Br. J. Clin. Pharmacol., 27:223, 1989.

179. Nakamura, K., et al.: Interethnic differences in genetic polymorphism of debrisoquin and mephenytoin hydroxylation between Japanese and Caucasian populations. Clin. Pharmacol. Ther., 38:402, 1985.

180. Steiner, E., et al.: A family study of genetic and environmental factors determining polymorphic hydroxylation of debrisoquin. Clin. Pharmacol. Ther., 38:394, 1985.

181. Idle, J.R., et al.: Some observations on the oxidation phenotype status of Nigerian patients presenting with cancer. Cancer Lett., 11:331, 1981.

182. Ayesh, R., et al.: Metabolic oxidation phenotypes as markers for susceptibility to lung cancer. Nature, 312:169, 1984.

183. Bertilsson, L., et al.: Debrisoquin hydroxylation polymorphism and personality. Lancet, 1:555, 1989.

184. Lewis, R.V., et al.: Timolol and atenolol: relationships between oxidation phenotype, pharmacokinetics and pharmacodynamics. Br. J. Clin. Pharmacol., 19:329, 1985.

185. Rahguram, T.C., et al.: Polymorphic ability to metabolize propranolol alters 4-hydroxypropranolol levels but not beta blockade. Clin. Pharmacol. Ther., 36:51, 1984.

186. Wang, T., et al.: Influence of genetic polymorphism on the metabolism and disposition of encainide in man. J. Pharmacol. Exp. Ther., 228:606, 1984.

187. Carey, E.L., et al.: Encainide and its metabolites. Comparative effects in man on electrocardiographic intervals. J. Clin. Invest., 73:539, 1984.

188. Barbey, J.T., et al.: Antiarrhythmic activity, electrocardiographic effects and pharmacokinetics of the encainide

metabolites O-desmethyl encainide and 3-methoxy-O-desmethyl encainide in man. Circul., 77:380, 1988.

189. Siddoway, L.A., et al.: Polymorphism of propafenone metabolism and disposition in man: clinical and pharmacokinetic consequences. Circul., 75:785, 1987.

190. Zoble, R.G., et al.: Pharmacokinetic and pharmacodynamic evaluation of propafenone in patients with ventricular arrhythmia. Clin. Pharmacol. Ther., 45:535, 1989.

191. Axelson, J.E., et al.: Food increases the bioavailability of propafenone. Br. J. Clin. Pharmacol., 23:735, 1987.

192. Brosen, K., Gram, L.F.: First-pass metabolism of imipramine and desipramine: Impact of the sparteine oxidation phenotype. Clin. Pharmacol. Ther., 43:400, 1988.

193. Mikus, G., et al.: The influence of the sparteine/debrisoquin phenotype on the disposition of flecainide. Clin. Pharmacol. Ther., 45:562, 1989.

194. Jurima, M., et al.: Genetic polymorphism of mephenytoin p(4')-hydroxylation: difference between Orientals and Caucasians. Br. J. Clin. Pharmacol., 19:483, 1985.

195. Wedlund, P.J., et al.: Mephenytoin hydroxylation deficiency in Caucasians: frequency of a new oxidative drug metabolism polymorphism. Clin. Pharmacol. Ther., 36:773, 1984.

196. Wedlund, P.J., et al.: Phenotypic differences in mephenytoin pharmacokinetics in normal subjects. J. Pharmacol. Exp. Ther., 234:662, 1985.

197. Meier, U.T., et al.: Mephenytoin hydroxylation polymorphism: characterization of the enzymatic deficiency in liver microsomes of poor metabolizers phenotyped in vivo. Clin. Pharmacol. Ther., 38:488, 1985.

198. Kupfer, A., Branch, R.A.: Stereoselective mephobarbital hydroxylation cosegregates with mephenytoin hydroxylation. Clin. Pharmacol. Ther., 38:414, 1985.

199. Bertilsson, L., et al.: Importance of genetic factors in the regulation of diazepam metabolism: relationship to S-mephenytoin, but not debrisoquin, hydroxylation phenotype. Clin. Pharmacol. Ther., 45:348, 1989.

200. Ward, S.A., et al.: Propranolol's metabolism is determined by both mephenytoin and debrisoquin hydroxylase activities. Clin. Pharmacol. Ther., 45:72, 1989.

13

Pharmacokinetic Variability—Disease

Pharmacokinetic data concerning specific drugs have come largely from studies in healthy, young adult subjects. This is paradoxical because drugs are used in sick people, of all ages. In the last decade, clinical scientists have directed their attention to this omission and have demonstrated the value of applying pharmacokinetics to the clinical setting. In parallel, regulatory agencies now require the pharmacokinetics of a new drug to be studied in the patient population in which it will be used.

Pharmacokinetic variability is greater in sick people than in healthy people. Disease affects various organ systems of the body and affects the way drugs are absorbed, distributed, excreted, and metabolized. Renal disease directly affects drug excretion, but also affects drug binding. Hepatic disease affects drug metabolism. Cardiovascular disease can substantially affect the transport of drugs to eliminating organs such as the liver and kidneys. These and similar considerations are the basis of this chapter.

RENAL DISEASE

Patients with renal disease need to be treated with a variety of drugs, both for their disease and intercurrent illness. Renal failure impairs the urinary excretion of drugs; drugs that are eliminated primarily by renal excretion accumulate excessively in a patient with renal insufficiency unless the dosage regimen is modified. Further complicating therapy in patients with renal disease are changes in drug distribution, potential effects on drug metabolism, and dialysis treatments.

Creatinine Clearance

Several methods are available to judge the degree of renal impairment in a patient. The most common way of assessing renal function is by de-termining the renal clearance of creatinine, the endogenous end product of muscle metabolism, and comparing this value to that observed in individuals of comparable size, sex, and age with normal renal function. Creatinine clearance may be measured directly or estimated indirectly from serum levels of creatinine.

Direct measurement of creatinine clearance is made by determining the amount of endogenous creatinine excreted in the urine over a 24-hr period and the creatinine concentration in the plasma during this period. Usually, blood samples are taken for creatinine determination immediately before and at the end of the urine collection period. Results of serum level determinations are averaged. The excretion rate of creatinine (expressed as mg/min) divided by the average creatinine concentration in the plasma (expressed as mg/ml) yields the endogenous creatinine clearance (in ml/min). Often, this value is normalized to a body surface area of 1.73 m^2. Normal values adjusted to 1.73 m^2 body surface area range from 140 to 180 L/24 hrs or 100 to 125 ml/min. Creatinine clearance values of 20 to 50 ml/min signify moderate renal failure; values < 10 ml/min signify severe renal failure.

Creatinine is poorly secreted and not subject to tubular reabsorption. Creatinine clearance is a useful measure of glomerular filtration rate (GFR) and although it tells us about only one aspect of renal function (i.e., filtration), it is an excellent indicator of the severity of renal disease.

This empiric observation led to the hypothesis called the intact nephron theory, which suggests that renal disease affects the entire nephron and does not selectively affect function. This hypothesis is an oversimplification of the disease process but it holds up well in clinical practice. The change in creatinine clearance should also reflect the effect

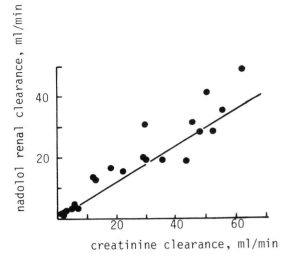

Fig. 13–1. Relationship between the renal clearance of nadolol, a β-blocker, and creatinine clearance in patients with varying degrees of renal function. (Data from Herrera, J., Vukovich, P.A., and Griffith, D.L.[2])

Table 13–1. Urinary Excretion of Nadolol After a Single 80-mg Oral Dose in Patients with Varying Degrees of Renal Function*

Patient group	Creatinine clearance (ml/min per 1.73 m^2)	Amount excreted (mg)
I	58	9.2
II	34	5.1
III	11	3.9
IV	2	0.6

*Data from Herrera, J., Vukovich, R.A., and Griffith, D.L.[2]

amount of unchanged nadolol excreted in the urine 120 hr after an oral dose of the drug to 4 groups of patients with different degrees of renal impairment. The amount of nadolol excreted decreases with decreasing renal function.

of renal disease on drug excretion, regardless of whether the drug is secreted or reabsorbed. This is usually the case.[1]

No other parameter of renal function other than GFR has been systematically evaluated as a quantitative index of drug excretion in patients with renal disease. It is not likely that assessment of renal blood flow or tubular function would prove more useful than GFR in developing dosage regimens for such patients.

Drug Excretion

Many studies have shown that there is a linear relationship between the renal clearance of a drug and creatinine clearance in patients with varying degrees of renal function. Figure 13–1 shows this relationship for nadolol, a relatively slowly eliminated β-blocker, in patients with hypertension.[2] The renal clearance of nadolol in essentially anephric patients is virtually zero. For nadolol and most other drugs, the following relationship applies:

Renal clearance

$$= A \times \text{Creatinine clearance} \quad (13-1)$$

where A is a drug-specific constant. For nadolol, A is equal to about 0.6.

Patients with renal disease also excrete less unchanged drug in the urine than patients with normal renal function. Table 13–1 shows the cumulative

Drug Elimination

The effect of renal disease on the elimination of a drug depends on the renal status of the patient and the elimination characteristics of the drug. The clearance of a drug eliminated only by renal excretion should be markedly affected in a patient with severe renal disease, but that of a drug eliminated only by hepatic metabolism should be unaffected, unless the disease process also affects drug metabolism.

The effect of changes in renal function on the elimination of 3 types of drugs is illustrated in

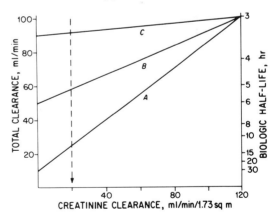

Fig. 13–2. Relationship between total clearance and renal function (creatinine clearance) for three drugs that are excreted in the urine to different degrees in patients with normal renal function. Vertical line shows clearances and half-lives when renal function is reduced to one-sixth of normal. Renal disease has the largest effect on drug A and the smallest effect on drug C. (From Gibaldi, M., and Levy, G.: Pharmacokinetics in clinical practice. I. Concepts. JAMA, *235:*1864, 1976. Copyright 1976, American Medical Association.)

Figure 13–2.[3] Drugs A, B, and C are 90%, 50% and 10% eliminated by renal excretion in patients with normal renal function. After parenteral administration of drug B to patients with normal renal function, the amount of unmetabolized drug ultimately found in the urine accounts for 50% of the dose. It is assumed that the nonrenal clearance of these drugs is unaffected by kidney disease and that renal clearance is linearly related to creatinine clearance, according to Equation 13–1. Under these conditions, as shown in Figure 13–2, the total clearance of the drug from blood or plasma is also a linear function of creatinine clearance:

Total clearance = A × Creatinine clearance

+ Nonrenal clearance
(13–2)

Figure 13–2 also shows how different the effect of renal impairment can be on the total clearance and half-life of different drugs. At a creatinine clearance of 20 ml/min per 1.73 m², the total clearance of drug A is decreased by 75%, that of drug B by 42%, and that of drug C by only 8.5%. The half-life of drug A increases from 3 hr in the patient with normal renal function to 30 hr in the anephric patient. The half-life of drug C hardly changes over this range of renal function.

Most cephalosporin, penicillin, and aminoglycoside antibiotics, ethambutol, flucytosine, vancomycin, lithium, and most diuretics are examples of drugs that, like drug A in Figure 13–2, are largely (> 80%) excreted unchanged.[4] Among the newer antibiotics, moxalactam[5] and cefoxitin[6] are also in this category. The total clearance of these drugs in the anephric patient will be less than 20% that measured in patients with normal renal function.

Digoxin, nadolol, and cimetidine are examples of drugs that, like drug B in Figure 13–2, are excreted unchanged in the urine to the extent of 40 to 75% of the dose.[4] Steady-state levels of these drugs are likely to be 2 to 4 times higher in anephric patients than in patients with normal renal function, unless the dosage is adjusted.

Drugs that are predominantly (i.e., > 80%) metabolized or otherwise eliminated by nonrenal mechanisms include most anticonvulsants, neuroleptics, and antidepressants, as well as digitoxin, chloramphenicol, and theophylline.

Current thinking suggests that individualized dosing of patients with renal disease be based on

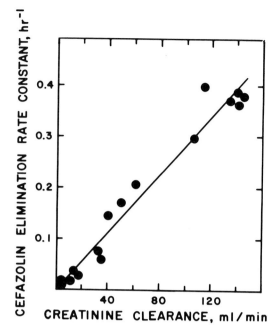

Fig. 13–3. Relationship between the elimination rate constant for cefazolin and renal function. (Data from Craig, W.A., et al.[7])

the relationship between total clearance and creatinine clearance expressed in Equation 13–2. Once we have cataloged the drug-specific constants (A and nonrenal clearance), we can estimate a patient's total clearance by simply plugging his creatinine clearance into Equation 13–2. This value can be compared to the total clearance of the drug in a population with normal renal function to determine if dosage adjustment is required.

Clearance correlations are used frequently today, but the historical developments in the field have favored the use of relationships between the elimination rate constant or half-life of a drug and creatinine clearance rather than between total clearance and creatinine clearance. Therefore, to use the drug literature, one must understand this alternative approach.

Total clearance is the product of the elimination rate constant (K) of the drug and its apparent volume of distribution (V). Accordingly, the elimination rate constant of a drug will be linearly related to creatinine clearance if the volume of distribution is unaffected by renal disease. In other words,

K = (A/V) Creatinine clearance

+ (Nonrenal clearance/V) (13–3)

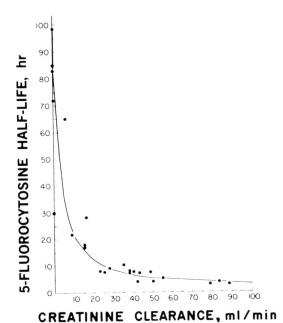

CREATININE CLEARANCE, ml/min

Fig. 13—4. Curvilinear relationship between the half-life of flucytosine (5-Fluorocytosine) and renal function. (Data from Schönebeck, J., et al.[10])

The relationship between renal function (creatinine clearance) and the overall elimination rate constant (K) of cefazolin, a cephalosporin antibiotic, after a single intramuscular (i.m.) dose to patients with different degrees of renal impairment is shown in Figure 13–3.[7] This kind of relationship has also been observed with nadolol,[2] cefoxitin,[6] amoxacillin,[8] and many other drugs.[1,9]

Because the half-life of a drug is reciprocally related to its elimination rate constant (i.e., $t_{1/2} = 0.693/K$), a curvilinear relationship between half-life and creatinine clearance is expected. The correlation between the half-life of flucytosine and creatinine clearance in patients with impaired kidney function and in nephrectomized or anuric patients is shown in Figure 13–4.[10]

Estimating Half-Life

The theory previously described permits one to estimate, with relatively little information, the half-life of a drug in a patient with renal disease. Knowledge of the pharmacokinetics of the drug in patients with normal renal function and of the patient's renal status is all that is required. The usual method is best described by example.

The problem is to estimate the half-life of ampicillin in a patient who has an endogenous creatinine clearance of 10 ml/min (i.e., one twelfth of normal). Ampicillin has an average half-life of 1.3 hr ($K = 0.693/t_{1/2}$ or 0.53 hr^{-1}) in patients with normal renal function. About 70% of a parenteral dose is excreted unchanged in the urine in normal subjects (i.e., $f = 0.7$). The renal excretion rate constant (k_e) and nonrenal elimination rate constant (k_{nr}) in normal subjects are calculated from the product of f and K, and the product of $(1 - f)$ and K, respectively. Thus $k_e = 0.37$ hr^{-1} and $k_{nr} = 0.16$ hr^{-1}. In the patient, the renal excretion rate constant is only one twelfth of normal or about 0.03 hr^{-1}. The nonrenal elimination rate constant is assumed to be unaffected by the disease. The overall elimination rate constant (K) is the sum of the renal and nonrenal elimination rate constants. Therefore, for this patient, $K = 0.19$ hr^{-1} and $t_{1/2} = 3.6$ hr. If the patient were anephric (i.e., $k_e = 0$), then $K = k_{nr}$ or 0.16 hr^{-1} and $t_{1/2} = 4.3$ hr. In principle, this approach can be applied to any drug.[1,9]

Dosage Regimens

The half-lives of some drugs are changed sufficiently in patients with impaired renal function to warrant a change in the usual dosage regimen to prevent accumulation of the drug in the body to toxic levels. Changes in regimen usually take the form of reducing the dose per dosing interval or increasing the length of the dosing interval. Either way, there is a reduction in the total daily dose. The dosage change is usually roughly proportional to the relative difference in half-life between the patient with renal disease and the patient with normal renal function.

For example, cephalexin is administered as a 250-mg to 1-g dose every 4 to 6 hr; its average half-life in patients with normal renal function is about 0.5 to 1 hr. In a patient with a creatinine clearance of 10 to 15 ml/min, the half-life of the drug is increased about 8-fold, because cephalexin is eliminated almost solely by urinary excretion. The dosing frequency suggested for the patient with this degree of renal impairment is the usual dose every 24 hr, a dosing interval 4 to 6 times longer than usual.[11] A similar approach has been suggested for amoxacillin[8] and procainamide.[4]

Because renal clearance accounts for more than 90% of the total clearance of moxalactam in patients with normal renal function, the dose of the drug must be reduced in patients with renal disease. One group of investigators suggested that a patient with a creatinine clearance of 50 ml/min receive half the usual dose of moxalactam at the usual time intervals and that a patient with a creatinine clearance of 10 ml/min be given 10% of the usual dose at the usual time intervals.[5]

The average half-life of digoxin is 1.6 days in patients with normal renal function but is increased to 4.4 days in anephric patients. The usual daily maintenance dose of digoxin ranges from 125 to 500 μg. The daily maintenance dose of digoxin in patients with little or no renal function, however, should be only one third to one half that used in patients with normal renal function.[12]

Renal excretion plays an important role in the elimination of all the histamine H_2-receptor antagonists currently available. About 75% of an iv dose of cimetidine is excreted unchanged in the urine. Urinary excretion accounts for about 70% of the elimination of ranitidine in patients with normal renal function. Sixty-five to 70% of an iv dose of famotidine and about two-thirds of an oral dose of nizatidine is excreted unchanged.

The pharmacokinetics of intravenous famotidine in patients with impaired renal function has been studied by Halstenson et al.[13] Patients were grouped on the basis of creatinine clearance (CrCl) as follows: mild renal impairment (CrCl = 30 to 60 ml/min); moderate-to-severe (CrCl = 10 to 30 ml/min); end-stage (CrCl < 10 ml/min). The average terminal half-life was about 9 hr for patients with mild or moderate-to-severe impairment but increased to about 18 hr in patients with end-stage renal impairment.

The clearance of famotidine decreased in a predictable fashion with decreasing renal function. Mean clearance was 109 ml/min in patients with mild impairment, 69 ml/min in those with moderate-to-severe failure, and 42 ml/min in anuric patients. Renal clearance accounted for nearly 60% of famotidine elimination in the mild group and about 30% in the moderate-to-severe group. Nonrenal clearance held constant at about 40 ml/min in all three groups.

The investigators concluded that because the apparent volume of distribution of famotidine does not vary with renal function, the dose in patients with renal impairment may be similar to that used for patients with normal renal function. However, because of decreased clearance in such patients, the dosing interval may need to be increased to avoid excessive drug accumulation and potential toxicity.

The angiotensin-converting enzyme (ACE) inhibition activity of enalapril resides largely in a diacid metabolite, enalaprilat, which is formed by hydrolysis of enalapril in the liver. Enalaprilat is extensively excreted unchanged. Lowenthal et al.[14] found that the total area under the enalaprilat concentration in serum versus time curve after a single oral dose of enalapril was 4 to 6 times greater in patients with creatinine clearance values ranging from 10 to 79 ml/min than in patients with normal renal function.

The prolonged reduction in blood pressure seen in patients with chronic renal failure is probably related to the elevated plasma levels of enalaprilat. Lowenthal et al. recommend that lower doses or less frequent dosing of enalapril be considered when treating hypertension in patients with renal insufficiency.

Patients with renal failure sometimes need loading doses because the time required to reach steady state with a particular drug may be much longer than in patients with normal renal function. This principle is particularly important when planning antibiotic or cardiac glycoside therapy.

The two methods for reducing maintenance dosage in patients with renal disease, lengthening the dosing interval or reducing the unit dose, are attractive because the required changes are easily calculated. However, when dosing interval extension is applied in severe renal disease to drugs with short half-lives, like the aminoglycoside antibiotics, prolonged periods of serum concentrations below the therapeutic range may result (Fig. 13–5).[15] On the other hand, administration of smaller doses with the usual frequency results in lower peak concentrations, which may be subtherapeutic, and higher trough concentrations, which may enhance the nephrotoxicity of the aminoglycoside antibiotics.[15]

With certain drugs it is best to combine dosage reduction with a change in the dosing interval. For example, the usual dose of carbenicillin required to maintain an average plasma concentration of 50 μg/ml in patients with normal renal function is about 1 g every 4 hr. The recommended dose to maintain equivalent levels in a patient with a creatinine clearance of 10 ml/min is 0.4 g every 8 hr.[16] This recommendation lowers the unit dose by 60% and doubles the dosage interval; it yields a drug concentration profile more similar to that observed in patients with normal renal function than would either dosage adjustment strategy alone.

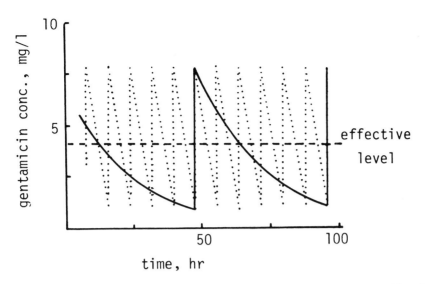

Fig. 13–5. Steady-state serum concentration profile for gentamicin in a patient with normal renal function who is given 1.7 mg/kg every 8 hr (stippled line) and in a patient with a creatinine clearance of 20 ml/min (one sixth of normal) who is given 1.7 mg/kg every 48 hr (solid line). (Data from Chennavasin, P., and Brater, D.C.[15])

Similar recommendations for aminoglycoside antibiotic dosage in renal failure have been reviewed by Chennavasin and Brater.[15]

It may also be prudent to change both the dose and dosing interval of vancomycin in patients with renal impairment. The use of this agent has increased dramatically in recent years because of the prevalence of infections caused by methicillin-resistant *Staph aureus* and the increased employment of prosthetic implants, which may become infected with *Staph epidermidis*. In patients with normal renal function, vancomycin is largely excreted unchanged.

Rodvold et al.[17] studied the kinetics of iv vancomycin in adult patients with various degrees of renal function, who were receiving the drug for treatment of gram-positive infections. Patients were categorized into three groups based on measured creatinine clearance: > 70, 40 to 70, and 10 to 39 ml/min per 1.73 m^2.

Vancomycin clearance decreased in a predictable manner, averaging 98 ml/min/1.73 m^2 in group 1, 53 in group 2, and 31 in group 3. Renal clearance accounted for about 90% of the total clearance of vancomycin in patients with normal renal function but for only 63% in patients with CrCl values less than 40 ml/min/1.73 m^2.

On the basis of these results, Rodvold et al. developed dosage guidelines. Their goal was to maintain peak levels of vancomycin in patients with impaired renal function similar to those seen in patients with normal renal function. They accomplished this by decreasing the daily dose while extending the dosing interval. They proposed the following algorithm for daily dose:

Daily Dose (mg/kg)

$$= 0.227 \ \text{CrCl} + 5.67 \quad (13\text{–}4)$$

where CrCl is expressed as ml/min per 70 kg. Practical dosing intervals ranged from every 8 hr to every 48 hr, based on renal function. The investigators suggested that vancomycin is to be given 3 times a day in patients with CrCl > 65 ml/min per 70 kg, once a day in patients with CrCl values of 20 to 39, and every other day in patients with CrCl values of 10 to 19.

A comprehensive guide to drug usage in adult patients with impaired renal function is available.[4] This guide consists of tables listing recommended dosing intervals of a wide variety of drugs for patients with mild, moderate, and severe renal failure. In most instances, the recommended dosing intervals are based on the clinical and pharmacokinetic principles discussed in the preceding paragraphs. More descriptive information on specific drugs is also available in two review articles concerned with drug prescribing in renal failure.[18,19] A nomogram for dosage adjustment in patients with renal failure is also available.[20]

Hemodialysis

Patients with renal failure may require intermittent hemodialysis, which can substantially augment the clearance of certain drugs in anephrics. Factors that influence drug removal during conventional hemodialysis are the molecular weight, lipid solubility, and binding of the drug, and the efficiency of the dialyzer.[21] Water-soluble drugs that have a molecular mass of less than 500 daltons and a small volume of distribution and that are poorly plasma protein bound are easily removed during dialysis.

One study in anephric patients found that the half-life of cephalexin was 6.3 hr on hemodialysis and 31 hr without dialysis.[11] The mean serum half-life of carbenicillin in anuric patients during hemodialysis was 4.3 hr compared to 14.6 hr off hemodialysis.[16] Large effects of hemodialysis have also been observed with nadolol,[2] cefoxitin,[6] amoxacillin,[8] cefamandole,[22] and other drugs.[21]

Dosage regimens for patients with renal failure that are developed without accounting for increased drug clearance during hemodialysis may result in periods of subtherapeutic drug levels. One report that recommends appropriately reduced dosing schedules for carbenicillin in anephric patients and in patients with severe renal impairment also advises that an additional 0.75 g or 1.5 g, depending on the desired steady-state level, should be given at the termination of each 6-hr hemodialysis to replace expected losses.[16]

Specific and sometimes complicated recommendations have been made to overcome the problem of drug removal during hemodialysis, but most clinical situations do not demand such rigorous approaches. It is common practice simply to replace one full maintenance dose for each dialysis period for drugs that are significantly cleared by conventional hemodialysis.[18]

Serum Creatinine

The difficulty in obtaining accurate 24-hr urine collections in patients for the purpose of estimating endogenous creatinine clearance has stimulated interest in other indicators of renal function that are easier to measure and might prove useful in predicting changes in drug elimination. One possibility is blood urea nitrogen (BUN). Although BUN is elevated in kidney disease, its level correlates poorly with creatinine clearance. On the other hand, serum creatinine, which is also elevated in patients with impaired renal function, appears to correlate well with creatinine clearance.

Two reports have compared 24-hr creatinine excretion and serum creatinine concentrations as indicators of renal function.[23,24] Both conclude that serum creatinine levels are superior to measured creatinine clearances for the detection of abnormal glomerular function and of changes in glomerular function in patients with chronic renal disease. Morgan and co-workers propose that direct measurement of creatinine clearance be abandoned as a routine measure of glomerular function.[23]

The use of serum creatinine concentrations to determine renal function has been reviewed in considerable detail by Lott and Hayton[25] and by Bjornsson.[26] Normal serum creatinine concentrations vary from 0.6 to 1.0 mg per 100 ml (mg/dl) in women and 0.8 to 1.3 mg/dl in men. In principle, the following equation describes the relationship between creatinine clearance (CrCl) and serum creatinine concentration (SCC) in a patient with stable renal function:

$$CrCl = k_o/SCC \qquad (13\text{--}5)$$

where k_o is the endogenous creatinine production rate. Serum creatinine remains constant unless there is a change in the rate of production of creatinine or in creatinine clearance.

It would be a simple matter to estimate creatinine clearance from SCC values if k_o were the same for everyone. Of course, this is not the case. The production rate of endogenous creatinine varies as a function of age, body weight, and sex.

Because creatinine production is proportional to lean body mass and inversely proportional to age, investigators have been able to develop formulas and nomograms for estimating creatinine clearance without the need for urine collection. The following equation is particularly useful;[27] it has been validated in hundreds of nonobese adult patients of both sexes with widely varying degrees of renal function:

$$CrCl = \frac{(140 - age)\ (body\ weight)}{72 \times SCC} \qquad (13\text{--}6)$$

Age is expressed in years, body weight in kg, and SCC in mg/dl. The same equation is used for male and female patients, but the value determined should be reduced by 15% for a female patient.[27]

According to Equation 13–6, a 20-yr-old, 70-kg male patient with a serum creatinine of 1 mg/dl has a creatinine clearance of 117 ml/min. The same patient with an elevated serum creatinine of 5 mg/dl has a creatinine clearance of 23 ml/min.

Table 13–2. Some Clinically Important Active or Toxic Drug Metabolites that Accumulate in Renal Failure

Drug	Metabolite
Allopurinol	Oxipurinol
Clofibrate	Chlorophenoxyisobutyric acid
Meperidine	Normeperidine
Procainamide	N-Acetylprocainamide
Propoxyphene	Norpropoxyphene

An 80-yr-old, 70-kg man with an apparently normal serum creatinine of 1 mg/dl has a creatinine clearance of only 58 ml/min.

Equation 13–6 applies to a remarkably large segment of the population. It overestimates measured creatinine clearance in the pregnant patient and may overestimate creatinine clearance in patients with edema or ascites.[18] Creatinine clearance is also overestimated in at least some patients with liver disease[28] and in obese patients, when total body weight is used in Equation 13–6.[29] Estimation of creatinine clearance from serum creatinine in obese patients is particularly difficult because substituting ideal body weight for total body weight in Equation 13–6 may also yield incorrect estimates of creatinine clearance.[29]

The estimation of creatinine clearance from serum creatinine in pediatric patients has also been evaluated, and clinically useful relationships have been developed.[30,31]

Effects on Metabolized Drugs

The rather simple theory used to explain and predict the influence of renal disease on drug elimination assumes that the pharmacokinetics of drugs eliminated by hepatic metabolism is unaffected by impairment of renal function. This is not always the case.

The incidence of adverse effects of certain highly metabolized drugs like phenytoin, clofibrate, and diazepam is higher in patients with renal disease than in patients with normal renal function. This may be related to changes in plasma protein binding that are evident in chronic renal failure and are discussed later in this chapter. Alternatively, drug metabolism may be inhibited or there may be the accumulation of metabolites that have pharmacologic activity but that are ordinarily excreted in the urine.

Patients with impaired renal function may experience severe and prolonged respiratory depression when treated with morphine, although morphine is extensively metabolized.[32] Improbably,

this has been attributed to accumulation of the drug during renal failure. Wolff et al.[33] studied the influence of renal function, as determined by the clearance of labeled EDTA, on morphine and morphine glucuronide pharmacokinetics in patients with various chronic renal diseases after a single iv dose of morphine. No relationship was found between total body clearance of morphine and renal function, but patients with renal insufficiency had impaired elimination of morphine glucuronides. The apparent clearance of the glucuronides was significantly correlated with EDTA clearance (r = 0.94).

These results suggest that the accumulation of a morphine metabolite, most likely morphine 6-glucuronide, rather than of morphine itself is the cause of enhanced activity and toxicity of morphine in patients with renal failure. Morphine 6-glucuronide crosses the blood-brain barrier, has a high affinity for the opioid receptor, and has opioid agonist activity.

The pharmacokinetic and clinical implications of drug metabolites in renal failure have been reviewed by Verbeeck and Branch.[34] Table 13–2 lists some clinically important active or toxic drug metabolites that accumulate in renal failure.

Several recent reports have addressed the regeneration of parent drug from glucuronide conjugates that accumulate in patients with renal failure. The net effect of this conversion is a decreased clearance of the parent drug. In the case of lorazepam,[34] diflusinal,[35] and clofibrate,[36] it appears that when the renal excretion of the glucuronide conjugate is impaired, the conjugate accumulates in plasma where it is hydrolyzed to regenerate parent drug.

Renal failure may also produce a more direct inhibition of drug metabolism. This has been elegantly demonstrated by Terao and Shen.[37] They found that first-pass metabolism of the l-isomer of propranolol was reduced in rats with chemically-induced acute renal failure. When livers from normal rats were perfused with diluted blood from normal rats, a very high extraction ratio was observed. Less than 3% of the dose escaped first-pass metabolism. The extraction of l-propranolol was significantly lower when livers from rats with acute renal failure were perfused with diluted blood from uremic rats. The percent of dose evading first-metabolism increased more than 3-fold, from 2.6% to 9.4%.

An interesting question arises from these observations. Does the basis for the impaired first-pass metabolism reside in the uremic liver or in the uremic blood? Terao and Shen found that when livers from normal rats were cross-perfused with uremic blood, first-pass metabolism was decreased to almost the same level as when livers from renal failure rats were perfused with uremic blood. The percent of dose evading first-pass metabolism was 7.3%. In contrast, livers from renal failure rats cross-perfused with normal blood exhibited l-propranolol extraction comparable to normal livers perfused with normal blood. The percent of dose evading first-pass metabolism was 3%.

The investigators concluded that the decrease in presystemic hepatic extraction of l-propranolol in the rat model of acute renal failure is due to the presence of an inhibitory factor in uremic blood. No apparent changes in the intrinsic activities of the hepatic transport and/or drug metabolizing enzyme systems were observed. They caution, however, that although the microsomal cytochrome P450 enzymes responsible for the biotransformation of propranolol did not appear to be affected by acute renal failure, this may not be the case in chronic renal failure.

Reduced drug metabolism had also been observed in patients with renal failure given encainide,[38] an antiarrhythmic agent eliminated almost entirely by oxidative metabolism. After a single iv and oral dose of encainide, its systemic and oral clearances were significantly lower in patients with renal failure than in healthy human subjects. Chronic oral dosing to steady state resulted in nearly a 2-fold increase in levels of O-desmethyl-encainide (ODE), the most important active metabolite, and a 3-fold increase in levels of 3-methoxy-ODE, another active metabolite, compared with levels measured in healthy subjects. The investigators concluded that patients with renal failure will require lower doses of encainide because of reduced clearance of encainide and increased accumulation of active metabolites.

End-stage renal disease also affects the disposition of sulindac. Sulindac is a prodrug. Ordinarily, it undergoes two major biotransformations: irreversible oxidation to an inactive sulfone metabolite and reversible reduction to a pharmacologically active sulfide metabolite.

Gibson et al.[39] determined areas under the plasma level-time curves (AUCs) after a single oral dose of sulindac to patients with end-stage renal failure. The AUC values for sulindac and the sulfone were similar to values measured in control subjects, but the AUC for the sulfide was only about one-third that found in controls.

Plasma protein binding of sulindac as well as binding of its two major metabolites was found to be lower in patients with renal failure. When corrected for protein binding, the AUC values for sulindac and the sulfone were twice that of controls, whereas that of the sulfide was about half the AUC determined in control subjects. The investigators concluded that end-stage renal failure impairs the reduction of sulindac to the active sulfide, whereas oxidation to the sulfone appears to be intact. These patients may require higher than normal doses of sulindac to achieve adequate control of rheumatic symptoms.

LIVER DISEASE

When hepatic metabolism is an important route of drug elimination, dysfunction of the liver could lead to changes in the pharmacokinetics of the drug. The clinical significance of the changes in drug metabolism, however, depends on the type and severity of the disease and on the pharmacokinetics of the drug. In a survey of some 30 investigations with many different drugs, only about two thirds of the studies showed a significant difference in drug elimination between patients with liver disease and patients or subjects with normal liver function.[40] No differences were reported for chlorpromazine, dicumarol, phenytoin, or salicylate. Other reports suggest that mild to moderate acute viral hepatitis has no effect on the disposition of warfarin[41] and that liver cirrhosis has little effect on the elimination of acetaminophen.[42]

The effects of liver disease on the pharmacokinetics of drugs are unpredictable, but clearly the elimination of some potent drugs is impaired in patients with chronic liver disease. The lack of predictability relates to the multiple effects that liver disease produces, effects on drug metabolizing enzymes, on drug binding, and on hepatic blood flow. It also relates to the complexity of hepatic metabolism; some enzyme systems seem to be far more sensitive to the effects of disease than other systems. Because of the lack of predictability, review articles that enumerate the effects of different hepatic diseases on the pharmacokinetics of specific drugs are useful to the physician and pharmacist in formulating dosage requirements for the individual patient.[43] A more recent guide to drug dosage in hepatic disease is also available.[44]

Considerable progress has been made during the last decade in our understanding of the effects of liver disease on drug disposition. A great deal of the literature has been reviewed by Howden et al.[45]

Antipyrine

Antipyrine has been used widely as a model drug to investigate the effects of liver disease on drug metabolism in man. Because antipyrine is negligibly bound to plasma proteins and tissues, and because it is eliminated almost exclusively by hepatic metabolism with a low hepatic extraction ratio, its half-life and clearance are considered sensitive indicators of liver function with respect to oxidative metabolism.

The usual procedure for calculating antipyrine clearance involves collection of 4 to 7 samples of blood or saliva during a 24 to 48 hr period after oral or iv administration of a single dose. To determine whether this procedure could be simplified, the usual method was compared in a large number of subjects with one based on the determination of antipyrine concentration in a single blood sample and an estimated volume of distribution.[46]

When the single sample was taken 18 to 27 hr after antipyrine administration, correlation coefficients between the one-point method and the customary method ranged from 0.97 to 0.99 and regression coefficients approximated unity. Useful correlations were obtained simply by assuming a volume of distribution of 40 L (total body water) for all subjects; more sophisticated estimates of total body water based on lean body weight, age, sex and height improved the correlation.

The term liver disease encompasses several distinct hepatic diseases, not a single disease entity. The particular disease and its severity are factors in drug metabolism. This is clearly seen in a study evaluating antipyrine half-life in patients with various liver diseases.[47] In general, the half-life of antipyrine was prolonged in these patients compared to that found in healthy subjects. Patients with chronic liver disease, however, showed a greater increase in half-life than those with acute, reversible conditions.

Compared to healthy subjects who had an average half-life of 12 hr, patients with cirrhosis and chronic active hepatitis had average antipyrine half-lives of 34 hr and 26 hr, respectively. Certain individuals in both groups had half-lives on the order of 50 hr. On the other hand, patients with acute hepatitis or obstructive jaundice showed relatively

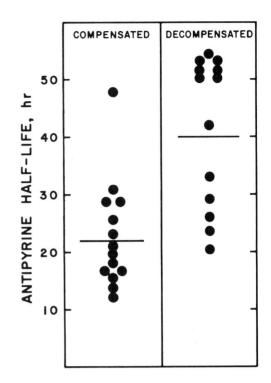

Fig. 13–6. Comparison of antipyrine half-life in patients with compensated liver disease (serum albumin >3 g/dl, prothrombin index >80%) and in patients with decompensated liver disease (serum albumin <3 g/dl, prothrombin index <80%). (Data from Branch, R.A., Herbert, C.M., and Read, A.E.[47])

small differences in antipyrine half-life from that found in normal subjects.

The most marked prolongation in antipyrine half-life was found in association with hypoalbuminemia and hypoprothrombinemia, suggesting that these changes were the result of or related to altered synthesis of microsomal enzyme protein.[47] Antipyrine half-lives in patients with "compensated" liver disease and in patients in whom the disease was "decompensated" are shown in Figure 13–6. Compensated patients had a serum albumin higher than 3 g/dl and a prothrombin index above 80%. Serum albumin and prothrombin index in the decompensated group were less than 3 g/dl and below 80%.

Mehta et al.[48] studied antipyrine kinetics before and after liver transplantation in 5 patients. After transplantation, there was a significant increase in antipyrine clearance and a marked decrease in antipyrine half-life. Mean clearance was 16.6 ml/min before and 36 ml/min after transplantation. Mean half-life decreased from 28 to 13 hr.

In another study, the total clearance of antipyrine

was determined in healthy subjects, in patients with cirrhosis, and in patients with severe liver disease before, during, and after hepatic encephalopathy.[49] The average antipyrine clearance in control subjects was about 51 ml/min. Patients with cirrhosis but no sign of encephalopathy showed an average antipyrine clearance of 17 ml/min. Antipyrine clearance measured in patients during hepatic encephalopathy (4.6 ml/min) was significantly lower than that of patients investigated 4 wk before or after encephalopathy (9.6 ml/min).

Table 13–3 shows the results of liver function tests and antipyrine clearance over a 5-month period in a patient with reversible hepatic encephalopathy. During the acute phase of the disease, results of all liver function tests were grossly abnormal; antipyrine clearance was depressed to 5.9 ml/min. Table 13–3 also shows that certain biochemical tests are poor indicators of the liver's ability to metabolize antipyrine. For example, 1 month after the first examination, galactose elimination and prothrombin index had returned to the normal range but antipyrine clearance was still only about one half of normal. Andreasen and Ranek suggest that the antipyrine clearance may serve as a quantitative measure of liver function and that it may be useful as a prognostic indicator of acute liver failure.[49]

Other Drugs with a Low Hepatic Extraction Ratio

The elimination of drugs that have a low hepatic extraction ratio and are largely cleared by metabolism in the liver is rate limited by the activity of hepatic drug metabolizing enzymes. The clearance of these drugs should be sensitive to changes in hepatic enzymes secondary to disease. A given liver disease, however, does not affect all enzyme pathways to the same extent. Therefore, the elimination of certain low extraction ratio drugs, such

as warfarin, salicylate, and phenytoin, is seemingly unimpaired by liver disease, at least in some cases.

Most drugs with low hepatic extraction ratios are like antipyrine in that their elimination is impaired in patients with moderate to severe hepatic disease. Many studies have been directed to the elimination of benzodiazepines in patients with hepatic dysfunction, particularly to the elimination of diazepam.[50]

The clearance of diazepam in patients with alcoholic cirrhosis is only about half that in age-matched control subjects. The half-life of the drug is increased about 4-fold over control values because of a decrease in clearance and an increase in apparent volume of distribution, consistent with reduced plasma protein binding of diazepam in the cirrhotics (Table 13–4).[51] These findings have been confirmed by other investigators.[52–54]

Branch and co-workers reported a significant correlation between the clearance of diazepam, or the dose of a constant rate intravenous infusion of diazepam required to produce a given degree of sedation, and the severity of the disease, as judged by serum albumin concentration.[53] Correlations between diazepam clearance and biochemical indices of the disease process were also found by Greenblatt and associates.[54]

In another study, Ochs et al.[55] gave a 5-mg dose of diazepam once daily for 3 weeks to patients with biopsy-proven cirrhosis and to healthy control subjects of similar age and weight. Steady-state levels of diazepam were 98 ng/ml in control subjects and 165 ng/ml in patients with liver disease. Corresponding levels of the active metabolite of diazepam, desmethyldiazepam, were about twice as high in patients with hepatic cirrhosis as in healthy subjects.

Sedation increased with time in all subjects during diazepam administration. Sedative effects, however, were significantly greater in cirrhotic

Table 13–3. Liver Function Tests and Antipyrine Clearance in a Patient with Reversible Hepatic Encephalopathy*

Date of examination	Hepatic encephalopathy	Galactose elimination (mmol/min)	Prothrombin (%)	Bilirubin (μmol/L)	Alanine amino-transferase (U/L)	Antipyrine clearance (ml/min)
July 7, 1973	Yes	1.1	12	540	430	5.9
July 25, 1973	No	1.6	57	454	130	13.5
August 9, 1973	No	1.7	129	107	70	29.3
December 4, 1973	No	2.2	94	15	10	54.5
Normal values		1.4–3.5	85–115	<17	5–25	50 ± 14

*Data from Andreasen, P.B., and Ranek, L.[49]

Table 13–4. Pharmacokinetic Parameters of Diazepam in Patients with Alcoholic Cirrhosis and in Age-Matched Control Subjects*

Parameter	Control	Alcoholic cirrhosis
Age, yr	44	46
Half-life, hr	27	106
Clearance, ml/min	27	14
Volume of distribution, l/kg	1.1	1.7
% Unbound in plasma	2.2	4.7

*Data from Klotz, U., et al.[51]

than in control subjects. Reduction of the daily diazepam dose by about 50% is probably appropriate for patients with hepatic cirrhosis.

Substantially impaired metabolism and changes in volume of distribution have also been found with chlordiazepoxide in patients with cirrhosis or acute viral hepatitis,[56] but not with oxazepam or lorazepam.[50] The elimination of diazepam and chlordiazepoxide primarily involves oxidative metabolism, whereas oxazepam and lorazepam are metabolized by glucuronic acid conjugation. In view of these differences, oxazepam and lorazepam are preferred for patients with liver disease.

The clearance of theophylline is also reduced in patients with liver disease,[57,58] particularly those with decompensated liver cirrhosis.[59] One study reported that patients with cirrhosis had a much longer half-life of theophylline (26 hr vs 7 hr) when compared to healthy subjects.[57] Another study found a significant correlation between theophylline clearance and serum bilirubin levels in patients with cirrhosis.[58] The maintenance dose of theophylline usually must be reduced in patients with liver disease to avoid toxicity.

In principle, one would expect liver disease to have little effect on the elimination of cimetidine because more than 60% of an iv dose is excreted unchanged in the urine. Nevertheless, the common use of cimetidine to treat peptic ulcers associated with chronic liver disease prompted a study to examine the effects of cirrhosis on the disposition of cimetidine.[60]

Cimetidine clearance after iv administration was similar in patients with chronic liver cirrhosis and in control subjects with ulcers, but nonrenal clearance was significantly smaller in patients with cirrhosis. Apparent volume of distribution of cimetidine was larger in cirrhotics but oral bioavailability was about the same in each group, about 70–75%. Irrespective of route of administration, patients in the control group excreted a smaller fraction of the dose as unmetabolized cimetidine.

Plasma levels of cimetidine after oral administration tended to be higher in patients with cirrhosis than in control patients. The time after a single oral dose during which plasma levels exceeded 0.5 mg/L was 205 min in controls and 295 min in cirrhotics. Clinically, liver disease would seem to require reduction of cimetidine dose only in the elderly or severely sick patient. The association between cimetidine and mental confusion occurs primarily in patients with organ failure and of advanced age.

The important role of hepatic metabolism in the activation and elimination of sulindac and its sulfide metabolite prompted Juhl et al.[61] to study the pharmacokinetics of sulindac in patients with confirmed alcoholic liver disease. Patients were divided into two groups based on their ability to eliminate indocyanine green (ICG), a marker of hepatic blood flow and hepatic function. Patients with ICG half-lives greater than 10 min were considered to have poor hepatic function; those with half-life values less than 10 min were classified as having fair hepatic function.

Serum levels of sulindac and its sulfide after a single oral dose of sulindac were considerably higher in patients with poor liver function than in healthy subjects. AUC values were 37 vs 13 μg-hr/ml for sulindac and 39 vs 10 μg-hr/ml for the sulfide. Average blood levels of the sulfide, the active form of the drug, were nearly 4 times higher in patients with poor hepatic function than in healthy subjects. The clinical consequences of these findings are uncertain, but the results suggest that sulindac be used cautiously in patients with poor hepatic function.

Fluoxetine is a novel antidepressant, chemically unrelated to the large group of tricyclic compounds widely used for the treatment of depression. The drug is well absorbed after oral administration, 94% bound to plasma proteins, and demethylated, presumably in the liver, to an active metabolite, norfluoxetine. The half-life of the parent drug is about 4 days and the half-life of the active metabolite is about 7 days.

Schenker et al.[62] studied the disposition of oral fluoxetine in healthy male subjects with normal liver function and in male patients with stable alcoholic cirrhosis. The total AUC following a single dose of fluoxetine was nearly twice as large in patients for both fluoxetine and its metabolite. The oral clearance of fluoxetine was 9.6 ml/min/kg in control subjects and 4.2 ml/min/kg in patients with cirrhosis.

The investigators suggested that at steady state both fluoxetine and norfluoxetine levels will be higher in patients with cirrhosis, unless the dosage is reduced. A 50% reduction would appear appropriate for the well-compensated cirrhotics examined in this study but a larger reduction may be needed in sicker patients. Unfortunately, conventional liver tests and ICG clearance did not correlate well with the apparent clearance of fluoxetine in individual patients, so extrapolation is not possible.

The pharmacokinetics of flecainide have also been studied in patients with documented cirrhosis of the liver.[62] All patients had abnormal values for most of the routine liver functions tests, and for albumin levels and prothrombin time. The mean, weight-adjusted, apparent clearance after a single oral dose of flecainide was reduced 60% in patients with cirrhosis compared with healthy control subjects. Renal clearance of flecainide was similar in each group. The average ratio of renal clearance to total clearance was 0.40 for healthy subjects and 0.83 for patients with cirrhosis of the liver, indicating that in patients with cirrhosis much less flecainide is eliminated by biotransformation than by renal excretion of unchanged drug.

Plasma levels of flecainide in patients with liver disease may accumulate to unacceptably high levels with usual therapeutic dosage regimens. According to McQuinn et al.,[63] in such cases, "the use of plasma level monitoring as a guide for dosage adjustments is very important." Particular caution must be exercised when flecainide is given to patients with liver disease along with other drugs known to inhibit drug metabolism.

Enalapril, like sulindac, requires bioactivation. The conversion of enalapril to enalaprilat appears to occur in the liver and it is important to know the pharmacokinetics and pharmacodynamics of enalapril in patients with cirrhosis. Ohnishi et al.[64] determined these parameters in biopsy-proven cirrhotic patients and healthy control subjects after oral administration of enalapril.

The peak concentration of enalapril after a single oral dose was nearly twice as high in the cirrhotic patients as in the controls and mean apparent clearance was much lower in the patients with liver disease (653 vs 1527 ml/min). Serum levels of enalaprilat, the active form of enalapril, in patients

with cirrhosis, were less than half those observed in control subjects.

The clinical implications of this study are unclear. Although the results suggest that the bioactivation of enalapril to enalaprilat is substantially impaired in patients with cirrhosis, the effects of the drug on blood pressure, heart rate, serum angiotensin-converting enzyme, and plasma renin activity appeared to be unaffected. The investigators cautioned that "the full therapeutic implication of the findings from this single-dose study must await further multiple-dose studies in patients with cirrhosis."

High Hepatic Extraction Ratio Drugs

Cirrhosis and other liver dysfunctions affect not only hepatic drug metabolizing enzymes but also liver blood flow.[65] Thus, hepatic disease can affect the disposition of high hepatic extraction ratio drugs in two ways. After oral administration, presystemic metabolism will be less in a cirrhotic patient than in a patient with normal hepatic function; the same oral dose may produce higher blood levels in the cirrhotic patient because systemic availability is greater. Once the drug is in the bloodstream, its clearance is lower in the cirrhotic patient than in the healthy individual because of reduced hepatic perfusion and decreased hepatic enzyme activity.

Indocyanine green (ICG) is eliminated so rapidly by the human liver that its clearance is often used as an indicator of hepatic blood flow rate. The disposition of intravenous ICG and lidocaine, another high hepatic extraction ratio drug, was studied in patients during and after recovery from an episode of acute viral hepatitis.[66] On the average, the clearance of both drugs was about 40% lower during the acute phase than after recovery. A similar decrease in ICG clearance has been found in patients with chronic liver disease.[67] These observations are consistent with the idea that a reduction in liver blood flow will decrease the clearance of drugs with high intrinsic hepatic clearance.

The importance of liver blood flow in the disposition of drugs with a high hepatic extraction ratio has been elegantly demonstrated by Feely et al.[68] with lidocaine in patients with orthostatic hypotension. They found that an abrupt change in position from supine to upright in healthy subjects resulted in an average decrease in mean arterial pressure (MAP) of only 2 mm Hg and a mean fall of about 5% in liver blood flow, estimated using ICG clearance. In patients with idiopathic orthostatic hypotension, however, a change in position resulted in a 24 mm Hg drop in MAP and a 30% decrease in liver blood flow.

The patients with orthostatic hypotension were studied on a second occasion to determine lidocaine clearance as a function of MAP and hepatic blood flow. Each subject received a 60 mg iv injection of lidocaine over 2 min, first in the supine position and then in the tilted (upright) position. MAP fell from 91 to 67 mm Hg when the table was tilted. Peak concentration of lidocaine was nearly twice as high in the upright than in the supine position. Lidocaine clearance decreased from 602 ml/min in the supine position to 475 ml/min in the upright position.

The clearance of propranolol is also lower in patients with alcoholic cirrhosis than in healthy subjects (580 ml/min vs 860 ml/min). After oral administration, systemic availability is 38% of the dose in control subjects and 54% in cirrhotic patients. The steady-state free drug concentration of propranolol following repetitive oral dosing is about 3 times higher in patients with cirrhosis than in control subjects, reflecting increased bioavailability, decreased clearance, and an increase in fraction free in the plasma.[69]

Similar results have been observed with metoprolol, another high hepatic extraction ratio β-blocker.[70] Bioavailability was 84% in patients with hepatic cirrhosis and 50% in a control group. The total body clearance of metoprolol was 0.61 L/min in cirrhotic patients and 0.80 L/min in the control subjects.

Dramatic increases in the systemic availability of oral analgesics have been observed in patients with cirrhosis. Intravenous and oral studies with pentazocine and meperidine in patients with moderate cirrhosis and in age-matched healthy subjects found that, compared to control subjects, there was a 46% decrease in the clearance of pentazocine and a 278% increase in bioavailability, and a 36% decrease in the clearance of meperidine and an 81% increase in bioavailability in cirrhotic patients.[71]

Consistent with theory, these studies suggest that the higher the intrinsic hepatic clearance of a drug, the larger is the increase in systemic availability of the drug in patients with cirrhosis. The decrease in clearance and increase in bioavailability have large effects on blood levels of the drug after oral administration. One eighth the dosage of pentazocine and one third the dosage of meperidine is required in cirrhotic patients to produce blood lev-

els comparable to those in healthy subjects after usual doses.[71]

Triamterene is a potassium-sparing diuretic that is efficiently metabolized by the liver and subject to a considerable first-pass effect on oral administration. Villeneuve et al.[72] studied the pharmacokinetics of triamterene in healthy control subjects and in patients with severe alcoholic cirrhosis. Each subject received a single 200 mg oral dose.

A profound difference was observed between the two groups. Mean oral clearance was 1617 ml/min in the control subjects but only 134 ml/min in patients with liver disease. The ratio of p-hydroxy-triamterene sulfate, a primary metabolite, to triamterene in plasma was 7.18 in the healthy subjects and 0.55 in the patients with cirrhosis.

The change in triamterene kinetics in patients with severe alcoholic cirrhosis resulted in prolongation of its natriuretic effect from 8 hr in control subjects to 48 hr in the patients. The overall diuretic response, however, as estimated by the cumulative increase in sodium excretion over 48 hr, was similar in both groups.

Nifedipine and related calcium channel blockers are less than completely available after oral administration because of first-pass metabolism. Kleinbloesem et al.[73] studied nifedipine in 7 patients with liver cirrhosis and in an equal number of age-matched healthy control subjects. All of the patients had varices and 3 had a portacaval shunt.

After an iv dose, nifedipine levels persisted far longer in patients with cirrhosis than in matched controls. The half-life of nifedipine was 420 min in patients and 111 min in controls. Clearance was decreased by more than 50%; mean values of 588 ml/min were calculated in controls and 233 ml/min in patients with cirrhosis. The unbound fraction of nifedipine in plasma was almost doubled in patients with liver disease (8.5 vs 4.4%), suggesting that the effect of cirrhosis on unbound clearance of nifedipine was even greater than on total clearance.

Large differences were also observed after oral administration of a controlled-release tablet containing 20 mg nifedipine. Absolute bioavailability was about 50% in the control subjects, with a range from 20 to 70%. A substantially greater bioavailability was determined in the patients with cirrhosis, particularly those with a shunt. Bioavailability ranged from 48 to 99% in patients that did not have a shunt, with a mean value of about 75%. Bioavailability was 100% in all 3 patients with a portacaval shunt. The large effects of a surgical portacaval shunt on the pharmacokinetics and oral bioavailability of lidocaine, another drug subject to extensive first-pass metabolism after oral administration, has been reported by others.[74]

Gengo et al.[75] found that cirrhosis has similar effects on the pharmacokinetics of nimodipine, a recently approved calcium channel blocker. The apparent oral clearance was 217 ml/min in the patients and 519 ml/min in healthy control subjects. The patients with cirrhosis also showed a greater fall in MAP after a single dose of nimodipine than did the control subjects. A statistically significant relationship was demonstrated in most patients between MAP and nimodipine levels in plasma.

Nitrendipine is also a dihydropyridine that blocks calcium transport through vascular smooth muscle cells and antagonizes calcium-induced contraction. Dylewicz et al.[75] studied the pharmacokinetics of nitrendipine after an iv injection and repeated oral administrations in healthy subjects and in patients with liver disease (cirrhosis, chronic hepatitis, or acute hepatitis). The systemic clearance of nifedipine was reduced from 1290 ml/min in control subjects to 853 and 840 ml/min, respectively, in patients with either liver cirrhosis or chronic hepatitis. The systemic clearance of nitrendipine in patients with acute hepatitis was similar to the values found in control subjects.

On repeated oral administration of nitrendipine, 20 mg once daily, steady-state levels were about 3 times greater than control values in patients with cirrhosis, about 2 times greater in patients with chronic hepatitis, and about the same as controls in patients with acute hepatitis.

Buspirone is an anxiolytic agent, unrelated to benzodiazepines. Buspirone is well absorbed after oral administration but first-pass metabolism is so extensive that less than 10% of the dose is available to the systemic circulation. The pharmacokinetics of buspirone after a single oral dose was evaluated in patients with cirrhosis and in healthy human subjects.[77] The average peak concentration and total AUC were about 16 times higher in the patients than in the controls. Based on the pharmacokinetic evidence from this study, one must conclude that buspirone should be used cautiously in patients with liver disease.

As noted elsewhere in the text, the antiarrhythmic agent encainide when given to extensive metabolizers of debrisoquine undergoes extensive first-pass metabolism after oral dosing to form two active metabolites, O-desmethylencainide (ODE) and 3-methoxy-ODE. Bergstrand et al.[78] reported that patients with cirrhosis had a lower systemic clearance (by a factor of 2) and oral clearance (by a factor of 8) of encainide compared with values measured in control subjects, resulting in a three-fold increase in oral bioavailability.

After a single oral dose of encainide or after repeated oral doses, encainide levels in plasma were much higher among the patients with cirrhosis. On the other hand, plasma levels of ODE and MODE in cirrhotics were comparable to those in healthy control subjects. The investigators concluded that although cirrhosis causes a large increase in steady-state levels of parent drug, a dosage adjustment is probably not required in patients with cirrhosis because no change occurs in the levels of the pharmacologically active metabolites.

The increase in bioavailability observed in patients with liver disease requires that oral doses of potent drugs with high hepatic extraction ratios be considered carefully for such patients and reduced when necessary.

Cholestasis

There are indications that cholestasis impairs the elimination of certain drugs. For example, the average half-life of rifampin was found to be 5.7 hr in patients with obstructive jaundice,[79] about twice as long as in patients without biliary obstruction. Other studies suggest that the elimination of meprobamate, pentobarbital, and tolbutamide may be altered in patients with certain forms of biliary stasis.[80] Studies with pancuronium, a neuromuscular blocking agent, in patients with total biliary obstruction indicate there is a doubling of half-life and a 50% decrease in the plasma clearance of the drug, compared to healthy subjects. Doses of pancuronium, beyond the initial dose, which may be required for prolonged surgery, should probably be reduced in such patients.[81]

Prediction of Disease Effects

Although liver dysfunction may have significant effects on the elimination of drugs, the degree of impairment of drug elimination in an individual being treated with a specific drug cannot be predicted. Unlike renal disease, for which creatinine clearance usually provides a quantitative index of the degree of impairment of drug excretion, indicators of impaired drug elimination are not apparent for hepatic disease. Although some correlations have been reported between certain biochemical indices of hepatic function and parameters of drug elimination, currently available laboratory tests do not generally reflect, in a useful, quantitative, and predictive manner, the ability of the liver to metabolize drugs.

There is sufficient information to support the idea that measurement of drug kinetics can be used to provide quantitative information of hepatic function in patients with liver disease. There is also a theoretical basis to indicate that drugs can be used to define not only hepatic metabolic function, but also to describe abnormal splanchnic blood flow.[82,83] However, the relationship between the severity of the disease and the degree of impairment of elimination of a specific drug remains elusive.

There is hope that the elimination of certain drugs, like antipyrine, may serve as an index of the liver's ability to metabolize other drugs. Although some progress has been made in this direction, Farrell et al.[84] forecast only limited success. The observation in man that different microsomal enzyme systems are influenced to a different extent by liver disease indicates functional heterogeneity of the hepatic drug-metabolizing system and may limit general correlations between drugs.

Crom et al.[85] have evaluated a method to simultaneously assess three major processes involved in hepatic drug metabolism (glucuronide conjugation, hepatic blood flow, and microsomal oxidative metabolism) using a single cocktail containing three model substrates (lorazepam, ICG, and antipyrine). In a panel of healthy adult subjects, they found that mean oral clearances of the substrates were not different when the agents were given alone or together. The investigators suggest that "this simple technique . . . has potential applications in the assessment of developmental changes in hepatic drug clearance, as well as the effects of environmental, therapeutic, and pathophysiologic factors on three major processes involved in hepatic drug clearance."

The investigators then used this technique to evaluate the hepatic drug clearance status in children with leukemia before and after receiving remission-induction therapy.[86] The clearance of antipyrine increased by about 67% and that of lorazepam increased by about 50% after remission. There was no significant difference in ICG clearance before and after treatment.

Although there were no important differences in liver function test results before and after therapy,

increases in the concentrations of albumin and apolipoprotein A in plasma, as well as a decrease in the levels of alpha$_1$-acid glycoprotein were noted. The investigators hypothesized that eradication of hepatic leukemic infiltration by acute lymphocytic leukemia remission therapy resulted in an improvement in microsomal metabolism of antipyrine and lorazepam.

More recently, Kawasaki et al.[87] measured the clearance of antipyrine, ICG, and galactose to evaluate changes in hepatic blood flow and hepatic drug metabolizing activity in patients with chronic liver disease. The clearance of galactose, like that of ICG, is related to hepatic blood flow. Galactose clearance decreased by about 30% and antipyrine and ICG clearance decreased by 60% and 85%, respectively, in patients with cirrhosis compared with healthy control subjects.

Clinical Significance

Questions regarding the clinical significance of the effects of liver dysfunction on drug elimination and, more specifically, whether or not the dosage regimen of a drug should be modified in a patient with liver disease are difficult ones to answer. Certainly, the incidence of adverse effects to drugs is expected to be higher in this population. Also, the accumulation of sedative and analgesic drugs in patients with liver disease increases the possibility of precipitating hepatic encephalopathy. An editorial on safe prescribing in liver disease in the British Medical Journal concludes that:[88]

little change in prescribing is necessary when liver disease is inactive, though doses should be kept low and particular care should be taken with sedative and antidepressant drugs. When active liver disease or signs of hepatic decompensation are present, it is likely that drug metabolism is deranged, and the greatest care indeed should be exercised in prescribing.

A commentary on the effect of liver disease on the elimination of sedatives and analgesics notes that:[89]

It would appear prudent to use such drugs cautiously in patients with parenchymal liver disease, titrating the dosage regimen in each patient to his clinical response, avoiding prolonged p.r.n. orders, and in selected instances monitoring of the drug plasma concentration.

A review of drug prescribing in hepatobiliary disease concludes with the following:[43]

The best advice to the physician at this present state of knowledge is to administer drugs to patients with liver disease carefully and to titrate the dose to the observed clinical response.

DISEASE EFFECTS ON DRUG BINDING

Drug distribution is significantly altered in certain diseases. Sometimes this is a result of changes in body composition (e.g., the accumulation of fluid), but far more often it results from changes in drug binding to plasma proteins. Changes in tissue binding are also likely, but our inability to measure these changes probably allows most to go undetected. Changes in drug binding and distribution are often accompanied by changes in drug elimination. The clearance of many drugs is a function of the free (unbound) fraction in plasma. The half-life of most drugs depends strongly on tissue binding and, to a lesser extent, on plasma protein binding. Relatively small changes in drug binding can dramatically affect the pharmacokinetics of a drug.

Albumin is considered to be the most important binding protein in plasma for acid and neutral drugs. More recent work has made it clear that α_1-acid glycoprotein (AAG) is of prime importance in the plasma binding of many basic drugs.

Drug binding to albumin is impaired in patients with renal or hepatic disease. This impairment is a result of a decreased concentration of protein in plasma (i.e., hypoalbuminemia) and the accumulation of endogenous inhibitors that interfere with drug binding. α_1-Acid glycoprotein is an acute phase reactant; its concentration in plasma rises in inflammation, malignancy, and stress, and falls in hepatic disease, nephrotic syndrome, and malnutrition.[90] Drug binding to AAG increases or decreases with AAG concentration in plasma.

Albumin Binding

Renal Disease. Plasma protein binding of acid drugs, including sulfonamides, phenytoin, thyroxine, clofibrate, salicylate, barbiturates, diazoxide, phenylbutazone, warfarin, and furosemide is impaired in patients with poor renal function.[91] The degree of impaired binding is often related to the severity of the renal disease. In many patients, reduced binding is observed despite the fact that serum albumin concentration is in the normal range. Plasma protein binding of most basic drugs is about the same in patients with uremia and in patients with normal renal function.[91]

Impaired drug binding in patients with renal disease is believed to be the result of decreased serum

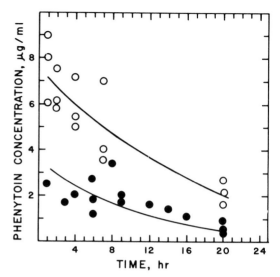

Fig. 13–7. Phenytoin concentrations in plasma of patients with uremia (●) or normal renal function (○) after a single 250-mg intravenous dose. (Data from Letteri, J.M., et al.[94])

albumin and accumulation of endogenous inhibitors that interfere with drug binding to albumin. Depner and Gulyassy found that treatment of uremic plasma with a resin improved drug binding, presumably by removing binding inhibitors.[92] They extracted a substance from the resin that, when added to plasma from human subjects with normal renal function, impaired drug binding. The binding inhibitor is believed to consist of relatively low molecular mass (1000 to 2000 daltons) peptides.[93]

The clearest consequence of impaired plasma protein binding is lower blood or plasma levels of drug in patients with impaired renal function. Figure 13–7 shows plasma levels of phenytoin after a single intravenous dose to patients with uremia and patients with normal renal function.[64] Typically, the fraction of total phenytoin concentration that is unbound in plasma is about twice as high in patients with poor renal function as it is in patients with normal renal function.

The plasma protein binding of warfarin and phenytoin was determined before and after kidney transplantation in patients with chronic renal disease.[95] Within 2 to 4 days after surgery, binding to plasma proteins increased dramatically and the free fraction of warfarin and phenytoin fell sharply, approaching values ordinarily seen in healthy control subjects, within two weeks of transplantation. Figure 13–8 shows the changes in serum creatinine and phenytoin binding after surgery.

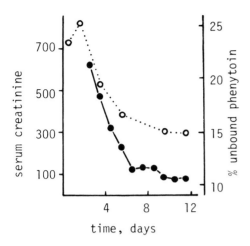

Fig. 13–8. Changes in serum creatinine levels (μmol/L) (●) and phenytoin binding (○) after a kidney transplant. (Data from Odar-Cederlof, S.[95])

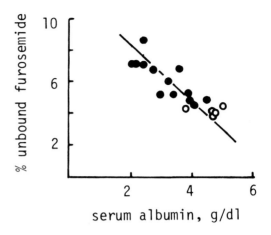

Fig. 13–10. Relationship between furosemide binding in plasma and serum albumin in normal subjects (○) and in patients with nephrotic syndrome or uremia (●). (Data from Rane, A., et al.[97])

Attention has also been given to the plasma protein binding of valproic acid and furosemide in patients with renal disease. At therapeutic plasma concentrations, unbound valproic acid was 8.4% in plasma of healthy subjects, but about 20% in patients with significant impairment of renal function.[96] Significant correlations were found in patients with renal disease between unbound valproic acid and serum creatinine, creatinine clearance, blood nitrogen, and blood uric acid (Fig. 13–9).

Rane and co-workers determined that the percent unbound furosemide in plasma was 36% higher in uremic patients and 65% higher in patients with nephrotic syndrome than in healthy control subjects.[97] When the data for the three study groups were combined, furosemide binding correlated with serum albumin concentration (Fig. 13–10).

Unlike several other basic drugs, the binding of diazepam is impaired in patients with renal disease.

Kobe and associates reported that unbound diazepam in plasma was 1.2% in healthy subjects and 4.7% in uremic subjects.[98] Grossman and co-workers[99] reported that about a doubling of the free fraction of diazepam in plasma occurs in patients with uremic or nephrotic syndrome compared to healthy control subjects. Despite its basic character, diazepam is largely bound to serum albumin rather than to AAG.

Liver Disease. Impaired plasma protein binding of drugs is often observed in patients with liver disease. The prevalent mechanism responsible for changes in binding in hepatic disease is reduced serum albumin concentration, but accumulation of endogenous biochemicals, such as bilirubin, also occurs and may contribute to the reduced binding. A review of protein binding and kinetics of drugs in liver disease was presented by Blaschke.[100]

One report found that the plasma protein binding of diazepam and tolbutamide was reduced in patients with alcoholic cirrhosis; free fraction in plasma was 50 to 150% higher in cirrhotic patients than in healthy subjects.[101] The binding of both drugs was dependent on serum albumin concentration. Another report indicated that unbound tolbutamide was about 30% higher during the acute phase of viral hepatitis than after clinical recovery.[102] Changes in binding were the result, in part, of elevated bilirubin levels.

Brodie and Boobis compared the binding of salicylate, sulfadiazine, and phenylbutazone in serum of patients with alcohol-induced liver disease to that in serum of chronic alcoholics with no evi-

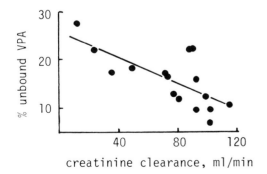

Fig. 13–9. Relationship between valproic acid (VPA) binding in plasma and renal function. (Data from Gugler, R., and Mueller, G.[96])

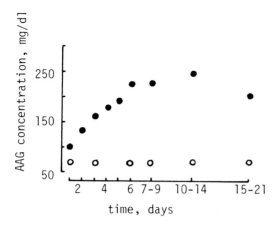

Fig. 13–11. α_1-Acid glycoprotein (AAG) concentrations in trauma patients after injury (●) and in healthy subjects (○) during a similar period of time. (Data from Edwards, D.J., et al.[111])

dence of liver disease.[103] Drug binding was normal in the chronic alcoholics but uniformly impaired in patients with alcoholic liver diseases.

Other investigators have reported decreased plasma protein binding of valproic acid[104] and furosemide[105] in patients with cirrhosis. In patients with liver disease, variations of the free fraction of valproic acid are correlated to albumin and bilirubin concentrations in serum.[104]

α_1-Acid Glycoprotein Binding

The variation in plasma albumin concentration as a result of disease is relatively narrow and is almost always in the direction of decreased concentrations. α_1-Acid glycoprotein (AAG) levels in plasma, on the other hand, show large fluctuations as a result of physiologic and pathologic changes. Decreases and increases in AAG concentrations have been observed, and parallel changes in the plasma binding of basic drugs have been reported.[106]

Quinidine binding in plasma increases shortly after gastric surgery in parallel with increases in the concentration of acute phase proteins including AAG.[107] Plasma protein binding of propranolol and chlorpromazine is increased in patients with inflammatory disease, specifically arthritis and Crohn's disease, consistent with a twofold increase in AAG concentrations, compared to control subjects.[108] Propranolol binding is also increased following myocardial infarction.[109]

Plasma AAG concentrations are considerably higher in patients with epilepsy than in age- and

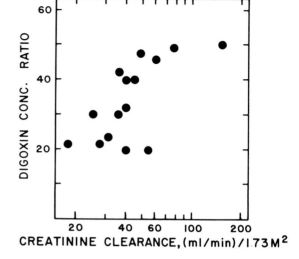

Fig. 13–12. Relationship between the myocardium-to-serum digoxin concentration ratio at necropsy and estimated antemortem renal function in individual patients. (Data from Jusko, W.J., and Weintraub, M.[112])

sex-matched control subjects (103 mg/dl vs 64 mg/dl); the binding of lidocaine is also greater in epileptics than in control subjects.[110] Lidocaine binding is also markedly increased in trauma patients, who manifest considerable elevations in AAG levels for several weeks after injury (Fig. 13–11).[111]

Tissue Binding

Since renal and hepatic diseases decrease the ability of plasma proteins to bind certain drugs because of the accumulation of endogenous binding inhibitors, one might expect a similar impairment of drug binding to other tissues in the body. With few exceptions, there is little information on this point.

Digoxin concentrations in serum and left ventricular tissues were measured at autopsy and related to estimated antemortem creatinine clearance in 15 patients.[112] A significant correlation was found between myocardium-to-serum concentration ratios of digoxin and creatinine clearance (Fig. 13–12). The uptake of digoxin by the myocardium was substantially reduced in patients with poor renal function.

Pharmacokinetic Implications

Changes in drug binding as a result of disease usually produce considerable change in the pharmacokinetic parameters of a drug. The most direct change occurs in the apparent volume of distribution.

The relationship between drug binding and volume of distribution is given by the following equation:

$$V = V_B + (f_B V_T/f_T) \qquad (13\text{–}7)$$

where V is the apparent volume of distribution, V_B is blood volume, V_T is extravascular volume, and f_B and f_T are the free (unbound) fractions of drug in the blood and extravascular (tissue) spaces. A decrease in albumin binding, because of renal disease, hepatic disease, hypoalbuminemia, or for some other reason, leads to an increase in V. Disease-related increases in the concentration of acute phase proteins enhance the plasma binding of basic drugs and lead to a decrease in V. A decrease in tissue binding of a drug also results in a decreased volume of distribution.

The apparent volume of distribution of furosemide is about 50% larger in patients with nephrotic syndrome[97] and in patients with cirrhosis[105] than in healthy control subjects, largely as a result of decreased plasma protein binding. Increased plasma binding of propranolol[113] and quinidine[114] results in a decrease in volume of distribution. Consistent with a decrease in tissue binding, the apparent volume of distribution of digoxin is considerably smaller in patients with renal disease than in patients with normal renal function.[115]

The effect of plasma protein binding on drug clearance is less direct. The clearance (Cl) of a drug eliminated solely by hepatic metabolism is given by the following equation:

$$Cl = HBF \frac{f_B Cl_I}{HBF + f_B Cl_I} \qquad (13\text{–}8)$$

where HBF is hepatic blood flow rate, f_B is the fraction free in the blood, and Cl_I is the intrinsic clearance of drug by the liver. A similar expression can be developed for a drug subject only to renal excretion.

Whether or not changes in plasma protein binding affect clearance depends on the hepatic extraction ratio of the drug (i.e., the ratio of HBF to f_B Cl_I). For drugs with low hepatic extraction ratios, such as warfarin, phenytoin, or tolbutamide, HBF $\gg f_B$ Cl_I. Under these conditions, Equation 13–8 reduces to the following relationship:

$$Cl = f_B Cl_I \qquad (13\text{–}9)$$

Assuming no changes in a patient's intrinsic metabolizing ability, clearance of a low hepatic extraction ratio drug will be higher in a patient with impaired plasma protein binding than in a patient with normal binding capacity. As a consequence, steady-state levels of the drug will be lower in the patient with impaired binding capacity.

For example, the clearance of tolbutamide was 28 ml/min during the acute phase of viral hepatitis, but only 20 ml/min in recovery. The clearance of unbound tolbutamide was about the same during and after the acute phase, indicating that metabolism (elimination) was not impaired. The increased clearance of tolbutamide during the acute phase of the illness is a result of decreased plasma protein binding (i.e., an increase in f_B).[102]

For drugs with a high hepatic extraction ratio, such as propranolol, imipramine, or meperidine, HBF $< f_B$ Cl_I. Under these conditions, Equation 13–8 reduces to the following:

$$Cl \simeq HBF \qquad (13\text{–}10)$$

Theory predicts that the clearance of drugs with high extraction ratios will be largely independent of plasma protein binding. Kornhauser and co-workers showed that propranolol clearance is independent of drug binding over a twofold range of free fraction values in blood.[116] Steady-state concentrations of high extraction ratio drugs should be similar in patients with altered drug binding capacity and in patients with normal binding capacity.

The effect of changes in binding on the half-life of a drug is difficult to predict, because half-life is a function of both volume of distribution and clearance. Half-lives of low hepatic extraction ratio drugs are likely to be sensitive to changes in plasma protein binding, because of the dependence of clearance on free fraction in the blood. The half-life of phenytoin in uremic patients is much shorter than in healthy subjects;[117] the half-life of diazepam was 37 hr in renal failure patients, compared to 92 hr in healthy control subjects.[118] The shorter half-life of phenytoin or diazepam in patients with renal disease is the result of decreased plasma protein binding and increased clearance.

Half-lives of high extraction ratio drugs are also sensitive to changes in plasma binding, because of the effects of binding on apparent volume of distribution. An increase in drug binding to plasma proteins leads to a smaller volume of distribution and a shorter half-life; a decrease in drug binding leads to a larger volume of distribution and a longer half-life. As the binding of propranolol increases from 90% ($f_B = 0.10$) to 95% ($f_B = 0.05$), the half-life of the drug decreases from 3.6 to 2.1 hr; over this range of drug binding the apparent volume of distribution decreases from 315 to 196 L.[119] As noted above, the clearance of propranolol is essentially independent of binding.

Changes in drug binding to tissues affects volume of distribution but not drug clearance. Therefore, a decrease in tissue binding leads to a decrease in volume of distribution and half-life; an increase in tissue binding leads to an increase in volume of distribution and half-life.

Clinical Significance

The pharmacokinetic consequences of changes in drug binding have been thoroughly explored, both theoretically and experimentally. The clinical implications of these changes in pharmacokinetics, if any, require further elaboration.

Changes in apparent volume of distribution may require changes in the loading dose of certain drugs given to patients with impaired drug binding. Particular attention has been given to the decreased volume of distribution of digoxin in patients with renal disease.[115] Ohnhaus and associates have recommended that the usual loading of digoxin (1.25 mg) be cut in half when digitalizing patients with severe renal failure.[120]

Much attention has been given to the clinical significance of the effects of altered binding on drug clearance and steady-state concentrations. Assuming no change in the patient's eliminating ability, the steady-state concentration of a drug with a low hepatic extraction ratio will be reduced in a patient with impaired plasma binding relative to the steady-state level in a patient with normal drug binding capacity.

On the other hand, steady-state levels of a drug with a high hepatic extraction ratio will be the same in patients with normal or impaired plasma protein binding. Does this mean that we should increase the dose of a low extraction ratio, largely metabolized drug in uremic patients to attain steady-state levels comparable to those in patients with normal plasma binding, or that we should not be concerned with binding changes for drugs with high hepatic extraction ratios? The answers to these questions are not easy to come by; we must rely on theory and limited clinical experience.

Theory, albeit with limited experimental support, suggests that drug effects will be more closely related to free (unbound) rather than total concen-

trations of drug in the blood or plasma. Accordingly, it is pertinent to examine concentrations of free drug at steady state in patients with impaired plasma binding.

Total drug concentration at steady state (C_{ss}) is given by the following expression:

$$C_{ss} = k_o/Cl \qquad (13\text{--}11)$$

where k_o is dosing rate (mg/min, mg/hr, or mg/day) and Cl is drug clearance. Free drug concentration ($C_{F,ss}$) is the product of free fraction in the blood and total drug concentration. Therefore:

$$C_{F,ss} = f_B k_o/Cl \qquad (13\text{--}12)$$

For drugs with low hepatic extraction ratios, eliminated solely by hepatic metabolism, clearance is given by Equation 13–9. Consequently:

$$C_{F,ss} = f_B k_o/f_B Cl_I = k_o/Cl_I \qquad (13\text{--}13)$$

Equation 13–13 indicates that free concentration at steady state for a drug with a low extraction ratio will be independent of changes in plasma protein binding. If this is the case, we should administer the same daily dose to patients with normal or impaired plasma binding and recognize that although total drug levels will be lower in the patients with impaired binding, free drug levels will be the same in both groups and so presumably will clinical effects.

Experimental support for this theory can be found in a study where phenytoin and clofibrate were given to healthy subjects and to patients with moderate hypoalbuminemia (plasma albumin of 1.2 to 3.9 g/dl), secondary to the nephrotic syndrome, but with relatively unimpaired renal function (creatinine clearance of > 50 ml/min) and with no evidence of liver disease.[121]

The percentage of unbound phenytoin in patients with the nephrotic syndrome was about twice that in control subjects (19.2% vs 10.1%). A strong linear correlation was observed between the free fraction of phenytoin and albumin concentration. Impaired binding was accompanied by a lower steady-state plasma concentration of phenytoin (2.9 μg/ml vs 6.8 μg/ml) because of an increase in the total clearance of the drug (0.8 ml/min per kg vs 0.37 ml/min per kg) in the nephrotic patient. The net effect however was *no significant difference* between the steady-state plasma concentration of free (unbound) phenytoin in healthy subjects (0.69 μg/ml) and that in patients with the nephrotic syndrome (0.59 μg/ml).

Similar results were obtained with clofibrate. Although binding was impaired (11.2% unbound vs 3.6% unbound) and steady-state plasma levels were reduced (46 µg/ml vs 131 µg/ml) in nephrotics compared to controls, the steady-state plasma concentrations of free (unbound) clofibrate were similar in healthy individuals (4.7 µg/ml) and in patients with nephrosis (5.1 µg/ml).

Gugler and associates recommend that, because the steady-state concentration of unbound drug in nephrotic patients is not different from that in subjects with normal plasma binding, the daily dose of drugs like phenytoin or clofibrate need not be changed for nephrotics.[121] This suggestion is important because it applies, in principle, to many drugs (compounds with low hepatic extraction ratios) under conditions of impaired plasma binding resulting from disease or drug-drug interactions.

The lower levels of some drugs in blood or plasma of patients with impaired plasma binding have important implications when therapeutic drug level monitoring is used. One must remember that a recommended therapeutic concentration range for a drug is based on the assumption of a certain degree of plasma protein binding. For drugs with low extraction ratios, a change in plasma binding usually means a change in therapeutic concentration range. For example, although the usual therapeutic concentration range for phenytoin in epileptic patients is 10 to 20 µg/ml, the therapeutic concentration range for an epileptic with severe renal failure, who has twice the free fraction of drug in plasma than the usual patient, is more likely to be 5 to 10 µg/ml. A less than adequate blood level of total drug may mean the patient requires a higher daily dose, but it may also mean that the patient is being adequately dosed but binds the drug less efficiently in plasma and does not need a change in dose.

The principles developed for phenytoin, clofibrate, and related drugs do not apply to drugs with a high hepatic extraction ratio. The clearance of these drugs approximates hepatic blood flow (HBF) and is independent of binding. Free drug concentration at steady state is given by the following equation:

$$C_{F,ss} = f_B k_o / HBF \qquad (13\text{--}14)$$

At a given dosing rate (k_o), total drug levels at steady state of a drug like propranolol or imipramine will be independent of a patient's plasma binding capacity, but free drug levels will be higher in a patient with impaired binding and lower in a patient with elevated binding. The steady-state concentration of a drug with a high hepatic extraction ratio may be more toxic or less effective in some patients than others depending on the patient's binding status.

The consequences of binding changes for propranolol or drugs with similar characteristics are of greater theoretical than clinical interest, because clinical problems have not been reported. This situation may relate to the fact that many of these drugs have a comfortable safety margin, that many of these drugs bind predominantly to AAG, the concentration of which is more likely to be elevated (greater binding) than reduced (less binding) in disease states, or that fluctuations in AAG concentration tend to be transient.

There is far more concern about drug usage in patients with hypoalbuminemia. In a comprehensive drug monitoring program, adverse reactions to phenytoin were recorded in 11.4% of 88 patients with serum albumin lower than 3 g/100 ml but in only 3.8% of 234 patients with a normal serum albumin.[122]

Surveillance of 240 medical inpatients receiving prednisone revealed a correlation between the frequency of side effects and serum albumin.[123] When serum albumin concentration was less than 2.5 g/dl, the frequency of prednisone side effects was doubled.

Of 6673 hospitalized medical patients monitored in a drug surveillance program, 1037 (15.5%) received chlordiazepoxide and 1202 (18.0%) received diazepam. Unwanted central nervous system (CNS) depression was noted in 7.1% of all diazepam recipients, but ranged from 2.9% in patients with normal serum albumin (> 4 g/dl) to 9.3% in those with hypoalbuminemia (< 3 g/dl). A similar trend was evident in patients receiving chlordiazepoxide.[124]

One reason for the higher rate of adverse drug effects in patients with hypoalbuminemia is that these patients may have had impaired elimination, in addition to reduced plasma protein binding. A reduced hepatic and/or renal function in conjunction with low serum albumin could cause increases in the steady state plasma concentrations of unbound drug with little or no change in total drug levels. In fact, the adverse reactions study with phenytoin includes all hypoalbuminemic patients without regard for the underlying disease.[122]

A more subtle pharmacokinetic reason for a

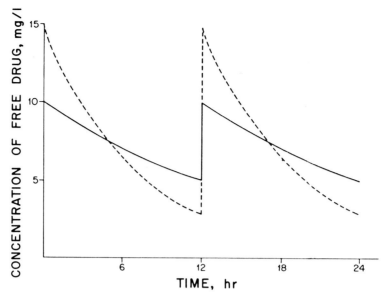

Fig. 13–13.   Effects of a change in fraction unbound (f) on free drug concentration in plasma at steady state when a 100 mg/kg dose is given intravenously every 12 hr. Continuous line: f = 0.01, apparent volume of distribution (V) = 0.2 L/kg, $t_{1/2}$ = 12 hr. Stippled line: f increases to 0.03, V increases to 0.25 L/kg, and $t_{1/2}$ decreases to 5 hr. (Data from Levy, G.[125])

higher incidence of adverse drug effects in patients with reduced plasma binding relates to the fact that although the clearance of unbound drug is often unchanged, the half-life of the drug is usually shorter. If a patient with impaired plasma binding is treated with the usual dosage regimen, the same average free drug concentration is found as that in patients with normal plasma binding, but a higher peak concentration is also found (Fig. 13–13).[125]

The steady-state peak-to-trough concentration ratio for unbound phenytoin is only 1.25 in healthy subjects, but doubles in nephrotic patients with hypoalbuminemia and reduced plasma protein binding.[126] Although theory and usage suggest no change in the total daily dose of drugs such as phenytoin, diazepam, or clofibrate for patients with reduced plasma binding, more frequent dosing of these drugs may be advisable.

CARDIOVASCULAR DISEASE

The influence of heart disease on drug pharmacokinetics has been reviewed by Williams and Benet.[127] A more recent review, concerned specifically with congestive heart failure, is also available.[128] According to Equation 13–8, plasma clearance is determined by the intrinsic clearance of the eliminating organ, blood flow to that organ, and plasma protein binding. Cardiovascular disease can alter one or more of these variables.

Decreased hepatic perfusion is usually found in patients with congestive heart failure because of reduced cardiac output. These changes reduce the clearance of propranolol, pentazocine, lidocaine, and related drugs highly extracted by the liver.

Changes in cardiac function may alter the concentrations of drug-binding proteins like AAG, alter blood or fluid pH, or result in the production of endogenous binding inhibitors. These effects could influence drug binding in plasma or tissues.

Congestive heart failure (CHF) also affects drug metabolism but the basis for this is not clear. Hepner and associates studied the elimination of aminopyrine, a model drug that, like antipyrine, has a low hepatic extraction ratio and is eliminated only by oxidative metabolism in the liver, in patients with congestive heart failure and in control patients.[129] Aminopyrine clearance was 30 ml/min in patients with CHF and 125 ml/min in control patients. Recovery of labeled carbon dioxide, a by-product of aminopyrine metabolism, in the breath was markedly decreased in CHF patients. Impaired drug metabolism in CHF has also been observed with other drugs.

Lidocaine. The elimination of lidocaine is sensitive to changes in HBF. Figure 13–14 shows lidocaine concentrations in the plasma during intravenous infusion of 1 mg/min to patients with acute myocardial infarction, but with minimal cir-

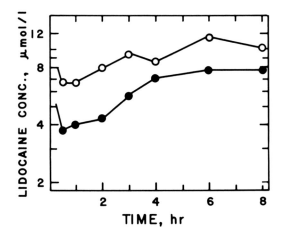

Fig. 13–14. Lidocaine concentrations in plasma after a loading dose and during a 1 mg/min intravenous infusion in patients with minimum circulatory disturbance and normal hepatic function (●) and in cardiothoracic surgical patients with overt circulatory disturbance and hepatic dysfunction (○). (Data from Aps, C., et al.[129])

culatory disturbance and normal hepatic function, and to cardiothoracic surgical patients with overt circulatory disturbance, including low cardiac output and hepatic dysfunction. Lidocaine levels are about 50% higher in the group with altered hemodynamics.[130] Similar findings have been reported by Prescott and co-workers.[131]

Other studies show a marked dependency of steady-state lidocaine levels on both cardiac index[132,133] and estimated HBF.[133] A nomogram has been developed for estimating the infusion rate of lidocaine necessary to attain a desired plateau concentration when cardiac output is known.[132] According to this method, a patient with a normal cardiac output of 80 ml/min per kg would require an infusion rate of 28 μg/kg per min (or about 2 mg/min for a 70-kg individual) to obtain a lidocaine concentration of 3 μg/ml. To achieve the same level in a patient with heart failure and a cardiac output of only 40 ml/min per kg requires a lidocaine infusion of 12 μg/kg per min (or about 0.8 mg/min for a 70-kg individual). The substantial decrease in lidocaine clearance in patients with reduced cardiac output makes it necessary to reduce the dose to avoid toxicity.

Propranolol. The elimination of propranolol, metoprolol, and several other β-blockers is dependent on HBF. These drugs are widely used to treat hypertension. Borderline hypertension patients often have high cardiac outputs, whereas permanent hypertension patients exhibit normal or reduced cardiac output. Weis and co-workers reported that propranolol clearance in permanent hypertension patients (cardiac output of 83 ml/min per kg) was only 50% of that observed in borderline hypertension patients (cardiac output of 111 ml/min per kg).[134]

Quinidine and Other Oral Antiarrhythmic Agents. Oral quinidine has been used for many years in the treatment of cardiac arrhythmias. In cardiac patients, about 20% of a dose is eliminated by renal excretion. Assuming the balance of the dose is metabolized in the liver, the hepatic extraction ratio of quinidine is about 0.20 to 0.25. The pharmacokinetics of quinidine were determined after intravenous administration to cardiac patients with and without CHF.[135] The half-life of quinidine was about the same in each group (6 to 7 hr), but renal clearance was about 50% smaller and total clearance about 35% smaller in CHF patients than in control cardiac patients, suggesting the need for a smaller maintenance dose of quinidine in patients with CHF. A particularly pronounced change in apparent volume of distribution of quinidine was noted; V = 1.8 L/kg for CHF patients and V = 2.7 L/kg for control subjects. The smaller V in patients with CHF suggests either enhanced plasma binding, possibly related to elevated levels of acute phase proteins, or impaired tissue binding.

Woosley[136] has summarized a large number of studies concerned with the pharmacokinetics and pharmacodynamics of lidocaine, quinidine, and other antiarrhythmic agents in patients with congestive heart failure. He observed that "changes in the pharmacokinetics of antiarrhythmic agents may be anticipated in patients with congestive heart failure (CHF), although the magnitude or direction of change is not always predictable."

Volume distribution may be as much as 50% smaller in patients with CHF and iv loading doses should be decreased proportionately. Decreased blood flow to the liver and kidneys and decreased hepatic drug metabolizing enzyme activity may seriously compromise the elimination of an antiarrhythmic drug.

Woosley stresses the fact that although it is widely assumed that antiarrhythmic therapy can benefit patients with highly symptomatic arrhythmias, "the pharmacokinetics of antiarrhythmic agents are made more variable and less predictable by heart failure, and the risk of toxicity is much greater than in patients with uncompromised cardiac function." He concludes by pointing out that "therapy for patients with CHF should be initiated with low doses of the agent selected and the dosage carefully titrated while the patient is monitored to confirm both the efficacy and the absence of adverse effects."

Prazosin. Prazosin is an antihypertensive agent that may be useful in CHF because of its vasodilatory effects. After oral administration of a 5-mg oral dose, the total area under the blood level versus time curve was about twice as large in patients with CHF than in healthy subjects; the half-life of prazosin was 6 hr in CHF patients and 2.5 hr in control subjects.[137] Similar findings were reported in a later study.[138] The results suggest impaired metabolism of prazosin in patients with CHF and, possibly, the need for smaller doses.

Theophylline. Reduced theophylline clearance and increased toxicity have been reported in patients with CHF.[139] Powell and co-workers report a theophylline clearance of 26.5 ml/hr per kg in patients with CHF compared to values of either 55 ml/hr per kg (smokers) or 39 ml/hr per kg (nonsmokers) in patients with uncomplicated asthma or chronic bronchitis.[140] Theophylline maintenance doses in patients with CHF must be reduced by about 50% to avoid adverse effects.

ACE Inhibitors. Angiotensin converting enzyme inhibitors have become mainline drugs in the treatment of congestive heart failure. Dickstein et al.[141] evaluated the pharmacokinetics of enalapril and enalaprilat after iv and oral administration of the parent drug and after iv administration of the active metabolite, in patients with stable, chronic CHF.

After oral administration of enalapril to these patients, the extent of absorption and the degree of conversion to enalaprilat were similar to values found in healthy control subjects, but absorption and hydrolysis were slower in patients with CHF. Peak levels of enalaprilat occurred about 2 hr later than expected and were about 30% higher than those found in control subjects. Enalaprilat concentrations were also consistently higher in CHF patients following iv administration of either enalapril or enalaprilat. Dickstein concluded that "the presence of CHF does not appreciably alter the pharmacokinetic behaviour of enalapril."

Loop Diuretics. Furosemide and bumetanide block active sodium chloride transport in the ascending limb of Henle's loop and have a much greater diuretic effect than the thiazides. They are widely used in the treatment of CHF, particularly in patients with pulmonary edema and in those who do not respond to thiazides.

The management of CHF is sometimes complicated by the failure of oral therapy to produce an effective diuresis and the need for iv administration to achieve the desired clinical response. Determinants of the diuretic response to furosemide are the total amount of drug delivered to the kidneys, the time course of that delivery, and the 'dose'-response or, more accurately, the urinary excretion rate-response relationship.

Oral furosemide has a bioavailability in healthy subjects of only 40 to 50%. Accordingly, more drug is needed to reach the same peak urinary excretion rate after oral administration than after iv injection. Furthermore, patients with CHF often show a shift in the dose-response relationship when compared with healthy subjects; a higher excretion rate of furosemide is required to produce the same sodium excretion rate. This resistance has been noted after both oral and iv administration.

Taking these factors into account still does not explain the very high resistance to oral furosemide in some patients with CHF. Some believe that the mechanism of this resistance is related to poor absorption of furosemide.

Brater et al.[142] studied the kinetics and dynamics of oral bumetanide and furosemide in patients with stable, compensated CHF and in healthy subjects. The mean time to reach peak concentration after a single dose was delayed in patients with CHF by 49 min for bumetanide and by 97 min for furosemide. Peak urinary excretion was 60% lower with bumetanide and 50% lower with furosemide in patients with CHF than in control subjects.

Only 23% of the oral dose of bumetanide was recovered in the urine in the patients compared with 30% in the controls; corresponding values for furosemide were 14 and 22%. The reason for the lower urinary recovery of unchanged drug in patients with CHF might be assigned to a change in the extent of absorption but the investigators concluded that the decreased recovery reflects renal impairment in patients with CHF rather than reduced bioavailability.

Bumetanide and furosemide appear to be absorbed more slowly in patients with CHF than in normal subjects. With furosemide there was a doubling of the time to peak urinary excretion rate. This delay was associated with a 50% decrease in peak urinary excretion rate, indicating not only a lag in absorption, but a decreased absorption rate as well.

Brater et al. suggested that "because the time course of delivery of any drug to the active site is an important determinant of overall response . . . , it is conceivable that this change in time course, but not extent, of absorption could in part be responsible for the diminished response to oral diuretics so often observed clinically in patients with CHF and other edematous disorders. The delayed rate of absorption might render excretion rates of diuretic attained in the urine sufficiently low to blunt overall response."

More recently, Vasko et al.[143] also studied the absorption of furosemide in patients with CHF who were receiving their usual oral dose of the loop diuretic. Each patient was evaluated twice, once while decompensated and again after attaining normal weight and while clinically compensated.

Most patients showed a substantially different serum level-time profile on the two occasions, with a considerable decrease in the time to peak drug concentration and a higher peak concentration when dry weight was achieved. The relative bioavailability of furosemide also tended to be larger in compensated patients than in decompensated patients but the difference was not statistically significant.

These findings indicate that the absorption of furosemide in patients with CHF improves as a patient's clinical status is upgraded, suggesting that the disease process in some way alters absorption. The principal changes in gastrointestinal physiology that have been noted in CHF are delayed gastric emptying, decreased GI motility, altered transit times, edema of intestinal epithelium, and decreased splanchnic blood flow. Vasko et al. suggested that their "results reinforce the clinical impression of physicians that absorption of furosemide in patients with decompensated congestive heart failure is abnormal and a prompt diuretic response requires intravenous therapy."

THYROID DISEASE

When thyroid function is altered, there are a series of physiologic changes that may affect drug absorption, excretion, and metabolism. The influence of thyroid dysfunction on drug pharmacokinetics has been reviewed by Shenfield[144] and more recently by O'Connor and Feely.[145]

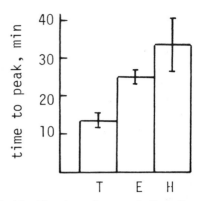

Fig. 13–15. Time-to-peak concentration after a single oral dose of acetaminophen in thyrotoxic (T) and hypothyroid (H) patients, and in the same patients when treated and euthyroid (E). (Data from Forfar, J.C., et al.[147])

Absorption

The bioavailability of riboflavin is increased in hypothyroidism and decreased in hyperthyroidism because of changes in gastrointestinal motility.[146] Enhanced absorption of riboflavin is also observed when gut motility is reduced by administration of an anticholinergic agent. Serum digoxin concentrations may be low in hyperthyroid patients because of hypermotility and decreased bioavailability.

Absorption of acetaminophen is faster in patients with untreated thyrotoxicosis than after treatment; the absorption of acetaminophen is relatively slow in hypothyroid patients (Fig. 13–15).[147] The absorption rates of propranolol and oxazepam are also increased in hyperthyroidism due to increased GI motility.[145]

Excretion

Renal plasma flow is reduced in hypothyroidism and increased in hyperthyroidism. The renal clearance of drugs may be affected in a similar way, but this is not firmly established. Most studies concerned with the effects of thyroid disease on renal clearance have examined digoxin elimination, but the results are conflicting.

There is considerable and controversial literature on cardiac glycosides and thyroid dysfunction. Clinically, hyperthyroid patients are less sensitive to these drugs. For many years, these differences were thought to be entirely pharmacologic in nature. In 1966, however, Doherty and Perkins reported their findings of relatively low blood levels of digoxin in hyperthyroid patients and relatively high blood levels in hypothyroid patients, compared to control patients.[148]

The findings in hyperthyroid patients have been confirmed by several investigators;[149,150] the results in hypothyroid patients have been confirmed by some[149] but not by others.[150] The basis for these pharmacokinetic changes is unexplained; they could relate to changes in renal or biliary excretion or in hepatic metabolism. Shenfield believes that pharmacokinetic changes alone cannot explain the clinical resistance to digoxin in hyperthyroidism and proposes that resistance is related to an increased number of $Na^+ K^+$-ATPase pumps.[144] This hypothesis is consistent with findings in neonates who are also relatively resistant to the effects of digoxin.

Other studies have shown that hyperthyroidism has no effect on the renal clearance of atenolol and nadolol.[145]

Metabolism

In general, the activity of hepatic microsomal drug metabolizing enzymes is reduced in hypothyroidism and increased in hyperthyroidism. The half-life of antipyrine was found to be about 8 hr in hyperthyroid and 17 hr in hypothyroid patients.[151] After treatment, half-life values were about 12 hr in each group, well within the normal range. Similar findings have been reported for the elimination of methimazole and propylthiouracil, antithyroid agents, in hypo- and hyperthyroid patients.[152]

Forfar and co-workers report that differences in the absorption rate of acetaminophen in patients with thyroid disease are paralleled by differences in metabolic clearance.[147] Relative to euthyroid patients, hypothyroid patients absorb and eliminate acetaminophen more slowly, whereas hyperthyroid patients absorb and eliminate the drug more rapidly. The rates of glucuronidation of acetaminophen and oxazepam are increased in hyperthyroidism.[145]

Thyroid disease seems to have a considerable effect on the elimination of propranolol.[153] In hyperthyroid patients receiving 160 mg/day, steady-state levels of propranolol rose from 38 ng/ml when hyperthyroid to 75 ng/ml when euthyroid. In hypothyroid patients receiving the same dose, there was a substantial fall in steady-state propranolol concentrations following treatment with thyroxine, from 117 ng/ml to 69 ng/ml.

While oxidative metabolism of antipyrine, propranolol, metoprolol, and theophylline is enhanced

in hyperthyroidism, the clearance of other drugs, including diazepam, warfarin, and phenytoin, is unchanged.[145]

INFLUENZA AND RELATED DISEASES

In 1978, Chang et al.[154] observed that the half-life of theophylline was prolonged during viral upper respiratory infection in children with chronic asthma. These findings were confirmed by Kraemer et al.[155] in 1982. Kraemer and his colleagues reported that during the 1980 influenza outbreak in King County, Washington, 11 children whose asthma had been well controlled with theophylline rapidly developed drug toxicity, with no change in dose, while suffering a bout of febrile viral illness. Toxicity included two cases of seizures. Theophylline concentrations in serum ranged from about 8 to 20 μg/ml before the viral illness and from 22 to 48 μg/ml during the illness, when the children were manifesting theophylline toxicity.

The apparent inhibition of theophylline metabolism during influenza may be related in part to the fever associated with the infection. Forsyth et al.[158] determined antipyrine clearance in saliva after a single oral dose to children ranging in age from 5 months to 5 years during a period of elevated body temperature (range 38.6° to 39.2°) secondary to upper or lower respiratory tract infection and again after the bout of fever.

Antipyrine clearance during the infection and fever was only about half that found during the control period. In an earlier study, Elin et al.[157] determined in adult subjects that etiocholanolone-induced fever also decreased the clearance of antipyrine compared to that observed during an afebrile control period, but the inhibition was less pronounced than that observed during natural fever in children.

The effects of viral infections on hepatic oxidative drug metabolism are believed to be mediated via the stimulation of interferon. A wide variety of interferon-inducing agents and interferon itself have been found to decrease hepatic concentrations of cytochrome P450-dependent drug metabolizing enzymes. Administration of influenza virus vaccine may also lead to elevated interferon levels, and several studies have demonstrated that flu vaccine depresses the metabolism of certain drugs subject to oxidative metabolism in the liver.[158,159]

Meredith et al.[160] studied the effects of influenza vaccine on the pharmacokinetics of intravenous chlordiazepoxide and lorazepam and oral theophylline, after a single dose of each drug, in healthy male subjects. Each subject was studied with one of the drugs 5 days before and either 1 or 7 days after a standard dose of a trivalent flu vaccine released for 1982.

The vaccine inhibited the metabolism of theophylline but not that of chlordiazepoxide, which is also oxidized, nor that of lorazepam, which is glucuronidated. The first day after vaccination, the clearance of theophylline was reduced by about 25%, compared with baseline. Impaired metabolism was no longer evident on day 7.

Levels of alpha-interferon were elevated in 3 of the 7 subjects for at least 6 to 8 hr after vaccination but returned to baseline within 24 hr. Plasma levels of gamma-interferon were elevated in all subjects for about 4 days after vaccination.

Meredith et al. concluded that the inhibition of theophylline is small and transient, seemingly related to the stimulation of interferon by the vaccine, and appears to be greater in subjects with high prevaccination theophylline clearances. No reasons are obvious to explain the apparently selective effects of flu vaccine on theophylline but not on chlordiazepoxide metabolism.

Other investigators have failed to detect an effect of influenza vaccination on theophylline metabolism, and there is now reason to believe that whether or not theophylline metabolism is inhibited depends on the composition of the vaccine. Winstanley et al.[161] found no effect of a highly purified subunit influenza vaccination on steady-state levels of theophylline in healthy subjects or in patients with chronic obstructive bronchitis.

These investigators proposed that "an ideal [influenza vaccine] would contain only those proteins that induce a protective antibody response—principally haemagglutinin (HA) and neuraminidase (N). Disruption of whole viron . . . produces a mixture of HA, N, viral RNA, matrix protein, and viral and egg lipid. These latter substances, although not important contributors to the antibody response, are potent interferon inducing agents."

Winstanley et al. suggest that highly purified subunit influenza vaccines are safe when given to patients receiving theophylline, but less purified flu vaccines should still be used with caution in such patients.

Grabowski et al.[162] found that a split virus influenza vaccine produces no detectable interferon activity in serum and no production of interferon in tonsil or peripheral lymphocyte cultures. They concluded that patients being treated with theophylline who receive split virus influenza vaccine need no modification of their theophylline dose.

Despite assurances of the safety of more purified flu vaccines, caution may still be prudent for patients on relatively high-dose theophylline therapy. Because of the nonlinear characteristics of theophylline metabolism, a relatively modest decrease in theophylline clearance may produce disproportionately large increases in steady-state theophylline levels, particularly in patients with serum levels in the range of 15 to 20 μg/ml.

BURN INJURY

Extensive and severe burns induce a variety of physiologic changes that could produce unpredictable changes in the pharmacokinetics of drugs.[163] Some investigators have found elevated glomerular filtration rates after burn trauma. This may contribute to the unusually rapid renal excretion of aminoglycoside antibiotics in burn patients.

In 14 burn patients treated for serious gram-negative infections, the use of usual doses of gentamicin, up to 5 mg/kg per day, resulted in subtherapeutic plasma concentrations; peak gentamicin concentrations were consistently below 4 μg/ml.[164] Gentamicin half-life in these patients was unusually short, particularly in the younger burn patients. Satisfactory gentamicin levels were achieved by increasing the daily dose, to as high as 12 mg/kg per day in the younger patients, and decreasing the dosing interval from 8 to 4 hr.

A follow-up study in 66 burn patients generally confirmed these initial results.[165] About 75% of the patients required doses greater than the recommended dose to achieve adequate drug levels in the serum. Dosing intervals of every 4 hr were required in about 25% of the patients and of every 6 hr in about 40% of the patients.

Larger-than-average doses of vancomycin also seem to be needed in some patients with serious burns. Brater et al.[166] measured the clearance of vancomycin from serum in patients with burns and found that it correlated closely ($r = 0.93$) with creatinine clearance. Five of the 10 patients with burn injury had creatinine clearances greater than 120 ml/min; these values ranged from 142 to 192 ml/min. The five highest values of vancomycin clearance occurred in the same 5 patients; these values ranged from 108 to 215 ml/min. The investigators suggested that a reasonable therapeutic strategy in a patient with burns would be to dose vancomycin based on the patient's creatinine clearance.

More recently, Garrelts and Peterie[167] determined vancomycin dosage requirements in patients with burns and medical/surgical patients with normal renal function who served as controls. The initial dosage regimen for most patients was 1.0 g vancomycin given iv every 12 hr. In each patient, however, the initial regimen was modified when necessary to achieve a peak serum level between 25 to 35 μg/ml and a trough level between 5 to 10 μg/ml.

The burn patients varied widely in the extent of total body surface area affected; estimates ranged from 4 to 46%, with a mean of 24%. Creatinine clearance was 131 ml/min in the patients with burns and 117 ml/min in the control patients. The difference was relatively small and not statistically significant. The average peak concentrations of vancomycin were 27 and 31 μg/ml in the burn and control groups, respectively. Mean trough levels were about 8 μg/ml in each group.

Despite the similarities between the two groups in age, weight, and creatinine clearance, burn patients required much larger doses of vancomycin to maintain serum levels comparable to control patients: 47 mg/kg/day versus 26 mg/kg/day. On average, patients with burn injuries required nearly 1 g/day more vancomycin than control patients.

Burn patients also had to be dosed more frequently than control patients to maintain trough levels within the specified range. Only 4 of 9 burn patients were dosed every 12 hr; the others needed doses every 8 hr or, in one case, every 6 hr. On the other hand, 7 of the 8 control patients could be given vancomycin every 12 hr and 1 patient received the drug every 18 hr.

Contrary to the results in the earlier study by Brater et al.,[166] Garrelts and Peterie concluded that the increased dosage requirement for vancomycin in patients with burns is not related to creatinine clearance. Accordingly, they believe that monitoring serum levels of vancomycin in patients with burn injuries is essential to avoid underdosing and therapeutic failure.

Acute stress ulceration of the stomach and duodenum is a life-threatening complication of burn injury. Attempts to control gastric acidity by iv administration of cimetidine have had mixed success. Martyn et al.[168,169] have considered the possibility that the usual dose of cimetidine may be ineffective in patients with burn injuries because

of enhanced clearance and subtherapeutic blood levels.

Studies in adults showed that both creatinine clearance and cimetidine clearance were much larger in patients with burns than in matched control subjects.[168] Creatinine clearance was 172 ml/min in burn patients compared with a value of about 125 ml/min in controls. Total clearance of cimetidine was 14.0 ml/min/kg in the patients and 8.2 ml/min/kg in the controls.

Martyn et al. also studied cimetidine pharmacokinetics in children with burn injuries.[169] Age ranged from 4 months to 17 years, with a mean of 6 years. Mean cimetidine clearance in these patients was 16.2 ml/min/kg, slightly higher than the mean value found in adult patients with burns and about twice as high as the mean value found in adult control subjects. Endogenous creatinine clearance normalized to 70 kg was 190 ml/min in the children with burns, again slightly higher than in adult patients with burns and much higher than in adult controls. The correlation coefficient between creatinine and cimetidine clearance was 0.93. These results support the hypothesis that the higher dosage requirements of cimetidine in children with burn injuries is due, at least in part, to the increased clearance of cimetidine in such patients.

CYSTIC FIBROSIS

Cystic fibrosis (CF) is an inherited disorder, characterized mainly by pancreatic insufficiency and progressive chronic lung disease. Evidence has been accumulating that suggests altered drug disposition in patients with CF. Specifically, there appears to be increased renal excretion of certain drugs and increased hepatic metabolism of others.

Knoppert et al.[169] studied theophylline metabolism following a single iv dose of aminophylline in young adults with stable, mild to moderate CF and in healthy control subjects of similar age. The total clearance of theophylline was 40 to 50% greater in patients with CF than in controls. The renal clearance of theophylline, which ordinarily accounts for about 10% of the total clearance, was increased by 45% and the nonrenal clearance by 41%, compared with control values.

The increased nonrenal clearance of theophylline in CF was the result of increased hepatic metabolism to each of its three main metabolites, 1-methyluric acid, 3-methylxanthine, and 1,3-dimethyluric acid. The formation clearances for each of these metabolites increased by more than 50%. Also, the renal clearance of each metabolite was greater in subjects with CF than in control subjects.

The increased renal clearance of theophylline observed in this study is consistent with earlier reports of increased renal clearance of dicloxacillin, methacillin, and tobramycin in patients with CF. The increased metabolic clearance of theophylline is largely related to enhanced N-demethylation and ring hydroxylation activity in patients with CF. In summary, there may be a need for larger doses of theophylline and other drugs in patients with CF to achieve adequate response.

CONCLUSIONS

Much more needs to be learned about how to best use drugs in patients, particularly critically ill patients. Dosing guidelines can be developed for many drugs in certain disease states when the patient's condition is stable. Far more individual judgment and empiricism is required in the acutely ill patient, when hemodynamics and end-organ function may fluctuate mercurially or decline precipitously. One thing is certain, we must never make the assumption that the same dose of a drug is adequate for every patient who requires it.

REFERENCES

1. Dettli, L., Spring, P., and Habersang, R.: Drug dosage in patients with impaired renal function. Postgrad. Med. J., 465:32, 1970.
2. Herrera, J., Vukovich, R.A., and Griffith, D.L.: Elimination of nadolol by patients with renal impairment. Br. J. Clin. Pharmacol., 2:227S, 1979.
3. Gibaldi, M., and Levy, G.: Pharmacokinetics in clinical practice. I. Concepts. JAMA, 235:1864, 1976.
4. Bennett, W.M.: Guide to drug dosage in renal failure. Clin. Pharmacokin., 15:326, 1988.
5. Bolton, W.K., et al.: Pharmacokinetics of moxalactam in subjects with various degrees of renal function. Antimicrob. Agents Chemother., 18:933, 1980.
6. Humbert, G., et al.: Pharmacokinetics of cefoxitin in normal subjects and in patients with renal insufficiency. Rev. Infect. Dis., 1:118, 1979.
7. Craig, W.A., et al.: Pharmacology of cefazolin and other cephalosporins in patients with renal insufficiency. J. Infect. Dis., 128:S347, 1973.
8. Humbert, G., et al.: Pharmacokinetics of amoxacillin: dosage nomogram for patients with impaired renal function. Antimicrob. Agents Chemother., 15:28, 1979.
9. Welling, P.G., Craig, W.A., and Kunin, C.M.: Prediction of drug dosage in patients with renal failure using data derived from normal subjects. Clin. Pharmacol. Ther., 18:45, 1975.
10. Schönebeck, J., et al.: Pharmacokinetic studies on the oral mycotic agent 5-fluorocytosine in individuals with normal and impaired kidney function. Chemotherapy, 18:321, 1973.
11. Linquist, J.A., Siddiqui, J.Y., and Smith, I.M.: Cephalexin in patients with renal disease. N. Engl. J. Med., 283:720, 1970.
12. Doherty, J.E., et al.: Studies with tritiated digoxin in anephric human subjects. Circulation, 35:298, 1967.
13. Halstenson, C.E., et al.: Disposition of famotidine in renal insufficiency. J. Clin. Pharmacol., 27:782, 1987.
14. Lowenthal, D.T., et al.: The effect of renal function on enalapril kinetics. Clin. Pharmacol. Ther., 38:661, 1985.
15. Chennavasin, P., and Brater, D.C.: Nomograms for drug use in renal disease. Clin. Pharmacokinet., 6:193, 1981.
16. Latos, D.L., Bryan, C.S., and Stone, W.J.: Carbenicillin therapy in patients with normal and impaired renal function. Clin. Pharmacol. Ther., 17:692, 1975.
17. Rodvold, K.A., et al.: Vancomycin pharmacokinetics in patients with various degrees of renal function. Antimicrob. Agents Chemother., 32:848, 1988.
18. Bennett, W.M.: Drug prescribing in renal failure. Drugs, 17:111, 1979.
19. Cheigh, J.S.: Drug administration in renal failure. Am. J. Med., 62:555, 1977.
20. Bjornsson, T.D.: Nomogram for drug dosage adjustment in patients with renal failure. Clin. Pharmacokin., 11:164, 1986.
21. Gibson, T.P., and Nelson, H.A.: Drug kinetics and artificial kidneys. Clin. Pharmacokinet., 2:403, 1977.
22. Gambertoglio, J.G., et al.: Cefamandole kinetics in uremic patients undergoing hemodialysis. Clin. Pharmacol. Ther., 26:592, 1979.
23. Morgan, D.B., Dillon, S., and Payne, R.B.: The assessment of glomerular function: creatinine clearance or plasma creatinine? Postgrad. Med. J., 54:302, 1978.
24. Wheeler, L.A., and Sheiner, L.B.: Clinical estimation of creatinine clearance. Am. J. Clin. Pathol., 72:27, 1979.
25. Lott, R., and Hayton, W.L.: Estimation of creatinine clearance from serum creatinine concentration—a review. Drug Intell. Clin. Pharm., 12:140, 1978.
26. Bjornsson, T.D.: Use of serum creatinine concentrations to determine renal function. Clin. Pharmacokinet., 4:200, 1979.
27. Cockcroft, D.W., and Gault, M.H.: Prediction of creatinine clearance from serum creatinine. Nephron, 16:31, 1976.
28. Hull, J.H., et al.: Influence of range of renal function and liver disease on predictability of creatinine clearance. Clin. Pharmacol. Ther., 29:516, 1981.
29. Dionne, R.E., et al.: Estimating creatinine clearance in morbidly obese patients. Am. J. Hosp. Pharm., 38:841, 1981.
30. Shull, B.C., et al.: A useful method for predicting creatinine clearance in children. Clin. Chem., 24:1167, 1978.
31. Traub, S.L., and Johnson, C.E.: Comparison of methods of estimating creatinine clearance in children. Am. J. Hosp. Pharm., 37:195, 1980.
32. Osborne, R.J., Joel, S.P., and Slevin, M.L.: Morphine intoxication in renal failure: the role of morphine-6-glucuronide. Br. Med. J., 292:1548, 1986.
33. Wolff, J., et al.: Influence of renal function on the elimination of morphine and morphine glucuronides. Eur. J. Clin. Pharmacol., 34:353, 1988.
34. Verbeeck, R.K., Branch, R.A., and Wilkinson, G.R.: Drug metabolites in renal failure: pharmacokinetic and clinical implications. Clin. Pharmacokinet., 6:329, 1981.
35. De Schepper, P.J., et al.: Pharmacokinetics of diflusinal elimination in patients with renal insufficiency. Br. J. Clin. Pharmacol., 4:645P, 1977.
36. Faed, E.M., and McQueen, E.G.: Plasma half-life of clofibric acid in renal failure. Br. J. Clin. Pharmacol., 7:407, 1979.

37. Terao, N., and Shen, D.D.: Reduced extraction of l-propranolol by perfused rat liver in the presence of uremic blood. J. Pharmacol. Exp. Ther., *233*:277, 1985.

38. Bergstrand, R.H., et al.: Encainide disposition in patients with renal failure. Clin. Pharmacol. Ther., *40*:64, 1986.

39. Gibson, T.P., et al.: Biotransformation of sulindac in end-stage renal disease. Clin. Pharmacol. Ther., *42*:82, 1987.

40. Wilkinson, G.R., and Schenker, S.: Drug disposition and liver disease. Drug. Metab. Rev., *4*:139, 1976.

41. Williams, R.L., et al.: Influence of acute viral hepatitis on disposition and pharmacologic effect of warfarin. Clin. Pharmacol. Ther., *20*:90, 1976.

42. Arnman, R., and Olsson, R.: Elimination of paracetamol in chronic liver disease. Hepatogastroenterology, *25*:283, 1978.

43. Roberts, R.K., Desmond, P.V., and Schenker, S.: Drug prescribing in hepatobiliary disease. Drugs, *17*:198, 1979.

44. Bass, N.M., and Williams, R.L.: Guide to drug dosage in hepatic disease. Clin. Pharmacokin., *15*:396, 1988.

45. Howden, C.W., Birnie, G.G., and Brodie, M.J.: Drug metabolism in liver disease. Pharmac. Ther., *40*:439, 1989.

46. Dossing, M., et al.: A simple method for determination of antipyrine clearance. Clin. Pharmacol. Ther., *32*:382, 1982.

47. Branch, R.A., Herbert, C.M., and Read, A.E.: Determinants of serum antipyrine half-lives in patients with liver disease. Gut, *14*:569, 1973.

48. Mehta, M.U., et al.: Antipyrine kinetics in liver disease and liver transplantation. Clin. Pharmacol. Ther., *39*:372, 1986.

49. Andreasen, P.B., and Ranek, L.: Liver failure and drug metabolism. Scand. J. Gastroenterol., *10*:293, 1975.

50. Wilkinson, G.T.: The effects of liver disease and aging on the disposition of diazepam, chlordiazepoxide, oxazepam and lorazepam in man. Acta Psychiat. Scand., (Suppl.) *274*:56, 1978.

51. Klotz, U., et al.: The effects of age and liver disease on the disposition and elimination of diazepam in man. J. Clin. Invest., *55*:347, 1975.

52. Andreasen, P.B., et al.: Pharmacokinetics of diazepam in disordered liver function. Eur. J. Clin. Pharmacol., *10*:115, 1976.

53. Branch, R.A., et al.: Intravenous administration of diazepam in patients with chronic liver disease. Gut, *17*:975, 1976.

54. Greenblatt, D.J., Harmatz, J.S., and Shader, R.I.: Factors influencing diazepam pharmacokinetics: Age, sex, and liver disease. Int. J. Clin. Pharmacol. Ther. Toxicol., *16*:177, 1978.

55. Ochs, H.R., et al.: Repeated diazepam dosing in cirrhotic patients: cumulation and sedation. Clin. Pharmacol. Ther., *33*:471, 1983.

56. Roberts, R.K., et al. The effect of age and parenchymal liver disease on the disposition and elimination of chlordiazepoxide (Librium®). Gastroenterology, *75*:479, 1977.

57. Piafsky, K.M., et al.: Theophylline disposition in patients with hepatic cirrhosis. N. Engl. J. Med., *296*:1495, 1977.

58. Mangione, A., et al.: Pharmacokinetics of theophylline in heart disease. Chest, *73*:616, 1978.

59. Staib, A.H., et al.: Pharmacokinetics and metabolism of theophylline in patients with liver disease. Int. J. Clin. Pharmacol., *18*:500, 1980.

60. Gugler, R., Muller-Liebenau, B., and Somogyi, A.: Altered disposition and availability of cimetidine in liver cirrhotic patients. Br. J. Clin. Pharmacol., *14*:421, 1982.

61. Juhl, R.P., et al.: Ibuprofen and sulindac kinetics in alcoholic liver disease. Clin. Pharmacol. Ther., *34*:105, 1983.

62. Schenker, S., et al.: Fluoxetine disposition and elimination in cirrhosis. Clin. Pharmacol. Ther., *44*:353, 1988.

63. McQuinn, R.L., et al.: Pharmacokinetics of flecainide in patients with cirrhosis of the liver. Clin. Pharmacol. Ther., *44*:566, 1988.

64. Ohnishi, A., et al.: Kinetics and dynamics of enalapril in patients with liver cirrhosis. Clin. Pharmacol. Ther., *45*:657, 1989.

65. Williams, R.L., and Mamelock, R.D.: Hepatic disease and drug pharmacokinetics. Clin. Pharmacokinet., *5*:528, 1980.

66. Williams, R.L., et al.: Influence of viral hepatitis on the disposition of two compounds with high hepatic clearance: Lidocaine and indocyanine green. Clin. Pharmacol. Ther., *20*:290, 1976.

67. Branch, R.A., James, J.A., and Read, A.E.: The clearance of antipyrine and indocyanine green in normal subjects and in patients with chronic liver disease. Clin. Pharmacol. Ther., *20*:81, 1976.

68. Feely, J., et al.: Effect of hypotension on liver blood flow and lidocaine disposition. N. Engl. J. Med., *307*:866, 1982.

69. Wood, A.J.J., et al.: The influence of cirrhosis on steady-state blood concentrations of unbound propranolol after oral administration. Clin. Pharmacokinet., *3*:478, 1978.

70. Regardh, C.-G., et al.: Pharmacokinetics of metoprolol in patients with hepatic cirrhosis. Clin. Pharmacokinet., *6*:375, 1981.

71. Neal, E.A., et al.: Enhanced bioavailability and decreased clearance of analgesics in patients with cirrhosis. Gastroenterology, *77*:96, 1979.

72. Villeneuve, J.P., Rocheleau, F., and Raymond, G.: Triamterene kinetics and dynamics in cirrhosis. Clin. Pharmacol. Ther., *35*:831, 1984.

73. Kleinbloesem, C.H., et al.: Nifedipine: kinetics and hemodynamic effects in patients with liver cirrhosis after intravenous and oral administration. Clin. Pharmacol. Ther., *40*:21, 1986.

74. Pomier-Layrargues, G., et al.: Effect of portacaval shunt on drug disposition in patients with cirrhosis. Gastroenterol., *91*:163, 1986.

75. Gengo, F.M., et al.: Nimodipine disposition and haemodynamic effects in patients with cirrhosis and age-matched controls. Br. J. Clin. Pharmacol., *23*:47, 1987.

76. Dylewicz, P., et al.: Bioavailability and elimination of nitrendipine in liver disease. Eur. J. Clin. Pharmacol., *32*:563, 1987.

77. Dalhoff, K., et al.: Buspirone pharmacokinetics in patients with cirrhosis. Br. J. Clin. Pharmacol., *24*:547, 1987.

78. Bergstrand, R.H., et al.: Encainide disposition in patients with chronic cirrhosis. Clin. Pharmacol. Ther., *40*:148, 1986.

79. Spring, P.: The pharmacokinetics of Rimactane in patients with impaired liver and kidney function. *In* A Symposium on Rimactane. Basel, Ciba, Ltd., 1968, pp. 32–34.

80. Carulli, N., et al.: Alteration of drug metabolism during cholestasis in man. Eur. J. Clin. Invest., *5*:455, 1975.

81. Somogyi, A.A., Shanko, C.A., and Triggs, E.J.: Disposition kinetics of pancuronium bromide in patients with total biliary obstruction. Br. J. Anaesth., *49*:1103, 1977.

82. McLean, A., duSouich, P., and Gibaldi, M.: Noninvasive kinetic approach to the estimation of total hepatic blood flow and shunting in liver disease. A hypothesis. Clin. Pharmacol. Ther., *25*:161, 1979.

83. Branch, R.A.: Drugs as indicators of hepatic function. Hepatol., *2*:97, 1982.

84. Farrell, G.C., Cooksley, W.G.E., and Powell, L.W.: Drug metabolism in liver disease: Activity of hepatic mi-

crosomal metabolizing enzymes. Clin. Pharmacol. Ther., 26:483, 1979.

85. Crom, W.R., et al.: Simultaneous administration of multiple model substrates to assess hepatic drug clearance. Clin. Pharmacol. Ther., 41:645, 1987.

86. Relling, M.V., et al.: Hepatic drug clearance in children with leukemia: changes in clearance of model substrates during remission-induction therapy. Clin. Pharmacol. Ther., 41:651, 1987.

87. Kawasaki, S., et al.: Hepatic clearances of antipyrine, indocyanine green, and galactose in normal subjects and in patients with chronic liver disease. Clin. Pharmacol. Ther., 44:217, 1988.

88. Anon.: Safe prescribing in liver disease. Br. Med. J., 1:193, 1973.

89. Schenker, S., Hoyumpa, A.M., Jr., and Wilkinson, G.R.: The effect of parenchymal liver disease on the disposition and elimination of sedatives and analgesics. Med. Clin. North Am., 59:887, 1975.

90. Schmid, K.: α_1-Acid glycoprotein. In The Plasma Proteins. Vol. I. Edited by T.W. Putnam. New York, Academic Press, 1975, pp. 184–228.

91. Reidenberg, M.M.: The binding of drugs to plasma proteins and the interpretation of measurements of plasma concentrations of drugs in patients with poor renal function. Am. J. Med., 62:466, 1977.

92. Depner, T.A., and Gulyassy, P.F.: Plasma protein binding in uremia: Extraction and characterization of an inhibitor. Kidney Int., 18:86, 1980.

93. Kinniburgh, D.W., and Boyd, N.D.: Isolation of peptides from uremic plasma that inhibit phenytoin binding to normal plasma proteins. Clin. Pharmacol. Ther., 30:276, 1981.

94. Letteri, J.M., et al.: Diphenylhydantoin metabolism in uremia. N. Engl. J. Med., 285:648, 1971.

95. Odar-Cederlof, I.: Plasma protein binding of phenytoin and warfarin in patients undergoing renal transplantation. Clin. Pharmacokinet., 2:147, 1977.

96. Gugler, R., and Mueller, G.: Plasma protein binding of valproic acid in healthy subjects and in patients with renal disease. Br. J. Clin. Pharmacol., 5:441, 1978.

97. Rane, A., et al.: Plasma binding and disposition of furosemide in the nephrotic syndrome and in uremia. Clin. Pharmacol. Ther., 24:199, 1978.

98. Kober, A., et al.: Protein binding of diazepam and digitoxin in uremic and normal serum. Biochem. Pharmacol., 28:1037, 1979.

99. Grossman, S.H., et al.: Diazepam and lidocaine plasma protein binding in renal disease. Clin. Pharmacol. Ther., 31:350, 1982.

100. Blaschke, T.F.: Protein binding and kinetics of drugs in liver diseases. Clin. Pharmacokinet., 2:32, 1977.

101. Thiessen, J.J., et al.: Plasma protein binding of diazepam and tolbutamide in chronic alcoholics. J. Clin. Pharmacol., 16:345, 1976.

102. Williams, R.L., et al.: Influence of acute viral hepatitis on disposition and plasma binding of tolbutamide. Clin. Pharmacol. Ther., 21:301,1977.

103. Brodie, M.J., and Boobis, S.: The effects of chronic alcohol ingestion and alcoholic liver disease on binding of drugs to serum proteins. Eur. J. Clin. Pharmacol., 13:435, 1978.

104. Urien, S., Albengres, E., and Tillement, J.-P.: Serum protein binding of valproic acid in healthy subjects and in patients with liver disease. Int. J. Clin. Pharmacol., 19:319, 1981.

105. Verbeeck, R.K., et al.: Furosemide disposition in cirrhosis. Clin. Pharmacol. Ther., 31:719, 1982.

106. Piafsky, K.M.: Disease-induced changes in the plasma binding of basic drugs. Clin. Pharmacokinet., 5:246, 1980.

107. Fremsted, D., et al.: Increased plasma binding of quinidine after surgery. Eur. J. Clin. Pharmacol., 10:441, 1976.

108. Piafsky, K.M., et al.: Increased plasma protein binding of propranolol and chlorpromazine mediated by disease-induced elevations of plasma α_1 acid glycoprotein. N. Engl. J. Med., 299:1435, 1978.

109. Routledge, P.A., et al.: Increased plasma propranolol binding in myocardial infarction. Br. J. Clin. Pharmacol., 9:438, 1980.

110. Routledge, P.A., et al.: Lignocaine disposition in blood in epilepsy. Br. J. Clin. Pharmacol., 12:663, 1981.

111. Edwards, D.J., et al.: Alpha$_1$-acid glycoprotein concentration and protein binding in trauma. Clin. Pharmacol. Ther., 31:62, 1982.

112. Jusko, W.J., and Weintraub, M.: Myocardial distribution of digoxin and renal function. Clin. Pharmacol. Ther., 16:449, 1974.

113. Evans, G.H., and Shand, D.G.: Disposition of propranolol. VI. Independent variation in steady state circulating drug concentration and half-life as a result of plasma drug binding in man. Clin. Pharmacol. Ther., 14:494, 1973.

114. Fremstad, D., et al.: Pharmacokinetics of quinidine related to plasma protein binding in man. Eur. J. Clin. Pharmacol., 15:187, 1979.

115. Reuning, R.H., Sams, R.A., and Notari, R.E.: Role of pharmacokinetics in drug dosage adjustment. I. Pharmacologic effect kinetics and apparent volume of distribution of digoxin. J. Clin. Pharmacol., 13:127, 1973.

116. Kornhauser, D.M., et al.: Biological determinants of propranolol disposition in man. Clin. Pharmacol. Ther., 23:165, 1978.

117. Odar-Cederlof, I., and Borga, O.: Kinetics of diphenylhydantoin in uraemic patients: Consequences of decreased plasma protein binding. Eur. J. Clin. Pharmacol., 7:31, 1974.

118. Ochs, H.R., et al.: Diazepam kinetics in patients with renal insufficiency or hyperthyroidism. Br. J. Clin. Pharmacol., 12:829, 1981.

119. Evans, G.H., Nies, A.S., and Shand, D.G.: The disposition of propranolol. III. Decreased half-life and volume of distribution as a result of plasma binding in man, monkey, dog and rat. J. Pharmacol. Exp. Ther., 186:114, 1973.

120. Ohnhaus, E.E., Lenzinger, H.R., and Galeazzi, R.L.: Comparison of two different loading doses of digoxin in severe renal impairment. Eur. J. Clin. Pharmacol., 18:467, 1980.

121. Gugler, R., et al.: Pharmacokinetics of drugs in patients with the nephrotic syndrome. J. Clin. Invest., 55:1182, 1975.

122. Boston Collaborative Drug Surveillance Program: Diphenylhydantoin side effects and serum albumin levels. Clin. Pharmacol. Ther., 14:529, 1973.

123. Lewis, G.P., et al.: Prednisone side-effects and serum-protein levels. Lancet, 2:778, 1971.

124. Greenblatt, D. J., and Koch-Weser, J.: Clinical toxicity of chlordiazepoxide and diazepam in relation to serum albumin concentration. Eur. J. Clin. Pharmacol., 7:259, 1974.

125. Levy, G.: Effect of plasma protein binding of drugs on duration and intensity of pharmacologic activity. J. Pharm. Sci., 65:1264, 1976.

126. Gugler, R., and Azarnoff, D.L.: Drug protein binding and the nephrotic syndrome. Clin. Pharmacokinet., 1:25, 1976.

127. Williams, R.L., and Benet, L.Z.: Drug pharmacokinetics

in cardiac and hepatic disease. Ann. Rev. Pharmacol. Toxicol., *20*:383, 1980.

128. Shammas, F.V., and Dickstein, K.: Clinical pharmacokinetics in heart failure. An updated review. Clin. Pharmacokin., *15*:94, 1988.

129. Hepner, G.W., Vesell, E.S., and Tantum, K.R.: Reduced drug elimination in congestive heart failure. Studies using aminopyrine as a model drug. Am. J. Med., *65*:271, 1978.

130. Aps, C., et al.: Logical approach to lignocaine therapy. Br. Med. J., *1*:13, 1976.

131. Prescott, L.F., Adjepon-Yanoah, K.K., and Talbot, R.G.: Impaired lignocaine metabolism in patients with myocardial infarction and cardiac failure. Br. Med. J., *1*:939, 1976.

132. Thomson, P.D., et al.: Lidocaine pharmacokinetics in advanced heart failure, liver disease, and renal failure in humans. Ann. Intern. Med., *78*:499, 1973.

133. Stenson, R.E., Constantino, R.T., and Harrison, D.C.: Interrelationship of hepatic blood flow, cardiac output, and blood levels of lidocaine in man. Circulation, *43*:205, 1971.

134. Weiss, Y.A., et al.: Comparison of the pharmacokinetics of dl-propranolol in borderline and permanent hypertension. Eur. J. Clin. Pharmacol., *10*:387, 1976.

135. Ueda, C.T., and Dzindzio, B.S.: Quinidine kinetics in congestive heart failure. Clin. Pharmacol. Ther., *23*:158, 1978.

136. Woosley, R.L.: Pharmacokinetics and pharmacodynamics of antiarrhythmic agents in patients with congestive heart failure. Am. Heart J., *114*:1280, 1987.

137. Jaillon, P., et al.: Influence of congestive heart failure on prazosin kinetics. Clin. Pharmacol. Ther., *25*:790, 1979.

138. Baughman, R.A., Jr., et al.: Altered prazosin pharmacokinetics in congestive heart failure. Eur. J. Clin. Pharmacol., *17*:425, 1980.

139. Ogilvie, R.I.: Clinical pharmacokinetics of theophylline. Clin. Pharmacokinet., *3*:267, 1978.

140. Powell, J.R., et al.: Theophylline disposition in acutely ill hospitalized patients. The effect of smoking, heart failure, severe airway obstruction, and pneumonia. Am. Rev. Resp. Dis., *118*:229, 1978.

141. Dickstein, K., et al.: The pharmacokinetics of enalapril in hospitalized patients with congestive heart failure. Br. J. Clin. Pharmacol., *23*:403, 1987.

142. Brater, D.C., et al.: Bumetanide and furosemide in heart failure. Kidney Int., *26*:183, 1984.

143. Vasko, M.R., et al.: Furosemide absorption altered in decompensated congestive heart failure. Ann. Intern. Med., *102*:314, 1985.

144. Shenfield, G.M.: Influence of thyroid dysfunction on drug pharmacokinetics. Clin. Pharmacokinet., *6*:275, 1981.

145. O'Connor, P., and Feely, J.: Clinical pharmacokinetics and endocrine disorders. Therapeutic implications. Clin. Pharmacokin., *13*:345, 1987.

146. Levy, G., MacGillivray, M.H., and Procknal, J.A.: Riboflavin absorption in children with thyroid disorders. Pediatrics, *50*:896, 1972.

147. Forfar, J.C., et al.: Paracetamol pharmacokinetics in thyroid disease. Eur. J. Clin. Pharmacol., *18*:269, 1980.

148. Doherty, J.E., and Perkins, W.H.: Digoxin metabolism in hypo- and hyperthyroidism. Studies with tritiated di-

goxin in thyroid disease. Ann. Intern. Med., *64*:489, 1966.

149. Croxson, M.S., and Ibbertson, H.K.: Serum digoxin in patients with thyroid disease. Br. Med. J., *2*:566, 1975.

150. Shenfield, G.M., Thompson, J., and Horn, D.B.: Plasma and urinary digoxin in thyroid dysfunction. Eur. J. Clin. Pharmacol., *12*:437, 1977.

151. Eichelbaum, M., et al.: Influence of thyroid status on plasma half-life of antipyrine in man. N. Engl. J. Med., *290*:1040, 1974.

152. Vesell, E.S., et al.: Accelerated plasma half-lives of antipyrine, propylthiouracil, and methimazole in thyroid dysfunction. Clin. Pharmacol. Ther., *17*:48, 1975.

153. Feely, J., Crooks, J., and Stevenson, I.H.: Plasma propranolol steady state concentrations in thyroid disorders. Eur. J. Clin. Pharmacol., *19*:329, 1981.

154. Chang, K.C., et al.: Altered theophylline pharmacokinetics during acute respiratory viral illness. Lancet, *1*:1132, 1978.

155. Kraemer, M.J., et al.: Altered theophylline clearance during an influenza B outbreak. Pediatrics, *69*:476, 1982.

156. Forsyth, J.S., Moreland, T.A., and Rylance, G.W.: The effect of fever on antipyrine metabolism in children. Br. J. Clin. Pharmacol., *13*:811, 1982.

157. Elin, R.J., Vesell, E.S., and Wolff, S.M.: Effects of etiocholanolane-induced fever on plasma antipyrine half-lives and metabolic clearance. Clin. Pharmacol. Ther., *17*:447, 1975.

158. Renton, K.W., Gray, J.D., and Hall, R.I.: Decreased elimination of theophylline after influenza vaccination. Can. Med. Assoc. J., *123*:288, 1980.

159. Kramer, P., and McClain, C.J.: Depression of aminopyrine metabolism by influenza vaccination. N. Engl. J. Med., *305*:1262, 1981.

160. Meredith, C.G., et al.: Effects of influenza virus vaccine on hepatic drug metabolism. Clin. Pharmacol. Ther., *37*:396, 1985.

161. Winstanley, P.A., et al.: Lack of effect of highly purified subunit influenza vaccination on theophylline metabolism. Br. J. Clin. Pharmacol., *20*:47, 1985.

162. Grabowski, N., et al.: The effect of split virus influenza vaccination on theophylline pharmacokinetics. Am. Rev. Respir. Dis., *131*:934, 1985.

163. Sawchuck, R.J., and Rector, T.S.: Drug kinetics in burn patients. Clin. Pharmacokinet., *5*:548, 1980.

164. Zaske, D.E., et al.: Increased dosage requirements of gentamicin in burn patients. J. Trauma, *16*:824, 1976.

165. Zaske, D.E., et al.: Rapid individualization of gentamicin dosage regimens in 66 burn patients. Burns, *7*:215, 1981.

166. Brater, D.C., et al.: Vancomycin elimination in patients with burn injury. Clin. Pharmacol. Ther., *39*:631, 1986.

167. Garrelts, J.C., and Peterie, J.D.: Altered vancomycin dose vs serum concentration relationship in burn patients. Clin. Pharmacol. Ther., *44*:9, 1988.

168. Martyn, J.A.J., Greenblatt, D.J., and Abernethy, D.R.: Increased cimetidine clearance in burned patients. JAMA, *253*:1288, 1985.

169. Martyn, J.A.J., et al.: Alteration by burn injury of the pharmacokinetics and pharmacodynamics of cimetidine in children. Eur. J. Clin. Pharmacol., *36*:361, 1989.

170. Knoppert, D.C., et al.: Cystic fibrosis: enhanced theophylline metabolism may be linked to the disease. Clin. Pharmacol. Ther., *44*:254, 1988.

14

Pharmacokinetic Variability— Drug Interactions

Antagonism or potentiation of the effects of one drug by another is a well-known phenomenon. We are now aware that in many cases these drug-drug interactions have a pharmacokinetic rather than pharmacologic basis. The absorption, distribution, excretion, or metabolism of a drug may be affected by the concomitant administration of a second drug, leading to differences in clinical effects.

Few topics in clinical pharmacology have attracted more attention than drug-drug interactions that may result in a loss of therapeutic effectiveness or an increase in adverse effects. Thousands of experimental, clinical, and epidemiologic studies have been reported. Hundreds of review articles on interactions between drugs have appeared, and more than a dozen books as well as a newsletter have been devoted to the subject. Many of these contributions contain important and useful information that increases our understanding of the mechanisms and clinical consequences of drug interactions.[1–8] On the other hand, some lack criticality and a clinical perspective.

The clinical problem presented by interactions between drugs has been vastly overestimated by some authors. In fact, only a relatively small number of the thousands of drug interactions listed in some published compilations are of clinical significance. Of these, most are predictable and preventable, usually by appropriate dosage adjustment, and few are potentially disabling or life threatening.[9]

Although drug interactions probably contribute less to the total incidence of iatrogenic disease than some authors have suggested in the past, this does not minimize the hazards of multiple drug therapy.

Epidemiologic studies demonstrate that the rate of adverse reactions to drugs increases from 4.2% when 5 or fewer drugs are given to 45% when 20 or more drugs are prescribed.[10] Another investigation, based on more than 10,000 patients hospitalized on a general medical service during a 5-year period, found that the average number of drugs received during hospitalization by each patient was 7.9, but the average number of drugs received by patients who experienced an adverse drug reaction was 13.4.[11] The adverse reaction rate was 4% in patients receiving 5 or fewer drugs, 10% in patients receiving 6 to 10 drugs, 28% in patients receiving 11 to 15 drugs, and 54% in patients receiving 16 to 20 drugs.

The risk of clinical consequences from drug-drug interactions is higher with some drug categories than with others. This is evident in Figure 14–1, which shows the percentage of hospitalized patients, categorized by drug group, who experienced adverse drug reactions.[11] Patients receiving anticoagulant or antihypertensive drugs were at a much greater risk than patients receiving other kinds of drugs. Of nine drug categories, the anticoagulants and antihypertensives were the only two for which the occurrence of adverse reactions increased significantly when the number of different drugs received by patients increased (Fig. 14–2).

Koch-Weser and Greenblatt proposed that clinically important drug interactions rarely involve drugs other than oral anticoagulants, cardiac glycosides, antiarrhythmics, sympathomimetic amines, antihypertensives, anticonvulsants, oral hypoglycemics, or cytotoxic drugs.[9] Common manifestations are hemorrhage, cardiac arrhyth-

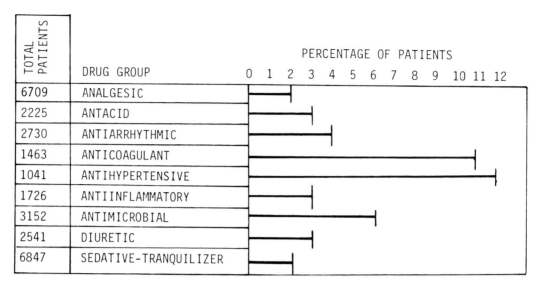

Fig. 14–1. Percentage of hospitalized patients, categorized by drug group, who experienced adverse drug reactions. (Data from May, F.E., Stewart, R.B., and Cluff, L.E.[11])

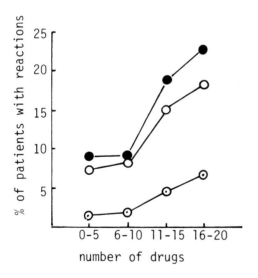

Fig. 14–2. Effects of the total number of drugs received by the patient on the percentage of patients experiencing an adverse drug reaction to a specific drug group. Key: (●) antihypertensives; (○) anticoagulants; (⊙) other drug groups (including analgesics, antacids, antiarrhythmics, anti-inflammatories, antimicrobial agents, diuretics, and sedatives-tranquilizers). (Data from May, F.E., Stewart, R.B., and Cluff, L.E.[11])

mias, severe hypertension or hypotension, convulsive seizures, or hypoglycemia. These are the interactions that prescribers should be made aware of.

This chapter largely concerns interactions between drugs and, to a small extent, drug interactions with environmental chemicals. Emphasis is given to the mechanisms of interaction and to clinically important interactions.

DRUG ABSORPTION

Interactions that interfere with drug absorption usually involve binding or chelation of drugs in the gastrointestinal tract or effects on gastric emptying or gastrointestinal motility.

One of the earliest reported drug-drug interactions was that between tetracycline antibiotics and antacids. Antacid drugs, particularly those containing aluminum, markedly decrease the absorption of most tetracyclines by forming an insoluble complex in the gastrointestinal tract.[12] The interaction is most pronounced when the drugs are given simultaneously.

Simultaneous administration of ferrous sulfate also impairs the absorption of tetracycline, oxytetracycline, methacycline, and doxycycline, probably by means of a chelation mechanism.[13] No interaction is observed when the iron salt is given 3 hr before or 2 hr after the tetracycline.[14]

Since these early studies, coadministration of antacids has been found to interfere with the absorption of other drugs including indomethacin,[15] nitrofurantoin,[16] diflusinal,[17] fluoride,[18] phenytoin,[19] and cimetidine.[20] Magnesium trisilicate reduces the absorption of nitrofurantoin by more than 50%.[16] These interactions are usually easily avoided by administering the antacid some time before or after the drug.

Sucralfate, a poorly absorbed complex of aluminum hydroxide and sulfated sucrose, used for treating peptic ulcers, interacts with some drugs in the gastrointestinal tract resulting in reduced absorption. One study found that concomitant administration of 1 g sucralfate reduced the absorption of 300 mg phenytoin capsules by 20% as measured by area under the curve from 0–48 hr.[21] Peak phenytoin levels were 3.7 μg/ml when it was given with placebo and 2.9 μg/ml when given with sucralfate.

More recently, the effect of sucralfate on the absorption of oral norfloxacin, a quinolone antibacterial agent, was evaluated.[22] On each occasion, subjects were given 400 mg norfloxacin alone, with 1 g sucralfate, or 2 hr after 1 g of sucralfate. When sucralfate was given concurrently, the bioavailability of norfloxacin was less than 2%. Administration of norfloxacin 2 hr after sucralfate resulted in a smaller but nevertheless substantial interaction. Bioavailability was 55 to 60% relative to the administration of norfloxacin alone.

Aluminum- and magnesium-containing antacids also dramatically decrease the absorption of norfloxacin and other oral quinolones. In each case, the mechanism appears to involve an interaction of the heavy metal ion with the quinolone nucleus, perhaps resulting in an insoluble complex. Considering norfloxacin concentrations in urine and minimum inhibitory concentrations (MICs) for relevant bacteria, the investigators concluded that administration of norfloxacin with antacids or sucralfate is likely to result in treatment failure for urinary tract infections. The investigators also pointed out that although the interaction with sucralfate "has not been studied with all quinolone antimicrobial agents, one would expect it to occur with all members of this class."

Absorption may also be reduced when drugs are given with adsorbents, such as kaolin or bismuth subsalicylate, or ion exchange resins, such as cholestyramine or colestipol. Antidiarrheal mixtures containing kaolin impair the absorption of lincomycin[23] and promazine.[24] Concomitant administration of 2 oz of a kaolin-pectin mixture re-

duces the absorption of digoxin by 40%.[25] Oral coadministration of a bismuth subsalicylate antidiarrheal mixture reduced the absorption of tetracycline[26] and doxycycline[27] by about 35 to 40%. A multiple dose regimen of bismuth subsalicylate mixture, typical of usage in traveler's diarrhea, reduced doxycycline absorption by about 50%.[27]

Ion exchange resins are now used for the treatment of elevated plasma cholesterol or bile acid levels. They are not absorbed but exert their effects by binding bile acids in the intestine, preventing their reabsorption. These resins also bind certain anionic and neutral drugs in the intestine and are known to interfere with the absorption of anticoagulants[28] and thyroxine.[29]

Brown et al.[30] gave either two 0.25 mg digoxin tablets or two 0.20 digoxin soft gelatin capsules (containing a nonaqueous solution of the drug) once a day, alone or with cholestyramine, 8 g once daily, to healthy adult subjects. Bioavailability was determined from steady-state 24-hour area under the serum concentration-time curve (AUC). The AUCs for tablets alone and with cholestyramine were 32.8 and 22.4 ng-hr/ml, respectively, while corresponding values for capsules were 31.7 and 24.7. Cholestyramine administration with digoxin tablets produced a 32% decrease in mean digoxin AUC, whereas a 22% decrease was measured when the resin was given with digoxin capsules. These differences suggest that digoxin capsules, the more rapidly dissolving form of digoxin, are perhaps less prone to drug interactions than digoxin tablets.

Certain drugs are metabolized in the gastrointestinal tract and only a fraction of the dose reaches the systemic circulation. Slow absorption, resulting from impaired gastric emptying, could result in a greater fraction of the dose undergoing metabolism in the gut and in a lower bioavailability. This mechanism may explain the effects of drugs with anticholinergic activity on the absorption of levodopa. Imipramine[31] and trihexyphenidyl[32] have been found to significantly reduce the bioavailability of levodopa in healthy human subjects. Concomitant administration of trihexyphenidyl with levodopa, a likely combination, may decrease the efficacy of levodopa.

Anticholinergics and other drugs that reduce gastric emptying usually decrease the rate but not the extent of drug absorption. Drugs, such as cimetidine, that reduce gastric acid output may decrease

Table 14–1. Effect of Antibiotic Therapy on Steady-State Digoxin Concentrations in Serum*

| Subject no. | Serum digoxin concentration (ng/ml) | |
	Control period	Antibiotic period
1	0.72	1.03
2	0.76	1.33
3	0.37	0.80

*Data from Lindenbaum, J., et al.[33]

the solubility of certain basic drugs in the stomach and impair absorption.

A particularly interesting interaction has been reported between digoxin and certain antibiotics.[33] Oral digoxin is slowly absorbed; a considerable fraction of the dose may reach the lower intestine where it is reduced to inactive metabolites by the bacterial flora. Bacterial metabolism limits the bioavailability of slowly dissolving preparations of digoxin in many patients and that of rapidly dissolving products in a much smaller number of patients. About 10% of patients receiving conventional oral digoxin tablets metabolize more than 40% of the dose to cardioinactive compounds in the lower intestine.

Certain oral antibiotics, including tetracycline and erythromycin, alter the bacterial flora and decrease the inactivation of digoxin.[33] Table 14–1 shows steady-state serum levels of digoxin before and during treatment with oral antibiotics. Digoxin levels were increased 43 to 116% by antibiotic treatment. It is possible that therapy with antimicrobial agents in certain patients occasionally precipitates digoxin toxicity.

Not all antimicrobial agents affect digoxin absorption in this manner; in fact, treatment with neomycin[34] or sulfasalazine[35] reduces the bioavailability of digoxin. When neomycin was given with maintenance doses of digoxin, steady-state serum digoxin concentrations were reduced, on the average, by 30%.[34] Similar effects on digoxin absorption have been observed after a 6-day treatment with sulfasalazine.[35] The mechanisms of these effects are not known.

Another interaction for which the mechanism is obscure is that observed with griseofulvin and phenobarbital.[36] Phenobarbital has no effect on the distribution or elimination of griseofulvin; however, phenobarbital reduces the plasma levels of griseofulvin and also reduces the cumulative urinary recovery of its principal metabolite, suggesting that phenobarbital interferes with the absorption of griseofulvin. A similar interaction has been re-

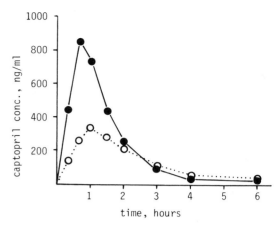

Fig. 14–3. Captopril concentrations in blood after a single 100-mg oral dose to fasted (●) and fed (○) healthy subjects. (Data from Singhvi, S.M., et al.[40])

ported to occur between heptabarbital and dicumarol.[37]

The effect of food on drug absorption has been considered in Chapter 3. In some cases, administration of a drug after a meal may seriously reduce clinical efficacy. The salivary suppression produced by propantheline is virtually abolished when it is given immediately after a meal.[38] The relative bioavailability of lincomycin is reduced to about 60% when given 1 hr before breakfast and to about 20% when given immediately after breakfast, compared to that observed after oral administration to fasting subjects.[39] The bioavailability of captopril, a potent angiotensin-converting enzyme inhibitor used in hypertension, is decreased 35 to 40% after a meal (Fig. 14–3).[40]

A potentially dangerous situation may arise because of delayed absorption of hypnotic agents in nonfasting patients. With the hypnotic capuride, a 42 min difference in onset of absorption has been observed between fasting and nonfasting subjects.[41] Failure to obtain early sleep could encourage additional doses and lead to toxicity.

Hydralazine blood levels were reduced almost 50% when the drug was given after a meal compared with levels measured in fasting subjects.[42] The higher blood levels in fasted subjects resulted in a greater change in mean arterial pressure (MAP). The maximum fall in MAP was 18 mm Hg in fasted subjects compared with 11 mm mg in subjects taking hydralazine after breakfast.

Food, particularly high-fat meals, have been found to have a profound effect on theophylline absorption after oral administration of some prolonged-release products. Both increased and decreased absorption have been reported depending on the product.

The unexpected and dramatic increase in the release rate of theophylline from a once a day product (Theo-24) when it was given with a high-fat meal sent regulatory agencies scrambling to revise guidelines for approval of prolonged-release products. In the US, a single-dose food study is now required as part of the submission for all controlled-release products.

Theo-24 is incompletely absorbed in fasted subjects. A high-fat meal not only increases the extent of absorption, but also dramatically increases the rate of absorption. About half the daily dose is absorbed over a 4-hr period, giving rise to excessively high blood levels of theophylline.[43]

Another slow-release product, Theo-Dur Sprinkle, specifically developed for pediatrics, is well absorbed in fasted subjects but bioavailability decreases by more than 50% when it is taken after a heavy breakfast.[44] A comprehensive review of food interactions with prolonged-release theophylline preparations is available.[45]

A meal may also have large effects on the absorption of drugs given in single-unit enteric-coated dosage forms. The mean time to a measurable plasma concentration of salicylate (lag time) after administration of enteric-coated aspirin tablets was 2.7 hr in fasted subjects and 7.9 hr when the tablets were given 30 min after breakfast, followed 4 hr later by lunch.[46] A 5-hr difference was also observed in the time to peak salicylate concentration in plasma. No effect was noted on the total amount of aspirin absorbed from enteric-coated tablets.

Under these conditions, gastric residence time (GRT), determined by a radio-telemetric device called a Heidelberg capsule, was 0.8 hr in fasted subjects and 5.9 hr in fed subjects. Female subjects had a significantly longer GRT than male subjects.[47] A strong (r = 0.94) correlation was observed between lag times of aspirin from enteric-coated tablets and GRTs.

In all cases, the lag time was greater than the GRT, consistent with the idea that the enteric coating remains intact in the stomach and a finite time in the small intestine is needed for the coating to disrupt and release aspirin. The average time for dissolution and absorption of enteric-coated aspirin after entering the small intestine (i.e., the lag time minus GRT) was about 2 hr for both fed and fasted subjects. The time to reach a peak level of salicylate

after gastric emptying was also independent of feeding status.

These studies confirm long-held beliefs that most of the variability in lag time following administration of enteric-coated tablets can be explained by differences in gastric residence time. Mojaverian et al.[46] concluded that "marked delays in the absorption of aspirin from enteric-coated tablets may be observed when they are consumed with food. This effect is particularly pronounced in women."

DRUG BINDING IN PLASMA

Competition between drugs for common binding sites on plasma proteins is an almost ubiquitous drug interaction. Mefenamic acid, ethacrynic acid, nalidixic acid, and diazoxide,[48] as well as phenylbutazone, thyroxine, sulfaphenazole, and clofibrate,[49] significantly displace warfarin from human serum albumin. Tolbutamide, indomethacin, and sulfamethoxypyridazine competitively inhibit the binding of phenylbutazone to serum albumin.[50] Various fatty acids displace both phenylbutazone and warfarin from human albumin.[50] Salicylic acid, sulfisoxazole, and phenylbutazone, at concentrations that are observed clinically, decrease phenytoin binding to plasma proteins.[51] Many more examples can be found in the literature.

These interactions between drugs usually produce considerable pharmacokinetic changes with respect to the drug that is displaced from plasma protein binding sites, but they are rarely of clinical importance. The following example may help to understand the reason for this.

A patient who has received drug A for a long period is now also given daily doses of drug B, which competitively inhibits the binding of A to plasma proteins. If the elimination of drug A is rate-limited by the intrinsic ability of the eliminating organs to clear it, rather than by renal or hepatic blood flow (HBF), the clearance of A from the blood or plasma will increase because of the increase in the fraction unbound. Therefore, the plasma levels of total A (bound and unbound) will decrease until a new and lower steady-state concentration is established. At the new steady-state, the free concentration of A is the same as the free concentration at the original steady-state, before treatment with drug B was initiated. It is conceivable that during the period from one steady-state to another, free drug level may be transiently elevated but this does not seem to be an important event.

This situation is almost the same as that described in Chapter 13 for the consequences of disease-related impairment of drug binding. It applies only when drug B simply displaces drug A from binding sites in the plasma but has no effect on the intrinsic clearance of A. Therefore, displacement interactions should be of little clinical significance. Although the total levels of A in the plasma are depressed when the two drugs are given together, there is no need to change the dosage of drug A because free levels are unchanged.[52]

Addition of valproic acid to an existing drug treatment regimen in epileptic patients results in a substantial fall in steady-state serum levels of phenytoin. One study found that phenytoin levels decline from about 20 to 15 μg/ml.[53] This is a result of displacement of phenytoin from plasma proteins by valproic acid. Unbound phenytoin increased from 9% in patients on phenytoin alone to 13 to 19% in patients with valproic acid levels less than 90 μg/ml and to greater than 20% in patients with valproic acid levels exceeding 90 μg/ml.[53]

Decreased binding also results in an increase in the clearance and apparent volume of distribution of phenytoin.[54,55] However, free phenytoin concentrations remain unchanged in the presence of valproic acid, despite the reduction in total phenytoin levels.[56] There is probably no need to adjust phenytoin dosage when valproate is added to the treatment regimen.

The effect of high-dose aspirin on the disposition of tenoxicam, a nonsteroidal antiinflammatory drug (NSAID) related to piroxicam, was studied in healthy human subjects.[57] In one study, subjects were given a single dose of tenoxicam, followed by a course of aspirin treatment; toward the end of the aspirin treatment period, a second dose of tenoxicam was given.

Aspirin was associated with a decrease in the half-life and with increases in the apparent volume of distribution and clearance of tenoxicam. Mean clearance was 97 ml/hr during the control period and 191 ml/hr during aspirin treatment. These changes suggested a competitive protein binding interaction between salicylate and tenoxicam. Binding studies indicated that percent unbound tenoxicam increased from 0.56% in the absence of aspirin to 1.24% in the presence of aspirin.

Although nearly all agree that pure plasma protein displacement interactions may be safely ignored, the chloral hydrate-warfarin interaction is frequently cited as an exception to this rule. Tri-

chloroacetic acid (TCA), a major metabolite of chloral hydrate, displaces warfarin from its binding sites on plasma albumin. Sellers and Koch-Weser[58] have concluded that this displacement results, for a short time, in elevated plasma levels of unbound warfarin, thereby increasing the anticoagulant activity of warfarin.

Administration of chloral hydrate to subjects on warfarin has been reported to increase its hypoprothrombinemic effect by 40 to 80%.[58] Triclofos, a hypnotic that also forms TCA, similarly prolongs prothrombin time in patients on chronic anticoagulant therapy with warfarin.[59]

Data from a comprehensive drug surveillance program were analyzed to determine the clinical importance of the interaction between chloral hydrate and warfarin.[60] Patients receiving continuous chloral hydrate therapy required significantly less warfarin (15.4 mg vs 22.3 mg) during the induction phase (second to fourth days) of anticoagulation than those receiving no chloral hydrate. Patients given occasional chloral hydrate required an intermediate dose of warfarin. All patients received a similar loading dose of warfarin on day 1 and similar maintenance doses from the fifth day onward. The results indicate that the interaction between these drugs is important; to prevent excessive hypoprothrombinemia, temporary reduction in warfarin requirement should be anticipated when chloral hydrate therapy is begun.

DRUG EXCRETION

The renal excretion of a drug may be affected by a coadministered drug that modifies urine pH, and thereby suppresses or promotes tubular reabsorption, one that interferes, competitively or noncompetitively, with tubular secretion, or one that alters glomerular filtration rate (GFR) or renal blood flow. Biliary excretion of a drug may be affected by a coadministered drug that inhibits transport in the hepatobiliary system or one that modifies bile flow rate.

Urine pH

The effects of urine pH on drug excretion have been discussed in Chapter 11. Changes in urine pH may be the result of certain diseases, dietary factors, or simultaneous administration of certain drugs. The ability of ammonium chloride to acidify and of sodium bicarbonate to alkalinize urine is well known; these materials are used in studies on the renal excretion of drugs to clarify renal excretion mechanisms.

Regular administration of usual doses of commonly used antacids can also affect urine pH.[61] Magnesium hydroxide (Milk of Magnesia) and calcium carbonate suspensions increased urine pH by 0.4 to 0.5 U, on the average, whereas aluminum-magnesium hydroxide suspension increased urine pH by an average of 0.9 U. Such elevations are sufficient to significantly alter the elimination of drugs such as salicylate or amphetamine.

Steady-state salicylate levels have been compared in subjects receiving aspirin or aspirin and sodium bicarbonate.[62] With aspirin alone, urine pH ranged from 5.6 to 6.1 and plasma salicylate concentration averaged 27 mg/dl. With aspirin and sodium bicarbonate, urine pH ranged from 6.2 to 6.9 and plasma salicylate concentration averaged only 15 mg/dl. The average difference in urine pH between studies was less than 1 U.

In another study, designed to determine if the common practice of giving antacids to patients on salicylate therapy has an effect on serum salicylate concentration, aluminum-magnesium hydroxide gel was given with aspirin to 3 children with rheumatic fever.[63] Urine pH increased and serum salicylate concentration decreased by 30 to 70%.

The hazards of unanticipated changes in urine pH in patients receiving intensive salicylate therapy are considerable. A salicylate dosage regimen yielding plasma concentration of 20 to 30 mg/dl in a patient with a urine pH of 6.5 is likely to produce plasma concentrations more than twice as high, and therefore in the toxic range, when urine pH decreases to about 5.5. Appropriate precautions are necessary, particularly in patients who may not recognize the typical symptoms of salicylism.

Patients receiving amphetamine or related drugs may also be placed at risk by relatively small changes in urine pH. The time course of amphetamine psychosis and amphetamine level in the plasma in amphetamine-dependent patients are shown in Figure 14–4.[64] Patients with alkaline urine had intense psychoses lasting more than 3 days after the last dose of amphetamine.

Probenecid

Probenecid is an old drug, indicated for the long-term management of patients with elevated uric acid levels associated with gout. Probenecid promotes the excretion of uric acid by blocking active reabsorption in the tubules; it also blocks the tubular secretion of other weak acids. Probenecid decreases the renal clearance of many drugs, including penicillins, cephalosporins, dapsone, rifampin, nitrofurantoin, sulfonamides, and thiazide diuretics.[65]

Methotrexate, an important drug for the treatment of neoplastic diseases, is largely eliminated by renal excretion; renal clearance accounts for about 95% of the total plasma clearance of the drug. Administration of probenecid reduces the renal clearance of methotrexate, from 108 to 69 ml/min, and prolongs and enhances serum methotrexate concentrations.[66] Smaller doses of methotrexate may be given with probenecid to achieve the same serum concentrations as when methotrexate is given alone. It may be possible to reduce the cost of treatment with methotrexate without decreasing its efficacy. This may also be true for some of the newer and costly antibiotics.

Because of its effect on renal excretion, probenecid is indicated as an adjunct to penicillin therapy and is used as an adjunct to cephalosporin antibiotic therapy. Probenecid is used primarily when high antibiotic levels in plasma and tissues are required (e.g., in the treatment of gonorrhea).

An interesting interaction has been reported between probenecid and ceftriaxone.[67] The pharmacokinetics of ceftriaxone are unusual because its plasma protein binding is concentration-dependent over the concentration range resulting from therapeutic doses. The percentage of free ceftriaxone in plasma increases from 4% to about 17% with a change in total plasma concentration from 0.5 to 300 μg/ml.

On the average, about half of an iv dose of ceftriaxone is excreted unchanged in the urine. But urinary excretion is variable and may range from 30 to 65% of the dose; the rest is excreted in the bile. Suspecting that tubular secretion and active biliary excretion played a role in the elimination of ceftriaxone, Stoekel et al. studied the effects of probenecid on its pharmacokinetics.

Unexpectedly, concurrent administration of probenecid *increased* the clearance of total (bound + unbound) ceftriaxone from 0.24 to 0.31 ml/min/kg and decreased its half-life from 8.1 to 6.5 hr. That probenecid *also* inhibited the elimination of ceftriaxone was evident from kinetic parameters based on free (unbound) ceftriaxone. Probenecid decreased the renal clearance of unbound ceftriaxone from 2.1 to 1.7 ml/min/kg and the nonrenal (biliary) clearance from 2.8 to 1.9 ml/min/kg.

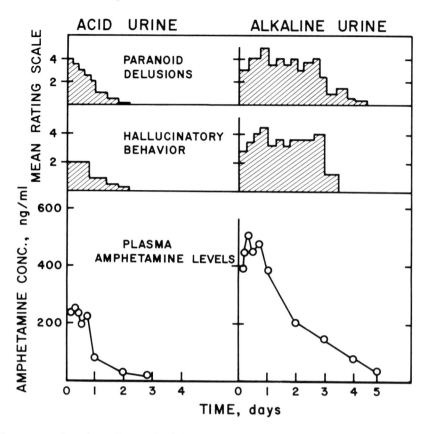

Fig. 14–4. Time course of amphetamine psychosis in patients with acid (pH 5.0 to 6.0) and alkaline (pH 6.5 to 7.1) urine, after a 150-mg oral dose. (Data from Anggard, E., et al.[64])

These findings suggested that probenecid substantially decreases the plasma protein binding of ceftriaxone. In vitro studies revealed that probenecid increased the average free fraction of ceftriaxone in plasma from 0.050 to 0.087, nearly a 75% change. Because the clearance of total ceftriaxone is strongly dependent on the free fraction in plasma, the substantial displacement of ceftriaxone from plasma protein binding sites by probenecid explains the increase in clearance of total drug even in the face of decreased renal and biliary clearance of unbound drug.

Cimetidine

As noted in an earlier section of the text, at least two transport systems have been characterized in the proximal renal tubule: one that handles anions and another that transports cations. The 'probenecid interaction' is the classic example of an acid drug inhibiting the tubular secretion of other acid drugs. Our understanding of the mutual active transport of basic drugs in the kidney, however, is far less developed. The hypothesis that basic

drugs can compete for active tubular secretion was evaluated in healthy subjects by comparing the pharmacokinetics of a single 1 g dose of oral procainamide before and during cimetidine administration.[68]

Cimetidine had a marked effect on the kinetics of both procainamide and its active metabolite, N-acetylprocainamide (NAPA). The total area under the procainamide concentration in plasma-time curve was increased by 44%; this change could be almost wholly accounted for by a decrease in renal clearance of procainamide from 347 ml/min during the control period to 197 ml/min during cimetidine administration. The average levels of NAPA in plasma also increased, by about 25%, during the cimetidine phase of the study, consistent with a decrease in the renal clearance of NAPA from 258 to 197 ml/min.

The results suggested that cimetidine inhibits the tubular secretion of both procainamide and NAPA. The report by Somogyi et al. appears to be the first example of this type of interaction with basic drugs in humans. The specific findings of the study are also of interest in that steady-state levels of procainamide would be expected to increase by nearly 50% during cimetidine administration, and NAPA levels are predicted to rise by 25% or more. Both compounds have a relatively narrow therapeutic index and there may be a need to reduce the dose of procainamide in patients also being treated with cimetidine, to avoid adverse effects.

More recently, van Crugten et al.[69] demonstrated in healthy human subjects that cimetidine also inhibits the renal clearance of ranitidine, another base, and cephalexin, a zwitterion. The renal clearance of ranitidine decreased by more than 40% with concurrent cimetidine, from 326 to 244 ml/min. A significant but smaller effect was observed with cephalexin. Renal clearance decreased in the presence of cimetidine from 267 to 208 ml/min. No effect of cimetidine was found on the renal clearance of cephalothin, an acid with a renal clearance > 500 ml/min. The investigators concluded that their findings "confirmed the hypothesis that cimetidine-mediated inhibition of renal drug clearance in humans is selective for a common cationic secretory transport mechanism in the proximal tubule of the kidney, rather than a nonspecific action on renal function."

Anti-Inflammatory Drugs

Certain anti-inflammatory drugs significantly affect renal function; this is related to their inhibition of prostaglandin synthesis. Clinically important interactions have been observed when these drugs are given with lithium.

Lithium is used widely in the treatment of patients with manic depression and other psychiatric disorders. It is eliminated almost exclusively by the kidneys. Lithium ions are filtered by the glomeruli, but 80% of the filtered load is reabsorbed by the renal tubules. The renal clearance of lithium is, therefore, about 20% of creatinine clearance or 15 to 30 ml/min in patients with normal renal function.

The effects of indomethacin on plasma lithium concentrations were studied in psychiatric patients and healthy subjects.[70] After steady-state plasma lithium levels had been reached, all subjects received indomethacin (50 mg 3 times a day) for 7 days. Indomethacin increased plasma lithium concentration, by 60% in the psychiatric patients and 30% in the healthy subjects, and suppressed the renal excretion of lithium (Fig. 14–5). In some

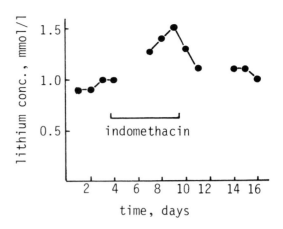

Fig. 14–5. Effect of indomethacin on steady-state lithium concentrations in plasma in a psychiatric patient. (Data from Frölich, J.C., et al.[70])

patients, the increase in plasma lithium levels was sufficient to lead to toxicity.

Diclofenac, another prostaglandin synthesis-inhibiting, nonsteroidal anti-inflammatory drug (NSAID), was found to decrease the renal clearance of lithium by 23% and to increase lithium plasma levels by 26%.[71] Care should be taken when using an inhibitor of prostaglandin synthesis in a patient being treated with lithium.

Aspirin and other NSAIDs also have the potential to reduce the antihypertensive effects of diuretics by directly competing for transport sites in the organic acid secretory system of the proximal renal tubules.[72] According to McGiff, "this secretory system serves as the major route of access of thiazide diuretics, furosemide, and potassium-sparing agents to their active sites within the renal tubules. As this route can be blocked by NSAIDs, diminished efficacy of the diuretic agent may occur . . . ."

Thyss et al.[73] reported serious and, in some cases, lethal methotrexate (MTX) toxicity when it was administered with ketoprofen, a recently approved NSAID. Toxicity was associated with unusually high serum levels of MTX. The investigators suggested that the mechanism of this interaction might involve "inhibition of renal prostaglandin synthesis by ketoprofen which would decrease renal perfusion rate and thus inhibit MTX clearance. An alternative suggestion, which is not mutually exclusive, would be competitive renal secretion of these two drugs, which are both eliminated to a large extent by the kidney."

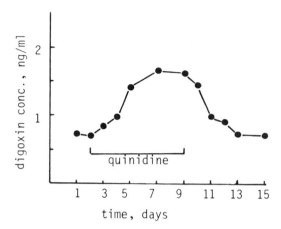

Fig. 14–6. Effect of quinidine on steady-state digoxin concentrations in serum. (Data from Doering, W.[77])

Furosemide

Furosemide is a potent diuretic that acts by inhibiting active chloride transport in the loop of Henle. Its effects on the kidney may alter the renal excretion of other drugs.

Studies in healthy subjects indicate that furosemide decreases inulin clearance, a measure of GFR; inulin clearance is also reduced in water-loaded subjects.[74] On the average, furosemide decreased inulin clearance from 130 to 80 ml/min. This change was paralleled by changes in the renal clearance of practolol, an early β-blocker no longer used today, gentamicin, and cephaloridine, but not of digoxin. Furosemide reduced the renal clearance of gentamicin from 142 to 110 ml/min and of cephaloridine from 213 to 136 ml/min. There is concern that furosemide may enhance the ototoxicity of aminoglycoside antibiotics and the nephrotoxicity of cephaloridine, particularly in patients with renal impairment.

Digoxin-Quinidine Interaction

Although digoxin and quinidine have been used in combination for more than 50 years in the treatment of cardiac arrhythmia, not until 1978 was it recognized that a major interaction occurs between these drugs, one that may put a patient at risk of digitalis toxicity. Since 1978 dozens of reports have been published on the subject.

In 1978, Ejvinsson reported on 12 patients who received the combination of digoxin and quinidine; all patients showed a rise in serum digoxin concentration.[75] Serum digoxin levels rose above the usual therapeutic concentration range in 6 patients. Leahey and co-workers found increased serum di-

goxin concentration in 25 of 27 patients receiving digoxin and quinidine, an incidence of 93%.[76] Gastrointestinal side effects, typical of digoxin toxicity, developed in 16 patients. Lowering the dose of digoxin alone substantially reduced the incidence of adverse effects. In 1979, Doering reported on 79 patients who demonstrated a significant average increase in digoxin concentration from 1.0 to 2.5 ng/ml when quinidine was added.[77] The time course of the interaction is shown in Figure 14–6.

An important question is why was this interaction overlooked for so long. Doherty suggests several reasons: quinidine alone and digoxin alone cause adverse effects; patients requiring both drugs are usually quite sick, which makes it difficult to determine whether symptoms are related to treatment or disease; the use of other drugs confuses the issue.[78]

The basis for the quinidine-digoxin interaction is unusually complicated. Steady-state concentrations of digoxin increase because quinidine decreases the clearance of digoxin. One report found that the total plasma clearance of digoxin in healthy subjects fell from 3.1 to 2.0 ml/min per kg in the presence of quinidine;[79] a 56% decrease in total clearance of digoxin was found in patients with atrial fibrillation.[80]

Part of the reason for the lower plasma clearance of digoxin is quinidine's effect on the renal clearance of digoxin. In healthy subjects quinidine reduced the renal clearance of digoxin from 1.6 to 1.1 ml/min per kg;[79] in patients with cardiac disease quinidine reduced the renal clearance of digoxin from 53 ml/min per 1.73 m² to 35 ml/min per 1.73 m².[81] Quinidine has no effect on creatinine clearance; it is thought that quinidine inhibits the tubular secretion of digoxin.

Renal clearance only accounts for about half of the elimination of digoxin. On the average, usual doses of quinidine decrease the renal clearance of digoxin by about 50% and increase steady-state levels by about 100%. Suppression of renal clearance can only account for about half of the increase in steady-state digoxin concentration. Therefore, quinidine must also inhibit the nonrenal clearance of digoxin to a similar degree.[80,82] The mechanism for the decrease in nonrenal clearance of digoxin is unknown. Quinidine may inhibit the biliary secretion of digoxin, the hepatic metabolism of digoxin, or both.

More direct evidence of the effect of quinidine on the nonrenal elimination of digoxin is available

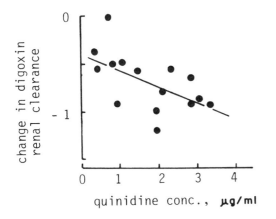

Fig. 14–7. Relationship between reduction in renal clearance (ml/min per kg) of digoxin and serum quinidine concentration. (Data from Leahey, E.B., et al.[82])

from a study of the quinidine-digoxin interaction in patients with end-stage renal failure (serum creatinine = 10.2–16.8 mg/dl).[83] In these patients, quinidine markedly decreased the total clearance of digoxin from 1.9 to 1.1 L/hr; the half-life of digoxin increased from 5.2 to 9.6 days. The renal clearance of digoxin is negligible in these patients and the decrease in total clearance of digoxin must be the result of an effect of quinidine on the nonrenal clearance of digoxin.

The effects of quinidine on digoxin are dose-related. Doses of less than 500 mg quinidine per day produced no appreciable effect on serum digoxin.[77] Leahey and co-workers reported that the decrease in renal clearance of digoxin was related to serum quinidine concentration (Fig. 14–7).[82] The change in nonrenal clearance was independent of serum quinidine.

The dependence of the digoxin-quinidine interaction on serum quinidine concentration is also seen in a case report concerned with sequential drug interactions.[84] A 94-year-old woman was stable when treated with a combination of quinidine, digoxin, and pentobarbital. Discontinuation of the barbiturate resulted in a 3-fold increase in serum digoxin levels, from about 1.4 to about 4.5 ng/ml, and symptoms of digitalis toxicity. Induction of quinidine metabolism by pentobarbital maintained serum levels of quinidine that were too low to significantly affect digoxin elimination. The elevated levels of quinidine on discontinuing the barbiturate substantially inhibited the clearance of digoxin.

Quinidine also decreases the apparent volume of distribution of digoxin, apparently by displacing

digoxin from extravascular binding sites (i.e., by decreasing the tissue binding of digoxin). In healthy subjects, quinidine decreased the volume of distribution of digoxin from 10.9 to 7.4 L/kg;[79] a decrease from 11.1 to 6.8 L/kg was observed in patients with atrial fibrillation.[80]

About 50% of digoxin in the body is found in skeletal muscle. Studies in patients with atrial fibrillation indicate that the ratio of digoxin concentration in skeletal muscle to that in serum decreases from 43 before quinidine treatment to 33 during quinidine treatment.[85] This change can largely account for the decrease in digoxin distribution volume in the presence of quinidine.

This additional effect of quinidine on the apparent volume of distribution of digoxin is interesting but unrelated to the elevation in serum digoxin concentration produced by quinidine. The clinical implications of this aspect of the digoxin-quinidine interaction are not clear.

More recently, it has come to light that some investigators find no evidence of digitalis toxicity when serum digoxin levels rise with concurrent quinidine. In fact, one study reported that the inotropic effects noted during digoxin therapy alone were markedly attenuated or completely antagonized when quinidine was added, despite a doubling of the serum digoxin concentration.[86] Positive inotropic effects reappeared on withdrawal of quinidine.

The conflicting reports may reflect the difficulty in defining the relationship between serum digoxin and myocardial effects in the presence of quinidine, because quinidine can produce symptoms similar to those of digoxin. This problem has been highlighted by Walker et al.[87] who reviewed inpatient data to determine the incidence of adverse effects in patients treated with digoxin alone, quinidine alone, and digoxin and quinidine.

The incidence of cardiac and gastrointestinal side effects nearly tripled when quinidine was added to digoxin therapy, compared with that recorded during treatment with digoxin alone, but most of the increased incidence of toxicity could be accounted for by the frequency with which quinidine itself produces similar symptoms. The investigators noted that "simple additivity of rates observed in this study suggests that there was little or no clinical interaction of digoxin and quinidine in the production of adverse reactions. Rather, these data reflect the general finding that patients receiving two drugs have more adverse reactions than those who receive only one.''

In an attempt to clarify the question, Warner et al.[88] studied the relationship between serum digoxin and digoxin effects in the presence of quinidine in dogs, using inhibition of myocardial cation transport as a measure of effect. The inotropic and toxic effects of digoxin are associated with an inhibition of myocardial Na,K-ATPase, which results in a reduction in monovalent cation transport. Cation transport is usually evaluated by measuring rubidium uptake.

Quinidine alone had no effect on myocardial cation transport, whereas digoxin inhibited rubidium uptake by the left ventricular myocardium in a concentration-dependent manner. A statistically significant correlation was found between rubidium uptake and serum digoxin concentration in dogs receiving digoxin alone as well as in those receiving digoxin with quinidine, but the slopes of these regression lines were different. At equivalent serum digoxin levels, dogs that were given digoxin and quinidine had less inhibition of Rb+ uptake than those that received only digoxin.

Warner et al. concluded that the increase in serum digoxin seen with quinidine was not accompanied by a proportional increase in digoxin effects. In fact, the excess digoxin concentration resulting from the interaction with quinidine appeared to have no effect on Rb+ uptake. It seems, therefore, that quinidine not only inhibits the elimination of digoxin, it also inhibits the inotropic effect of digoxin. Although extrapolation of these findings to the clinical setting must be done carefully, questions are raised concerning the value of serum digoxin as a predictor of the effects of digoxin in the presence of quinidine.

The results suggest that reducing the dosage of digoxin in proportion to changes in serum levels when digoxin is used with quinidine may be inappropriate. Inhibition of myocardial Rb+ uptake is related to the effects of digoxin on contractility and ventricular arrhythmias. Patients receiving both digoxin and quinidine may have less inotropic effect and less likelihood of developing tachyarrhythmia at a given serum digoxin concentration than patients on digoxin alone.

On the other hand, the effects of digoxin on the sinus and AV node is indirect, mediated through the autonomic nervous system and unrelated to myocardial cation transport. The same is true for the gastrointestinal toxicity of digoxin, which is neu-

rally mediated. Until the clinical effects of digoxin in the presence of quinidine are further clarified, Warner et al. recommend that digoxin dosing be based on clinical evaluation, as well as on serum digoxin concentration measurements.

Digoxin and Other Antiarrhythmic Drugs

Leahey and co-workers compared the effects of quinidine on digoxin with those of other type I membrane active antiarrhythmic drugs, including procainamide and disopyramide, which are used frequently in the United States as alternatives to quinidine, and mexiletine, which is widely used in Europe.[89] Quinidine increased serum digoxin concentration and prolonged the P-R interval on the electrocardiogram, a finding consistent with earlier studies, but none of the other drugs affected serum digoxin levels or P-R interval.

On the other hand, verapamil, a calcium channel blocker used for treating patients with angina and arrhythmias, affects digoxin in the same way as quinidine.[90] In healthy subjects, verapamil decreased the total plasma clearance of digoxin from 3.3 to 2.2 ml/min per kg by inhibiting both renal and nonrenal clearance. Unlike quinidine, verapamil had no effect on the apparent volume of distribution of digoxin. Amiodarone, a long-acting antiarrhythmic drug, also inhibits the elimination of digoxin.[91]

Renal Blood Flow

Drug-related changes in renal blood flow can affect the urinary excretion of drugs, particularly drugs subject to tubular secretion. The effect of vasodilator therapy on the renal clearance of digoxin was studied in patients with congestive heart failure (CHF).[92] Intravenous nitroprusside or hydralazine increased cardiac index, para-aminohippurate (PAH) clearance, renal blood flow, and the renal clearance of digoxin. The results are summarized in Table 14–2. If this improvement in renal hemodynamics is achieved during chronic treatment with vasodilators, then maintenance digoxin doses may need to be increased to maintain therapeutic drug concentrations in serum.

Biliary Excretion

Difficulties in measuring drug concentrations in bile have all but precluded clinical or human experimental investigations on drug-drug interactions that affect biliary excretion. The few interactions that we are aware of derive from indirect evidence.

Table 14–2.   Effects of Vasodilators on Hemodynamics, Renal Function, and Digoxin Excretion*

Variable	Control	Nitroprusside	Hydralazine
Cardiac index (L/min per m²)	2.00	2.65	3.28
Paraaminohippurate clearance (ml/min)	200	289	425
Renal blood flow (ml/min)	337	480	718
Digoxin renal clearance (ml/min)	104	152	147

*Data from Cogan, J.J., et al.[92]

Probenecid significantly inhibits the elimination of indomethacin; plasma clearance of indomethacin was 174 ml/hr per kg in the control period and 107 ml/hr per kg in the presence of probenecid.[93] There was no change in the renal clearance of indomethacin during probenecid treatment; but probenecid decreased nonrenal clearance from 168 ml/hr per kg to 104 ml/hr per kg. It is likely that probenecid inhibits the biliary excretion of indomethacin.

A more general interaction has been reported between drugs that are excreted, either in the bile or directly, into the gastrointestinal tract and non-absorbable ion exchange resins that bind drugs in the gut and prevent reabsorption. The effect of cholestyramine on the pharmacokinetics and pharmacodynamics of a single intravenous dose of phenprocoumon, the oral anticoagulant of choice in Europe, was studied in healthy subjects.[94] Cholestyramine treatment led to increased elimination in all subjects; half-life decreased from 5 days to 3.1 days and clearance increased from 17 ml/day per kg to 29 ml/day per kg. Cholestyramine reduced the area under the anticoagulant effect versus time curve from 660 to 344 U. Concomitant use of these drugs should probably be avoided. Higher doses of phenprocoumon would be required in the presence of cholestyramine to achieve satisfactory anticoagulation. From a different point of view, cholestyramine may be useful in the treatment of phenprocoumon overdosage.

DRUG METABOLISM

Interactions between two drugs that affect the metabolism of one or both constitute most of the clinically important drug interactions. Many drugs stimulate or induce the activity of hepatic drug metabolizing enzymes, thereby reducing blood levels and clinical effects of drugs given concurrently. We now recognize that a wide range of drugs can inhibit drug metabolizing enzymes and lead to accumulation and toxicity of coadministered drugs. The effects of drug metabolizing enzyme inducers or inhibitors may be particularly pronounced when drugs subject to presystemic hepatic metabolism are given at the same time. Drug metabolism may be affected not only by other drugs but also by environmental chemicals; these interactions are sometimes important.

Induction of Drug Metabolizing Enzymes

A wide range of chemically unrelated substances can stimulate the activity of mixed function oxidases by enzyme induction. The molecular mechanism of enzyme induction is not fully understood nor have the molecular characteristics essential for induction been defined. Enzyme inducers are lipophilic, bind to cytochrome P-450 enzymes, and have relatively long half-lives, but not all drugs with these characteristics are enzyme inducers.

Induction is usually associated with an increase in liver weight and in the amounts of microsomal protein, cytochrome P-450, and other oxidative enzymes in the liver. The enzyme systems involved in conjugation, such as glutathione transferase and glucuronyl transferase, can also be induced. The time course of induction varies with the inducing agent. A powerful enzyme inducer such as rifampin can produce measurable changes in the activity of drug metabolizing enzymes within 48 hr, but less potent inducers may require a longer time.

Enhancement of drug metabolism by ethanol, tobacco smoking, and diet also involves enzyme induction. Induction of drug metabolizing enzymes usually leads to a reduction in drug efficacy, but it may also enhance the toxicity of certain drugs with active metabolites. The clinical implications of enzyme induction have been reviewed by Park and Breckenridge.[95]

Anticonvulsant Drugs.   Phenobarbital, phenytoin, and carbamazepine are potent inducers of drug metabolizing enzymes and are often used in combination in the treatment of patients with epilepsy. Patients treated with anticonvulsant drugs have, in general, an above average ability to metabolize many drugs and often require higher than average dosages. Pharmacokinetic interactions with antiepileptic drugs have been reviewed by Perucca.[96]

A study comparing epileptic patients receiving phenytoin alone or phenytoin with phenobarbital or carbamazepine with healthy subjects found that epileptic patients had much higher cytochrome P-450 levels in liver biopsies and metabolized antipyrine considerably faster than control subjects.[97]

In a more recent investigation, antipyrine kinetics were studied in patients with epilepsy who were to have phenytoin, carbamazepine, or valproic acid discontinued as part of a planned simplification of therapy.[98] Antipyrine was given before and 4 weeks after discontinuation of one drug.

Removal of carbamazepine was associated with a nearly 50% decrease in antipyrine clearance in those patients who were also treated with either valproic acid or ethosuximide, neither of which is an enzyme-inducing agent. There was no change in antipyrine clearance after removal of carbamazepine in those patients treated with phenytoin and/or barbiturates. Removal of phenytoin was associated with a 10 to 15% decrease in antipyrine clearance in those patients who were also receiving carbamazepine, with or without barbiturates. As expected, removal of valproic acid had no effect on antipyrine clearance.

When carbamazepine was the only enzyme inducing agent being taken, its removal resulted in a marked decrease in antipyrine clearance. However, if an enzyme inducer (e.g., phenytoin, barbiturates) was also being taken, the removal of carbamazepine had no effect on antipyrine clearance.

These results suggest that carbamazepine has no additional effect on antipyrine clearance beyond that of phenytoin and/or barbiturates. Phenytoin, on the other hand, has enzyme inducing activity over and above that of carbamazepine, or carbamazepine and barbiturates, and appears to be a more powerful inducer of hepatic enzyme activity than is carbamazepine. Although differences between carbamazepine and phenytoin may exist, carbamazepine is nevertheless a strong inducer, capable of reducing the efficacy of drugs given concurrently (see Fig. 14–9).

Consistent with the findings on antipyrine kinetics, the investigators also found that removal of phenytoin resulted in elevated blood levels of carbamazepine and valproic acid, and removal of carbamazepine resulted in increased levels of valproic acid and ethosuximide. It also follows from these results that, for a given dose of anticonvulsant, serum levels may be higher in those patients re-

ceiving monotherapy than in those treated with additional drugs. This has been demonstrated with valproic acid by Chiba et al.[99] in children. Plasma clearance of valproate was 13 ml/hr/kg in patients receiving only valproic acid and 23.5 ml/hr/kg in those treated with valproic acid and other anticonvulsants.

Blood level studies of quinidine in healthy subjects before and at the end of a 4-week course of phenobarbital or phenytoin showed that the anticonvulsant drugs decreased the half-life and the total area under the concentration-time curve after a single oral dose by more than 50%. Quinidine half-life ranged from 3.0 to 6.1 hr during the control period but fell to 1.6 to 2.6 hr during the anticonvulsant drug period.[100] In two patients, the concomitant use of primidone or phenytoin resulted in inadequate blood levels of quinidine with standard dosages of the drug (i.e., 300 mg every 4 hr). In another patient, oral doses of quinidine sulfate up to 800 mg every 4 hr were required to obtain therapeutic plasma quinidine concentrations.[100]

The pharmacokinetics of diazepam after intravenous administration were determined in healthy subjects and in epileptic patients receiving chronic anticonvulsant drug therapy, including combinations of carbamazepine, valproate sodium, phenytoin, clonazepam, or primidone.[101] Large differences in half-life and clearance were observed. The half-life of diazepam was only 13 hr in the patients with epilepsy compared to a value of 34 hr in control subjects. The clearance of diazepam increased from 20 ml/min in control subjects to 52 ml/min in epileptic patients. Considerably larger doses of antianxiety drugs may be required for adequate clinical effects in patients being treated for epilepsy.

Some of the literature on oral contraceptives suggests that OCs are not predictably effective in preventing conception in women taking anticonvulsant medication.[102] Failure rates are higher in groups of women taking enzyme-inducing anticonvulsants than in control groups. Evidence shows that the most common cause of failure in these women is insufficient steroid (estrogen or progestin) levels to block ovulation. These reduced levels are probably the result of increased steroid metabolism as a consequence of induction of microsomal oxidative enzymes by the antiepileptic drugs.

Drugs subject to first-pass metabolism after oral administration appear to be particularly susceptible to the enzyme inducing effects of anticonvulsants.

A good example is provided by studies with felodipine, an investigational dihydropyridine calcium channel blocker.[103] Felodipine undergoes extensive first-pass hepatic metabolism and ordinarily has an oral bioavailability of about 15%.

Felodipine disposition was studied in patients on chronic anticonvulsant therapy for control of seizures and normal subjects matched for age and sex. Plasma felodipine levels after an oral dose were dramatically lower in the patients with epilepsy. Mean peak concentrations in plasma were about 9 nmol/L in controls and 1.6 nmol/L in patients. The relative bioavailability of felodipine in the patients with seizure disorders was less than 10% of that in the control subjects. Therefore, the mean oral bioavailability of felodipine in subjects receiving anticonvulsants is about 1%. "Patients on anticonvulsant medication will require substantially higher doses of felodipine to achieve plasma concentrations equivalent to those in non-induced subjects."[103]

Phenytoin. Phenytoin can induce the metabolism of many drugs, including antipyrine, hydrocortisone, dexamethasone, dicumarol, digitoxin, and thyroxine; it does not, however, stimulate its own metabolism.[95]

Phenytoin is usually used with other drugs in the treatment of epilepsy. Although it has little effect on phenobarbital, phenytoin does stimulate the metabolism of clonazepam and primidone. Long-term treatment with phenytoin lowers the blood levels of clonazepam after a single oral dose by more than 50%.[104] Phenytoin stimulates clonazepam metabolism to a considerably greater extent than does phenobarbital.

Primidone is a widely used anticonvulsant drug; it is converted to two active metabolites, phenylethylmalonamide (PEMA) and phenobarbital. Whether or not primidone has pharmacologic activity of its own is not known. The steady-state serum concentration ratio of derived phenobarbital to unmetabolized primidone is higher in patients treated with a combination of primidone and phenytoin than in patients treated with primidone alone (2.2 vs 1.6);[105] a twofold difference in serum concentration ratio was found in another investigation.[106] Phenytoin also increases the steady-state serum concentration ratio of derived PEMA to primidone.[106]

Phenytoin accelerates the metabolism of most corticosteroids; it has a clinically important effect on the elimination of prednisolone. Phenytoin de-

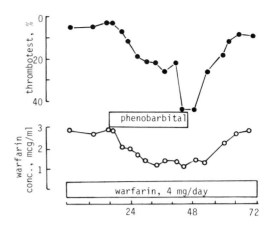

Fig. 14–8. Warfarin-phenobarbital interaction. Phenobarbital (120 mg/day) reduces plasma warfarin levels and antagonizes its anticoagulant effect. (Data from Breckenridge, A.M., and Orme, M.L.E.[110])

creased the half-life of prednisolone by about 50% and increased its clearance from plasma by about 80%.[107] The average oral dose, given at midnight, required to suppress the 8 A.M. plasma level of endogenous hydrocortisone (cortisol) to 5 μg/dl was doubled following treatment with phenytoin.

Drugs that influence the activity of hepatic drug metabolizing enzymes may have particularly pronounced effects on coadministered drugs subject to presystemic metabolism. Phenytoin treatment increases the systemic clearance of meperidine by about 25%, from 1017 ml/min to 1280 ml/min. Phenytoin also increases the extent of hepatic first-pass metabolism of meperidine after oral administration; bioavailability is reduced from 61% to 43%. To achieve comparable blood levels of meperidine, about twice the oral dose is required in patients treated with phenytoin as is needed in patients who are not induced.[108] This means that patients on phenytoin tend to have high levels of normeperidine, the metabolite of meperidine closely associated with its adverse effects. It may be preferable to give intravenous rather than oral meperidine to these patients.

Unexpectedly, phenytoin also appears to increase the metabolism of theophylline. This was first noted in a case study. A 49-year-old man with asthma and epilepsy who was receiving 400 mg/day phenytoin responded poorly to apparently adequate doses of theophylline. This observation prompted a study of the effects of phenytoin on the elimination of theophylline in adult nonsmoking healthy subjects.[109] Phenytoin dosage was adjusted in each individual to achieve a serum level of 10 to 20 µg/ml before the test dose of theophylline was given.

Phenytoin administration reduced the half-life of theophylline from 10 to 5 hr. The results suggest that the dosage of theophylline should be increased by 50 to 100% when phenytoin is added to long-term theophylline therapy or when theophylline is initiated in patients being treated with phenytoin. This report is of additional interest because phenobarbital, which is thought to stimulate the same drug-metabolizing enzymes as does phenytoin, has no effect on theophylline metabolism.

Phenobarbital. This barbiturate has been the most extensively studied enzyme-inducing agent; it is a potent inducer in most species. Phenobarbital can stimulate a wide range of metabolic pathways and has been shown to reduce the effects of many drugs in man.

Probably the most widely studied interaction of barbiturates is with oral anticoagulants. Figure 14–8 shows plasma warfarin levels and anticoagulant effect before, during, and after phenobarbital treatment. A significant decline in warfarin levels and anticoagulant effect is evident within 6 days; the maximum effect is usually seen after 2 to 3 weeks.[110]

Phenobarbital administration has also been shown to stimulate the metabolism of dicumarol. Patients who had been on dicumarol for an average of about 4 years were found to require an average increase of 33% in their daily dose to maintain adequate anticoagulation when phenobarbital therapy was initiated.[111]

The barbiturate-oral anticoagulant interaction is clinically significant. A physician may respond to the reduced anticoagulant effect by increasing the dose of warfarin or dicumarol. No problems ensue as long as both the barbiturate and the anticoagulant are continued. The patient is at risk, however, when the barbiturate is stopped, because the rate of drug metabolism will return to normal levels over a week or two and the plasma concentrations of the anticoagulant will increase. Unless the dose is reduced, serious or fatal hemorrhage may occur.

An additional complication of the interaction between barbiturates and oral anticoagulants is the considerable interpatient variability in the degree of induction. Whenever possible this drug combination should be avoided because, even with careful monitoring, optimal anticoagulant control will be difficult.

Few reports have considered the effects of hepatic enzyme induction with phenobarbital on the disposition of high clearance drugs. To this end, Rutledge et al.[112] studied the kinetics of verapamil before and after 21 days of phenobarbital (180 mg/day) in healthy subjects. The mean apparent clearance of unbound drug after an oral dose of verapamil was increased after treatment with phenobarbital from 950 to 3600 ml/min/kg, but the systemic clearance of unbound verapamil, determined after an iv dose, was about the same before and after phenobarbital. The findings suggest that much larger oral doses of verapamil may be required in patients regularly receiving phenobarbital. The lack of effect on the systemic clearance of verapamil suggests that phenobarbital has little effect on hepatic blood flow rate in humans.

Phenobarbital and other barbiturates are known to induce enzymes involved in the metabolism of steroids, including those used in oral contraceptive products. Pregnancies have been reported in patients taking phenobarbital in conjunction with oral contraceptives,[113] but it has not been established whether the interaction is with the estrogen or the progestogen. The clinical implications of drug-stimulated biotransformation of hormonal steroid contraceptives has been reviewed by Hempel and Klinger.[114]

The ability of phenobarbital to stimulate liver enzymes has been used to advantage in the treatment of unconjugated hyperbilirubinemia in neonates.[115] In some infants, the induction of glucuronyl transferase results in a significant decrease in bilirubin levels. The induction of this enzyme has also been used as a method of minimizing the hazard of Rh-incompatibility and neonatal jaundice by dosing a mother who has developed rhesus antibodies with phenobarbital to induce the enzymes in the liver of her unborn child.[116]

Other Barbiturates. Enzyme induction appears to be a characteristic shared by most if not all barbiturates. Differences in potency may exist but their importance is not known. Human investigations indicate that phenobarbital reduces the anticoagulant effect of warfarin to a slightly greater extent than does secobarbital.[117]

When the metabolism of a drug is rate-limited by the rate of hepatic blow flow, changes in the activity of hepatic drug metabolizing enzymes may have little effect on systemic clearance. This has been demonstrated with verapamil[112] and with alprenolol.[118] The systemic clearance of alprenolol,

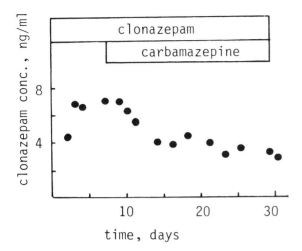

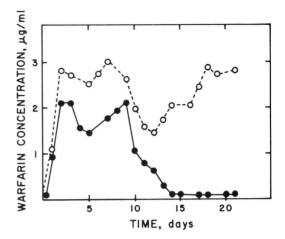

Fig. 14–9. Effect of carbamazepine on clonazepam levels in plasma. (Data from Lai, A.A., Levy, R.H., and Cutler, R.E.[119])

Fig. 14–10. Warfarin concentrations in plasma after daily doses of warfarin alone (○) or daily doses of warfarin and rifampin (●) in a healthy subject. The daily dose of warfarin was the same in both studies, the studies were 4 wk apart, and the daily dose of rifampin was 600 mg. (Data from O'Reilly, R.A.[123])

a β-blocking drug widely used in Europe, was determined after intravenous administration before and during treatment with pentobarbital. Clearance was not significantly different, averaging 1.2 L/min in the control period and 1.5 L/min in the barbiturate period. One might incorrectly conclude from these results that pentobarbital interacts little or not at all with alprenolol. The effect of pentobarbital on the metabolism of alprenolol is clearly evident, however, after oral administration of the β-blocker. The bioavailability decreases from 26% of the dose during the control phase to only 7% during the pentobarbital period because of a large increase in presystemic metabolism of alprenolol, secondary to induction of drug metabolizing enzymes.[118] If one wishes to determine whether or not a compound is an inducer or inhibitor of drug metabolizing enzymes, it is better to study its effects after oral rather than intravenous administration of a test drug.

Carbamazepine. The clearance of many drugs given with carbamazepine is increased because carbamazepine, like phenytoin, is a potent inducer of drug metabolizing enzymes. As noted above, discontinuing carbamazepine in patients with epilepsy who were also treated with either valproic acid or ethosuximide resulted in a nearly 50% decrease in antipyrine clearance.[98] Removal of carbamazine also resulted in increased levels of valproic acid and ethosuximide in these patients.

Carbamazepine has also been reported to increase the elimination of phenytoin, warfarin, and clonazepam.[95] The effect of carbamazepine on

steady-state levels of clonazepam are shown in Figure 14–9.[119]

Autoinduction

There are many examples of changes in pharmacokinetics during repeated dosing of a drug compared with a single dose. In a very small number of cases, changes appear to be related to a slow induction of drug-metabolizing enzymes involved in the biotransformation of the inducer itself. This has been called autoinduction.

Carbamazepine is the principal example of a drug that displays autoinduction. It is now well established that during long-term therapy, carbamazepine induces its own metabolism.[120] During repeated dosing, the clearance of carbamazepine increases at least 2-fold and blood levels decline by 50%. Induction occurs over 3 to 4 weeks; thereafter, blood levels are relatively stable. Concomitant treatment with phenobarbital or phenytoin at this time further induces the metabolism of carbamazepine.

A recent report suggests that cyclophosphamide may also induce its own metabolism. Moore et al.[121] studied the disposition of cyclophosphamide and its active metabolite phosphoramide mustard in patients receiving high-dose intravenous cyclophosphamide daily for 2 days before bone marrow transplantation.

Total clearance of cyclophosphamide increased from 93 ml/min on the first day of treatment to 178 ml/min on the second day. An increased rate of formation of phosphoramide mustard with higher peak concentrations was also seen. Peak levels were 19 μmol/L on day 1 and 36.5 μmol/L on day 2.

Moore et al. gave an iv test dose of dexamethasone each day, hypothesizing that, if increased cyclophosphamide clearance was due to microsomal enzyme induction, increased clearance of dexamethasone should also be observed on day 2. Dexamethasone, like antipyrine, is metabolized by hepatic mixed-function oxidases and exhibits increased clearance in the presence of hepatic enzyme induction. Dexamethasone clearance was 369 ml/min on day 1 and 526 ml/min on day 2. The investigators concluded that "high-dose cyclophosphamide causes an increase in its own clearance and that of dexamethasone through an apparent induction of hepatic-metabolizing enzymes detectable 24 hours after initial exposure to cyclophosphamide."

Rifampin. Since the introduction of rifampin into clinical practice for the treatment of tuberculosis, there have been many reports of interactions with other drugs, most of which relate to rifampin being a potent enzyme-inducing agent. Drug interactions with rifampin have been reviewed by Zilly and co-workers.[122]

The interaction between rifampin and warfarin is a particularly dramatic example of rifampin's ability to stimulate drug metabolism. Administration of 600 mg daily doses of rifampin to subjects on warfarin abolishes the anticoagulant effect and reduces plasma warfarin levels to near zero (Fig. 14–10).[123]

Clinical reports indicate menstrual disturbances and an unusually high incidence of pregnancy in patients with tuberculosis treated with rifampin and also on oral contraceptives. These findings suggest stimulated elimination of one or both of the components of oral contraceptive products.[122] Back and co-workers found a 50% decrease in blood levels and half-life of norethindrone, a commonly used progestin in oral contraceptives, during rifampin treatment compared to that found during a control period.[124]

Rifampin also stimulates the metabolism of glucocorticoids, hexobarbital, diazepam, metoprolol, quinidine, and other drugs.[122] Increased clearance and decreased effects of glucocorticoids, resulting from treatment with rifampin, may lead to rejection episodes in renal transplant patients.[125] Rifampin

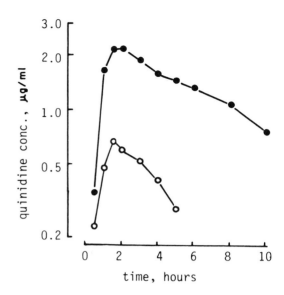

Fig. 14–11. Plasma quinidine concentrations (log scale) after a single 6 mg/kg oral dose of quinidine sulfate before (●) or after oral rifampin, 500 mg daily for 7 days (○). (Data from Twum-Barima, Y., and Carruthers, S.G.[129])

was found to decrease the half-life of hexobarbital from 407 min to 171 min and increase its clearance 3-fold.[126] The half-life of diazepam in tuberculosis patients treated with several drugs including rifampin was only 14 hr compared to a value of 58 hr in age- and sex-matched control subjects.[127] Metoprolol concentrations after an oral dose are decreased about one third from control levels during treatment with rifampin.[128] Rifampin markedly increases the clearance and presystemic metabolism of oral quinidine and virtually abolishes the clinical effect of standard dosages of the drug (Fig. 14–11).[129]

More recent drug interaction studies with rifampin have demonstrated a two-fold increase in the clearance of phenytoin[130] and a decrease in steady-state levels of sulfapyridine, from 17 to 7 μg/ml, following sulfasalazine administration.[131] Peak levels of chloramphenicol at steady state in 2 patients with *Hemophilus influenzae* fell from 21.5 and 38.5 μg/L before rifampin to 3.1 and 8 μg/L, respectively, after initiation of rifampin therapy.[132] These investigators concluded that "if the American Academy of Pediatrics' recommendation is followed and index patients receive rifampin during treatment of serious *H influenza* Type b infections, there is a risk that serum concentrations of chloramphenicol will be reduced to subtherapeutic levels, resulting in treatment failure."

Although enzyme-inducing drugs like rifampin ordinarily decrease the efficacy of coadministered drugs, enhanced toxicity may be found if stimulation of drug metabolizing enzymes leads to the production of active or toxic metabolites. A higher than expected number of cases of isoniazid-related hepatitis have been described in patients treated with isoniazid and rifampin.[133] Hepatitis may be the result of a hepatotoxic metabolite of isoniazid, the production of which is stimulated by the enzyme-inducing effects of rifampin.

Inhibition of Drug Metabolizing Enzymes

Much of the research in drug metabolism during the past decade has been concerned with enzyme inhibition. A surprisingly large number of drugs have been found to inhibit the metabolism of other drugs in man. Inhibition mechanisms include substrate competition, interference with drug transport, depletion of hepatic glycogen, and functional impairment of enzyme activity by hepatotoxicity. Competition for the same substrate-binding site is probably the most prevalent mechanism for drug interactions in man.

Interactions between drugs that lead to impaired metabolism are probably more important than those that result from stimulated metabolism. The clinical consequence of enzyme induction is usually a decrease in the efficacy of the drug. This is undesirable but usually not life-threatening. Inhibition of drug metabolism may lead to serious adverse effects because of accumulation of drugs to toxic concentrations. The therapeutic problems associated with enzyme inhibition have been reviewed by Park and Breckenridge.[95] A more recent, comprehensive review article that should be noted is a survey of the pharmacokinetic interactions of cimetidine.[134]

Chloramphenicol. Chloramphenicol has been shown to be a potent inhibitor of the metabolism of tolbutamide, phenytoin, and dicumarol in man.[135] Treatment with chloramphenicol for several days results in a marked rise in the steady-state serum concentrations of tolbutamide and phenytoin. A case of chloramphenicol-induced nystagmus in a phenytoin-treated patient has also been reported.[136] Another case report documents a serious phenytoin intoxication resulting from the simultaneous administration of chloramphenicol; blood levels of phenytoin as high as 50 μg/ml were observed (Fig. 14–12).[137]

Disulfiram. Disulfiram is used to treat chronic

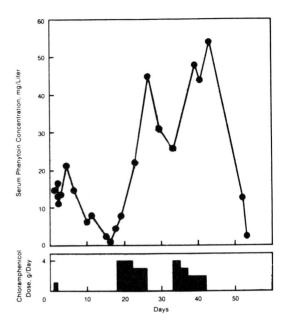

Fig. 14–12. Changes in serum phenytoin concentrations associated with intermittent administration of chloramphenicol during hospitalization of a patient receiving 300 mg/day phenytoin until day 43. (From Rose, J.Q., et al.: JAMA, 237:2630, 1977. Copyright 1977, American Medical Association.)

alcoholism; it acts by inhibiting the enzyme aldehyde dehydrogenase, which is involved in the conversion of ethanol to acetic acid. When alcohol is taken by a patient receiving disulfiram there is an accumulation of acetaldehyde, which produces undesirable central effects. Disulfiram also inhibits other drug metabolizing enzymes.

Disulfiram impairs the metabolism of antipyrine,[138] warfarin,[139] and phenytoin.[140] It also increases the anticoagulant effect of warfarin. Disulfiram decreases the plasma clearance of chlordiazepoxide by 50% and of diazepam by 40%.[141] This interaction is important because benzodiazepines are frequently used with disulfiram in the treatment of chronic alcoholics. Disulfiram has little effect on the elimination of oxazepam, which is metabolized by glucuronide conjugation rather than by oxidation.[141]

Allopurinol. Allopurinol and its metabolite oxypurinol decrease the production of uric acid by inhibiting xanthine oxidase, the enzyme that converts hypoxanthine to xanthine and xanthine to uric acid. It is indicated in the treatment of gout. Xanthine oxidase is also involved in the metabolism of mercaptopurine, an antineoplastic drug. Concurrent use of allopurinol and mercaptopurine may result in greatly increased mercaptopurine activity and toxicity.

Although the interaction between mercaptopurine (MP) and allopurinol is well known, it has not been studied in much detail. In light of this, Zimm et al.[142] considered the effects of allopurinol on the pharmacokinetics of oral and iv mercaptopurine in patients with acute lymphoblastic leukemia.

After an iv dose, plasma levels of MP decline rapidly; mean clearance is about 750 ml/min. MP levels were slightly elevated when the drug was given intravenously after allopurinol pretreatment, but there were no significant changes in clearance or half-life. On the other hand, pretreatment with allopurinol profoundly affected the kinetics of MP after oral administration.

MP is subject to considerable first-pass metabolism after oral administration. Pretreatment with allopurinol increased oral bioavailability from 12 to 59%, producing a 500% increase in the plasma levels of MP compared with those observed during the control period. Zimm et al. ascribe the results to inhibition of first-pass metabolism of oral MP related to the effects of allopurinol on liver and intestinal xanthine oxidase.

They suggested that "the interaction between 6-MP and allopurinol appears to represent a unique example of inhibition of first-pass metabolism in cancer chemotherapy." When oral MP is given with allopurinol, dosage reduction is appropriate but changes in dose do not appear to be needed when MP is given intravenously.

Allopurinol also inhibits drug metabolizing enzymes other than xanthine oxidase. It decreases the elimination of antipyrine and dicumarol,[143] phenprocoumon,[144] and theophylline.[145] Administration of an oral dose of allopurinol, 300 mg every 12 hr, decreased the clearance and increased the half-life of theophylline by about 25%.

Phenylbutazone. Although the use of phenylbutazone has declined a great deal in recent years, the interaction between warfarin and phenylbutazone is a classic one because it was one of the earliest examples of inhibition of metabolism, albeit unrecognized, and because of its complexity. The anticoagulant effect of warfarin is greatly enhanced when phenylbutazone is given to patients stabilized on warfarin; unless the dosage of warfarin is reduced, bleeding and hemorrhage can result. For many years, this interaction was thought to be the result of displacement of warfarin from plasma protein binding sites by phenylbutazone.

We now recognize that the mechanism is much more complex.[146,147]

Warfarin is a racemic mixture of two enantiomers, R- and S-warfarin, which are really two different drugs. S-warfarin is 5 times more potent than R-warfarin and the metabolism of the two enantiomers is quite different. In man, phenylbutazone either has no effect or slightly increases the metabolism of R-warfarin, but it significantly inhibits the metabolism of the S-isomer. The accumulation of the more potent S-warfarin is believed to account for the toxicity observed when warfarin and phenylbutazone are given at the same time. Confusion arose initially because accumulation was limited to the S-isomer and was masked by the plasma binding displacement effect of phenylbutazone.

Sulfinpyrazone. Sulfinpyrazone is a derivative of phenylbutazone. It was originally used to lower elevated uric acid levels but is now of interest for its effects on platelets. Several drug interactions have been reported with sulfinpyrazone, involving displacement from plasma protein, inhibition and induction of hepatic microsomal metabolism, and effects on renal tubular secretion. Clinically, the most important interactions are potentiation of the effects of oral anticoagulants, phenytoin, and tolbutamide probably resulting from enzyme inhibition.[148]

Toon et al.[149] determined that sulfinpyrazone increases the anticoagulant effect of racemic warfarin primarily by inhibiting the cytochrome P-450-mediated oxidation of S-warfarin, the biologically more potent enantiomer. Curiously, the clearance of R-warfarin was greater when sulfinpyrazone was given concurrently. The increased clearance of R-warfarin, however, arises not from induction of drug metabolizing enzymes but from competitive displacement of warfarin from plasma protein binding sites.

These investigators also reported that sulfinpyrazone treatment did not affect the anticoagulant response to phenprocoumon, an agent which is widely used outside the U.S., and did not appear to change the pharmacokinetics of the racemic drug or of its two enantiomers.[150] Inhibition of 7-hydroxylation of S-phenprocoumon by sulfinpyrazone occurred, but was masked by an increase in the free fraction in plasma of both enantiomers. This interaction, however, was not sufficient to measurably change the anticoagulant effect of phenprocoumon.

Sulfonamides. Certain sulfa drugs also inhibit drug metabolizing enzymes. Severe hypoglycemia has been observed in patients receiving tolbutamide and sulfaphenazole, because of an unusual accumulation of tolbutamide. Sulfaphenazole increased the half-life of tolbutamide from the usual 4 to 8 hr to values ranging from 24 to 70 hr.[151] Sulfamethizole has similar, though less pronounced, inhibitory effects on the metabolism of several drugs, including tolbutamide, phenytoin, and warfarin.[152]

Coadministration of warfarin and trimethoprim-sulfamethoxazole (TMP-SMZ) results in a marked increase in the anticoagulant effect but little change in the plasma concentration of warfarin. This finding might suggest a pharmacodynamic rather than a pharmacokinetic basis for the interaction. A complex mechanism like that found in the phenylbutazone-warfarin interaction, however, masks the underlying basis for this interaction.

Trimethoprim-sulfamethoxazole displaces warfarin from plasma proteins, which tends to lower blood levels, but also inhibits the metabolism of warfarin, which tends to elevate blood levels; the net effect is little change in steady-state levels of total warfarin in plasma. The inhibition of warfarin metabolism is stereoselective; TMP-SMZ has no effect on the clearance or anticoagulant effect of R-warfarin, but it decreases the clearance of the S-isomer by about 20% and increases the anticoagulant effect by about 65%.[153]

Metronidazole. A stereoselective interaction in man has also been observed between warfarin and metronidazole, a widely used drug indicated for the treatment of anaerobic infections, amebiasis, trichomoniasis, and other protozoal infections. Metronidazole increases the apparent half-life of racemic warfarin from 35 to 46 hr and increases its anticoagulant effect by 40%. This effect is almost completely the result of inhibition of the metabolism of S-warfarin. Metronidazole has no effect on the half-life or anticoagulant activity of R-warfarin.[154]

Isoniazid. In vitro studies suggest that isoniazid is a noncompetitive inhibitor of drug metabolism. Some patients receiving isoniazid show an impaired capacity to metabolize phenytoin and may become intoxicated.[155] In one study, 6 of 32 patients receiving both drugs developed phenytoin toxicity; all were slow inactivators of isoniazid.[156] No cases of phenytoin intoxication were found among the 18 fast inactivators of isoniazid. Animal experiments indicate that the rate of phenytoin me-

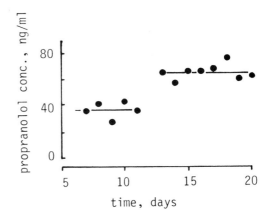

Fig. 14–13. Effect of chlorpromazine on steady-state concentrations of propranolol in plasma. The subject was maintained on 80-mg oral propranolol every 8 hr. On day 11, chlorpromazine, 50 mg every 8 hr was initiated and maintained. (Data from Vestal, R.E., et al.[160])

tabolism is inversely related to isoniazid concentrations.

The clinical problem of phenytoin toxicity induced by isoniazid appears to be prevalent in patients who are slow inactivators of isoniazid. Most of these patients show significant impairment in phenytoin metabolism when these drugs are given together.

The clinical importance of the interaction between phenytoin and isoniazid has been documented in a more recent report.[157] Of 22 hospitalized medical patients who received phenytoin and isoniazid for at least 5 days, 6 (27%) experienced central nervous system (CNS) toxicity. In contrast, only 30 of 1093 patients (3%) who received phenytoin without isoniazid had CNS toxicity. The risk of adverse effects from phenytoin is greatly increased in patients also receiving isoniazid, probably because of isoniazid-induced impairment of phenytoin metabolism. A recent report suggests that isoniazid also inhibits the metabolism of carbamazepine; coadministration can result in carbamazepine intoxication.[158]

Wright et al.[159] also studied the isoniazid-carbamazepine interaction in a patient with neurologic disorders. Addition of isoniazid to long-term, stable carbamazepine therapy resulted in a rapid and considerable (about 50%) decrease in the metabolic clearance of carbamazepine, leading to carbamazepine toxicity and requiring discontinuation of both drugs. It was later found that the patient was genetically a slow acetylator and probably had high serum levels of isoniazid.

On reinitiating drug therapy with more conservative doses, the apparent inhibition of carbamazepine metabolism by isoniazid was confirmed. About 3 weeks later, the patient had elevated serum levels of liver enzymes suggestive of isoniazid hepatotoxicity. The investigators proposed that carbamazepine stimulated the metabolism of isoniazid to form hepatotoxic reactive intermediates.

Neuroleptics. Recent investigations indicate that phenothiazines and other neuroleptic drugs inhibit the elimination of a wide variety of drugs including propranolol, phenytoin, and perhaps some tricyclic antidepressants. The effects of chlorpromazine, 50 mg every 8 hr, on the disposition and effectiveness of propranolol was studied in healthy subjects.[160] Chlorpromazine decreased the presystemic metabolism of propranolol and increased steady-state plasma propranolol levels by 70% (Fig. 14–13). Elevated levels of propranolol in plasma resulted in increased isoproterenol antagonism and lower plasma renin activity.

Phenytoin toxicity has been reported in 2 patients during concurrent administration of thioridazine, another phenothiazine drug.[161] More than 2-fold increases in steady-state plasma desipramine concentrations have been found in patients also receiving antipsychotic agents, including perphenazine, haloperidol, or thiothixene.[162] High plasma concentrations of imipramine and desipramine have been observed in patients simultaneously treated with oral imipramine and intramuscular fluphenazine decanoate.[163]

β-Blockers. There is evidence that β-blockers may be inhibitors of drug metabolizing enzymes. This is of interest because of the widespread use of these drugs.

Propranolol has been found to inhibit the metabolism of antipyrine; antipyrine half-life is increased from 11 to 14 hr and clearance is decreased from 0.7 to 0.5 ml/min per kg.[164] Another group of investigators reported that both propranolol and metoprolol inhibit antipyrine metabolism, but propranolol has a greater effect.[165] Studies with rat liver microsomes suggest that inhibition of oxidative drug metabolism by β-blockers is related to their lipid solubility; propranolol was the most potent of the drugs studied; timolol, oxprenolol, and labetalol were slightly less potent than propranolol.[166]

Propranolol lowers the systemic clearance of li-

docaine by about 40%. Since lidocaine is highly extracted by the liver, its systemic clearance is dependent on hepatic blood flow. Therefore, the effects of propranolol might be due to a decrease in hepatic blood flow, inhibition of hepatic microsomal enzymes, or both. To answer this question, Bax et al.[167] administered oral lidocaine to healthy subjects with and without propranolol pretreatment (80 mg twice daily for 3 days).

Propranolol increased the mean peak lidocaine concentration in plasma from 502 to 875 ng/ml and increased the area under the lidocaine curve (AUC) from 58 to 117 μg-min/ml. Propranolol pretreatment decreased iv indocyanine green clearance, an index of hepatic blood flow, by 11% but this change was not statistically significant. Based on these data, the investigators concluded that propranolol lowers the systemic clearance of lidocaine mainly by direct inhibition of its hepatic metabolism rather than by lowering hepatic blood flow.

Other investigators have reported that propranolol decreases the systemic clearance of bupivicaine by 35%, an effect that could result in the accumulation of this local anesthetic to toxic levels.[168] These investigators also ascribed the effects of propranolol to inhibition of hepatic metabolism, rather than to changes in hepatic blood flow.

Miners et al.[169] studied the effects of propranolol at two dose levels, 120 mg/day and 720 mg/day, on the disposition of theophylline. The low dose of propranolol decreased theophylline by 30%, whereas the high dose resulted in a 52% decrease in clearance. Low-dose propranolol decreased the formation clearances of the two demethylated metabolites of theophylline, 1-methyluric acid and 3-methylxanthine, by 40 to 45% and the formation clearance of the 8-hydroxylated metabolite, dimethyluric acid, by 27%. High-dose propranolol had a greater effect. The formation clearances of the demethylated metabolites decreased by 70 to 75% and the formation clearance of the hydroxylated metabolite decreased by 44%. The investigators concluded that the results were "consistent with a dose-dependent and selective inhibitory effect of propranolol on the separate forms of cytochrome P-450 involved in theophylline demethylation and 8-hydroxylation."

Oral Contraceptives. Oral contraceptive steroids decrease the plasma clearance of antipyrine[170] and inhibit N-demethylation of aminopyrine.[171] In another study, women using low-dose estrogen oral contraceptive steroids (OCS) on a long-term basis were matched for age and weight with female control subjects not using OCS. Subjects on OCS had a longer antipyrine half-life than control subjects (17 hr vs 10.5 hr). Both estrogens and progestins are competitive inhibitors of cytochrome P-450 and both probably contribute to this interaction.

Plasma metoprolol concentrations after an oral dose are about 70% higher in young women using oral contraceptives than in matched control subjects not using oral contraceptive steroids.[172] The half-life of diazepam is considerably longer (69 hr vs 47 hr) and its plasma clearance much lower (0.27 ml/min per kg vs 0.45 ml/min per kg) in women using oral contraceptive steroids than in control subjects.[173] The clinical significance of these interactions is probably small, but the widespread use of oral contraceptives warrants caution in patients receiving the combination of potent drugs and oral contraceptive steroids.

Other studies have shown that oral contraceptives markedly decrease the plasma clearance of unbound prednisolone in healthy women subjects, from 576 to 214 ml/min.[174] The investigators proposed "very careful monitoring of women taking birth control pills who are concurrently undergoing prednisolone therapy . . [and] expect lower doses of prednisolone to yield clinical efficacy in these subjects."

Valproic Acid. Although valproic acid is a relatively recent addition to the treatment of convulsive disorders and epilepsy, its capacity for interacting with other drugs is well documented. Valproic acid displaces drugs from plasma proteins and inhibits drug metabolism.

The phenobarbital-valproic acid interaction has been carefully studied. Elevated blood levels of phenobarbital and sedation are seen when valproic acid is given to patients treated with phenobarbital.[175] Dosage reductions of phenobarbital of 40 to 50% are required to avoid these effects. Patel and associates report that when a single dose of phenobarbital was given before and during treatment with valproic acid (250 mg twice a day), the half-life of phenobarbital rose from 96 to 142 hr and its clearance fell from 4.2 to 3.0 ml/hr per kg; renal clearance was unchanged but metabolic clearance fell from 3.3 to 2.0 ml/hr per kg; the percentage of the phenobarbital dose excreted unchanged in the urine rose from 22 to 33%.[176] These findings indicate that valproic acid inhibits phenobarbital metabolism.

Valproic acid also inhibits the elimination of

Table 14–3. Effect of Valproic Acid (VPA) Treatment on Ethosuximide Concentrations in Serum*

| Patient | Ethosuximide serum concentration (µg/ml) | |
	Before VPA	With VPA
1	91	115
2	84	126
3	46	53
4	59	138
5	87	130
Mean	73	112

*Data from Mattson, R.H., and Cramer, J.A.[177]

ethosuximide. The addition of valproic acid to an ethosuximide dosage regimen in patients treated for seizures resulted in increased serum concentrations of ethosuximide in 4 of 5 patients (Table 14–3).[177] All patients felt sedated and the average initial dose of 27 mg/kg was lowered to 20 mg/kg.

The teratogenic effects of valproic acid on the human fetus, particularly when combined with other anticonvulsants, may also be related to valproic acid's ability to inhibit enzymes involved in the detoxification of active agents. Kerr and Levy[178] proposed that valproic acid inhibits epoxide hydrolase, a microsomal enzyme required to detoxify unstable reactive arene oxide metabolites that are formed by the oxidative metabolism of phenytoin and carbamazepine.

They found that therapeutic concentrations of valproic acid inhibit the metabolism of carbamazepine epoxide by human liver microsomal epoxide hydrolase and strongly recommended that combination drug therapy with valproic acid should be avoided during pregnancy. This preliminary communication was followed by a more detailed report.[179]

Cimetidine. This histamine H_2-receptor antagonist is an effective drug in the treatment of peptic ulcer and certain other gastrointestinal disorders. It is among the most widely prescribed drugs in the world.

Cimetidine has been shown to inhibit microsomal drug metabolizing enzymes in animals and man, mostly likely through binding of the imidazole ring of cimetidine to cytochrome P-450. Related drugs, like ranitidine, without the imidazole ring do not appear to inhibit drug metabolizing enzymes. Because of the widespread use of cimetidine, there is considerable potential for interactions to occur with other drugs.[180]

The single dose pharmacokinetics of warfarin

were studied in healthy subjects before and after 2 weeks of repeated dosing (1.6 g/day) with cimetidine.[181] Cimetidine reduced the clearance of warfarin from 3.4 to 2.5 ml/min. In an additional 7 subjects maintained on a daily warfarin dose, administration of cimetidine caused a significant increase in plasma warfarin concentrations and anticoagulant effect.[181] Cimetidine also increased the anticoagulant effects of nicoumalone and phenindione.[181] This interaction is clinically relevant; physicians should take care when prescribing cimetidine for patients on anticoagulant therapy.

The effects of cimetidine on the clearance of several benzodiazepines are shown in Table 14–4.[180] Cimetidine inhibited the elimination of diazepam, desmethyldiazepam, and chlordiazepoxide by 30 to 60% but had no effect on the elimination of oxazepam or lorazepam. During chronic dosing with oral diazepam, concomitant administration of cimetidine increased steady-state diazepam concentrations by 30 to 80%, a consequence of reduced diazepam plasma clearance.[182]

Cimetidine also inhibits the metabolism of theophylline and phenytoin. Table 14–5 shows the half-lives and clearances of theophylline during a control period and after 1 and 8 days of cimetidine treatment.[183] Cimetidine significantly inhibits theophylline clearance even on the first day of cimetidine administration. This effect persists or increases as cimetidine is continued in usual therapeutic doses.

The effects of cimetidine on serum phenytoin concentrations were studied in patients requiring the anticonvulsant drug for various neurologic or cardiovascular indications.[184] Steady-state levels rose from 5.7 to 9.1 μg/ml after 3 weeks on cimetidine, then fell to 5.8 μg/ml within 2 weeks after withdrawal of cimetidine. In another study, steady-state serum levels of phenytoin in epileptic patients increased from 13.6 μg/ml before cimetidine to 17.2 μg/ml after 6 days of cimetidine.[185] Patients with relatively high serum phenytoin concentrations, in the order of 15 to 20 μg/ml, are at risk of phenytoin toxicity when cimetidine is added to the treatment regimen.

Other investigators studied the effects of cimetidine, 300 mg 4 times daily for 7 days, on the pharmacokinetics and pharmacodynamics of quinidine.[186] Cimetidine increased the average plasma levels of quinidine by almost 60% and increased the effect of quinidine on several electrocardiographic parameters, including QT intervals. The interaction between cimetidine and quinidine may lead to quinidine toxicity. ECG monitoring and/or dosage reduction of quinidine may be appropriate in patients treated with both drugs.

In another study,[187] patients receiving lidocaine were divided into two groups. About two-thirds of the patients were given cimetidine, 300 mg every 6 hours, in addition to lidocaine, and the rest of the patients received only lidocaine. In all but one of the patients receiving both drugs, lidocaine serum levels were higher than any of those found in the control group. The average difference between the two groups was 75% at steady state. Nearly half of the patients given both drugs were found to have lidocaine levels above 5 μg/ml, a warning point, and 2 patients had symptoms of lethargy and confusion, attributed to lidocaine. No patient in the control group had excess levels. The investigators recommended careful monitoring of serum lidocaine during cimetidine administration.

Cimetidine inhibits hepatic microsomal oxidative drug metabolism but has little effect on conjugation. This distinction was clearly demonstrated by Abernethy et al.,[188] who found that cimetidine impaired the elimination of antipyrine and diazepam, drugs subject to hepatic cytochrome P-450-mediated oxidation, but had no effect on lorazepam, which is glucuronidated, or acetaminophen (APAP), which is predominantly metabolized by glucuronidation and sulfation.

The small fraction of an acetaminophen dose subject to oxidative metabolism and inhibition by

Table 14–4. Effect of Cimetidine on the Half-Life and Clearance of Several Benzodiazepines*

Benzodiazepine	Half-Life, hr		Clearance, ml/min	
	Control	Cimetidine	Control	Cimetidine
Diazepam	34	51	20	11
Desmethyldiazepam	52	73	12	9
Chlordiazepoxide	10	24	0.38	0.14
Oxazepam	13	11	107	93
Lorazepam	21	19	—	—

*Data from Somogyi, A., and Gugler, R.[180]

Table 14–5. Effects of Cimetidine on Theophylline Pharmacokinetics after 1 Day or 8 Days of Cimetidine Administration*

Theophylline variable	Control	Cimetidine administration	
		(1 day)	(8 days)
Half-life, hr	7.6	10.0	11.7
Clearance, ml/min	46.0	37.2	31.5

*Data from Reitberg, D.P., Bernhard, H., and Schentag, J.J.[183]

cimetidine is of little consequence after therapeutic doses of APAP, but may be important following an overdose. Ordinarily, the reactive metabolites resulting from oxidation of APAP are quickly conjugated with glutathione and excreted. When large amounts of acetaminophen are ingested, however, the amount of reactive material formed overwhelms the availability of the glutathione pool and hepatotoxicity may result. Cimetidine inhibits the formation of reactive metabolites and may be useful in APAP overdose. Studies in mice have shown that the average lethal dose of acetaminophen is increased about twofold when it is given with cimetidine.[188] More recently, it hs become clear that too high a dose of cimetidine is needed in man to protect against APAP toxicity.

Several studies have compared cimetidine and ranitidine with respect to drug interactions. For example, Schwartz et al.[189] found that pretreatment with cimetidine decreased the oral clearance of nifedipine following a single dose of the calcium antagonist from 66 to 33 L/hr, whereas ranitidine had no effect. Sambol et al.[190] compared the influence of famotidine and cimetidine on phenytoin elimination. Cimetidine decreased the plasma clearance of phenytoin by 16%, but famotidine had no effect.

Cimetidine is known to cause gynecomastia and sexual dysfunction in some men. This may be related to inhibition of the cytochrome P-450-dependent metabolism of estradiol. Galbraith and Michnovicz[191] found that cimetidine reduced the extent of 2-hydroxylation of estradiol in male subjects from a mean of about 30 to 20% after 2 weeks of oral treatment (800 mg twice daily). At the same time, the urinary excretion of 2-hydroxyestrone decreased by about 25% and the serum levels of estradiol increased by about 20%.

Another male subject, given cimetidine at a lower dose, 400 mg twice a day, showed a reduction in the 2-hydroxylation of estradiol from 37 to

24%. In a separate study, ranitidine, 150 mg twice daily, was found to have no effect on the 2-hydroxylation of estradiol. The investigators suggested that "this mechanism may help to account for the signs and symptoms of estrogen excess reported with the long-term use of cimetidine."

Calcium Channel Blockers. Many reports have been published concerning interactions of various drugs with calcium channel blockers. Both diltiazem[192] and verapamil[193] decrease the nonrenal clearance of digoxin and may elevate steady-state digoxin concentrations by 20 to 30%. Nifedipine, on the other hand, has no effect on the elimination of digoxin.

To better understand the effects of calcium antagonists on the disposition of other drugs, Bauer et al.[194] studied antipyrine and indocyanine green (ICG) kinetics in healthy subjects before and after pretreatment with nifedipine (10 mg 3 times daily), diltiazem (30 mg 4 times daily), and verapamil (80 mg 3 times daily).

Diltiazem and verapamil, but not nifedipine, significantly decreased the clearance of antipyrine by about 25%. ICG clearance was about 700 ml/min during the control period but increased to about 900 ml/min when either nifedipine or verapamil was given. These results suggest that nifedipine primarily increases liver blood flow with little effect on hepatic oxidative metabolism, whereas diltiazem has only a modest effect on liver blood flow but significantly inhibits oxidative metabolism. Interactions of verapamil with other drugs may involve either or both of these mechanisms.

Other investigators have determined that diltiazem also inhibits the metabolism of theophylline.[195] The calcium antagonist decreased the clearance of theophylline from 52 to 42 ml/min/1.73 m^2 in nonsmokers, and from 65 to 51 ml/min/1.73 m^2 in cigarette smokers.

Both verapamil and diltiazem present a clinical problem when given with carbamazepine. Verapamil, 120 mg 3 times daily, when given to patients with epilepsy, treated with carbamazepine, resulted in elevated plasma levels of carbamazepine and neurotoxicity.[196] Two patients, rechallenged with a lower dose of verapamil, 120 mg twice daily, again showed signs of carbamazepine toxicity. Withdrawal of verapamil was associated with a decline in plasma carbamazepine from 12 to 7 μg/ml. A case report concerning a patient on carbamazepine also described elevated blood levels of the anticonvulsant and neurotoxicity when diltiazem was given concurrently but not when nifedipine was administered.[197]

Quinolone Antibiotics. A large group of synthetic fluroquinolones, related chemically to nalidixic acid, are under investigation. At this time, two compounds, norfloxacin and ciprofloxacin, are approved for use in the United States. Several others are in clinical trials, awaiting approval.

A potential disadvantage of some of the quinolones is their ability to inhibit the metabolism of drugs given concurrently.[198] The earliest reports indicated that enoxacin increased blood levels of theophylline when the drugs were given concomitantly. Beckmann et al.[199] reported that enoxacin inhibited the formation of all three primary metabolites of theophylline.

In another study, Wijnands et al.[200] found that pefloxacin and ciprofloxacin also inhibited the metabolism of theophylline but much less so than enoxacin. These investigators suggested that the inhibition involved the 4-oxo metabolite of the quinolones, which is formed in larger amounts after enoxacin than after pefloxacin or ciprofloxacin.

The ciprofloxacin-theophylline interaction was also studied by Schwartz et al.[201] Theophylline clearance after 2 days of ciprofloxacin, 750 mg twice daily, was decreased in 8 of 9 subjects; clearance was decreased by an average of 31%, after 4 days of ciprofloxacin. Theophylline clearance returned to baseline 2 days after discontinuing ciprofloxacin. Norfloxacin also inhibits theophylline metabolism but to a smaller extent than does ciprofloxacin.[202] Mean theophylline clearance decreased by 15% after a course of norfloxacin.

Clearly, the quinolones inhibit theophylline metabolism but they differ widely in the magnitude of their effects, perhaps related to the ease of formation of a particular metabolite. Ofloxacin and lomefloxacin appear to have a negligible effect on theophylline metabolism.

Most likely, quinolones will also be found to inhibit the metabolism of other drugs. One report indicates that enoxacin decreases the mean clearance of R-warfarin by about 30% but has no effect on the clearance of the more potent S-enantiomer. Consequently, enoxacin may be given with racemic warfarin without seeing any effect on anticoagulant response.[203]

Propoxyphene. A case study concerning a massive overdose of acetaminophen reported, unexpectedly, little liver damage.[204] The authors speculated that this outcome may have resulted because large quantities of propoxyphene were also ingested with acetaminophen. In vitro studies have shown that propoxyphene is an inhibitor of cytochrome P-450 hepatic oxidative drug metabolism. Recent reports have provided clinical evidence of this.

An elderly man stabilized on doxepin for depression was given propoxyphene 65 mg every 6 hours for relief of arthritic pain. The addition of propoxyphene produced a more than 2-fold increase in doxepin levels and progressive lethargy. Doxepin levels declined and attentiveness improved when propoxyphene was discontinued.[205] As a follow-up to this observation, the effects of propoxyphene on the metabolism of antipyrine were studied. A short course of propoxyphene, 65 mg every 4 hours, decreased antipyrine clearance by 20%.

Other investigators concerned with the clearance of benzodiazepines during regular administration of propoxyphene reported that propoxyphene decreased the clearance of alprazolam and diazepam by 40% and 13%, respectively, but had no effect on the elimination of lorazepam.[206] To summarize, propoxyphene significantly impairs the clearance of alprazolam, metabolized mainly by aliphatic hydroxylation, has far less effect on the oxidation of diazepam via an N-demethylation pathway, and has no effect on the conjugation of lorazepam with glucuronic acid.

Erythromycin. The most widely known interaction of erythromycin is with theophylline; concurrent administration for at least 5 days increases serum theophylline levels about 2-fold, requiring a theophylline dosage reduction.[207] More recently, other investigators have reported several case studies of a carbamazepine-erythromycin interaction.[208] In 4 patients with head trauma, serum levels of carbamazepine doubled or tripled when erythromycin treatment, 1 g/day in divided doses, was initiated.

Another report suggests that erythromycin may also have a significant effect on the elimination of cyclosporine.[209] Cylosporine levels in a woman receiving the drug after renal transplantation rose from 122 to 666 ng/ml within a few days of starting erythromycin treatment for a urinary tract infection. Five days after discontinuing erythromycin, the patient's cyclosporine levels declined to 222 ng/ml.

Other Interactions. A wide range of other drugs have been reported to inhibit the metabolism of certain drugs given concurrently. Ketoconazole, like several other related antifungal drugs and like cimetidine, has an imidazole ring and is a likely candidate to inhibit oxidative metabolism. Clinical evidence of this has been presented by Brown et al.[210]

Methoxsalen (8-methoxypsoralen), a natural product used in the treatment of psoriasis, is a potent inhibitor of caffeine metabolism.[211] Methoxsalen increased the mean area under the concentration-time curve after a single oral dose of caffeine from 34 to 106 mg-hr/ml. Assuming caffeine is completely bioavailable after oral administration, methoxsalen decreased caffeine clearance from 110 to 34 ml/min. The investigators pointed out that "patients receiving methoxsalen . . . are often treated with other drugs, such as sulindac, indomethacin, and analogs of retinoic acid. Our results suggest that elimination of these or other microsomally metabolized drugs may be altered by methoxsalen."

Omeprazole, a selective inhibitor of gastric acid secretion, is still another imidazole derivative. Treatment over 6 days with a single daily dose of 40 mg omeprazole decreased diazepam clearance by more than 50%. Plasma levels of desmethyldiazepam, diazepam's major metabolite, were smaller after omeprazole indicating reduced metabolite formation. Omeprazole has also been found to cause a small (15%) but consistent reduction in phenytoin clearance but appears to have no effect on theophylline clearance.[212]

Propafenone, a class Ic antiarrhythmic agent under active investigation, also appears to be a potent inhibitor of drug metabolism. After a case report suggesting that propafenone potentiates the anticoagulant effects of phenprocoumon, Kates et al.[213] set out to determine if there was an interaction between propafenone and warfarin. Propafenone increased mean steady-state levels of warfarin nearly 40% and significantly prolonged prothrombin time compared with the effects of warfarin alone.

Propafenone also inhibits the metabolism of metoprolol.[214] The investigators pointed out that although the therapeutic index of metoprolol is large, the marked rise in plasma metoprolol levels when propafenone is added might cause serious adverse effects in susceptible patients. "It seems necessary therefore to reduce the dose of metoprolol when propafenone is administered simultaneously."

A life-threatening interaction has been reported

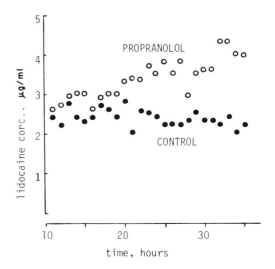

Fig. 14–14. Effect of coadministered propranolol on serum lidocaine levels during a continuous intravenous infusion of lidocaine. (Data from Ochs, H.R., Carstens, G., and Greenblatt, D.J.[216])

between tamoxifen, an adjuvant used in the treatment of breast cancer, and warfarin.[215] A 43-year-old woman was stabilized on a daily warfarin dose of 5 mg and a prothrombin time of 19 seconds. Seven weeks later, tamoxifen 40 mg daily was added to her treatment. The next day her prothrombin time was 38 seconds. Eventually, she was restabilized on 1 mg warfarin daily to maintain a prothrombin time of 20 to 25 seconds.

A review of medical records suggested that this problem had occurred in 5 other patients who received tamoxifen and warfarin concurrently. It is likely that tamoxifen inhibits the metabolism of warfarin, but further studies are needed to firmly nail down the mechanism of this interaction.

Changes in Hepatic Blood Flow

The clearance of drugs such as lidocaine and propranolol, that have a high hepatic extraction (> 0.5), will be sensitive to changes in the blood flow rate to the liver. Interactions may occur when they are given with other drugs that affect cardiac output or directly affect hepatic blood flow (HBF).

Propranolol-induced β-blockade results in a reduction in cardiac output and HBF. Consistent with this effect, propranolol also reduces the elimination of lidocaine because the clearance of lidocaine is HBF rate-limited.[216] Single dose studies indicate that the clearance of iv lidocaine falls from 18 ml/min per kg during a control period to 11 ml/min per kg during a propranolol treatment period. Propranolol also causes a 30% increase in steady-state serum lidocaine levels during continuous intravenous infusion (Fig. 14–14).[216] This difference may be clinically important because the therapeutic index of lidocaine is narrow. A lower dosage of lidocaine may be required in patients who are also being treated with β-blockers. It is also important to note that propranolol not only reduces HBF, but also inhibits hepatic metabolism. Increases in lidocaine levels are probably related to both effects of propranolol.

A single dose of cimetidine significantly reduces the clearance of indocyanine green in man;[217] this is consistent with the known effect of cimetidine on HBF in the dog, an effect related to its histamine blocking action. Therefore, cimetidine can affect the clearance of drugs with high hepatic excretion ratios in two ways, by decreasing the HBF rate and by inhibiting hepatic drug metabolizing enzymes.

Cimetidine decreased the systemic clearance of intravenous propranolol by about 25%.[217] Steady-state levels of propranolol on oral dosing were increased from 23 to 45 ng/ml during treatment with cimetidine.[218] Cimetidine also reduced the systemic clearance of lidocaine from 766 ml/min to 576 ml/min.[219] Lidocaine toxicity was noted in 5 of 6 subjects during the cimetidine infusion but in only 1 of 6 subjects during a placebo infusion. Lidocaine concentrations were 50% higher when subjects received cimetidine.

Whether or not changes in the rate of liver blood flow play an important role in these interactions with cimetidine is difficult to say in light of the inhibitory effects of cimetidine on the intrinsic hepatic clearance of propranolol and lidocaine.

Low concentrations of caffeine and theophylline block the vasodilatory effects of adenosine and, in this manner, may modulate hepatic blood flow. To test this hypothesis, Onrot et al.[220] studied the effects of these xanthines on liver perfusion using ICG clearance as an index of hepatic blood flow.

Thirty min after dosing with 250 mg oral caffeine, ICG clearance was reduced by an average of 19%, from 630 to 510 ml/min. Dosing with theophylline, 4.3 mg/kg iv infused over 1 hr, also resulted in a fall in ICG clearance from 550 to 470 ml/min. The investigators suggested that "the observed fall . . . may affect the disposition of concomitantly administered drugs or absorbed nutrients that are highly extractable." They concluded that "because of their widespread use in Western society, caffeine and theophylline may be major determinants of liver blood flow in the general population."

In principle, blood levels of a drug subject to presystemic hepatic metabolism on oral administration are independent of HBF. Elevated blood levels, however, may be observed if HBF rate is transiently increased during absorption but thereafter declines to baseline.[221] This phenomenon may explain the elevated blood levels of propranolol when it is given with food[222] or with hydralazine,[223] a potent vasodilator. A 25-mg oral dose of hydralazine given simultaneously with oral propranolol increased plasma propranolol levels by 60%; a 50-mg oral dose of hydralazine increased plasma propranolol concentrations by about 80%.[223]

An alternative mechanism to explain the interaction between hydralazine and propranolol is inhibition of the first-pass metabolism of the beta-blocker by hydralazine. To select between these mechanisms, Schneck and Vary[224] measured the urinary excretion rate and profile of propranolol metabolites after oral administration of radiolabeled propranolol 40 mg, alone or with 25 or 50 mg hydralazine.

The investigators reasoned that if hydralazine inhibits the metabolism of propranolol, the urinary excretion rate of propranolol metabolites would be expected to decrease and, if there were selective inhibition of the propranolol metabolic pathways, there would be a change in the composition of propranolol metabolites in urine. On the other hand, if hydralazine affects only liver blood flow, there would be no change in the profile of propranolol metabolites in urine.

Coadministration of hydralazine substantially increased the plasma levels of propranolol, by 60% after the 25 mg dose and by 120% after the 50 mg dose, but hydralazine had no effect on the fraction of the propranolol dose recovered in the urine as basic, acidic, or polar metabolites; these fractions accounted for 99% of the dose.

Furthermore, hydralazine did not alter the pattern of metabolites measurable by high-performance liquid chromatography (i.e., naphthoxylactic aid, propranolol glucuronide, and 4-hydroxypropranolol) and did not decrease the urinary excretion rates of propranolol metabolites. These results support an interaction mechanism involving an increase in hepatic blood flow during the absorption of propranolol when it is given with hydralazine.

Other investigators have reported that hydralazine also increases blood levels of metoprolol, another drug highly extracted by the liver.[225] Steady-state concentrations of metoprolol in plasma increased nearly 40% and peak levels of metoprolol increased by about 90% in hypertensive pregnant women when hydralazine 25 mg twice daily was added to a regimen of metoprolol 50 mg twice daily.

Stereochemical Considerations in Drug Interactions

Most investigators now agree that effects on individual enantiomers must be considered when studying an interaction involving a racemic drug. As noted above, the interaction between enoxacin and warfarin is not clinically important because only the R-form of warfarin is inhibited, not the more potent S-enantiomer.[203] Considering only the effects on racemic warfarin, we would arrive at the implausible conclusion that the interaction results in an increase in warfarin serum levels but no change in anticoagulant activity.

Stereoselective interactions have also been reported with cimetidine. Toon et al.[226] discovered that cimetidine, like enoxacin, inhibits the metabolism of R-warfarin, but not that of S-warfarin, and has little effect on the anticoagulant activity of a dose of racemic warfarin. These investigators also found that although cimetidine had no effect on beta-blockade after a single dose of metoprolol, it did increase the bioavailability of oral metoprolol through inhibition of first-pass metabolism.[227] The interaction was stereoselective, with the major effect being on the less pharmacologically active enantiomer of metoprolol.

Drug Interactions as a Probe to Identify Metabolic Pathways Regulated by the Debrisoquin Phenotype

Poor metabolizers (PMs) of debrisoquin may be at risk of adverse effects during treatment with drugs that share its genetic polymorphism. Patients at risk have usually been identified by phenotyping with debrisoquin or sparteine, which displays the same genetic polymorphism as debrisoquin. Drugs that cosegregate with debrisoquin or sparteine have been identified by pharmacokinetic studies in panels of phenotyped subjects.

The low frequency of PMs in the U.S. population (less than 10%) has made it difficult to identify, early in the course of development, those drugs likely to cause adverse effects in patients with im-paired oxidative metabolism. Few centers have available panels of phenotyped subjects and in those that do, very few PMs are included in the panel. The development of an alternative screening method not requiring the preselection of PMs would be an important contribution.

An agent that could be given safely and acted as a potent and selective inhibitor of debrisoquin 4-hydroxylase activity might be useful in this regard. Ideally, this agent would inhibit the elimination of only those drugs significantly metabolized by the cytochrome P-450 isozyme regulating debrisoquin hydroxylation. One compound that may be suitable for this purpose is quinidine.

Speirs et al.[228] reported that quinidine was a potent inhibitor of the 4-hydroxylation of debrisoquin and the 1′-hydroxylation of bufuralol by human liver microsomes. Quinidine was about 100 times more potent in this respect than quinine, its diastereoisomer. Quinidine also inhibited the O-deethylation of phenacetin but 1000-fold higher concentrations were required than those needed to inhibit the aforementioned hydroxylation processes.

Other studies have shown that the polymorphic isozyme directing debrisoquin hydroxylation is important in the metabolism of bufuralol. The dealkylation of phenacetin, on the other hand, is known to be catalyzed by an isozyme other than that involved in the hydroxylation of debrisoquin. Other oxidation pathways that do not appear to be associated with the debrisoquin/sparteine isozyme are the hydroxylation of mephenytoin and tolbutamide, and the N-demethylation of aminopyrine.

Speirs and his colleagues concluded that "quinidine at subpharmacological doses may be used to investigate the contribution of the isozyme of cytochrome P-450 catalysing the 4-hydroxylation of debrisoquin in the elimination of a new drug. If the elimination of such a compound is significantly impaired following the co-administration of quinidine then it could be concluded that this isozyme is likely to catalyse a quantitatively important proportion of the elimination of the drug and would indicate that its elimination may well be impaired in PM subjects." This conclusion has been supported by a report showing that quinidine nearly abolished the oxidation of sparteine.[229]

The debrisoquin/sparteine isozyme is known to be involved in the metabolism of more than 30 drugs. The metabolism of all that have been studied, including metoprolol, propafenone, encainide, and dextromethorphan is inhibited by quinidine.[230] A great deal more must be done, however, before we can be sure that quinidine will interact only with a drug having a metabolic pathway that co-segregates with debrisoquin hydroxylation. In the meantime, it would make sense to study the interaction between quinidine and new compounds subject to oxidative metabolism, at least at the level of human liver microsomes. If an interaction is observed, it might be prudent to set up a panel of EMs and PMs for further study.

ENVIRONMENTAL CHEMICALS

Although genetic factors contribute substantially to the large degree of intersubject variability found in apparently healthy, drug-free individuals, certain environmental factors also contribute to this variability. Relatively few of these factors have been isolated, but during the past 2 decades a lot has been learned about the effects of excessive or chronic alcohol consumption, cigarette smoking, and diet on drug metabolism.

Alcohol

The damaging effects of chronic alcoholism on the human liver are well documented. The hepatic metabolism of many drugs is impaired in patients with alcoholic cirrhosis. Excessive or chronic alcohol consumption, however, also affects drug metabolism in people who have no signs of liver disease.

Acute ethanol intoxication inhibits drug metabolism.[231] This effect is clearly seen in studies with chlordiazepoxide.[232] The elimination of chlordiazepoxide after intravenous administration was determined before and after acute ingestion of ethanol, 0.8 g/kg followed by 0.5 g/kg every 5 hr for 30 hr. Plasma clearance of chlordiazepoxide fell about one third, from 27 ml/min in the control period to 17 ml/min during ethanol intoxication. Plasma ethanol concentrations were maintained in a range of 50 to 150 mg/dl during the study. Ethanol also decreased the plasma protein binding of chlordiazepoxide; percentage unbound rose from 5.3 to 6.6%. Therefore, plasma clearance of unbound chlordiazepoxide decreased almost 50%, from 468 ml/min to 264 ml/min. The results suggest that pharmacokinetic as well as pharmacologic factors contribute to the more profound sedation observed when chlordiazepoxide is taken with ethanol.

Drug metabolism studies with alcohol are complicated by the fact that ethanol not only inhibits drug metabolism but also stimulates drug metabolism, at least on chronic administration.[233] Regular administration of ethanol for one month to alcoholic and nonalcoholic subjects resulted in an enhanced elimination of meprobamate, phenobarbital, and ethanol itself. The half-life of meprobamate was reduced from 17 to 7 hr in alcoholic subjects and from 14 to 8 hr in nonalcoholic subjects. The half-life of pentobarbital in nonalcoholic subjects decreased from 35 to 26 hr. Approximately 4 to 8 weeks after the end of the ethanol treatment, the rate of elimination of ethanol and meprobamate had returned to normal.

Cigarette Smoking

Tobacco smoke is a complex mixture composed primarily of gases, but it also contains particulate matter. The particulate matter consists of water-soluble compounds, including nicotine, and fat-soluble compounds, including polycyclic aromatic hydrocarbons.

Polycyclic aromatic hydrocarbons, and perhaps other constituents of tobacco smoke, are potent inducers of certain drug metabolizing enzymes, particularly the enzyme aryl hydrocarbon hydroxylase. The enzymes affected by tobacco smoke are involved in the metabolism of many drugs; chronic smoking has been reported to increase the metabolism of nicotine, phenacetin, antipyrine, theophylline, imipramine, pentazocine, and propranolol. The effects of smoking on drug metabolism and actions have been reviewed by Miller,[234] Jusko,[235] and Dawson and Vestal.[236]

Propoxyphene was rated ineffective for the relief of mild to moderate pain or headache in 10% of nonsmokers, 15% of light smokers, and 20% of heavy smokers.[237] Of the 7 reported adverse reactions to propoxyphene, 6 occurred in nonsmokers. The reduced efficacy of propoxyphene in smokers is consistent with enhanced metabolism and suggests the need for higher dosage in these patients.

The incidence of drowsiness in patients receiving diazepam or chlordiazepoxide is also related to smoking history.[234] About 8% of nonsmokers or light smokers but only 3% of heavy smokers reported drowsiness with diazepam. The incidence of drowsiness with chlordiazepoxide was 10% in nonsmokers, 6% in light smokers, and 3.5% in heavy smokers. No heavy smoker experienced drowsiness with doses of diazepam up to 20 mg/day. Whether these results are related to stimulated

Table 14–6. Phenacetin Concentrations in the Plasma after Oral Administration of a 900-mg Dose to Cigarette Smokers and Nonsmokers*

Time after administration (hr)	Plasma phenacetin levels (μg/ml)	
	Nonsmokers	Smokers
1	0.81	0.33
2	2.24	0.48
3.5	0.39	0.09
5	0.12	0.02

*Data from Pantuck, E.J., Kuntzman, R., and Conney, A.H.[239]

metabolism or increased tolerance to benzodiazepines in smokers is not established.

Clinically, the dosage requirements for pentazocine as a supplement to nitrous oxide anesthesia are greater in smokers than nonsmokers. Studies in healthy subjects suggest that stimulated metabolism is the reason for differences in dosage requirements because smokers metabolize pentazocine more efficiently than nonsmokers.[238]

The metabolism of phenacetin is also accelerated in smokers.[239] Plasma phenacetin levels after oral administration are much lower in smokers than in nonsmokers (Table 14–6). The low plasma concentrations of phenacetin in smokers are probably the results of increased presystemic gastrointestinal or hepatic metabolism.

The interaction between theophylline and tobacco smoke is one of the most clinically important effects of smoking because of the low therapeutic index of theophylline. The half-life of theophylline is short in smokers, averaging about 4 hr, compared to nonsmokers, who show values of about 7 hr.[240] The clearance of theophylline was 44.5 ml/min per 1.73 m² in nonsmokers and 100 ml/min in smokers.[241] These differences suggest a 2-fold difference in theophylline dosage requirements in smokers and nonsmokers to achieve comparable blood levels, the smokers requiring more theophylline.

The increased metabolism of theophylline in smokers seems to be associated with reduced toxicity during clinical use of this bronchodilator. There is a significant relationship between the incidence of adverse reactions to theophylline and smoking history.[242] The incidence of theophylline toxicity was 13% in nonsmokers, 11% in light smokers, and 7% in smokers.

Vestal and his colleagues[243,244] determined that the effects of smoking on theophylline disposition are independent of age and persist even when the metabolism of theophylline is inhibited by cimetidine or accelerated by phenytoin. Their study group consisted of young (19 to 31 years) and elderly (65 to 75 years) smokers and nonsmokers.

Theophylline clearance was 68 ml/hr/kg in young smokers and 46 ml/hr/kg in young nonsmokers. Similar differences were observed in the elderly panel: 55 ml/hr/kg in smokers and 31 ml/hr/kg in nonsmokers. Young smokers treated with cimetidine also had a higher theophylline clearance than young nonsmokers similarly treated: 48 vs 32 ml/hr/kg. The same was true in the old subjects. Theophylline clearance in subjects treated with phenytoin was again consistently higher in smokers than in nonsmokers. Old and young smokers had values of 106 and 120 ml/hr/kg, respectively; corresponding values in nonsmokers were 49 and 78 ml/hr/kg.

In a related study, Crowley[245] again found that phenytoin enhanced the metabolism of theophylline in both smokers and nonsmokers. In a panel of young adults, before treatment with phenytoin, theophylline clearance was 48 ml/hr/kg in nonsmokers and 90 ml/hr/kg in smokers. Phenytoin increased theophylline clearance by 40% in nonsmokers and by 48% in smokers.

In spite of the pronounced increase in theophylline clearance as a result of smoking, the drug metabolizing enzymes concerned with theophylline metabolism can be induced further. The investigators concluded that "the induction of theophylline clearance by phenytoin is additive to that caused by cigarette smoking and provides support for the suggestion that theophylline metabolism is influenced by multiple polymorphisms."

When cigarette smokers are hospitalized, they are often forced to stop smoking. With this in mind, Lee et al.[246] studied the effects of brief abstinence from tobacco on theophylline elimination in healthy subjects. Abstinence from smoking for 1 week resulted in a 38% decrease in the clearance of theophylline. The results indicate that at least partial normalization of the enzyme-inducing effects of smoking may be realized in a short time after stopping. The investigations recommended that "for smokers who are taking theophylline chronically, their dose of theophylline will need to be reduced by one fourth to one third after brief tobacco abstinence."

Smoking also accelerates the metabolism of caffeine. This may explain the higher coffee consumption in smokers than in nonsmokers. To better understand the implications of this interaction, Benowitz et al.[247] investigated the effects of smoking and short-term abstinence from smoking on the rate and pattern of caffeine metabolism in habitual smokers who were regular coffee drinkers. Participants were heavy smokers whose habit ranged from 30 to 50 cigarettes per day and who regularly consumed 3 to 8 cups of coffee per day.

Blood levels of caffeine following a series of 6 test doses given every 2 hr were about 50% higher 3 to 4 days after smoking was stopped than just before stopping. The mean peak caffeine concentrations during the smoking and abstinence phases were 2.9 and 3.8 μg/ml, respectively. Cessation also resulted in a significant decrease in the urinary recovery of two metabolites of caffeine. The urinary excretion patterns found in this study suggest that smoking accelerated the demethylation pathways of caffeine metabolism but had little effect on the xanthine oxidase pathway.

In another study,[248] caffeine consumption and plasma caffeine concentrations were measured before and for 6 months after a panel of subjects gave up smoking. Volunteers were recruited for a stop smoking program and evaluated before and at 12 and 26 weeks afterward. Of the 95 subjects who started the program, 64 were available for evaluation at 12 weeks; 30 of these subjects had resumed smoking during this period.

Although coffee consumption was unchanged from baseline, both in those who resumed smoking and those who remained abstinent, plasma levels of caffeine increased markedly after 12 weeks in the former smokers, from 6.6 to 17.9 μmol/L, but hardly at all in those who resumed smoking. The findings were almost identical at 26 weeks. Mean plasma caffeine levels increased by nearly 300% in those who remained abstinent, whereas caffeine consumption during this period actually decreased by about 25%. Caffeine levels in plasma were unchanged in those who did not succeed in their efforts to quit smoking.

The investigators recommended that "doctors offering antismoking treatment should advise patients that continued consumption of coffee at the same level may exacerbate the tobacco withdrawal syndrome and contribute to increased health risks; these patients should reduce their consumption."

Epidemiologic data have linked smoking to earlier menopause and increased osteoporosis, both of which are associated with a relative deficiency of estrogen. Michnovitz et al.[249] have considered the possibility that the apparent anti-estrogen effects of smoking may be related to increased hepatic metabolism of natural estrogens. They found a significant increase in estradiol 2-hydroxylation, on the order of 50%, in premenopausal women who smoked compared with those who did not smoke. The investigators concluded that "smoking exerts a powerful inducing effect on the 2-hydroxylation pathway of estradiol metabolism, which is likely to lead to decreased bioavailability at estrogen target tissues."

Diet

Dietary factors have been shown to be determinants of drug-metabolizing enzyme activity in laboratory animals, but little is known of the effects of diet or specific foods on drug metabolism in man. When the diets of healthy subjects were changed from their usual diets to a low carbohydrate-high protein diet, the half-life of antipyrine decreased from 16 to 10 hr and that of theophylline decreased from 8 to 5 hr. When diets were again changed from low carbohydrate-high protein to high carbohydrate-low protein, the mean antipyrine half-life increased from 10 to 16 hr and the mean theophylline half-life increased from 5 to 8 hr. Supplementing standard diets with carbohydrate caused an increase in drug half-life, whereas a protein supplement caused a decrease in drug half-life.[250]

Certain vegetables, including brussels sprouts, cabbage, turnips, broccoli, cauliflower, and spinach, contain chemicals that induce aryl hydrocarbon hydroxylase enzyme activity. A test diet containing brussels sprouts and cabbage reduced plasma phenacetin concentrations after oral administration to healthy subjects by 50% compared to those observed in the same subjects maintained on a control diet containing no enzyme-inducing vegetables.[251]

Charcoal-broiled beef also enhances drug metabolism. The average peak concentration of phenacetin in plasma after a 900-mg oral dose fell from 1630 ng/ml when healthy subjects were fed a control diet to 350 ng/ml after they were maintained on a diet containing charcoal-broiled beef.[252] Charcoal-broiled beef also induces the metabolism of antipyrine and theophylline; the half-lives of these 2 drugs were each decreased about 20% when healthy subjects were fed a diet containing charcoal-broiled beef.[253] These effects are probably related to the fact that charcoal-broiled beef contains large quantities of polycyclic aromatic hydrocarbons.

In 1984, Nutt and his colleagues[254] presented evidence suggesting that competition between large neutral amino acids (resulting from the administration of phenylalanine, leucine, or isoleucine) and levodopa for transport from plasma to brain may be partly responsible for the fluctuating clinical response, called the 'on-off phenomenon,' frequently seen in patients with Parkinson's disease treated with levodopa.

More recently, these investigators considered the use of a low-protein diet as a therapeutic strategy for treating parkinsonian patients handicapped by a fluctuating response to levodopa.[255] A diet containing 1.6 g/kg protein was compared with a 0.8 g/kg diet with protein evenly distributed between meals, and a 0.8 g/kg diet with protein restricted to the evening meal.

The mean percent of the time patients were responding satisfactorily to levodopa (i.e., 'on' time) was 51% for the high-protein diet, 67% for the low-protein diet distributed over three meals, and 77% for the low-protein diet restricted to the evening meal. The mean plasma levels of large neutral amino acids were 732 nmol/ml for the high-protein diet, 640 for the distributed low-protein diet, and 542 for the restricted low-protein diet.

Nutt et al. concluded that "for patients with a fluctuating response who have not responded to dosage adjustment, lower protein intake will augment the effects of levodopa. The low-protein distributed diet is effective and easiest to implement."

A decrease in diet protein depresses creatinine clearance and renal plasma flow. Dietary protein also affects the renal tubular transport of certain endogenous compounds, but there is little understanding of the role of diet in the renal excretion of drugs. Studies with allopurinol suggest that this kind of interaction merits more attention.[256]

The pharmacokinetics of allopurinol and oxypurinol, its active metabolite, were studied in healthy subjects. Each subject received, in random order, a low-protein (19 g/day) or high-protein (268 g/day) diet for 14 days. Before the study and on day 12 of each diet, 24-hour urine and plasma samples were obtained to determine creatinine clearance. On day 13 of each diet, each subject received a 600-mg oral dose of allopurinol.

Compared with baseline values, renal function was decreased by the low-protein diet and increased by the high-protein diet. Creatinine clearance increased from 96 ml/min on the low-protein

diet to 138 ml/min on the high-protein diet. The same was true of urea and uric acid renal clearance.

Small differences were observed in the kinetics of allopurinol. Consistent with the difference in creatinine clearance, the renal clearance of allopurinol was about 30% smaller, compared with control values, when protein was restricted. The area under the curve (AUC) for allopurinol was about 45% greater during the low-protein diet than during the high-protein diet. Since the renal clearance of allopurinol accounts for only a small percentage of its total body clearance, the increase in allopurinol AUC may reflect a decrease in the xanthine-oxidase dependent metabolism of allopurinol to oxypurinol during protein restriction.

In contrast to the relatively small effect of dietary protein on allopurinol, a pronounced effect was observed on the pharmacokinetics of oxypurinol. Renal clearance of the metabolite during protein restriction was only one-third that observed during the high-protein diet; the AUC and half-life of oxypurinol were three times greater.

The decrease in the renal clearance of oxypurinol during protein restriction was about twice as large as the change in creatinine clearance. Based on the size of this difference, the investigators proposed that the mechanism of the interaction must also involve a change in tubular function associated with protein restriction.

They hypothesized that oxypurinol, a weak acid chemically similar to uric acid, may be reabsorbed by the uric acid system in the renal tubules. A high-protein diet, which is similar to the typical American diet, inhibits reabsorption and produces the characteristic pharmacokinetic profile of oxypurinol. Protein restriction, on the other hand, allows extensive tubular reabsorption of oxypurinol, which would result in a decreased renal clearance and more persistent oxypurinol levels in plasma.

In support of this hypothesis, urea and uric acid renal clearances were about 60% smaller during protein restriction than during the high-protein diet, whereas creatinine clearance was only 30% smaller. If this hypothesis is correct, it adds a new mechanism to the ways in which dietary factors can alter clinical pharmacokinetics.

Other Chemicals

Certain chemicals found in the work environment can stimulate drug metabolizing enzymes.[257] The half-life of antipyrine in men occupationally exposed to a mixture of insecticides (mainly Lindane and DDT) was significantly shorter than in 33 control subjects (8 hr vs 12 hr).[258] Others have shown a decrease in the half-life of phenylbutazone in workers exposed to chlorinated pesticides.[259]

Other chemicals in the work environment may inhibit drug metabolism. Plasma warfarin half-life and anticoagulant effect were determined in anesthesiology residents at the start of their training period. Average warfarin half-life in these subjects was 32 hr and average prothrombin response was 1340 U. After 4 months in the operating room, average warfarin half-life had increased to 49 hr and prothrombin response to 1550 U.[260] The change in warfarin kinetics and effect appears to be the result of inhibition of warfarin metabolism, related to the repeated exposure of these subjects to an operating room environment.

CONCLUSIONS

In view of the effects of age, sex, body size, genetic factors, disease, and interactions on drug blood levels resulting from usual dosage regimens, one cannot be surprised that a wide range of individual responses to therapy is found with all drugs. One can also understand the need for and interest in individualization of dosage regimens.

REFERENCES

1. Tatro, D.S.: Drug Interaction Facts. Philadelphia, Facts and Comparisons Division, J.B. Lippincott Co., 1988.
2. Hansen P.D., and Horn, J.R.: Drug Interaction Newsletter. Spokane, WA, Applied Therapeutics, Inc.
3. Somogyi, A., and Muirhead, M.: Pharmacokinetic interactions of cimetidine 1987. Clin. Pharmacokin., *12*:321, 1987.
4. Gugler, R., and Jensen, J.C.: Drugs other than H₂-receptor antagonists as clinically important inhibitors of drug metabolism *in vivo*. Pharmac. Ther., *33*:133, 1987.
5. Anon.: Drug interactions update. Med. Lett. Drugs Ther., *26*:11, 1984.
6. Shinn, A.F.: Evaluation of Drug Interactions. 1988/89 Ed. Washington, DC, American Pharmaceutical Association, 1988.
7. Hansen, P.D.: Drug Interactions. Decision Support Tables. Spokane, WA, Applied Therapeutics Inc., 1987.
8. Hansen, P.D. and Horn, J. R.: Drug Interactions. 6th Ed. Philadelphia, Lea & Febiger, 1989.
9. Koch-Weser, J., and Greenblatt, D.J.: Drug interactions in clinical perspective. Eur. J. Clin. Pharmacol., *11*:405, 1977.
10. Smith, J.W., Seidl, L.G., and Cluff, L.E.: Studies on the epidemiology of adverse drug reactions. V. Clinical factors influencing susceptibility. Ann. Intern. Med., *65*:629, 1966.
11. May, F.E., Stewart, R.B., and Cluff, L.E.: Drug interactions and multiple drug administration. Clin. Pharmacol. Ther., *22*:323, 1977.
12. Kunin, C.M., and Finland, M.: Clinical pharmacology of the tetracycline antibiotics. Clin. Pharmacol. Ther., *2*:51, 1961.
13. Neuvonen, P.J., et al.: Interference of iron with absorption of tetracyclines in man. Br. Med. J., *1*:532, 1970.
14. Gothoni, G., et al.: Iron-tetracycline interactions: Effect of time interval between the drugs. Acta Med. Scand., *191*:409, 1972.
15. Galeazzi, R.L.: The effect of an antacid on the bioavailability of indomethacin. Eur. J. Clin. Pharmacol., *12*:65, 1977.
16. Naggar, V.F., and Khalil, S.A.: Effect of magnesium trisilicate on nitrofurantoin absorption. Clin. Pharmacol. Ther., *25*:857, 1979.
17. Verbeeck, R., et al.: Effect of aluminum hydroxide on diflusinal absorption. Br. J. Clin. Pharmacol., *7*:519, 1979.
18. Spencer, H., et al.: Effect of aluminum hydroxide on fluoride metabolism. Clin. Pharmacol. Ther., *28*:529, 1980.
19. Carter, B.L., et al.: Effects of antacids on phenytoin bioavailability. Ther. Drug. Monit., *3*:333, 1981.
20. Gugler, R., Brand, M., and Somogyi, A.: Impaired cimetidine absorption due to antacids and metoclopramide. Eur. J. Clin. Pharmacol., *20*:225, 1980.
21. Smart, H.L., et al.: The effects of sucralfate upon phenytoin absorption in man. Br. J. Clin. Pharmacol., *20*:238, 1985.
22. Parpia, S.H., et al.: Sucralfate reduces the gastrointestinal absorption of norfloxacin. Antimicrob. Agents Chemother., *33*:99, 1989.
23. Wagner, J.G.: Biopharmaceutics: Absorption aspects. J. Pharm. Sci., *50*:539, 1961.
24. Sorby, D.L., and Liu, G.: Effects of adsorbents on drug absorption. II. Effect of an antidiarrhea mixture in promazine absorption. J. Pharm. Sci., *55*:504, 1966.
25. Brown, D.B., and Juhl, R.P.: Decreased bioavailability of digoxin due to antacids and kaolin-pectin. N. Engl. J. Med., *295*:1034, 1976.
26. Albert, K.S., et al.: Decreased tetracycline bioavailability caused by a bismuth subsalicylate antidiarrheal mixture. J. Pharm. Sci., *68*:586, 1979.
27. Ericsson, C.D., et al.: Influence of subsalicylate bismuth on absorption of doxycycline. JAMA, *247*:2266, 1982.
28. Robinson, D.S., Benjamin, D.M., and McCormack, J.J.: Interaction of warfarin and nonsystemic gastrointestinal drugs. Clin. Pharmacol. Ther., *12*:491, 1971.
29. Northcutt, R.C., et al.: The influence of cholestyramine on thyroxine absorption. JAMA, *208*:1857, 1969.
30. Brown, D.D., et al.: A steady-state evaluation of the effects of propantheline bromide and cholestyramine on the bioavailability of digoxin when administered as tablets or capsules. J. Clin. Pharmacol., *25*:360, 1985.
31. Morgan, J.P., et al.: Imipramine-medicated interference with levodopa absorption from the gastrointestinal tract in man. Neurology, *25*:1029, 1975.
32. Algeri, S., et al.: Effect of anticholinergic drugs on gastrointestinal absorption of L-dopa in rats and in man. Eur. J. Clin. Pharmacol., *35*:293, 1976.
33. Lindenbaum, J., et al.: Inactivation of digoxin by the gut flora; Reversal by antibiotic therapy. N. Engl. J. Med., *305*:789, 1981.
34. Lindenbaum, J., Maulitz, R.M., and Butler, V.P., Jr.: Inhibition of digoxin absorption by neomycin. Gastroenterology, *71*:399, 1976.
35. Juhl, R.P., et al.: Effect of sulfasalazine on digoxin bioavailability. Clin. Pharmacol. Ther., *20*:387, 1976.
36. Riegelman, S., Rowland, M., and Epstein, W.L.: Griseofulvin-phenobarbital interaction in man. JAMA, *213*:426, 1970.
37. Aggeler, P.M., and O'Reilly, R.A.: Effect of heptabar-

bital on the response to bishydroxycoumarin in man. J. Lab. Clin. Med., *74*:229, 1969.

38. Gibaldi, M., and Grundhofer, B.: Biopharmaceutical influences on the anticholinergic effects of propantheline. Clin. Pharmacol. Ther., *18*:457, 1975.

39. McCall, C.E., Steigbigel, N.H., and Finland, M.: Lincomycin: Activity in vitro and absorption and excretion in normal young men. Am. J. Med. Sci., *254*:144, 1967.

40. Singhvi, S.M., et al.: Effect of food on the bioavailability of captopril in healthy subjects. J. Clin. Pharmacol., *22*:135, 1982.

41. Johnson, P.C., Braun, G.A., and Cressman, W.A.: Nonfasting state and the absorption of a hypnotic. Arch. Intern. Med., *131*:199, 1973.

42. Shepherd, A.M.M., Irvine, N.A., and Ludden, T.M.: Effect of food on blood hydralazine levels and response in hypertension. Clin. Pharmacol. Ther., *36*:14, 1984.

43. Hendeles, L., et al.: Food-induced dose-dumping from a once-a-day theophylline product as a cause of theophylline toxicity. Chest, *87*:758, 1985.

44. Pedersen, S., and Moller-Petersen, J.: Erratic absorption of a slow-release theophylline sprinkle product caused by food. Pediatrics, *74*:534, 1984.

45. Jonkman, J.H.G.: Food interactions with sustained-release theophylline preparations. Clin. Pharmacokin., *16*:162, 1989.

46. Mojaverian, P., et al.: Effect of food on the absorption of enteric-coated aspirin: correlation with gastric residence time. Clin. Pharmacol. Ther., *41*:11, 1987.

47. Mojaverian, P., et al.: Effects of gender, posture, and age on gastric residence time of an indigestible solid: pharmaceutical considerations. Pharm. Res., *5*:639, 1988.

48. Sellers, E.M., and Koch-Weser, J.: Displacement of warfarin from human albumin by diazoxide and ethacrynic, mefenamic, and nalidixic acids. Clin. Pharmacol. Ther., *11*:524, 1970.

49. Solomon, H.M., and Schrogie, J.J.: The effect of various drugs on the binding of warfarin-^{14}C to human albumin. Biochem. Pharmacol., *16*:1219, 1967.

50. Solomon, H.M., Schrogie, J.J., and Williams, D.: The displacement of phenylbutazone-^{14}C and warfarin-^{14}C from human albumin by various drugs and fatty acids. Biochem. Pharmacol., *17*:143, 1968.

51. Lunde, P.K.M., et al.: Plasma protein binding of diphenylhydantoin in man. Clin. Pharmacol. Ther., *11*:846, 1970.

52. MacKichan, J.J.: Protein binding drug displacement interactions, fact or fiction? Clin. Pharmacokin., *16*:65, 1989.

53. Friel, P.N., Leal, K.W., and Wilensky, A.J.: Valproic acid-phenytoin interactions. Ther. Drug. Monit., *1*:243, 1979.

54. Frigo, G.M., et al.: Modification of phenytoin clearance by valproic acid in normal subjects. Br. J. Clin. Pharmacol., *8*:553, 1979.

55. Perucca, E., et al.: Interaction between phenytoin and valproic acid: Plasma protein binding and metabolic effects. Clin. Pharmacol. Ther., *28*:779, 1980.

56. Sansom, L.N., Beran, R.C., and Schapel, G.J.: Interaction between phenytoin and valproate. Med. J. Aust., *2*:212, 1980.

57. Day, R.O., et al.: The effect of concurrent aspirin upon plasma concentrations of tenoxicam. Br. J. Clin. Pharmacol., *26*:455, 1988.

58. Sellers, E.M., and Koch-Weser, J.: Potentiation of warfarin-induced hypoprothrombinemia by chloral hydrate. N. Engl. J. Med., *283*:827, 1970.

59. Sellers, E.M., Lang, M., and Koch-Weser, J.: Enhance-

ment of warfarin-induced hypoprothrombinemia by triclofos. Clin. Pharmacol. Ther., *13*:911, 1972.

60. Boston Collaborative Drug Surveillance Program. Interaction between chloral hydrate and warfarin. N. Engl. J. Med., *286*:53, 1972.

61. Gibaldi, M., Grundhofer, B., and Levy, G.: Effect of antacids on pH of urine. Clin. Pharmacol. Ther., *16*:520, 1974.

62. Levy, G., and Leonards, J.R.: Urine pH and salicylate therapy. JAMA, *217*:81, 1971.

63. Levy, G., et al.: Decreased serum salicylate concentrations in children with rheumatic fever treated with antacid. N. Engl. J. Med., *293*:323, 1975.

64. Anggard, E., et al.: Pharmacokinetic and clinical studies on amphetamine dependent patients. Eur. J. Clin. Pharmacol., *3*:3, 1970.

65. Offerhaus, L.: Drug interactions at excretory mechanisms. Pharmacol. Ther., *15*:69, 1981.

66. Aherne, G.W., et al.: Prolongation and enhancement of serum methotrexate concentrations by probenecid. Br. J. Clin. Pharmacol., *1*:1097, 1978.

67. Stoeckel K., et al.: Effect of probenecid on the elimination and protein binding of ceftriaxone. Eur. J. Clin. Pharmacol., *34*:151, 1988.

68. Somogyi, A., McLean, A., and Heinzow, B.: Cimetidine-procainamide pharmacokinetic interaction in man: evidence of competition for tubular secretion of basic drugs. Eur. J. Clin. Pharmacol., *25*:339, 1983.

69. van Crugten J., et al.: Selectivity of the cimetidine-induced alterations in the renal handling of organic substrates in humans. Studies with anionic, cationic and zwitterionic drugs. J. Pharmacol. Exp. Ther., *236*:481, 1986.

70. Frölich, J.C., et al.: Indomethacin increases plasma lithium. Br. Med. J., *1*:1115, 1979.

71. Reimann, I.W., and Frolich, J.C.: Effects of diclofenac on lithium kinetics. Clin. Pharmacol. Ther., *30*:348, 1981.

72. McGiff, J.C.: Interactions of nonsteroidal anti-inflammatory drugs and antihypertensives. JAMA, *260*:850, 1988.

73. Thyss, A., et al.: Clinical and pharmacokinetic evidence of a life-threatening interaction between methotrexate and ketoprofen. Lancet, *1*:256, 1986.

74. Tilstone, W.J., et al.: Effects of furosemide on glomerular filtration rate and clearance of practolol, digoxin, cephaloridine, and gentamicin. Clin. Pharmacol. Ther., *22*:389, 1977.

75. Ejvinsson, G.: Effect of quinidine on plasma concentrations of digoxin. Br. Med. J., *1*:279, 1978.

76. Leahey, E.B., Jr., et al.: Interaction between quinidine and digoxin. JAMA, *240*:533, 1978.

77. Doering, W.: Quinidine-digoxin interaction. Pharmacokinetics, underlying mechanism and clinical implications. N. Engl. J. Med., *301*:400, 1979.

78. Doherty, J.E.: The digoxin-quinidine interaction. Annu. Rev. Med., *33*:163, 1982.

79. Hager, W.D., et al.: Digoxin-quinidine interaction. Pharmacokinetic evaluation. N. Engl. J. Med., *300*:1238, 1979.

80. Schenck-Gustafsson, K., and Dahlquist, R.: Pharmacokinetics of digoxin in patients subjected to the quinidine-digoxin interaction. Br. J. Clin. Pharmacol., *11*:181, 1981.

81. Mungall, D.R., et al.: Effects of quinidine on serum digoxin concentration. A prospective study. Ann. Intern. Med., *93*:689, 1980.

82. Leahey, E.B., et al.: Quinidine-digoxin interaction: Time course and pharmacokinetics. Am. J. Cardiol., *48*:1141, 1981.

83. Fenster, P., et al.: Digoxin-quinidine interaction in patients with chronic renal failure. Circulation, 66:1277, 1982.

84. Chapron, D.J., Mumford, D., and Pitegoff, G.I.: Apparent quinidine-induced digoxin toxicity after withdrawal of pentobarbital. Arch. Intern. Med., 139:363, 1979.

85. Schenck-Gustafsson, K., et al.: Effect of quinidine on digoxin concentration in skeletal muscle and serum in patients with atrial fibrillation. N. Engl. J. Med., 305:209, 1981.

86. Das, G., Barr, C.E., and Carlson, J.: Reduction of digoxin effect during the digoxin-quinidine interaction. Clin. Pharmacol. Ther., 35:317, 1984.

87. Walker, A.M., et al.: Drug toxicity in patients receiving digoxin and quinidine. Am. Heart J., 105:1025, 1983.

88. Warner, N.J., et al.: Myocardial monovalent cation transport during the quinidine-digoxin interaction in dogs. Circ. Res., 54:453, 1984.

89. Leahey, E.B., et al.: The effect of quinidine and other oral antiarrhythmic drugs on serum digoxin. Ann. Intern. Med., 92:605, 1980.

90. Pedersen, K.E., et al.: Digoxin-verapamil interaction. Clin. Pharmacol. Ther., 30:311, 1981.

91. Moysey, J.O., et al.: Amiodarone increases plasma digoxin concentrations. Br. Med. J., 282:272, 1981.

92. Cogan, J.J., et al.: Acute vasodilator therapy increases renal clearance of digoxin in patients with congestive heart failure. Circulation, 61:973, 1981.

93. Baber, N., et al.: The interaction between indomethacin and probenecid. A clinical and pharmacokinetic study. Clin. Pharmacol. Ther., 24:298, 1978.

94. Meinertz, T., et al.: Interruption of the enterohepatic circulation of phenprocoumon by cholestyramine. Clin. Pharmacol. Ther., 21:731, 1977.

95. Park, B.K., and Breckenridge, A.M.: Clinical implications of enzyme induction and inhibition. Clin. Pharmacokinet., 6:1, 1981.

96. Perucca, E.: Pharmacokinetic interactions with antiepileptic drugs. Clin. Pharmacokinet., 7:57, 1982.

97. Sotaniemi, E.A., et al.: Drug metabolism in epileptics: in vivo and in vitro correlations. Br. J. Clin. Pharmacol., 5:71, 1978.

98. Patsalos, P.N., Duncan, J.S., and Shorvon, S.D.: Effect of removal of individual antiepileptic drugs on antipyrine kinetics, in patients taking polytherapy. Br. J. Clin. Pharmacol., 26:253, 1988.

99. Chiba, K., et al.: Comparison of steady-state pharmacokinetics of valproic acid in children between monotherapy and multiple antiepileptic drug treatment. J. Pediatrics, 106:653, 1985.

100. Data, J.L., Wilkinson, G.R., and Nies, A.S.: Interaction of quinidine with anticonvulsant drugs. N. Engl. J. Med., 294:699, 1976.

101. Dhillon, S., and Richens, A.: Pharmacokinetics of diazepam in epileptic patients and normal volunteers following intravenous administration. Br. J. Clin. Pharmacol., 12:841, 1981.

102. Mattson, R.H., et al.: Use of oral contraceptives by women with epilepsy. JAMA, 256:238, 1986.

103. Capewell, S., et al.: Reduced felodipine bioavailability in patients taking anticonvulsants. Lancet, 2:480, 1988.

104. Khoo, K., et al.: Influence of phenytoin and phenobarbital on the disposition of a single oral dose of clonazepam. Clin. Pharmacol. Ther., 28:368, 1980.

105. Reynolds, E.H., et al.: Interaction of phenytoin and primidone. Br. Med. J., 2:594, 1975.

106. Porro, M.G., et al.: Phenytoin: An inhibitor and inducer of primidone metabolism in an epileptic patient. Br. J. Clin. Pharmacol., 14:294, 1982.

107. Petereit, L.B., and Meikle, A.W.: Effectiveness of prednisolone during phenytoin therapy. Clin. Pharmacol. Ther., 22:912, 1977.

108. Pond, S.M., and Kretschzmar, K.M.: Effect of phenytoin on meperidine clearance and normeperidine formation. Clin. Pharmacol. Ther., 30:680, 1981.

109. Marquis, J.F., et al.: Phenytoin-theophylline interaction. N. Engl. J. Med., 307:1189, 1982.

110. Breckenridge, A.M., and Orme, M.L'E.: Clinical implications of enzyme induction. Ann. NY Acad. Sci., 179:421, 1971.

111. Goss, J.E., and Dickhaus, D.W.: Increased bishydroxycoumarin requirements in patients receiving phenobarbital. N. Engl. J. Med., 273:1094, 1965.

112. Rutledge, D.R., Pieper, J.A., and Mirvis, D.M.: Effects of chronic phenobarbital on verapamil disposition in humans. J. Pharmacol. Exp. Ther., 246:7, 1988.

113. Hempel, E., et al.: Medikamentose enzymindaktion und hormonale kontrazeption. Zentralbl. Gynaekol., 95:1451, 1973.

114. Hempel, E., and Klinger, W.: Drug stimulated biotransformation of hormonal steroid contraceptives: Clinical implications. Drugs, 12:442, 1976.

115. Yaffe, S.J., et al.: Enhancement of glucuronide-conjugating capacity in hyperbilirubinemic infants due to apparent enzyme induction by phenobarbital. N. Engl. J. Med., 275:1461, 1966.

116. Maurier, H.M., et al.: Reduction in concentration of total serum bilirubin in offspring of women treated with phenobarbitone during pregnancy. Lancet, 2:122, 1968.

117. Udall, J.A.: Clinical implications of warfarin interactions with five sedatives. Am. J. Cardiol., 35:67, 1975.

118. Alván, G., et al.: Effect of pentobarbital on the disposition of alprenolol. Clin. Pharmacol. Ther., 22:316, 1977.

119. Lai, A.A., Levy, R.H., and Cutler, R.E.: Time course of interaction between carbamazepine and clonazepam in normal man. Clin. Pharmacol. Ther., 24:316, 1978.

120. Bertilsson, L., and Tomson, T.: Clinical pharmacokinetics and pharmacological effects of carbamazepine and carbamazepine-10,11-epoxide. An update. Clin. Pharmacokin., 11:177, 1986.

121. Moore, M.J., et al.: Rapid development of enhanced clearance after high-dose cyclophosphamide. Clin. Pharmacol. Ther., 44:622, 1988.

122. Zilly, W., Breimer, D.D., and Richter, E.: Pharmacokinetic interactions with rifampin. Clin. Pharmacokinet., 2:61, 1977.

123. O'Reilly, R.A.: Interaction of chronic daily warfarin therapy and rifampin. Ann. Intern. Med., 83:506, 1975.

124. Back, D.J., et al.: The effect of rifampicin on norethisterone pharmacokinetics. Eur. J. Clin. Pharmacol., 15:193, 1979.

125. Buffington, G.A., et al.: Interaction of rifampin and glucocorticoids. Adverse effect on renal allograft function. JAMA, 236:1958, 1976.

126. Breimer, D.D., Zilly, W., and Richter, E.: Influence of rifampicin on drug metabolism: Differences between hexobarbital and antipyrine. Clin. Pharmacol. Ther., 21:470, 1977.

127. Ochs, H.R., et al.: Diazepam interaction with antituberculosis drugs. Clin. Pharmacol. Ther., 29:671, 1981.

128. Bennett, P.N., John, V.A., and Whitmarsh, V.B.: Effect of rifampicin on metoprolol and antipyrine kinetics. Br. J. Clin. Pharmacol., 13:387, 1982.

129. Twum-Barima, Y., and Carruthers, S.G.: Quinidine-rifampin interaction. N. Engl. J. Med., 304:1466, 1981.

130. Kay, L., et al.: Influence of rifampicin and isoniazid on the kinetics of phenytoin. Br. J. Clin. Pharmacol., 20:323, 1985.

131. Shaffer, J.L., and Houston, J.B.: The effect of rifampin on sulphapyridine plasma concentrations following sulphasalazine administration. Br. J. Clin. Pharmacol., *19*:526, 1985.

132. Prober, C.G.: Effect of rifampin on chloramphenicol levels. N. Engl. J. Med., *312*:788, 1985.

133. Pessayre, D., et al.: Isoniazid-rifampin fulminant hepatitis. A possible consequence of the enhancement of isoniazid hepatotoxicity by enzyme induction. Gastroenterology, *72*:284, 1977.

134. Somogyi, A., and Muirhead, M.: Pharmacokinetic interactions of cimetidine 1987. Clin. Pharmacokin., *12*:321, 1987.

135. Christensen, L.K., and Skovsted, L.: Inhibition of drug metabolism by chloramphenicol. Lancet, 2:1397, 1969.

136. Ballek, R.E., Reidenberg, M.M., and Orr, L.: Inhibition of diphenylhydantoin metabolism by chloramphenicol. Lancet, *1*:150, 1973.

137. Rose, J.Q., et al.: Intoxication caused by interaction of chloramphenicol and phenytoin. JAMA, *237*:2630, 1977.

138. Vesell, E.S., Passananti, G.T., and Lee, C.H.: Impairment of drug metabolism by disulfiram in man. Clin. Pharmacol. Ther., *12*:785, 1971.

139. O'Reilly, R.A.: Interaction of disulfiram (Antabuse) in man. Ann. Intern. Med., *78*:73, 1973.

140. Svendsen, T.L., et al.: The influence of disulfiram on the half-life and metabolic clearance rate of diphenylhydantoin and tolbutamide in man. Eur. J. Clin. Pharmacol., *9*:439, 1976.

141. MacLeod, S.M., et al.: Interaction of disulfiram with benzodiazepines. Clin. Pharmacol. Ther., *24*:583, 1978.

142. Zimm, Z., et al.: Inhibition of first-pass metabolism in cancer chemotherapy: interaction of 6-mercaptopurine and allopurinol. Clin. Pharmacol. Ther., *34*:810, 1983.

143. Vesell, E.S., Passananti, G.T., and Greene, F.E.: Impairment of drug metabolism in man by allopurinol and nortriptyline. N. Engl. J. Med., *283*:1484, 1970.

144. Janhnchen, E., Meinertz, T., and Gilfrich, N.J.: Interaction of allopurinol with phenprocoumon in man. Klin. Wochenschr., *55*:759, 1977.

145. Manfredi, R.L., and Vessell, E.S.: Inhibition of theophylline metabolism by long-term allopurinol administration. Clin. Pharmacol. Ther., *29*:224, 1981.

146. Lewis, R.J., et al.: Warfarin. Stereochemical aspects of its metabolism and the interaction with phenylbutazone. J. Clin. Invest., *53*:1607, 1974.

147. Schary, W.L., Lewis, R.J., and Rowland, M.: Warfarin-phenylbutazone interaction in man: A long term multiple dose study. Res. Commun. Chem. Pathol. Pharmacol., *10*:663, 1975.

148. Pedersen, A.K., et al.: Clinical pharmacokinetics and potentially important drug interactions of sulphinpyrazone. Clin. Pharmacokinet., *7*:42, 1982.

149. Toon, S., et al.: The warfarin-sulfinpyrazone interaction: stereochemical considerations. Clin. Pharmacol. Ther., *39*:15, 1986.

150. Heimark, L.K., et al.: The effect of sulfinpyrazone on the disposition of pseudoracemic phenprocoumon in humans. Clin. Pharmacol. Ther., *42*:312, 1987.

151. Rowland, M., and Matin, S.B.: Kinetics of drug-drug interactions. J. Pharmacokinet. Biopharm., *1*:553, 1973.

152. Lumholtz, B., et al.: Sulfamethizole-induced inhibition of diphenylhydantoin, tolbutamide, and warfarin metabolism. Clin. Pharmacol. Ther., *17*:731, 1975.

153. O'Reilly, R.A.: Stereoselective interaction of trimethoprim-sulfamethoxazole with the separated enantiomorphs of racemic warfarin in man. N. Engl. J. Med., *302*:33, 1980.

154. O'Reilly, R.A.: The stereoselective interaction of warfarin and metronidazole in man. N. Engl. J. Med., *295*:354, 1976.

155. Kutt, H., et al.: Diphenylhydantoin intoxication: a complication of isoniazid therapy. Am. Rev. Respir. Dis., *101*:377, 1970.

156. Brennan, R.W., et al.: Diphenylhydantoin intoxication attendant to slow inactivation of isoniazid. Neurology, *20*:687, 1970.

157. Miller, R.R., Porter, J., and Greenblatt, D.J.: Clinical importance of the interaction of phenytoin and isoniazid. A report from the Boston Collaborative Surveillance Program. Chest, *75*:356, 1979.

158. Valsalan, V.C., and Cooper, G.L.; Carbamazepine intoxication caused by interaction with isoniazid. Br. Med. J., *285*:261, 1982.

159. Wright, J.M., Stokes, E.F., and Sweeney, V.P.: Isoniazid-induced carbamazepine toxicity and vice versa. A double drug interaction. N. Engl. J. Med., *307*:1325, 1982.

160. Vestal, R.E., et al.: Inhibition of propranolol metabolism by chlorpromazine. Clin. Pharmacol. Ther., *25*:19, 1979.

161. Vincent, F.M.: Phenothiazine-induced phenytoin intoxication. Ann. Intern. Med., *93*:56, 1980.

162. Nelson, J.C., and Jatlow, P.I.: Neuroleptic effect on desipramine steady-state plasma concentrations. Am. J. Psychiatry, *137*:1232, 1980.

163. Siris, S.G., et al.: Plasma imipramine concentrations in patients receiving concomitant fluphenazine decanoate. Am. J. Psychiatry, *139*:104, 1982.

164. Greenblatt, D.J., Franke, K., and Huffman, D.H.: Impairment of antipyrine clearance in humans by propranolol. Circulation, *57*:1161, 1978.

165. Bax, N.D.S., Lennard, M.S., and Tucker, G.T.: Inhibition of antipyrine metabolism by β-adrenoceptor antagonists. Br. J. Clin. Pharmacol., *12*:779, 1981.

166. Deacon, C.S., et al.: Inhibition of oxidative drug metabolism by β-adrenoceptor antagonists is related to their lipid solubility. Br. J. Clin. Pharmacol., *12*:429, 1981.

167. Bax, N.D.S., et al.: The impairment of lignocaine clearance by propranolol—major contribution from enzyme inhibition. Br. J. Clin. Pharmacol., *19*:597, 1985.

168. Bowdle, T.A., Freund, P.R., and Slattery J.T.: Propranolol reduces bupivicaine clearance. Anesthesiol., *66*:36, 1987.

169. Miners, J.O., et al.: Selectivity and dose-dependency of the inhibitory effect of propranolol on theophylline metabolism in man. Br. J. Clin. Pharmacol., *20*:219, 1985.

170. Abernethy, D.R., and Greenblatt, D.J.: Impairment of antipyrine metabolism by low-dose oral contraceptive steroids. Clin. Pharmacol. Ther., *29*:106, 1981.

171. Field, B., Lu, C., and Hepner, G.W.: Inhibition of hepatic drug metabolism by norethindrone. Clin. Pharmacol. Ther., *25*:196, 1979.

172. Kendall, M.J., et al.: Metoprolol pharmacokinetics and the oral contraceptive pill. Br. J. Clin. Pharmacol., *14*:120, 1982.

173. Abernethy, D.R., et al.: Impairment of diazepam metabolism by low-dose estrogen-containing oral-contraceptive steroids. N. Engl. J. Med., *306*:791, 1982.

174. Legler, U.F., and Benet, L.Z.: Marked alterations in dose-dependent prednisolone kinetics in women taking oral contraceptives. Clin. Pharmacol. Ther., *39*:425, 1986.

175. Wilder, B.J., et al.: Valproic acid: Interaction with other anticonvulsant drugs. Neurology, *28*:892, 1978.

176. Patel, I.H., Levy, R.H., and Cutler, R.E.: Phenobarbital-valproic acid interaction. Clin. Pharmacol. Ther., *27*:515, 1980.

177. Mattson, R.H., and Cramer, J.A.: Valproic acid and etho-suximide interaction. Ann. Neurol., 7:583, 1980.

178. Kerr, B.M., and Levy, R.H.: Inhibition of epoxide hydrolase by anticonvulsants and risk of teratogenicity. Lancet, 1:610, 1989.

179. Kerr, B.M., et al.: Inhibition of human liver microsomal epoxide hydrolase by valproate and valpromide: in vitro/in vivo correlation. Clin. Pharmacol. Ther., 46:82, 1989.

180. Somogyi, A., and Gugler, R.: Drug interactions with cimetidine. Clin. Pharmacokinet., 7:23, 1982.

181. Serlin, M.J., et al.: Cimetidine interactions with oral anticoagulants in man. Lancet, 2:317, 1979.

182. Klotz, U., and Reimann, I.: Elevation of steady-state diazepam levels by cimetidine. Clin. Pharmacol. Ther., 30:513, 1981.

183. Reitberg, D.P., Bernhard, H., and Schentag, J.J.: Alteration of theophylline clearance and half-life by cimetidine. Ann. Intern. Med., 95:582, 1981.

184. Neuvonen, P.J., Tokola, R.A., and Kaste, M.: Cimetidine-phenytoin interaction: Effect on serum phenytoin concentration and antipyrine test. Eur. J. Clin. Pharmacol., 21:215, 1981.

185. Hetzel, D.J., et al.: Cimetidine interaction with phenytoin. Br. J. Clin. Pharmacol., 282:1512, 1981.

186. Hardy, B.G., et al.: Effect of cimetidine on the pharmacokinetics and pharmacodynamics of quinidine. Am. J. Cardiol., 52:172, 1983.

187. Knapp, A.B., et al.: The cimetidine-lidocaine interaction. Ann. Intern. Med., 98:174, 1983.

188. Abernethy, D.R., et al.: Differential effect of cimetidine on drug oxidation (antipyrine and diazepam) vs conjugation (acetaminophen and lorazepam): prevention of acetaminophen toxicity by cimetidine. J. Pharmacol. Exp. Ther., 224:508, 1983.

189. Schwartz, J.B., et al.: Effect of cimetidine or ranitidine administration on nifedipine pharmacokinetics and pharmacodynamics. Clin. Pharmacol. Ther., 43:673, 1988.

190. Sambol, N.C., et al.: A comparison of the influence of famotidine and cimetidine on phenytoin elimination and hepatic blood flow. Br. J. Clin. Pharmacol., 27:83, 1989.

191. Galbraith, R.A., and Michnovicz, J.J.: The effects of cimetidine on the oxidative metabolism of estradiol. N. Engl. J. Med., 321:269, 1989.

192. Rameis, H., Magometschnigg, D., and Ganzinger, U.: The diltiazem-digoxin interaction. Clin. Pharmacol. Ther., 36:183, 1984.

193. Pedersen, K.E., et al.: Digoxin-verapamil interaction. Clin. Pharmacol. Ther., 30:311, 1981.

194. Bauer, L.A., et al.: Changes in antipyrine and indocyanine green kinetics during nifedipine, verapamil, and diltiazem therapy. Clin. Pharmacol. Ther., 40:239, 1986.

195. Nafziger, A.N., May, J.J., and Bertino, J.S., Jr.: Inhibition of theophylline elimination by diltiazem therapy. J. Clin. Pharmacol., 27:862, 1987.

196. Macphee, G.J.A., et al.: Verapamil potentiates carbamazepine neurotoxicity: a clinically important inhibitory interaction. Lancet, 1:700, 1986.

197. Brodie, M.J., and Macphee, G.J.A.: Carbamazepine neurotoxicity precipitated by diltiazem. Br. Med. J., 292:1170, 1986.

198. Edwards, D.J., et al.: Inhibition of drug metabolism by quinolone antibiotics. Clin. Pharmacokin., 15:194, 1988.

199. Beckman, J., et al.: Enoxacin—a potent inhibitor of theophylline metabolism. Eur. J. Clin. Pharmacol., 33:227, 1987.

200. Wijnands, W.J.A., Vree, T.B., and van Herwaarden, C.L.A.: The influence of quinolone derivatives on theophylline clearance. Br. J. Clin. Pharmacol., 22:687, 1986.

201. Schwartz, J., et al.: Impact of ciprofloxacin on theophylline clearance and steady-state concentrations in serum. Antimicrob. Agents Chemother., 32:75, 1988.

202. Ho, G., Tierney, M.G., and Dales, R.E.: Evaluation of the effect of norfloxacin on the pharmacokinetics of theophylline. Clin. Pharmacol. Ther., 44:35, 1988.

203. Toon, S., et al.: Enoxacin-warfarin interaction: pharmacokinetic and stereochemical aspects. Clin. Pharmacol. Ther., 42:33, 1987.

204. Pond, S.M., et al.: Massive intoxication with acetaminophen and propoxyphene: unexpected survival and unusual pharmacokinetics of acetaminophen. J. Toxicol. Clin. Toxicol., 19:1, 1982.

205. Abernethy, D.R., et al.: Impairment of hepatic drug oxidation by propoxyphene. Ann. Intern. Med., 97:223, 1982.

206. Abernethy, D.R., et al.: Interaction of propoxyphene with diazepam, alprazolam and lorazepam. Br. J. Clin. Pharmacol., 19:51, 1985.

207. Shinn, A.F., and Shrewsbury, R.P.: Evaluation of Drug Interactions, 3rd ed, St. Louis, C.V. Mosby Co., 1985.

208. Wroblewski, B.A., Singer, W.D., and Whyte, J.: Carbamazepine-erythromycin interaction. Case studies and clinical significance. JAMA, 255:1165, 1986.

209. Ptachcinski, R.J., et al.: Effect of erythromycin on cyclosporine levels. N. Engl. J. Med., 313:1416, 1985.

210. Brown, M.W., et al.: Effect of ketoconazole on hepatic oxidative drug metabolism. Clin. Pharmacol. Ther., 37:297, 1985.

211. Mays, D.C., et al.: Methoxsalen is a potent inhibitor of the metabolism of caffeine. Clin. Pharmacol. Ther., 42:621, 1987.

212. Gugler, R., and Jensen, J.C.: Drugs other than H_2-receptor antagonists as clinically important inhibitors of drug metabolism in vivo. Pharmacol. Ther., 33:133, 1987.

213. Kates, R.E., Yee, Y.-G., and Kirsten, E.: Interaction between warfarin and propafenone in healthy volunteer subjects. Clin. Pharmacol. Ther., 42:305, 1987.

214. Wagner, F., et al.: Drug interaction between propafenone and metoprol. Br. J. Clin. Pharmacol., 24:213, 1987.

215. Tenni P., Lalich, D.L., and Byrne, M.J.: Life threatening interaction between tamoxifen and warfarin. Br. Med. J., 298:93, 1989.

216. Ochs, H.R., Carstens, G., and Greenblatt, D.J.: Reduction in lidocaine clearance during continuous infusion and by coadministration of propranolol. N. Engl. J. Med., 303:373, 1980.

217. Feely, J., Wilkinson, G.R., and Wood, A.J.J.: Reduction of liver blood flow and propranolol metabolism by cimetidine. N. Engl. J. Med., 304:692, 1981.

218. Reimann, I.W., Klotz, U., and Frolich, F.C.: Cimetidine increases propranolol steady-state plasma levels in man (abstr.). Eighth International Congress of Pharmacology, Tokyo, 1981.

219. Feely, J., et al.: Increased toxicity and reduced clearance of lidocaine by cimetidine. Ann. Intern. Med., 96:592, 1982.

220. Ontrot, J., et al.: Reduction of liver plasma flow by caffeine and theophylline. Clin. Pharmacol. Ther., 40:506, 1986.

221. McLean, A.J., et al.: Food, splanchnic blood flow, and bioavailability of drugs subject to first-pass metabolism. Clin. Pharmacol. Ther., 24:5, 1978.

222. Melander, A., et al.: Enhancement of the bioavailability of propranolol and metoprolol by food. Clin. Pharmacol. Ther., 22:108, 1977.

223. McLean, A.J., et al.: Interaction between oral propranolol and hydralazine. Clin. Pharmacol. Ther., 27:726, 1980.

224. Schneck, D.W., and Vary, J.E.: Mechanism by which

hydralazine increases propranolol bioavailability. Clin. Pharmacol. Ther., *35*:447, 1984.

225. Lindeberg, S., et al.: The effect of hydralazine on steady-state plasma concentrations of metoprolol in pregnant hypertensive women. Eur. J. Clin. Pharmacol., *35*:131, 1988.

226. Toon, S., et al.: Comparative effects of ranitidine and cimetidine on the pharmacokinetics and pharmacodynamics of warfarin in man. Eur. J. Clin. Pharmacol., *32*:165, 1987.

227. Toon, S., et al.: The racemic metoprolol H₂-antagonist interaction. Clin. Pharmacol. Ther., *43*:283, 1988.

228. Speirs, C.J., et al.: Quinidine and the identification of drugs whose elimination is impaired in subjects classified as poor metabolizers of debrisoquine. Br. J. Clin. Pharmacol., *22*:739, 1986.

229. Brinn, R., et al.: Sparteine oxidation is practically abolished in quinidine-treated patients. Br. J. Clin. Pharmacol., *22*:194, 1986.

230. Gibaldi, M.: Drug interactions—a probe to identify drug metabolism pathways controlled by the debrisoquine phenotype. Perspect. Clin. Pharmacol., *7*:89, 1989

231. Rubin, E., et al.: Inhibition of drug metabolism by acute ethanol intoxication: A hepatic microsomal mechanism. Am. J. Med., *49*:801, 1970.

232. Desmond, P.V., et al.: Short-term ethanol administration impairs the elimination of chlordiazepoxide (Librium) in man. Eur. J. Clin. Pharmacol., *18*:275, 1980.

233. Misra, P.S., et al.: Increase of ethanol, meprobamate and pentobarbital metabolism after chronic ethanol administration in man and rats. Am. J. Med., *51*:346, 1971.

234. Miller, R.R.: Effects of smoking on drug action. Clin. Pharmacol. Ther., *22*:749, 1977.

235. Jusko, W.J.: Role of tobacco smoking in pharmacokinetics. J. Pharmacokinet. Biopharm., *6*:7, 1978.

236. Dawson, G.W., and Vestal, R.E.: Smoking and drug metabolism. Pharmacol. Ther., *15*:207, 1982.

237. Boston Collaborative Drug Surveillance Program: Decreased clinical efficacy of propoxyphene in cigarette smokers. Clin. Pharmacol. Ther., *14*:259, 1973.

238. Vaughan, D.P., Beckett, A.H., and Robbie, D.S.: The influence of smoking on the intersubject variation in pentazocine elimination. Br. J. Clin. Pharmacol., *3*:279, 1976.

239. Pantuck, E.J., Kuntzman, R., and Conney, A.H.: Decreased concentration of phenacetin in plasma. Science, *175*:1248, 1972.

240. Jenne, J., et al.: Decreased theophylline half-life in cigarette smokers. Life Sci., *17*:195, 1975.

241. Hunt, S.N., Jusko, W.J., and Yurchak, A.M.: Effect of smoking on theophylline disposition. Clin. Pharmacol. Ther., *19*:546, 1976.

242. Pfeifer, H.J., and Greenblatt, D.V.: Clinical toxicity of theophylline in relation to cigarette smoking. Chest, *73*:455, 1978.

243. Vestal, R.E., et al.: Aging and drug interactions I. Effect of cimetidine and smoking on the oxidation of theo-

phylline and cortisol in healthy men. J. Pharmacol. Exp. Ther., *241*:488, 1987.

244. Crowley, J.J., et al.: Aging and drug interactions II. Effect of phenytoin and smoking on the oxidation of theophylline and cortisol in healthy men. J. Pharmacol. Exp. Ther., *245*:513, 1988.

245. Crowley, J.J., et al.: Cigarette smoking and theophylline metabolism: effects of phenytoin. Clin. Pharmacol. Ther., *42*:334, 1987.

246. Lee, B.L., Benowitz, N.L., and Jacob, P., III: Cigarette abstinence, nicotine gum, and theophylline disposition. Ann. Intern. Med., *106*:553, 1987.

247. Brown, C.R., et al.: Changes in rate and pattern of caffeine metabolism after cigarette abstinence. Clin. Pharmacol. Ther., *43*:488, 1988.

248. Benowitz, N.L., Hall, S.M., and Modin, G.: Persistent increase in caffeine concentrations in people who stop smoking. Br. Med. J., *298*:1075, 1989.

249. Michnovicz, J.J., et al.: Increased 2-hydroxylation of estradiol as a possible mechanism for the anti-estrogenic effect of cigarette smoking. N. Engl. J. Med., *315*:1305, 1986.

250. Kappas, A., et al.: Influence of dietary protein and carbohydrate on antipyrine and theophylline metabolism. Clin. Pharmacol. Ther., *20*:643, 1976.

251. Pantuck, E.J., et al.: Stimulatory effect of bussels sprouts and cabbage in human drug metabolism. Clin. Pharmacol. Ther., *25*:88, 1979.

252. Conney, A.H., et al.: Enhanced phenacetin metabolism in human subjects fed charcoal-broiled beef. Clin. Pharmacol. Ther., *20*:633, 1976.

253. Kappas, A., et al.: Effect of charcoal-broiled beef on antipyrine and theophylline metabolism. Clin. Pharmacol. Ther., *23*:445, 1978.

254. Nutt, J.G., et al.: The ''on-off'' phenomenon in Parkinson's disease. Relation to levodopa absorption and transport. N. Engl. J. Med., *310*:483, 1984.

255. Carter, J.H., et al.: Amount and distribution of dietary protein affects clinical response to levodopa in Parkinson's disease. Neurol., *39*:55, 1989.

256. Berlinger, W.G., Park, G.D., and Spector, R.: The effect of dietary protein on the clearance of allopurinol and oxypurinol. N. Engl. J. Med., *313*:771, 1985.

257. Alvares, A.P.: Interactions between environmental chemicals and drug biotransformation in man. Clin. Pharmacokinet., *3*:462, 1978.

258. Kolmodin, B., Azarnoff, D.L., and Sjöqvist, F.: Effect of environmental factors on drug metabolism: Decreased plasma half-life of antipyrine in workers exposed to chlorinated hydrocarbon insecticides. Clin. Pharmacol. Ther., *10*:638, 1969.

259. Kolmodin-Hedman, B.: Decreased plasma half-life of phenylbutazone in workers exposed to chlorinated pesticides. Eur. J. Clin. Pharmacol., *5*:195, 1973.

260. Ghoneim, M.M., et al.: Alteration of warfarin kinetics in man associated with exposure to an operating-room environment. Anesthesiology, *43*:333, 1975.

15

Individualization and Optimization of Drug Dosing Regimens

Drug therapy is so routine that even physicians and pharmacists sometimes take for granted the unusual complexity of the process. The scheme in Figure 15–1 shows some of the steps involved in the initiation and management of drug therapy.[1] The major tasks are defining the therapeutic objective, selecting the drug and its dosage regimen, and evaluating whether or not the objective has been met. Selecting a drug is an exercise in therapeutics, but selecting the dosage regimen is a quantitative task that usually requires an understanding of clinical pharmacokinetics. The evaluation of how well the therapeutic objective has been achieved and the decision to modify the dosage regimen or turn to another drug also requires the knowledge base of clinical pharmacology and clinical pharmacokinetics.

INDIVIDUALIZING DOSAGE REGIMENS

Not so long ago essentially all patients needing a certain drug were prescribed the same dose. Pharmacodynamic and pharmacokinetic variability had no place in the initiation of drug therapy. During 1970 to 1972, Koch-Weser surveyed phenytoin dosages prescribed for seizure prevention to 200 ambulatory patients and found that 92% of the patients received the usual dose of 300 mg/day.[2] This observation is remarkable because phenytoin is the quintessential example of a drug with substantial interpatient variability in clinical response.

Today, a clinician initiating a dosage regimen considers the patient's age, size, disease status, and concomitant drug therapy. It is now common to find higher than usual mg/kg doses of theophylline prescribed for children or smokers and lower than usual dosages prescribed for patients with congestive heart failure (CHF). Dosages of most antibiotics, digoxin, lithium, and other drugs are routinely reduced for patients with impaired renal function. More conservative dosages of hypnotics, antianxiety drugs, and other psychotropic agents are prescribed for the elderly. The information on drug characteristics in different patient populations is now being applied to the individual patient.

OPTIMIZING DOSAGE REGIMENS

Incorporating the patient's characteristics in the process of initiating a drug dosage regimen is an important step toward optimization of drug therapy, but it does not guarantee the success of the therapy. We still need to evaluate the outcome of the treatment and we still find in some cases that the therapeutic objective has not been achieved. There are many reasons for failure, including the need for larger or smaller dosages of the drug. This is not surprising because few schemes to individualize the initial dosage regimen take into account the pharmacokinetics of the drug in the individual patient or the individual's responsiveness to the drug. Individualization of the initial dosing regimen is usually based on population rather than individual data. To the extent that the patient deviates from the population average, his response will deviate from the therapeutic objective.

Traditionally, the management of drug therapy has been accomplished by monitoring the incidence and intensity of both desired therapeutic effects and undesired adverse effects; an inadequate therapeutic response calls for a higher dosage, drug-related toxicity calls for a lower dosage. The patient with

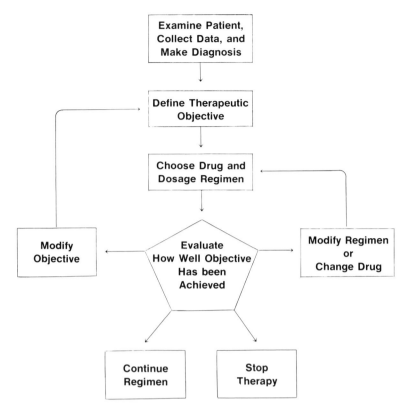

Fig. 15-1. Steps in the initiation and management of drug therapy. (From Rowland, M., and Tozer, T.N.[1])

rheumatoid arthritis who shows inadequate reduction of inflammation and continued pain in response to treatment with a nonsteroidal anti-inflammatory drug and the patient with asthma who experiences insufficient bronchodilation in response to treatment with theophylline probably need higher dosages. But what do we mean by inadequate and insufficient? The words are imprecise because our ability to measure therapeutic outcome is usually imprecise. Individual management of drug dosage regimens based on clinical efficacy requires an inordinate degree of skill and an unreasonable share of the physician's time and attention.

Our ability to measure excessive drug dosage is also limited. At one time we thought that tinnitus during salicylate therapy and nausea during theophylline therapy were harbingers of drug toxicity. The emergence of these signs would permit us to reduce drug dosage before the onset of more serious toxicity. Today, we recognize that some patients do not hear or discern the ringing in the ears characteristic of high serum concentrations of salicylate and can develop life-threatening metabolic acidosis. Fatal theophylline-induced convulsive seizures

have been observed in patients who displayed no signs of nausea.

The problems illustrated by theophylline and salicylate are common; they suggest that traditional management of drug therapy based on clinical outcome can rarely be applied in its purest form. The closest we come to it is in the management of oral anticoagulant, oral antidiabetic, or uricosuric therapy. Although we do not directly assess the therapeutic objectives in these cases, we do substitute and closely monitor a laboratory test (i.e., prothrombin time, urine glucose, or uric acid levels) that is closely related to the objective. There is a continual and intensive search for biochemical correlates of drug effects, but this desirable alternative is available for few drugs.

Titrating a drug dosing regimen to a target concentration range in blood or plasma is yet another strategy. It is not as precise as titrating to a biochemical end point, but when combined with an assessment of clinical outcome it is often superior to clinical evaluation alone.

During the past 30 years, plasma concentrations of drugs have been measured during their therapeutic use. This has been made possible by the development of methods of analysis (e.g., gas chromatography, mass spectrometry, high-pressure liquid chromatography, and radioimmunoassay) that allow determination of low drug concentrations. A review article on this subject offers the following comments:[3]

Measurement of serum levels of a drug become useful guides for dosage adjustments only when the therapeutically effective range of serum concentrations has been defined by careful clinical studies. At present, this has been accomplished for few important drugs. Compared to the large individual variations in the optimal dosages of these drugs, the width of their therapeutic serum concentration ranges is relatively narrow. Concentrations of these drugs below the therapeutic range can exert beneficial effects but are inadequate in most patients. Within the therapeutic range the intensity of the desired effect of the drug increases with its serum concentration. In occasional patients, high therapeutic concentrations may have minor toxic actions. As serum concentrations rise above the therapeutic range, the frequency and severity of toxic effects increase progressively. Some patients can tolerate serum concentrations above the usual therapeutic levels, and a few may even require them for a fully satisfactory response. Thus, some overlap between therapeutic and toxic serum concentrations is the rule, and it is considerable for certain drugs, such as the digitalis glycosides. Whenever concentrations above the usual therapeutic range are produced for therapeutic purposes, patients must be closely monitored for the appearance of serious toxicity.

Evans[4] has pointed out that the idea of a therapeutic range for serum concentrations of drugs is frequently misunderstood. Some assume that the therapeutic range for most drugs has been well-defined from carefully controlled trials and that drug concentrations in the therapeutic range will result in the desired clinical response with no adverse effects. Evans presents a more precise definition of therapeutic range as ''a range of drug concentrations within which the probability of the desired clinical response is relatively high and the probability of unacceptable toxicity is relatively low.''

Drug level determinations cannot substitute for clinical judgment and must always be interpreted in the context of available clinical data. By reducing the number of unknown variables, however, the availability of such data permits the physician to apply his clinical skills to the maximum by focusing more directly on the disease process and on the physiologic status of the patient.

The experience of the past decade with determination of serum drug levels in the clinical setting has been extensive and exciting. New journals have been devoted to therapeutic drug concentration monitoring[5] and clinical pharmacokinetics.[6] Several books on the subject are available.[4,7,8] Many of the reports in the clinical pharmacology and pharmacy literature today are concerned with applications of pharmacokinetics. As is true of many sound concepts, however, therapeutic drug concentration monitoring for optimization of drug therapy must be placed in perspective.

Koch-Weser has pointed out that routine determination of serum concentrations of all drugs is not the sine qua non of good patient care.[9] Drugs can be and have been used effectively without any knowledge of their concentrations in the body; determination of serum concentrations does not guarantee skillful drug therapy.

According to Richens and Warrington, the general indications for plasma drug level monitoring are as follows:[10]

1) When there is a wide interindividual variation in the rate of metabolism of the drug, leading to marked differences in steady-state plasma levels. This can be particularly important in children, in whom differences in body weight and metabolic rate are wide.
2) When saturation kinetics occur, causing a steep relationship between dose and plasma level within the therapeutic range (e.g., phenytoin).
3) When the therapeutic ratio of a drug is low; i.e., when therapeutic doses are close to toxic doses (e.g. aminoglycoside antibiotics).
4) When signs of toxicity are difficult to recognize clinically, or where signs of overdosage or underdosage are indistinguishable.
5) When gastrointestinal, hepatic or renal disease is present, causing disturbance of drug absorption, metabolism or excretion.
6) When patients are receiving multiple drug therapy with the attendant risk of drug interaction.
7) When there is doubt about the patient's reliability in taking his tablets.

An important illustration of the potential benefits of monitoring plasma drug levels is found in a report on digoxin toxicity from the Boston Collaborative Drug Surveillance Program.[11] Adverse reactions to digoxin in hospitalized medical patients were monitored for 2 years at 2 Boston hospitals. Dose-related adverse reactions were confirmed in 10% of 272 patients at 1 hospital but in only 4% of 291 patients at the other. The only important difference between these hospitals was that serum digoxin concentrations were measured in more patients receiving digoxin at the second hospital (40%) than at the first (12%). Mean digoxin levels were lower at the second hospital than at the first, probably reflecting the use of serum digoxin concentration monitoring for therapeutic guidance. The authors conclude that the use of serum digoxin assays in clinical practice can decrease the frequency of adverse reactions to this drug.

CLINICAL EXPERIENCE WITH INDIVIDUALIZATION AND OPTIMIZATION BASED ON PLASMA DRUG LEVELS

There are few well-controlled prospective studies to show that individualization of initial drug dosing regimens and monitoring of plasma drug levels to optimize drug dosages result in better drug therapy. If this kind of evidence were a requirement, however, cardiac bypass surgery, liver transplants, and most other clinical procedures would not be available. In the absence of controlled, prospective studies, the value of individualization and optimization of certain drug therapies must be judged on clinical experience. The balance of this chapter concerns specific drugs for which individualization of dosage regimens and/or routine or selective monitoring of plasma concentrations have been found by some investigators to be helpful in guiding therapy and minimizing adverse effects.

Antiarrhythmic Drugs

Most antiarrhythmic agents have a narrow therapeutic window, requiring careful titration of dosage. Investigators first proposed the use of plasma level monitoring for antiarrhythmic drugs nearly 40 years ago by characterizing the relation between antiarrhythmic response and plasma concentrations of quinidine.[12] Since that pioneering work other investigators have sought a relationship between drug level and response for other antiarrhythmic drugs.[13]

In a recent review, Woosley[14] stated that "plasma concentration monitoring of antiarrhythmic agents is valuable, but it is often misused or overemphasized in therapeutic decision-making . . . For maximum value, there must be a reliable, accurate relation between the plasma drug concentration and drug action, a relation closer than that between dosage and drug action."

Procainamide. Procainamide is usually given orally for prophylaxis of arrhythmias. It has a short half-life (2.5 to 5.0 hr) and a narrow therapeutic concentration range. About 40 to 60% of a dose of procainamide is excreted in the urine. Oral and intravenous dosages of the drug must be reduced in patients with impaired renal function.

The clinical pharmacokinetics of procainamide and the use of serum procainamide levels as therapeutic guides have been reviewed.[15,16] The usually effective antiarrhythmic plasma procainamide concentrations are 4 to 8 μg/ml; in some patients, higher concentrations are more effective. Toxic manifestations are uncommon at plasma concentrations less than 12 μg/ml, but are seen often with concentrations more than 16 μg/ml.[17] Serious toxic effects include marked hypotension, disturbances in conduction, major active ventricular arrhythmias, and cardiac arrest.

Blood samples for monitoring plasma procainamide concentrations are taken when steady state is attained; this usually occurs within 24 hr of initiating oral therapy but may require up to 2 days in patients with little renal function or when a prolonged-release product is used. Typically, two blood samples are obtained during a steady-state dosing interval; one sample is collected at the end of a dosing interval and the other 2 hr later to approximate the peak drug concentration.

Therapeutic plasma levels of procainamide were established before it was known that N-acetylprocainamide (NAPA), a principal metabolite, could contribute to the therapeutic and toxic effects of procainamide. The relationship between plasma NAPA levels and antiarrhythmic activity has not been established. Some investigators have claimed that NAPA's activity is similar to that of procainamide at equal plasma concentrations; others have reported that higher levels of NAPA, on the order of 10–20 μg/ml, are needed to suppress arrhythmias.

Patients with poor renal function who are genetically rapid acetylators will have the highest ratios of NAPA to procainamide concentrations in plasma. These patients may show a good clinical response even when procainamide levels are below those usually associated with efficacy.[7]

Quinidine. Quinidine is useful for both prophylaxis and treatment of a variety of atrial and ventricular arrhythmias. It is usually administered orally but may be given by intramuscular or intravenous injection. About 60 to 80% of an intravenous dose of quinidine is metabolized in the liver; it has a half-life of about 6 to 7 hr. Maintenance dosages of quinidine may need to be reduced by one third to one half in patients with CHF.[18] When usual dosages of quinidine are given to patients on enzyme-inducing drugs, such as phenobarbital, phenytoin, or rifampin, low, subtherapeutic blood levels of quinidine are likely to result. Higher than usual dosages of quinidine are required in these patients, but these dosages must be reduced if the enzyme-inducer is withdrawn. The clinical pharmacokinetics of quinidine has been reviewed by Ochs and associates.[19]

Confusion has existed concerning the therapeutic concentration range of quinidine. Quinidine concentrations that are determined with a nonspecific assay method will be higher than actual quinidine concentrations. With these older methods, the therapeutic range for quinidine is higher than the range determined with more specific methods. Quinidine concentrations of about 3 to 8 μg/ml are considered therapeutic when nonspecific assay methods are used.

As assay specificity for quinidine improves, therapeutic effects are associated with lower plasma concentrations. With a high performance liquid chromatography assay procedure or the EMIT method, both of which are in common use, antiarrhythmic effects are associated with serum quinidine levels of 2 to 5 μg/ml.[20]

The frequency of gastrointestinal disturbances increases with quinidine levels above 5 μg/ml; cardiovascular disturbances are a concern at concentrations exceeding 8 μg/ml. Cardiovascular toxicity of quinidine includes re-entrant arrhythmias that could lead to heart block. Several metabolites of quinidine have cardiovascular effects in laboratory animals, but their clinical significance is not known.

Woosley[14] observed that "restriction of dosages to maintain plasma levels below a predetermined limit is of value with drugs such as quinidine, which have variable clearance . . . However, careful dose titration and electrocardiographic monitoring are essential because plasma concentration monitoring is of only limited value in guiding therapy." Woosley believes that the most important role for plasma concentration monitoring is to ensure adequate dosing in those patients who rapidly clear quinidine.

Quinidine, like most antiarrhythmic agents, is basic and largely bound to alpha-1-acid glycoprotein (AAG); as noted elsewhere in the text, the concentration of AAG in plasma may vary widely. Under these circumstances free rather than total drug concentrations may be more closely related to pharmacologic effect.

Garfinkel et al.[21] found serum concentrations of quinidine of about 11 μg/ml with no evidence of adverse effects in a patient who had undergone cardiac surgery following an acute myocardial infarction. AAG levels at this time were elevated considerably and the free fraction of quinidine was only 0.03; values in healthy subjects range from 0.07 to 0.13. The patient showed no signs or symptoms of toxicity presumably because the concentration of free quinidine was in the therapeutic range.

Lidocaine. Lidocaine is the most frequently used intravenous antiarrhythmic agent for the short-term management of ventricular arrhythmias; it is usually the drug of choice following acute myocardial infarction. Lidocaine is also used prophylactically after myocardial infarction to prevent or reduce the likelihood of primary ventricular fibrillation or tachycardia.

The half-life of lidocaine is about 2 hr but may be considerably longer in patients with reduced cardiac output and/or hepatic blood flow rate. In some patients, the clearance of lidocaine decreases with continuous infusion; dosage reduction may be required during therapy. Coadministration of cimetidine or propranolol, which decreases liver blood flow and inhibits hepatic metabolism, may also require dosage reduction of lidocaine. The clinical pharmacokinetics of lidocaine has been reviewed by Benowitz and Meister.[22]

Plasma levels of lidocaine less than 1.5 μg/ml are usually ineffective. The usual therapeutic lidocaine concentration range is 1.5 to 4.0 μg/ml, but levels up to 8 μg/ml may be needed in refractory patients. These higher concentrations may be associated with central nervous system (CNS) toxicity and cardiovascular depression. Lidocaine levels exceeding 8 μg/ml may be associated with seizures and serious cardiovascular disturbances.

The usefulness of monitoring plasma lidocaine concentrations is controversial. There is general agreement that no need exists for monitoring when the lidocaine infusion is no longer than 12 hr in duration. Richens and Warrington note that:[10]

Plasma concentrations of ligocaine (lidocaine) are of limited value in clinical practice. The drug is almost always given intravenously, so variability in absorption does not occur. It is given only to patients under close supervision, and is rarely continued for more than a few days. It is therefore much easier to monitor the pharmacologic effects of the drug than with long term oral antidysrhythmic therapy.

According to Benowitz and Meister,[22] measurements of plasma lidocaine concentrations may be useful in the following situations: (1) in patients in shock who may have markedly reduced clearance; (2) during prolonged infusion (>24 hr), especially in patients with cardiac or hepatic failure; and (3) in assisting in the clinical diagnosis of lidocaine toxicity in the presence of ambiguous signs and symptoms.

One study examined serum lidocaine levels and lidocaine effects in 33 patients in a coronary care unit.[23] Deglin and co-workers concluded that it is difficult to adjust lidocaine dosage during therapy on the basis of clinical assessment of the patient and rhythm monitoring alone. On the 8 occasions in which the diagnosis of a lidocaine toxic reaction was clinically considered, serum levels were greater than 8 µg/ml in 4 but less than 5 µg/ml in 3. In another study, 38 of 69 blood samples that the house staff predicted would be within the therapeutic range were indeed between 1.2 and 5 µg/ml, but 10 were between 5 and 9 and 7 samples were above 9 µg/ml. Each of these 7 patients exhibited signs consistent with lidocaine toxicity; however, in every instance there were associated disease symptoms, including hypoxia, inadequate cerebral perfusion, CNS depression, tremor, and orthostatic hypotension, that masked the adverse drug reactions.[23]

Plasma protein binding of lidocaine varies considerably because, like quinidine, it is largely dependent on circulating levels of AAG. Although free concentration of lidocaine may be more useful than total concentration, available methods for determining binding are too time consuming to be of value.

As an alternative, Routledge et al. examined whether AAG measurements could be used to estimate lidocaine binding indirectly.[24] A free lidocaine index was developed on the basis of measurements of plasma lidocaine and AAG in plasma samples from patients admitted to coronary care and given lidocaine prophylactically. The free fraction of lidocaine in plasma was determined by equilibrium dialysis.

Levels of AAG in plasma ranged from 50 to 250 mg/dl. Free fraction (F) was related to AAG and total lidocaine levels (T) as follows:

$$1/F = 1.45 + 0.023 \text{ (AAG)} - 0.129 \text{ (T)}$$

This relationship was used to calculate the free lidocaine index, defined as $F \times T$. A highly significant relationship ($r = 0.93$) was found between

Table 15–1. Recommended Lidocaine Infusion Rates According to Clinical Classification of Heart Failure*

Clinical class	Infusion rate (µg/kg per min)	
	Minimum	Maximum
I	35	88
II	12	35
III, IV	5	12

*From Zito, R.A., and Reid, P.R.: Lidocaine kinetics predicted by indocyanine green clearance. N. Engl. J. Med., *298*:1160, 1978. (Reprinted by permission of The New England Journal of Medicine.)

predicted and observed values of free concentration of lidocaine.

Although there is controversy regarding the need for monitoring plasma lidocaine concentrations, there is general agreement that better guidelines are desirable for individualizing the initial infusion rate of lidocaine. Zito and Reid showed a close relationship ($r = 0.95$) between the clearances of the indocyanine green (ICG) and lidocaine.[25] Because ICG clearance can be determined rapidly and easily, a test dose of ICG might be given before lidocaine therapy to estimate the clearance and the required infusion rate of lidocaine. As these results could not be confirmed by Bax and co-workers,[26] however, the value of this method is uncertain.

With some drugs there is a strong correlation between clearance at steady state and the concentration in blood or plasma at a certain time after a bolus test dose.[27] The critical time for sampling after a single test dose depends on the half-life of the drug. This one-point method of predicting clearance and steady-state concentration of a drug appears to apply to lidocaine.[28] A close relationship was observed between the plasma lidocaine concentration at 1 hr after a loading dose of 225 mg over 20 min and 2 mg/min thereafter and the patient's lidocaine clearance after 12 hr of infusion. Using this relationship prospectively, it was possible to alter the infusion rate to achieve a mean plasma lidocaine concentration of 3.69 ± 0.14 (s.d.) µg/ml at 12 hr in 6 subjects, close to the desired concentration of 3.5 µg/ml.[29] This approach may reduce the incidence of inadequate or excessive plasma lidocaine concentrations.

Lidocaine infusion rates may also be individualized based on population data from patients with different degrees of heart failure (Table 15–1).[25] Lopez and co-workers compared plasma lidocaine levels in a control group and in an experimental group who received an adjusted lidocaine regimen

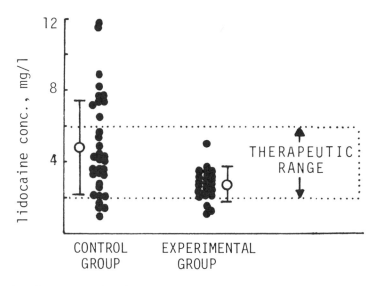

Fig. 15–2. Plasma lidocaine concentrations in a control group, dosed based on clinical judgment, and an experimental group who received an adjusted lidocaine dosage regimen based on the presence or absence of heart failure. Vertical bars denote the mean ± 1 standard deviation for each group. (Data from Lopez, L.M., et al.[30])

based on the presence or absence of heart failure.[30] Each group received a 1- to 2-mg/kg loading dose. Control patients were dosed using a conventional approach, receiving an infusion rate of 1 to 4 mg/min based on clinical judgment. Patients in the experimental group with no heart failure (Class I) received 35 to 88 μg/min per kg body weight; patients with Class II heart failure received 12 to 35 μg/min per kg body weight. The results are shown in Figure 15–2. This approach has merit, at least for some patients, and may be able to be extended to patients with Class III or IV heart failure.

Vozeh et al.[31] evaluated the performance of a computerized dosing approach to achieve a serum lidocaine concentration of 3.5 μg/ml, about the middle of the therapeutic range, in patients treated for acute ventricular arrhythmias. In all patients a blood sample to determine lidocaine levels was taken 2 hr after starting therapy. In about one-third of all patients, this information as well as population pharmacokinetic parameters served as input for a statistical program called Bayesian forecasting.[32] In the others, the physician considered the measured levels and altered the regimen as he or she deemed appropriate.

Both groups were similar with respect to average lidocaine concentrations 12 hr after starting therapy but interpatient variability was considerably larger in the control group. The 95% confidence intervals were 2.3 to 4.7 μg/ml in the computer-assisted group and 1.5 to 6.1 in the control group. Nine of the 41 patients in the control group had levels outside the recommended therapeutic range of 2 to 5 μg/ml, compared with only 1 of 22 patients in the Bayesian group. The investigators concluded that "Bayesian forecasting outperforms the physician in early adjustment of lidocaine dosage based on serum concentration measurements."

Flecainide. Flecainide is a class 1C orally effective antiarrhythmic agent. Therapeutic doses cause characteristic changes in the ECG. During the development of flecainide, correlations between trough plasma levels and suppression of ventricular ectopic beats were reported. Suggested minimal therapeutic levels of flecainide range from 200 to 400 ng/ml.

More recently, Salerno et al.[33] considered whether the side effects of flecainide correlated with drug plasma levels. They found that flecainide trough levels in plasma were higher when cardiovascular side effects were observed (mean 1063 ng/ml, range 296 to 2050 ng/ml) than when no adverse effects occurred (mean 609 ng/ml, range 89 to 1508 ng/ml).

The investigators defined the lower end of the therapeutic-toxic window as the flecainide level where there is at least 50% probability of efficacy and the upper end as the level where there is less than 10% probability of cardiovascular side effects. Under these conditions, they suggested a therapeutic range of 381 to 710 ng/ml.

The investigators concluded that "the risk of cardiovascular side effects increases at higher plasma levels of flecainide and is associated with greater increases in the PR and QRS intervals from baseline than are routinely observed during flecainide dosing . . . Fortunately, the close relationship of both therapeutic efficacy and cardiovascular side effects with level of flecainide and ECG intervals should make it possible to administer flecainide therapy with acceptable safety."

Another report, based on intravenous dosing regimens of flecainide concluded that plasma levels between 200 and 1000 ng/ml are associated with antiarrhythmic effects in most patients, but some require and tolerate higher levels and others manifest toxicity at "therapeutic" levels.[34]

Antibiotics

Evaluation of antibiotic therapy by monitoring plasma concentrations of drugs is controversial. According to Rylance and Moreland:[35]

Blood levels of the antibacterial drugs may be presumed to be meaningful measures of drug effect only if bacteraemia is present. Otherwise, the blood concentration is only one of many determinants of drug effect. Other factors, which apply to other drugs too but to antibacterials in particular, are the blood flow to the infected site, the degree of drug protein binding, and penetration of the drug into abscesses, cells, and interstitial fluids.

For optimal effect, drug levels should exceed the mean inhibitory concentration (MIC) for the likely or known causative organism by as great a margin as possible without undue risk of toxicity. However, it should be remembered that the MIC refers to a drug level in vitro, and although levels in excess of this are found in the blood, the levels in the infected tissue may be considerably lower. In addition, the controversy about whether high, but poorly sustained (peak), or lower, but adequate (continuous), levels should be achieved has not been resolved. Although a 'peak' regimen may aid in diffusion of drugs into poorly vascularised areas, and there is evidence that it is effective provided that the interval between doses is not unduly long, it remains unclear which method should be adopted and whether the mode of action of a drug (for example, bacterial wall synthesis inhibition or intracellular protein synthesis inhibition) should determine the type of regimen to be used.

Neu, in his review of practices in antimicrobial dosing, observed that erratic adherence to pharmacokinetic concepts has been the order of the day.[36] The only general guideline in effect today is that new antibiotics similar to established antibiotics but eliminated more slowly tend to be given less frequently. Interesting ideas regarding the use of pharmacokinetics in the development of dosage regimens for antibiotics in general,[37] and for cephalosporins in particular,[38] have been presented but await testing. Of the many antibiotics and other antibacterial drugs available, a case for monitoring plasma drug levels can only be made for the aminoglycoside antibiotics and, in some circumstances, chloramphenicol.[35]

Aminoglycoside Antibiotics. An extensive review of the clinical pharmacokinetics of aminoglycoside antibiotics has been presented by Pechere and Dugal.[39] Comprehensive commentaries on therapeutic drug concentration monitoring for aminoglycosides are also available.[40-44]

The aminoglycoside antibiotics are effective in treating pneumonia, urinary tract, soft tissue, burn wound, and other systemic infections caused by gram-negative organisms. In life-threatening infections, they are often combined with either β-lactam antibiotics or clindamycin. Gentamicin and tobramycin are among the most widely used antibiotics in hospitalized patients. Amikacin is used less frequently but is often useful against gentamicin- and tobramycin-resistant isolates. All aminoglycosides are ototoxic and nephrotoxic and have a relatively low therapeutic index.

The major elimination route for the aminoglycosides is renal excretion, largely by way of glomerular filtration. The half-lives of gentamicin, tobramycin, and amikacin in patients with normal renal function are variable but average about 2.5 hr. Patients with impaired renal function eliminate the aminoglycosides more slowly and require reduced dosage. Infants less than 7 days of age and elderly patients also require lower dosages.

Therapeutic aminoglycoside concentration monitoring appears to be useful for optimizing efficacy; whether it is also useful for reducing toxicity is controversial. It is generally held that appropriate treatment of serious systemic infections with gentamicin or tobramycin requires steady-state peak concentrations of 6 to 10 μg/ml and trough concentrations of 0.5 to 1.5 μg/ml. The corresponding values for amikacin are 20 to 30 μg/ml and 1 to 8 μg/ml, depending on the infection. It has been argued that monitoring of plasma aminoglycoside levels is needed because some patients, perhaps as many as 30 to 50% of all patients with normal renal function, require higher daily doses of gentamicin or tobramycin than the recommended 3 to 5 mg/kg per day to attain therapeutic concentrations.[40,43]

Moore et al.[45] examined the association of ami-

Table 15–2. Suggested Changes in Dose or Dosing Interval Based on Measured Serum Aminoglycoside Concentration*

Measured serum concentrations compared to desired values		Suggested change in dosing regimen	
Trough	Peak	Dose	Dosing Interval
Desired	Desired	No change	No change
Higher	Higher	Decrease or no change	Increase
Higher	Lower	Increase	Increase
Lower	Lower	Increase or no change	Decrease
Lower	Higher	Decrease	Decrease
Desired	Higher	Decrease	No change
Desired	Lower	Increase	No change
Higher	Desired	No change or increase	Increase
Lower	Desired	No change or decrease	Decrease

*From Cipolle, R.J., Zaske, D.E., and Crossley, K.[43]

noglycoside levels with mortality from gram-negative bacteremia. Each patient received a single aminoglycoside combined with a penicillin or cephalothin. Aminoglycoside levels in plasma were measured 24 to 48 hr after the start of treatment and were considered to be therapeutic when peak concentration of gentamicin or tobramycin exceeded 5 μg/ml and when the peak concentration of amikacin exceeded 20 μg/ml.

Twelve of the 89 patients died during antibiotic therapy or within 24 hr of its termination. Various factors were found to significantly influence mortality. Stepwise linear discriminant analysis of these factors indicated that the severity of the underlying illness was the strongest discriminator between death and survival. Next in importance was peak aminoglycoside concentration.

Plasma aminoglycoside levels were available for 84 patients, 10 of whom had died. Only 1 death occurred in 41 patients with early therapeutic levels of gentamicin, tobramycin, or amikacin, whereas 9 deaths were recorded in 43 patients with subtherapeutic concentrations; the corresponding mortalities were 2.4% and 20.8%. The results suggest that achieving adequate aminoglycoside levels, particularly within the first 48 hr of antibiotic therapy, in patients with gram-negative bacteremia may significantly improve the patient's chances of survival.

The relationship between plasma aminoglycoside concentration and toxicity is not clear. One school of thought proposes that among the risk factors for aminoglycoside toxicity are age, renal impairment, prior exposure to aminoglycosides, duration of treatment, total daily dose, cumulative dose, and elevated peak and trough plasma concentrations. The advocates of this school believe that aminoglycoside toxicity is reduced when peak

concentrations of gentamicin or tobramycin are kept below 12 to 15 μg/ml and when trough concentrations do not exceed 2 μg/ml; the corresponding concentrations for amikacin are 30 μg/ml and 8 μg/ml. Cipolle et al.[43] recommend therapeutic aminoglycoside concentration monitoring during therapy and dosage adjustments, according to Table 15–2, when the peak or trough concentration deviates from the guideline. Some studies that support this idea include the work of Echeverria and co-workers who found that peak serum gentamicin concentrations greater than 12 μg/ml were significantly associated with ototoxicity in children,[46] and the work of Smith and associates who found that peak levels of amikacin greater than 38.5 μg/ml or of gentamicin greater than 10 μg/ml and trough levels of amikacin above 10 μg/ml were associated with nephrotoxicity.[47]

Other studies have failed to find a relationship between plasma aminoglycoside concentration and toxicity and support another school of thought that questions the value of therapeutic aminoglycoside concentration monitoring in reducing the risk of toxicity. An investigation of 201 critically ill patients during 267 courses of gentamicin or tobramycin reported that no clinical parameters, including plasma levels, were of value in predicting nephrotoxicity.[48] These investigators observed:

Early concentration versus toxicity studies are difficult to interpret since oto- and nephrotoxicity were correlated with serum peak concentrations measured after serum creatinine was already rising. Since serum creatinine rise is a result of established nephrotoxicity, these studies did not establish serum concentration ranges which produce toxicity.

Schentag et al.[48] also noted that the controversy regarding the ability of peak aminoglycoside concentrations to predict nephrotoxicity also applies to the value of trough concentrations to predict toxicity.

Advocates of this school believe that the nephrotoxicity of aminoglycosides is associated with an unusual ability of the kidneys to accumulate the drug that is characteristic of certain patients. If these patients could be identified, they could be treated with alternative antibiotics (e.g., third-generation cephalosporins). Careful examination of plasma level data suggests that, during therapy but before nephrotoxicity, trough levels of aminoglycosides rise more rapidly in these patients than in other patients. This hypothesis, however, requires further study.

Although plasma level monitoring of aminoglycosides is controversial, target plasma concentrations related to efficacy or to both efficacy and toxicity are often used to guide initial dosage recommendations. Nomograms based on an individual's creatinine clearance and lean body weight are available for gentamicin and tobramycin[49] and for amikacin.[50]

Some investigators carry out a pharmacokinetic study on an initial test dose of aminoglycoside to determine the clearance, half-life, and apparent volume of distribution of the drug in the patient. These parameters are then used to determine the required daily dosage and frequency of dosing for the individual.[43] Desired concentrations of gentamicin are attained in significantly more patients with this individualized pharmacokinetic method than with nomograms based on patient characteristics.[51]

Vancomycin. The increasing prevalence of infections caused by methicillin-resistant strains of *Staphylococcus aureus* has dramatically increased the use of vancomycin. Because of its potential to cause nephrotoxicity and ototoxicity, there has been considerable interest in developing appropriate dosing guidelines for vancomycin. Ototoxicity has been observed when peak serum levels of vancomycin are greater than 80 to 100 μg/ml; trough levels higher than 20 to 30 μg/ml have been associated with nephrotoxicity. Peak levels of 30 to 40 μg/ml and trough levels of 5 to 10 μg/ml are recommended.[52]

Several approaches have been developed to achieve optimal levels of vancomycin. These methods have been evaluated by Zokufa et al.[52] and Ackerman.[53] Zokufa and his colleagues found that most methods underpredicted vancomycin clearance. They concluded that a simple approach using a dose of 8 mg/kg (rounded to the nearest 50 mg) and a dosing interval based on creatinine clearance seemed to work best, and that this approach should be considered, at least for initial dosing of vancomycin. Even this method, however, is likely to produce trough and peak concentrations outside the therapeutic range in a large number of patients.

Both Ackerman and Zokufa et al. agree that early serum concentration monitoring and adjustment of initial algorithm- or nomogram-derived doses is necessary to assure safe and effective vancomycin serum concentrations. Whether or not routine monitoring of serum vancomycin concentrations is justified, however, is controversial.

Rodvold et al.[54] have concluded that routine monitoring of vancomycin concentrations is justified for most patients and that it is particularly important in critically ill patients. In their hospital, they monitor vancomycin levels once the patient has reached steady-state and once a week thereafter. More frequent monitoring occurs when the patient's status is changing. Edwards and Pancorbo,[55] on the other hand, have argued that the relationship between serum vancomycin levels and either efficacy or adverse events is not sufficiently compelling, given the costs, to recommend routine monitoring. They qualify their conclusion, however, by suggesting that in patients ''demonstrating a poor therapeutic response, [and] those in whom unusually high MIC values have been documented, measurement of vancomycin concentrations may be justified.''

Anticonvulsants

For most epileptic patients, long-term drug therapy is the only practical form of treatment. Therapy usually continues for at least 3 years and often for a lifetime. In many clinics and institutions, monitoring of plasma anticonvulsant levels is a part of the routine management of patients with epilepsy. It is generally held that monitoring has led to a more rational approach to drug therapy for convulsive disorders, resulting in better control of seizures, less drug toxicity, and use of fewer drugs. Dozens of reviews and commentaries on the clinical pharmacokinetics and therapeutic drug concentration monitoring of anticonvulsants are available.[50,57,58]

Carbamazepine. Originally developed for relief of pain associated with trigeminal neuralgia, carbamazepine was approved in 1974 for the treatment of convulsive disorders. It is used in both adults and children for prophylaxis of grand mal and complex partial seizures. Carbamazepine is poorly water-soluble; oral doses are slowly but completely absorbed. It is extensively metabolized; less than 2% of a dose is found unchanged in the urine.

An epoxide with anticonvulsive activity is carbamazepine's principal plasma metabolite. Carbamazepine stimulates its own metabolism and, as a result, observed steady-state plasma concentrations are only about half of the concentrations predicted based on carbamazepine clearance after a single dose. Clinically, this is of little consequence because carbamazepine therapy is initiated with small doses that are gradually increased to a maintenance level over 3 to 4 weeks.

The half-life of carbamazepine at steady state is reported to be variable (5 to 27 hr); the recommended daily dose for adults varies 2-fold (7 to 15 mg/kg) and is usually given twice a day. Children metabolize the drug more rapidly than adults and may need to receive the drug 3 or 4 times a day. Adult patients taking other anticonvulsants (enzyme-inducing agents) may also need a higher daily dosage and more frequent administration.

Therapeutic drug concentration monitoring of carbamazepine has been reviewed by MacKichan and Kutt.[59] The therapeutic concentration range of carbamazepine is reported to be 4 to 12 μg/ml. It has been suggested that plasma concentrations of both carbamazepine and its epoxide metabolite might correlate better with therapeutic and toxic effects but knowledge of the activity of the metabolite is limited.

Theodore et al.[60] studied the relation of plasma levels of carbamazepine and carbamazepine epoxide as well as their ratio to drug toxicity and seizure control in patients with complex partial seizures. Patients receiving only carbamazepine showed a significant correlation between the levels of parent drug and its epoxide. In turn, the serum concentration of each, as well as their sum and ratio, was significantly correlated with toxicity scores and seizure frequency. The investigators concluded that measurement of epoxide levels did not provide additional information useful for monitoring clinical response to carbamazepine therapy.

When patients were taking other anticonvulsants, the ratio of epoxide to parent drug was higher than that seen in patients on monotherapy, largely due to lower levels of carbamazepine. The investigators recommended that rather than assume the decrease in carbamazepine levels resulting from

coadministration of enzyme inducing agents would be compensated by increased levels of epoxide, it is more appropriate to increase the carbamazepine dose to maintain plasma levels in the therapeutic range. "The contribution of carbamazepine epoxide to the therapeutic effect of carbamazepine is uncertain, and the role of carbamazepine epoxide plasma levels has not been established."[60]

Generally, carbamazepine concentrations of 4 to 8 μg/ml are considered adequate in patients receiving other anticonvulsant drugs; concentrations of 8 to 12 μg/ml are recommended in patients on monotherapy with carbamazepine. Carbamazepine serum levels exceeding 12 μg/ml are associated with a high incidence of incapacitating neurologic side effects. Concentrations exceeding 8 μg/ml are associated with carbamazepine toxicity when other anticonvulsants are also prescribed.[61]

Plasma carbamazepine concentrations may be monitored indirectly by determining carbamazepine concentration in saliva and relating it to plasma concentration. There has been interest in therapeutic drug concentration monitoring in saliva because it offers a noninvasive alternative to venepuncture and because, under some circumstances, it provides a measure of free rather than total drug concentration in plasma.[62]

In most cases, the relationship between saliva concentration and free or total drug concentration in plasma has been found to be too variable to be of predictive value. Carbamazepine may be one of the few drugs that is suitable for therapeutic monitoring in saliva.[63] Saliva sampling is likely to be of clinical value when venepuncture is difficult or undesirable (e.g., in children). In 11 studies, the correlation coefficient between saliva and plasma concentrations ranged from 0.83 to 0.97, averaging 0.92. Carbamazepine concentration in saliva is about 30% that in plasma, consistent with the fact that the free fraction (fraction unbound to plasma proteins) in plasma is about 0.3. The therapeutic carbamazepine concentration range in saliva is suggested to be 1.2 to 3.5 μg/ml.[63]

Enthusiasm for monitoring free rather than total serum concentrations of carbamazepine was dampened by a report from Froscher et al.[64] These investigators studied more than 200 patients receiving carbamazepine monotherapy and considered the relationship of free and total drug levels with therapeutic outcome and side effects. They found no closer correlation between free concentration and seizure reduction or side effects than between total concentration and effectiveness or side effects. Whether monitoring free drug is advantageous when more than one anticonvulsant is used has not been determined.

Ethosuximide. Ethosuximide is specifically indicated for the treatment of patients with absence (petit mal) seizures. It is extensively metabolized but no active metabolites have been reported. Highly variable half-lives of ethosuximide have been observed, ranging from 14 to 72 hr. The average half-life of ethosuximide is 30 hr in children and 50 to 60 hr in adults. Most patients can be dosed with ethosuximide once a day.

The use of plasma ethosuximide levels as a guide to drug therapy has been reviewed by Stoehr and Sherwin.[65] Plasma concentrations of 40 to 100 μg/ml have been associated with ethosuximide efficacy. No relationship has been established between toxicity and plasma levels of ethosuximide but most patients who fail to respond at concentrations of about 100 μg/ml do not benefit from higher concentrations. There have been conflicting reports on the value of saliva concentration monitoring of ethosuximide.[63]

Phenobarbital. In general, phenobarbital is effective in all convulsive disorders except petit mal seizures; it has been used as an anticonvulsant drug since 1912. About two thirds of a dose of phenobarbital is metabolized and the rest is excreted in the urine. The half-life of phenobarbital ranges from 50 to 120 hr in adults and from 40 to 70 hr in children. Because of its long half-life, phenobarbital is usually given to adults once a day at bedtime. Children sometimes require twice-a-day dosing. Approximately 2 to 3 weeks may be required to reach steady-state levels of phenobarbital in plasma.

Therapeutic drug concentration monitoring of phenobarbital has been reviewed by Saunders and Penry.[66] Plasma concentrations of 15 to 40 μg/ml are usually required for adequate therapeutic effect. Plasma phenobarbital levels exceeding 60 μg/ml result in lethargy, stupor, or coma, but habitual barbiturate abusers may tolerate much higher concentrations. In fact, the upper limit of the therapeutic concentration range of phenobarbital is not clearly defined because of the wide variation in tolerance to the sedative and hypnotic effects of the drug. Whether or not tolerance develops to the anticonvulsant effect of phenobarbital is not known. It is generally agreed that the value of monitoring phenobarbital levels is less than that for phenytoin.

Primidone. Uncertainty exists regarding the anticonvulsant effect of primidone as distinct from the effects of its principal metabolites. Primidone is extensively metabolized; both of its major metabolites, phenobarbital and phenylethylmalonamide, have anticonvulsant activity.

Levels of 5 to 12 μg/ml have been suggested as the therapeutic plasma concentration range for primidone.[66] These levels, however, are usually associated with plasma phenobarbital concentrations within the phenobarbital therapeutic concentration range (15 to 40 μg/ml). At this time, there seems to be no clear indication for measuring primidone concentration in plasma, but there may be some value in monitoring plasma phenobarbital levels during primidone therapy.

Phenytoin. No drug has a greater need for therapeutic drug concentration monitoring and individualized dosing than phenytoin. A relationship between drug concentration in plasma and daily dose is almost nonexistent because phenytoin is poorly absorbed, highly plasma protein bound, and subject to nonlinear, capacity-limited metabolism. Despite these problems, it is the most frequently prescribed anticonvulsant drug for the management of grand mal and partial seizures.

The value of therapeutic drug concentration monitoring for phenytoin has been reviewed by Winter and Tozer[67] and by Finn and Olanow.[68] Optimum phenytoin efficacy is achieved in most patients with serum concentrations in the range of 10 to 20 μg/ml. Only 20% of a typical patient population will have steady-state serum phenytoin concentrations in the therapeutic range if given the usual 300-mg daily dose.[67] An additional 30% will have levels between 5 and 10 μg/ml and may derive some benefit from the drug; however, this dose is clearly subtherapeutic for at least 27% of the patients and produces excessive serum concentrations that are likely to result in adverse effects in 16% of the patients. Daily phenytoin dosages as small as 125 mg or as large as 600 mg may be required to produce therapeutic concentrations in a given patient.

Tables 15–3 and 15–4 show the relationship between plasma phenytoin concentration and the degree of seizure control; Table 15–3 also shows the poor correlation between dose and efficacy of phenytoin.[69] Relatively small changes in plasma phen-

Table 15–3. Number of Epileptic Seizures During 2 Months in Relation to Mean Prescribed Dose and Plasma Concentration of Phenytoin*

No. of seizures	No. of patients	Prescribed dose (mg/kg per day)	Phenytoin concentration (μg/ml)
0	84	5.0	13.4
1	19	5.7	8.8
2	23	4.8	7.3
3–5	11	4.4	4.5
>5	11	6.4	6.2

*Data from Lund, L.[69]

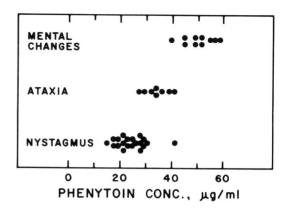

Fig. 15–3. Phenytoin levels in blood at the time patients experienced certain adverse effects of the drug. (Data from Kutt, H., et al.[70])

ytoin levels can dramatically affect the frequency of seizures.

Concentration-related CNS toxicity of phenytoin is generally observed at serum concentrations above 20 μg/ml. As serum levels rise, so do the frequency and severity of side effects (Fig. 15–3).[70] Nystagmus is generally the earliest side effect detected, and is seen at levels of 15 to 30 μg/ml. Ataxia usually occurs at levels greater than 30 μg/ml; somnolence and diminished mental capacity are seen at levels exceeding 40 μg/ml.

The most common adverse effect of phenytoin therapy is gingival hyperplasia, which may lead to impaired mastication and malocclusion. This condition is said to occur in more than 40% of the patients taking the drug and may be more common in children. Gingival hyperplasia during phenytoin therapy appears to be a direct effect of phenytoin on gingival tissue. The relationship between serum phenytoin concentration and the severity of gingival hyperplasia is shown in Table 15–5.[71]

Despite the wide variation in serum levels of phenytoin in response to a given dose, there are few guidelines for initiating phenytoin dosage and most patients are started on 300 mg/day. Children metabolize phenytoin more rapidly than do adults and may require 2 or 3 times larger mg/kg daily doses (up to 15 mg/kg per day) than do adults. The dosage of phenytoin may need to be increased during pregnancy because of the increased clearance of the drug during this period.

Because most patients are started on the same initial dosage of phenytoin and because this dosage regimen is likely to produce serum phenytoin levels that are outside the therapeutic concentration range in about three fourths of the patients, most patients benefit from a determination of phenytoin concentration in serum 2 weeks after initiating therapy. When the plasma levels are low and seizure control is inadequate or when plasma levels are high and there are signs of phenytoin toxicity, it is usually desirable to modify the dosage regimen.

Unlike the dosage adjustment for most drugs, that for phenytoin in response to plasma levels outside the therapeutic range and clinical signs is not a simple matter of ratio and proportions. Ordinarily, one might think that a patient showing less than optimal seizure control and a serum level of 8 μg/ml would require a doubling of the dosage to bring the levels up to a range of 15 to 20 μg/ml. This is not so for phenytoin because it is eliminated by capacity-limited metabolism. A doubling of the dosage under these conditions in most patients would produce excessive, potentially toxic serum phenytoin levels. Some patients may need as little as a 50-mg increment to the usual daily dose to

Table 15–4. Relationship Between Degree of Seizure Control and Plasma Phenytoin Concentration Interval*

Phenytoin concentration (μg/ml)	No. of patients	No. of patients without seizures during 2 mo	Seizure-free (%)
0 to 9.9	95	41	43
10.0 to 19.9	33	24	72
above 20.0	20	19	95

*Data from Lund, L.[69]

Table 15–5. Dose and Serum Levels of Phenytoin in Patients with Gingival Hyperplasia*

Grade of hyperplasia	No. of patients	Dose (mg/kg)/day	Phenytoin concentration (μg/ml)
0	75	3.0	3.0
I	26	3.4	3.8
II	99	4.4	9.5
III	27	5.7	18.4

*Data from Kapur, R.N., et al.[71]

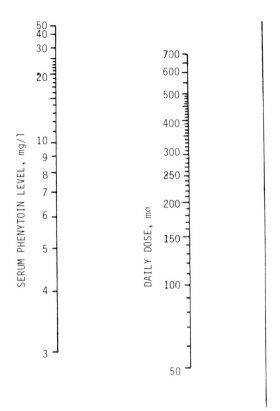

Fig. 15–4. Nomogram for predicting the daily dose of phenytoin required to achieve a desired serum level when a reliable serum level on a given daily dose is known. A line is drawn connecting the observed serum level (left-hand scale) with the administered dose (center scale) and extended to the right-hand vertical line. From this point of intersection, another line is drawn to the desired serum level (left-hand scale). The dose needed to produce this level is read off the center scale. (From Rambeck, B., et al.: Predicting phenytoin dose. A revised nomogram. Ther. Drug Monit., *1*:325, 1979.)

bring the levels within the therapeutic concentration range. The same problem occurs when the dosage of phenytoin is reduced; in most patients, halving the dose will result in a greater than 50% decrease in serum phenytoin levels.

Many schemes have been proposed to estimate the change in phenytoin dosage required to bring the serum level to the therapeutic range once a reliable serum concentration on a given daily dose of phenytoin has been determined.[67,72–74] One nomogram is shown in Figure 15–4. Richens proposes that all patients be started on a small dose of phenytoin, 200 mg/day, and that the steady-state serum concentration of phenytoin be determined after 2 to 3 weeks.[76] If the drug level and clinical signs

indicate a need for dosage change, this can be carried out by means of the nomogram in Figure 15–4.

All of the schemes proposed to adjust phenytoin dosage during therapy are imperfect.[72,73] Individual predictions may err on the high or low side; nevertheless, most seem to give better results than clinical judgment alone.

Of all the drugs for which therapeutic drug concentration monitoring has been advocated, phenytoin is the most compelling. Phenytoin is also one of a small number of drugs that is considered suitable for therapeutic monitoring in saliva. Many investigators have reported strong correlations between phenytoin concentrations in saliva and plasma.[63] In general, the average ratio of saliva to plasma concentrations is about 0.1, consistent with the fact that only about 10% of phenytoin concentration in plasma is not bound to plasma proteins. The therapeutic concentration range for phenytoin in saliva is 1 to 2 μg/ml. The main indications for using saliva phenytoin concentrations in therapeutic drug monitoring are in children and in patients with renal failure or hypoalbuminemia, where plasma protein binding is impaired so that total plasma concentration gives a false estimate of free drug concentration unless binding is determined.

The measurement of free rather than total phenytoin concentration is sometimes justified. Some hospitals have made available a routine monitoring service for determining free phenytoin levels in plasma. Peterson et al.[77] have examined the value of such services. Free phenytoin levels were determined when specifically requested by a physician, or when a determination of total phenytoin levels was requested but the patient's chart suggested the possibility of impaired plasma protein binding.

The percentage of free phenytoin in plasma in the study population ranged from 9 to 29%, with a median value of 14%. Total phenytoin concentration was in the therapeutic range (10 to 20 μg/ml) in only 30% of the patients, and below the range in more than half of the patients. On the other hand, because of the large number of patients demonstrating impaired binding of phenytoin, free levels were within the therapeutic range in about half of the cases and above the range in about 20% of the patients. The investigators concluded that the "use of the total phenytoin assay indicated that most patients needed increases in dosage, whereas the free phenytoin assay level showed that most patients probably required no alteration in dosage or even a reduction."

The variability in plasma protein binding of phenytoin reported by Peterson and his colleagues is large; other investigators have found less variability, particularly in patients who are not hospitalized. For example, Rimmer et al.[78] observed that the percentage of free phenytoin in plasma in epileptic patients attending an outpatient clinic ranged from 12 to 18%.

These investigators concluded that "there appears to be very little variability in protein binding of phenytoin in epileptic patients and thus total plasma phenytoin concentration closely reflects the free (unbound) drug concentration. Routine estimation of free plasma phenytoin concentration is therefore unnecessary and should be reserved for those patients where alteration in binding is likely."

In another study, Theodore et al.[79] examined the relationship between total or free phenytoin levels and adverse effects in patients with seizure disorders. They also found relatively little variability in phenytoin binding to plasma protein. They reported a significant correlation ($r = 0.84$) between free and total phenytoin concentration. No relationship was found between the daily dose of phenytoin and drug toxicity, but significant partial correlations with adverse effects were seen for total ($r = 0.49$) and free ($r = 0.59$) phenytoin.

These investigators concluded that "free phenytoin measurements were only marginally better predictors of drug toxicity than were total plasma phenytoin levels. Therefore we suggest that neither clinical nor pharmacological considerations warrant routine monitoring of free phenytoin levels."

It is usually assumed that the type of epileptic seizure plays little or no role in defining the therapeutic concentration range for phenytoin or other anticonvulsants. Schmidt et al.[80] examined this assumption by monitoring plasma concentration of phenytoin in patients with various types of epileptic seizures. The mean plasma concentration needed for complete control of tonic-clonic seizures alone was 14 μg/ml, whereas a mean level of 23 μg/ml was necessary to control simple or complex partial seizures alone or together with tonic-clonic seizures. A similar trend was observed in patients treated with phenobarbital and with carbamazepine.

The investigators concluded that "higher plasma concentrations of phenytoin, phenobarbital, and carbamazepine are necessary for control in epilepsy with simple or complex partial seizures compared with epilepsy with tonic-clonic seizures alone. The efficacy of plasma concentrations of phenytoin, phenobarbital, and carbamazepine varies with the type of seizure."

Almost since the beginning of therapeutic drug monitoring, there has been concern that pharmacists or physicians would attempt to treat the blood level rather than the disease. For example, should the dose of an anticonvulsant be increased in patients with epilepsy who were free of seizures but had subtherapeutic serum levels? An attempt to answer this question was described by Woo et al.,[81] who randomized patients with tonic-clonic seizures treated with monotherapy (phenytoin or phenobarbital) and seizure-free for at least 3 mos to two groups, group one in which the dose and the level were maintained in the subtherapeutic range, and group two in which the dose was increased until the level was in the therapeutic range.

Over a period of 24 mos, there were no significant differences between the two study groups in the occurrence of seizures, but patients in group two had an increased incidence of neurotoxic side effects from the increased dose. The investigators concluded that "it is unnecessary to increase the dose of the antiepileptic drug despite a subtherapeutic serum concentration in relatively well-stabilized patients . . . "

Valproic Acid. This drug has a broad spectrum of antiepileptic activity; there is evidence that it acts by inhibiting enzymes involved in the degradation of gamma-aminobutyric acid (GABA) in the CNS.

Valproic acid is highly bound to plasma proteins, but binding is concentration-dependent; its volume of distribution may vary from 0.1 to 0.5 L/kg. Valproate is essentially eliminated by metabolism. The clearance (5 to 30 ml/hr per kg) and half-life (4 to 17 hr) of valproic acid are variable. Children appear to eliminate the drug more rapidly than adults. Phenytoin, phenobarbital, primidone, and carbamazepine significantly increase the clearance of valproic acid.

Optimal daily dosage of valproate may vary from 15 to 100 mg/kg; the dosing interval may vary from 6 to 24 hr. Children may require higher and more frequent dosage than adults. Patients on other anticonvulsant drugs may require larger doses than patients on valproic acid alone. Patients with severe hepatic disease require smaller than average doses.

The clinical pharmacokinetics of valproic acid has been reviewed by Gugler and von Unruh[82] and the use of plasma levels to guide valproate therapy by Cloyd and Leppik.[83] Data from several studies suggest that adequate seizure control requires serum valproate levels of at least 40 to 50 μg/ml.

The relationship between adverse effects and serum levels is not clear, but hepatotoxicity has been associated with serum valproic acid levels above 100 μg/ml. The most common side effects of valproate therapy, nausea, vomiting, and drowsiness, do not seem to be related to serum valproate levels. The therapeutic concentration range of valproic acid is considered to be 50 to 100 μg/ml.

Because the binding of valproic acid is variable, many investigators believe it would be more useful to monitor free rather than total drug concentrations in plasma.[84] Unfortunately, the correlation between saliva and total or free plasma valproate levels is poor. Other methods to determine free drug concentration in plasma are available but poorly validated and in limited use.

The development of ultrafiltration techniques has facilitated the determination of free drug concentration in serum. These advances prompted Froscher et al.[64] to reevaluate the clinical significance of free level monitoring of valproic acid. In keeping with the results of other studies, they found a close correlation between free and total levels of valproate and therefore no better correlation between free valproic acid and clinical endpoints than between total drug levels and the same endpoints.

Anti-Inflammatory Drugs

A large number of nonsteroidal anti-inflammatory and analgesic drugs are now available. All are indicated for the treatment of acute and chronic rheumatoid arthritis and osteoarthritis. Naproxen, tolmetin, and salicylate are also indicated for juvenile arthritis. The newer drugs seem to be similar in mechanism of pharmacologic effect to salicylate but most are considered more potent or less toxic than aspirin. Knowledge of pharmacokinetic characteristics has played a small role in therapy with these drugs because therapeutic outcome is difficult to assess and no clear concentration-response relationship has been defined. The half-life of these drugs is believed to be related to duration of effect; naproxen, which has a longer half-life than ibuprofen (13 hr vs 2 hr), is given twice a day rather than 3 or 4 times a day; piroxicam, with a still longer half-life is given once a day. Only in the

case of salicylate has there been interest in monitoring serum drug concentrations during therapy; this interest is largely directed at avoiding side effects.

Salicylate. Salicylate is the active anti-inflammatory component of many drugs including aspirin, choline salicylate, choline and magnesium salicylates, magnesium salicylate, salsalate (salicylsalicylic acid), and sodium salicylate. Pharmacologically significant plasma levels of salicylate are also found in patients taking antidiarrheal mixtures containing bismuth subsalicylate.

At low therapeutic salicylate concentrations in plasma (10 mg/dl) about 90% is bound, whereas at high concentrations (40 mg/dl) only about 75% is bound to plasma proteins. Accordingly, the apparent volume of distribution of salicylate is concentration-dependent.

Only about 10% of a small dose of salicylate (300 mg or less) is excreted unchanged in the urine, but the fraction excreted is greater when higher doses are given because the metabolism of salicylate is capacity-limited. Accordingly, the apparent half-life of salicylate increases with dose and plasma concentration.

The renal excretion of high levels of salicylate is dependent on urine pH. Larger doses are needed for a patient with alkaline urine than for a patient with acid urine to achieve the same plasma levels of salicylate.

The monitoring of plasma concentrations of salicylate has been recently reviewed.[85,86] It can be seen in Figure 15–5 that plasma salicylate concentrations correlate with clinical and adverse effects of the drug; there is considerable overlap, however, between the effective concentration region and the region of concentration associated with adverse effects and toxicity. Assessment of a therapeutic concentration range for salicylate is complicated by concentration-dependent changes in plasma binding, changes in albumin levels, and concomitant drug therapy.

Some physicians determine maximum tolerated salicylate doses by gradually increasing the amount given until tinnitus is observed, then decreasing the daily dosage by 600 mg. In one study, 67 patients with rheumatoid arthritis were given gradually increasing doses of buffered aspirin until tinnitus was noted.[87] In 52 patients experiencing tinnitus, the average serum salicylate was 29.5 mg/dl (range 19.6 to 45.8). The majority of patients noted tinnitus when taking a daily dose of 4.5 to 7.2 g of

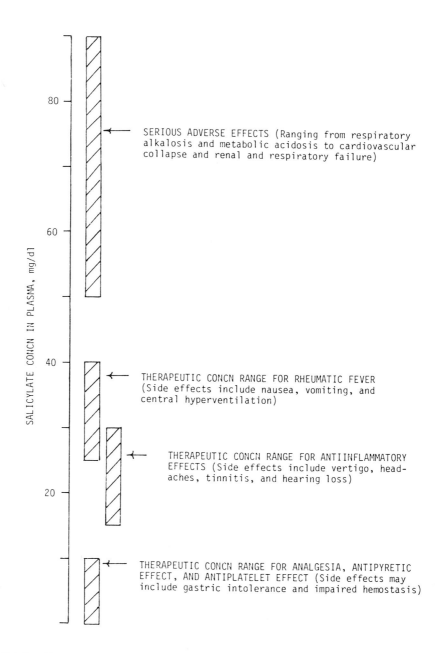

Fig. 15—5. Relationships between plasma salicylate concentrations, effects, and complications. (Data from Dromgoole, S.H., and Furst, D.E.[87])

aspirin (15 to 24 tablets per day), but some patients experienced tinnitus at doses as low as 3.6 g/day and as high as 10.8 g/day. Despite high daily doses, 15 patients did not note tinnitus. The average serum salicylate concentration in this group was 43.8 mg/dl (range 31 to 67.7). All 15 patients had pre-existing impaired hearing.

Reversible bilateral hearing loss is known to occur at serum salicylate levels exceeding 30 mg/dl. Patients with normal hearing, however, apparently experience tinnitus before any significant salicylate-induced hearing loss occurs. On the other hand, patients with pre-existing hearing loss apparently cannot hear the high-tone tinnitus characteristic of salicylate ototoxicity. These patients are at risk if salicylate therapy is guided by the clinical adage, ''Push to tinnitus, then back off slightly.''

It has been recommended that if there is any suggestion on history or physical examination of a hearing loss, serum salicylate levels rather than tinnitus should be used to guide salicylate dosage.[87] Moreover, any patient over the age of 50 yr who does not note tinnitus on a daily dose of 6 g of aspirin should have his serum salicylate level determined.

Although aspirin and other salicylate-containing compounds continue to be useful drugs, the dwindling incidence of rheumatic fever and the increasing use of alternative nonsteroidal anti-inflammatory drugs in the treatment of arthritic disease has resulted in far fewer indications for using high doses of salicylate and for measurement of plasma salicylate concentrations.

Indomethacin. In addition to its use in rheumatoid arthritis, indomethacin is also approved as an alternative to surgery in newborns with patent ductus arteriosus (PDA). Reasoning that inadequate blood levels of indomethacin may play a role in infants failing to respond to the drug, Brash et al.[88] studied the pharmacokinetics of iv indomethacin in 35 premature infants with symptomatic PDA.

Most infants responded to indomethacin with ductus constriction. Lack of efficacy in 6 patients was associated with a significantly higher clearance of indomethacin and a shorter half-life. Indomethacin levels in plasma less than 250 ng/ml at 24 hr after an iv dose were observed in 6 of 7 unsuccessful infusions. In contrast, 32 of 38 successful infusions resulted in indomethacin levels above 250 ng/ml at 24 hr.

Some reports have suggested that the ductus in older infants is less likely to respond to indomethacin. This does not appear to be a case of true resistance. The clearance of indomethacin increases with age and rapid clearance is a critical factor in treatment failure.

Cardiac Glycosides

Cardiac glycoside preparations officially recognized in the United States include powdered digitalis, digitoxin, digoxin, and deslanoside. They are indicated in the treatment of CHF and in the management of certain arrhythmias. Deslanoside is approved only for intravenous administration. Both intravenous and oral forms of digoxin are available. Digoxin is the most widely used form of digitalis.

All the cardiac glycosides are potent and have narrow therapeutic indices. Toxic manifestations include gastrointestinal and CNS symptoms and disturbances of cardiac rhythm. The use of individualized dosage and therapeutic drug concentration monitoring has been considered for digoxin and digitoxin.

Digoxin. One survey has shown that 22% of all medical patients receive digoxin; about 18% of these patients experience one or more side effects.[89] Another study indicates a 23% incidence of digoxin toxicity in treated patients.[90] The mortality rate in toxic patients is 40%, whereas the mortality rate in nontoxic patients is only 17%. The use of digoxin has decreased in recent years because of changes in treatment and availability of other drugs, but it remains a widely used drug. The incidence of digitalis toxicity has also decreased during the past decade because of a better understanding of the pharmacokinetic and pharmacologic characteristics of digoxin.

Oral digoxin is incompletely absorbed; absorption may be erratic in certain patients and with certain dosage forms. Bioavailability is considered to be a factor contributing to interpatient variability in clinical response. Digoxin is poorly bound to plasma proteins, only to the extent of about 25% and has a large apparent volume of distribution (500 to 600 L). The volume of distribution of digoxin is 30 to 50% smaller in patients with renal failure. Digoxin distributes slowly; 8 to 12 hr may be required to reach equilibration between blood and tissues. In patients with normal renal function, the half-life of digoxin varies from 32 to 48 hr. About 50 to 70% of an intravenous dose is excreted unchanged in the urine; the balance is subject to metabolism and biliary excretion.

Rapid digitalization calls for a loading dose, usually 1.0 to 1.5 mg divided into 2 or more doses given every 6 to 8 hr, followed by daily maintenance doses, usually 0.125 to 0.5 mg once a day. Smaller loading doses may be appropriate in patients with severe renal failure because of a reduced apparent volume of distribution. Dosage calculations for digoxin and other digitalis glycosides should be based on ideal rather than total body weight because these drugs are not taken up by adipose tissue. Larger loading and maintenance doses per kg body weight are used in infants and children up to 10 years of age. Maintenance dosage should be reduced in patients with impaired renal function and may require reduction in the elderly. Digoxin should be administered cautiously to certain patients who seem more sensitive to the effects of the drug (e.g., patients with low serum potassium).

More than 50 studies on the relationship between serum digoxin concentration and digoxin toxicity have been reported.[91] Based on these investigations the therapeutic serum digoxin concentration range is considered to be 0.5 to 2.5 ng/ml. Maintenance of serum digoxin levels between 1.0 and 1.5 ng/ml during therapy is considered ideal by some investigators. Digoxin toxicity is likely if serum levels are greater than 3 ng/ml and unlikely if the levels are less than 1 ng/ml. Similar guidelines apply to infants and young children, but infants tolerate higher serum digoxin concentrations than adults do without developing signs of digitalis toxicity.[92]

One of the earliest studies examining the relationship between digoxin toxicity and serum levels found that patients with cardiac rhythm disturbances from digoxin intoxication tended to be older and to have diminished renal function compared to a nontoxic group.[93] Despite comparable mean daily digoxin doses, intoxicated patients had a mean serum digoxin concentration of 3.7 ng/ml, whereas nontoxic patients had a mean level of 1.4 ng/ml. Of the patients with no evidence of toxicity, 90% had serum digoxin concentrations of 2.0 ng/ml or less; 87% of the toxic group had levels above 2.0 ng/ml.

In another study, serum digoxin concentrations were determined in 143 patients who were divided into 4 groups on the basis of clinical considerations, as follows: I, not toxic but in CHF (subtherapeutic); II, not toxic and not in CHF (therapeutic); III, possibly toxic; IV, definitely toxic.[94] Significant differences between the means were found among the different groups for the following variables: digoxin level, dose per kg body weight, and creatinine clearance. These data are shown in Table 15–6. Of all the independent variables, digoxin level was the best predictor of both subtherapeutic and toxic patients.

The two studies cited above and, in fact, the majority of studies have demonstrated that there is a significant difference between the mean values of serum digoxin concentration in patients with and without digitalis toxicity, but also that there is a variable overlap between the two groups. Toxicity has been observed in some patients with serum digoxin levels less than 1.5 ng/ml; other patients have tolerated levels exceeding 3 ng/ml with no manifestations of digitalis toxicity. Toxicity at low serum levels of digoxin has frequently but not always been associated with hypokalemia or myxedema. The absence of toxicity with apparently high serum levels of digoxin has sometimes been the result of determining digoxin concentration during the distributive rather than the postdistributive phase of the drug concentration versus time curve; blood for serum digoxin level determinations

Table 15–6. Laboratory Data for Patients Receiving Digoxin*†

Variable	Patient group			
	Subtherapeutic	Therapeutic	Possibly toxic	Definitely toxic
Weight (kg)	72.7	65.3	64.0	60.7
Creatinine clearance (ml/min)	62.4	60.9	47.2	41.5
Dose (mg/day)	0.234	0.260	0.292	0.316
Digoxin level (ng/ml)	0.95	1.49	2.53	3.32
Dose (ng/kg)	0.003	0.004	0.005	0.005

*Any two mean values not underscored by the same line are significantly different at the 95% level.
†Data from Huffman, D.H., et al.[94]

should be drawn at steady state, 12 to 24 hr after the daily dose.

Several commentaries have stressed the pitfalls in the interpretation of serum digoxin concentrations.[95–97] Another commentary, presenting a more balanced view, concludes that although not every patient receiving digoxin requires the measurement of a blood level, the serum digoxin level is a useful clinical tool when used with good judgment.[98]

Interest exists in using patient and population parameters to individualize the initial dosage regimen of digoxin, but these efforts have met with only limited success. Several studies have suggested that little of the variability in serum digoxin concentrations can be accounted for by dose, age, body weight, or renal function.[99–101] Nevertheless, these considerations may augment clinical judgment in patients with renal failure and in elderly patients.

Nicholson and co-workers have described a simple method for prescribing digoxin based on clinical information and patient characteristics.[102] Using this method, they found that about 72% of all patients are expected to achieve mean steady-state serum digoxin concentrations within the therapeutic range, 7% above the range, and 21% below. A sophisticated computer method for forecasting the dosage required to obtain desired serum digoxin levels based on patient characteristics and early determinations of serum digoxin concentrations has also been described.[103]

Snidero et al.[104] have documented the overuse of digoxin serum assays for ambulatory patients in Italy. These results probably reflect the general overuse of digoxin therapeutic drug monitoring in most western countries. Hallworth and Brodie[105] have clearly stated that "routine serum digoxin measurement is not necessary if the patient is clinically stable and renal function is unaltered."

These investigators examined nearly 1600 requests for digoxin measurement in 886 patients over a 1-year period in a general hospital in Glasgow. In a subset of 334 patients who had more than one blood sample assayed for digoxin, 51.5% were within the therapeutic range at the first measure compared with 56.3% at the last measure. These results cast doubt on whether measurements had influenced patient management.

Digitoxin. Digitoxin is far less prescribed in the United States than digoxin, but it is an important drug in other parts of the world. It has a much longer half-life than digoxin (120 to 216 hr) and

is largely metabolized. Digitoxin may be a more useful drug than digoxin in patients with impaired renal function because dosage adjustments are unnecessary. Like digoxin, digitoxin is usually given as a divided loading dose, followed by daily maintenance doses.

The therapeutic serum digitoxin concentration range is considered to be 15 to 25 ng/ml; concentrations exceeding 35 to 40 ng/ml are frequently associated with adverse effects.[106] As with digoxin, there is considerable variation and overlap in serum digitoxin concentrations associated with toxicity and therapeutic response.

Cyclosporine

Cyclosporine is a selective immunosuppressant that has revolutionized organ transplantation. Comprehensive reviews of this agent are available.[107,108] Several excellent commentaries specifically concerned with therapeutic drug monitoring have also been published.[109–112] Yee and Kennedy[107] have presented an algorithm for dosing cyclosporine based on measurements of trough concentrations at steady state. These guidelines are helpful in some patients but there is no general consensus as to how to apply cyclosporine concentration data to patient care. Some success has been reported in linking cyclosporine serum levels to the prevention of graft-versus-host disease, a major cause of morbidity and mortality after bone marrow transplantation.[113]

Methotrexate

The clearance of methotrexate varies widely in children; a 7-fold difference has been reported in one study.[114] In another study, investigators found a 50 to 100% greater probability of clinical relapse in children with acute lymphocytic leukemia (ALL) in remission who rapidly cleared methotrexate, compared with those patients who eliminated methotrexate more slowly.[115]

More recently, Evans et al.[116] reported the results of their efforts to determine whether an optimal range of serum concentrations of methotrexate could be identified for patients with ALL receiving high-dose methotrexate therapy. The mean systemic clearance of methotrexate was 78 ml/min but varied considerably. Median steady-state levels in individual patients ranged from about 9 to 24 μM.

During a follow-up period that averaged 3.5 years from diagnosis, there were 34 relapses among the 108 patients, about two-thirds of which were hematologic relapses. Probability analysis revealed that patients with median steady-state serum levels below 16 μM were about 3 times more likely to have a relapse of any kind during therapy and 7 times more likely to have a hematologic relapse than those with concentrations above 16 μM. Patients with low methotrexate concentrations were also more likely to have an early relapse.

The investigators concluded that "the results of this study indicate that the relative exposure to methotrexate . . . can have a significant influence on the probability of relapse in children with acute lymphocytic leukemia." They also noted that "although this study has not established a 'therapeutic' serum concentration or dosage of methotrexate in standard-risk ALL, we have identified a concentration that is more frequently associated with therapeutic failure (i.e., a 'subtherapeutic' range)."

Metoclopramide

Metoclopramide is a dopamine antagonist that stimulates upper gastrointestinal motility and enhances gastric emptying. Metoclopramide also has antiemetic activity and is used to treat nausea and vomiting associated with cancer chemotherapy, particularly with cisplatin.

To better understand and improve the effectiveness of metoclopramide for cisplatin-induced emesis, Meyer et al.[117] studied the relationship between serum metoclopramide levels and control of nausea and vomiting in patients with cancer. All patients received metoclopramide, 2 mg/kg intravenously every 2 hours for a total of 4 doses starting one-half hr before cisplatin was given.

Although the dose of metoclopramide was adjusted for body weight, serum levels varied a great deal, ranging from 200 to 2000 ng/ml. A clear relationship between metoclopramide concentration and antiemetic response emerged. Serum levels greater than 850 ng/ml immediately before the third dose of metoclopramide were associated with control of emesis in 78% of the patients and partial control in 18%. Control of emesis was not observed in any patient with serum levels of metoclopramide less than 850 ng/ml, but partial control was established in 42% of these patients. Increasing the dose of metoclopramide for nonresponders produced higher metoclopramide levels and improved clinical response in 4 of 5 patients. The investigators recommended that "if an assay for serum metoclopramide is available, we suggest that a level greater than 850 ng/ml will be needed just before the third dose for most patients."

Oral Anticoagulants

The oral anticoagulants include the coumarin derivatives, dicoumarol, phenprocoumon, and warfarin, and the indanedione derivatives, anisindione and phenindione. In the United States, warfarin is used almost exclusively. Phenprocoumon is a drug of choice in the United Kingdom and other parts of the world. The dosage of these drugs is always individualized according to prothrombin-time determinations. The usual therapeutic goal is to prolong prothrombin time by 1.5 to 2.5 times the control value or to reduce prothrombin activity to 15 to 35% of normal.

A higher incidence of bleeding in patients treated with warfarin in the U.S. than those treated in the UK prompted a major reexamination of anticoagulant targets. According to Hirsch,[118] "on the basis of current evidence, it would be reasonable to aim for a therapeutic range of 1.3 to 1.4 times control (equivalent to a prothrombin time of 14 to 17 seconds) with the rabbit-brain thromboplastin in common use in North America . . . " He also noted that "patients with venous thrombosis can be treated effectively and more safely by using a therapeutic range . . . of 1.3 to 1.4 times the control value rather than the formerly recommended range of 2.0 to 2.5 times control."

There are large interindividual differences in the clinical response to oral anticoagulants. The usual adult dose of warfarin varies from 2 to 10 mg a day; that of phenprocoumon from 0.75 to 6 mg a day. These differences are the result of variation in receptor affinity, in the availability of vitamin K and vitamin K-dependent clotting factors, and in the pharmacokinetics of the drug.[119–121]

Because of the long half-life of warfarin, treatment is usually started with a loading dose, typically 10 to 15 mg a day for 2 to 4 days. Thereafter, the daily maintenance dose is adjusted on a trial-and-error basis until the desired effect on blood coagulation has been achieved. Dosage titration is time consuming; until the optimum dosage is found, the patient is at risk either from the condition for which the anticoagulant is prescribed or from hemorrhage.

Routledge and co-workers investigated the possibility that a patient's response to a loading dose of warfarin might be used to predict his required daily maintenance dose.[122] They observed a strong correlation (r = 0.90) between the maintenance dose needed to achieve a thrombotest of 8 to 12%

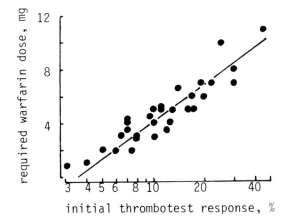

Fig. 15–6. Relationship between thrombotest response to an initial loading dose of warfarin (10 mg/day for 3 days) and the daily maintenance warfarin dose required to achieve anticoagulation at a thrombotest of 8 to 12%. (Data from Routledge, P.A., et al.[122])

and the log of the patient's thrombotest values 64 to 66 hr after the start of the warfarin loading regimen (Fig. 15–6). The theoretical basis for this relationship has been considered by Sawyer.[123] The relationship seems strong enough to have practical value in predicting warfarin dosage requirements in individual patients.

Psychotropic Drugs

Drugs used in the treatment of psychiatric disorders are often collectively called psychoactive or psychotropic agents. Antipsychotic or neuroleptic agents, like the phenothiazines, thioxanthenes, or butyrophenones, are used to treat psychoses, the most severe psychiatric illnesses; they have beneficial effects on mood and thought, but also carry the risk of neurotoxic effects that mimic neurologic diseases. Mood-stabilizing drugs (lithium salts) and mood elevating drugs (antidepressants) are used to treat affective disorders. Antianxiety-sedative agents, particularly the benzodiazepines, are used to treat anxiety states.

Although individualized dosage for the benzodiazepines is not common this is not the case for other psychotropic drugs. Among the antipsychotic agents, chlorpromazine dosage varies from 20 to 1000 mg a day and haloperidol dosage varies from 1 to 100 mg a day. The usual adult dose of amitriptyline is 50 to 300 mg a day. Dosage adjustments of these drugs are made on the basis of psychiatric response and adverse effects; pharmacokinetic factors or serum drug concentration

measurements are rarely considered.[124] The adjustment of lithium dosage is an exception.

Many investigators have examined the relationship between serum levels of tricyclic antidepressants and clinical response. Whether serum drug concentration monitoring during tricyclic antidepressant therapy is worthwhile for some patients remains controversial. The application of pharmacokinetic principles to this large and diverse class of drugs has been limited by serum concentrations so low they are difficult to measure, active metabolites, indefinite clinical endpoints, and an incomplete understanding of pharmacologic mechanisms.

Antipsychotic Drugs. Dahl[125] and Sramek et al.[126] have presented reviews concerning the clinical utility of plasma level monitoring of antipsychotic drugs. Dahl noted that there have been some reports suggesting a relationship between therapeutic response and antipsychotic drug 'concentration' determined by means of a chemically nonspecific radioreceptor assay (RRA) that measures dopamine receptor-blocking activity in plasma. He pointed out, however, that most studies "have failed to demonstrate such a relationship, and the RRA does not seem to provide the generally useful tool for plasma concentration monitoring of antipsychotic drugs that was hoped for initially."

Other studies, using chemically specific assay methods, have, in most cases, also failed to demonstrate useful correlations. Among other problems, this approach does not consider the contribution of active metabolites to pharmacologic effect, which appears to be prevalent following the administration of most antipsychotic drugs.

According to Dahl, "reasonably controlled studies of plasma concentration-response relationships using randomly allocated, fixed dosages of chlorpromazine, fluphenazine, haloperidol, perphenazine, sulpiride, thioridazone, and thiothixene have been published but often involve relatively few patients . . . Plasma level monitoring of thioridazine and its metabolites . . . appears to have no clinical value . . .

"Non-responders and good responders to chlorpromazine treatment . . . have plasma drug concentrations in the same range . . . Therapeutic plasma haloperidol concentrations . . . in the range of 5 to 20 μg/L have been reported by some investigators, but others have found no such relationship . . . Unfortunately, there is no evidence that plasma concentration monitoring of antipsychotic drugs may significantly reduce the incidence of tardive dyskinesia."[125]

Sramek et al.[126] pointed out that "the most impressive evidence to date for the presence of a neuroleptic therapeutic window is for haloperidol." This may relate to the relatively simple metabolic pathway of this drug compared with other antipsychotic agents. Volavka and Cooper[127] cautioned that "a therapeutic window for haloperidol may exist, but the evidence for it is inconsistent."

Virtually all studies agree that a haloperidol level of at least 5 ng/ml is required for efficacy in responsive patients. Some studies, however, suggest a need for levels of at least 20 ng/ml. One study suggested that benefit would derive with haloperidol levels as high as 50 ng/ml, whereas others report no benefit at levels above 15 ng/ml.[127] Perry et al.[128] recently reported that a serum haloperidol concentration in the range of 9 to 15 ng/ml was associated with a clinically important decrease in the rating scale used to evaluate the severity of schizophrenia. "Serum concentrations above this limit do not appear to either decrease or increase the probability of response."

Lithium. Lithium, in the form of lithium carbonate or lithium citrate, is an important drug for the treatment of mania and for the prevention of recurrent attacks of manic-depressive illness. Almost all of an oral dose of lithium is eliminated in the urine. The half-life of lithium is variable, averaging about 24 hr in patients with normal renal function. Because lithium distributes slowly from the blood and because lithium toxicity can occur with doses at or near therapeutic levels the daily dosage must be subdivided. Lithium carbonate capsules or tablets are usually given 3 times a day; an extended-release tablet is available for twice-a-day dosage.

The daily dosage of lithium varies widely depending on the severity of the disorder, the patient's response, and the ability to excrete lithium; a range of 150 to 3500 mg of lithium carbonate a day has been reported.[129] A more typical dosage range for responsive patients with normal renal function is 900- to 1800-mg lithium carbonate a day.

Determination of serum lithium concentration is a routine part of lithium therapy; it may be performed as often as twice a week during the acute phase of treatment until the clinical condition of the patient is stabilized. Effective serum levels during the acute manic phase are considered to be 1.0

Table 15–7. Dosages Required to Achieve a Steady-State Serum Lithium Level of 0.6 to 1.2 meq/L Based on the Serum Level of Lithium 24 hr after a Single Loading Dose of 600 mg Lithium Carbonate*

Initial serum level	Dosage required (mg)
<0.05	1200, three times a day
0.05 to 0.09	900, three times a day
0.10 to 0.14	600, three times a day
0.15 to 0.19	300, four times a day
0.20 to 0.23	300, three times a day
0.24 to 0.30	300, twice a day
>0.30	300, twice a day (with caution)

*Data from Cooper, Bergner, and Simpson.[131]

to 1.5 meq per L; recommended maintenance serum lithium concentrations are 0.6 to 1.5 meq per L. Side effects may occur at serum lithium levels below 1.5 meq per L; mild to moderate toxicity may occur at levels from 1.5 to 2.5 meq. Serum lithium concentrations above 3 meq per L are associated with serious CNS disturbances and renal toxicity.[129,130]

A predictive technique has been described that enables the estimation of a patient's lithium dosage requirement on the basis of a single blood sample collected 24 hr after the administration of a 600 mg initial dose of lithium carbonate.[131,132] The lithium dosage required to achieve a steady-state serum level of 0.6 to 1.2 meq per L based on the 24-hr serum lithium concentration after a single loading dose is shown in Table 15–7.

Recent review articles[133,134] suggest that the thinking on serum lithium monitoring has not changed in any important way. Schou,[133] in 1988, again concluded that "serum lithium monitoring is important for dosage adjustment during the start of treatment and for control after dosage changes." Lobeck,[134] who critically reviewed several methods to optimize the dose of lithium, concluded that "because of the number of factors influencing lithium disposition and the potential of these factors to change, even the best of methods would not eliminate the need routinely to monitor serum lithium concentration and clinical condition. Considering the shortcomings of the currently available methods, careful monitoring is imperative."

Cyclic Antidepressants. Several classes of drugs are useful in the pharmacologic treatment of depression. The tricyclics, including amitriptyline, desipramine, doxepin, imipramine, nortriptyline, protriptyline, and trimipramine, are the most widely used antidepressants. Maprotiline is a closely related drug but chemically has a tetracyclic ring structure. Imipramine is also used in the treatment of childhood enuresis.

The tricyclics undergo considerable presystemic hepatic metabolism after oral administration; doxepin is subject to the greatest first-pass effect and protriptyline to the least. Presystemic metabolism contributes to the large intersubject variability in blood levels of tricyclics. All of these drugs are considerably bound to plasma proteins ($> 90\%$) but have large volumes of distribution (10 to 30 L/kg) and low blood levels. The tricyclics are eliminated essentially by hepatic metabolism. Half-lives are relatively long; doxepin and imipramine have the shortest half-lives (10 to 25 hr) and protriptyline has the longest half-life (50 to 100 hr). All of these compounds produce active metabolites. Desipramine and nortriptyline are the demethylated metabolites of imipramine and amitriptyline, respectively. 2-Hydroxy imipramine, 2-hydroxy desipramine, and 10-hydroxy nortriptyline also have antidepressant activities.

Because of the long half-lives of these drugs, they may be given once a day, preferably at bedtime. Dosage of tricyclics must be individualized on the basis of clinical response and side effects; determination of serum tricyclic levels may or may not be useful in this process. Dosage probably should be reduced in the elderly because of a decrease in clearance. Patients on barbiturates and those who smoke may require a higher daily dosage.

The use of serum levels as a guide to treatment has been the subject of many review articles and commentaries.[135-140] These papers summarize and report a conflicting picture of the value of therapeutic drug concentration monitoring of tricyclic antidepressants. For example, reports on a relationship between serum concentration and clinical response have been published for imipramine, nortriptyline, amitriptyline, desipramine, doxepin, and protriptyline. Failure to observe a relationship has also been reported for all these drugs except protriptyline.[135]

A major problem with investigations on depression is the lack of definition of depression and the fact that more than one disease may be involved.[137,141] The diagnostic classification of the patient appears to be important in this context; consistent serum level-effect relationships have so far been established only in patients with endogenous depression.[140]

Table 15–8. Relationship Between Plasma Nortriptyline Concentration and Amelioration Score in Depressed Patients*

Nortriptyline concentration (ng/ml)	No. of patients	Amelioration score
<49	5	0.4
50 to 79	10	6.2
80 to 109	4	6.1
110 to 139	5	5.0
>140	5	1.2

*Data from Asberg, M., et al.[142]

The case for therapeutic drug concentration monitoring seems to be strongest for nortriptyline. Most careful investigations have concluded that there is a clinically useful relationship between plasma nortriptyline levels and therapeutic response but that the relationship is a curvilinear one. The therapeutic concentration range for nortriptyline is considered to be 50 to 150 ng/ml; generally, patients with lower or higher levels do not respond as well (Table 15–8).[142] This is unusual; ordinarily, the upper boundary of a therapeutic concentration range is related to the emergence of toxicity. With nortriptyline, the upper boundary reflects loss of efficacy rather than toxicity.

Amitriptyline has been studied in more than 300 patients, but the results are less consistent than for nortriptyline. In general, a minimum concentration of 80 to 120 ng/ml of total tricyclic antidepressant (i.e., amitriptyline plus nortriptyline) seems to be required for efficacy. An upper plasma level limit, above which the therapeutic effect is poor, has been suggested by some studies but not by others.[140]

More recently, Breyer-Pfaff et al.[143] reported the findings of a double-blind study in 29 depressed patients receiving amitriptyline 150 mg/day for 4 weeks. The severity of depression was assessed before treatment and after 2 and 4 weeks, and plasma levels of amitriptyline, nortriptyline, and 10-hydroxy nortriptyline were monitored weekly. Response, reflected by percent reduction in Hamilton Depression Rating Scale score, was better at steady-state amitriptyline + nortriptyline concentrations of 125 to 210 ng/ml than at lower or higher plasma levels. No influence of the 10-hydroxy metabolite of nortriptyline was discerned. The investigators concluded that "plasma level monitoring may be helpful when patients do not respond to conventional amitriptyline doses."

Several studies, involving small numbers of subjects, have suggested a relationship between imipramine + desipramine concentrations, up to 250 ng/ml, and therapeutic effectiveness in patients treated with imipramine. More recently, Rigal et al.[144] monitored imipramine and desipramine levels in 51 depressed inpatients treated with imipramine 4 mg/kg per day. Combined steady-state blood levels ranged from 60 to 585 ng/ml with a mean value of 271 ng/ml. No correlation was observed between the dose of imipramine and plasma concentrations.

Consistent with earlier reports, Rigal et al. found a positive correlation between the combined levels of imipramine and desipramine and effectiveness, with a leveling off at around 250 ng/ml. They also found that the imipramine/desipramine ratio was an important parameter. Of the patients responding to imipramine, 86% had ratios between 0.4 and 1.0. Conversely, most patients with a ratio below 0.4 or above 1.0 were nonresponders.

There are also conflicting reports as to the relationship of plasma levels to effectiveness in patients treated with desipramine. For example, Simpson et al.,[145] in studying patients with depression dosed with desipramine 150 mg/day, reported that desipramine levels in plasma ranged from about 10 to > 400 ng/ml in both responders and nonresponders. The results provided no support for routine monitoring of desipramine levels.

More encouraging results were reported by Nelson et al.[146] These investigators studied the relationship between desipramine plasma concentration and antidepressant response in 30 depressed inpatients treated for 3 weeks with desipramine 100 to 300 mg/day.

Eleven of the patients were evaluated as responders. These patients had a mean desipramine level of 184 ng/ml, significantly greater than that found in nonresponders (mean value, 71 ng/ml). The plasma level that best separated responders and nonresponders was 115 ng/ml. Eight of 9 patients with levels above 115 ng/ml responded to desipramine, whereas only 3 of 22 patients with levels below 115 ng/ml responded to the drug. Ten nonresponders were converted to responders by increasing daily dosage to produce desipramine levels of 125 ng/ml or above.

More recently, these investigators evaluated desipramine plasma levels and response in elderly melancholic patients.[147] Again, desipramine levels in responders (median, 126 ng/ml) were significantly higher than those in nonresponders (median, 81 ng/ml). Among elderly patients with levels above 115 ng/ml, 4 of 5 responded, and below this level, only

2 of 13 responded. Five patients not responding during the initial 3-week trial, responded when desipramine dosage was increased and the plasma levels were above 115 ng/ml.

Other antidepressants have been studied less systematically and less extensively; more information is required before drug level monitoring can be considered.

Several studies have examined the relationship between plasma tricyclic concentrations and toxicity.[135] The common side effects of the tricyclic antidepressant correlate poorly with plasma levels. The serious CNS, respiratory, and cardiovascular toxicities of tricyclics can be related to plasma concentration but are seen only at levels far above those found with therapeutic dosage regimens. Measurement of plasma tricyclic concentrations may be useful following overdosage. Levels of 1000 ng/ml or greater have been used to define a serious overdosage.

Thousands of people in the U.S. poison themselves each year with tricyclic antidepressant drugs. Acute overdoses with antidepressants account for more than one-third of all poison-related admissions to intensive care units. Seizures, ventricular arrhythmias, and death are the most serious sequelae.

It is generally held that seizures and arrhythmias occur most frequently when the combined serum concentration of the antidepressant and its major metabolite exceeds 1000 ng/ml. It is also held that this combined level is reflected in a QRS duration of 100 msec or longer on routine electrocardiography. With this construct in mind, Boehnert and Lovejoy[148] undertook a prospective study of 49 patients presenting within 24 hours of an acute overdose of tricyclic antidepressant drugs (amitriptyline, nortriptyline, imipramine, desipramine, doxepin, and protriptyline) to determine relationships of serum drug levels, QRS duration, and the incidence of seizures and ventricular arrhythmias.

Patients were divided into two groups on the basis of QRS interval: 13 patients (Group A) had a duration of less than 100 msec and 36 patients (Group B) had a QRS duration of 100 msec or longer. There were no deaths in either group and there were no seizures or ventricular arrhythmias in Group A, but 12 patients in Group B had seizures and 5 had ventricular arrhythmias. Patients had a first seizure or arrhythmia within 6 hours of their overdose or not at all. No patient had seizures or arrhythmias more than 24 hours after ingestion.

Consistent with the more serious overdose situation in Group B, mean serum antidepressant levels were about twice as large in group B as in Group A, 1473 vs 792 ng/ml.

Although the difference in maximum serum drug levels between the groups was statistically significant, the range of values in each group was considerable. Two patients in Group A had serum levels greater than 1000 ng/ml, and 11 patients in Group B had serum levels below 1000 ng/ml. There was no statistically significant association between serum antidepressant levels and the occurrence of seizures or arrhythmias when 1000 ng/ml was used as a cutoff point.

The investigators concluded that "the fact that such a simple bedside procedure—electrocardiography—can predict the likelihood of both seizures and ventricular arrhythmias in acute tricyclic antidepressant overdose is noteworthy. The facts that the electrocardiogram is more accurate and its results are more rapidly available than serum drug measurements make it an invaluable tool in assessing the clinical risk in acute antidepressant overdose."

Some investigators strongly advocate the monitoring of serum nortriptyline or serum amitriptyline plus nortriptyline levels in selected patients during therapy; others are more cautious; still others contend that the costs of these tests outweigh their value. Burrows and co-workers concluded that until further studies have been carried out, "routine monitoring of plasma levels of tricyclic antidepressant is not warranted. The majority of patients (70 to 80%) respond satisfactorily to a standard dose of 150 mg/day of the commonly prescribed tricyclics. The cost of plasma assay is still rather expensive and the dangers of relying on a 'magical' if not inaccurate plasma level measurement, rather than clinical judgment, is still real."[149]

Gram and his colleagues advocate a different position.[140] They note that "there is a solid rationale for using drug level monitoring as a guide for dose regulation in tricyclic antidepressant treatment." They also point out that "drug level monitoring cannot replace diagnostic evaluation and clinical control of the patients but it should be considered as a significant addition to the treatment procedure in order to enhance efficacy and safety." Further investigations, better diagnostic classification and evaluation of outcome, and simpler methods of drug analysis are required before a con-

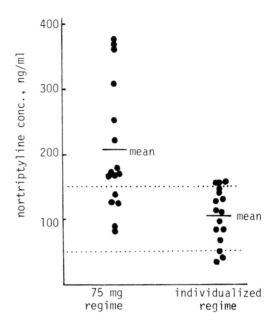

Fig. 15–7. Comparison of steady-state nortriptyline concentrations in plasma from patients who received 75 mg/day with those from patients who received an individualized dosage ranging from 20 to 90 mg/day. Horizontal lines delineate the therapeutic concentration range. (Data from Dawling, S., et al.[150])

clusion can be reached regarding the value of serum tricyclic level monitoring.

Those who hold that there is a relationship between plasma tricyclic concentrations and efficacy strongly support efforts to optimize the initial dosage regimen in order to reduce the need for drug level monitoring and reduce the time required to achieve a desirable plasma tricyclic concentration range. An approach to predict dosage at the outset of therapy is to determine the pharmacokinetics of the drug after giving a single initial or test dose to the patient. This information is then used to calculate the daily dosage and dosage interval required to achieve a desired range of plasma drug concentrations. This approach has been used with aminoglycoside antibiotics, theophylline, and phenytoin, as well as with tricyclic antidepressants.

Success in predicting steady-state concentrations of tricyclics based on the clearance determined after a single dose has been reported for imipramine, nortriptyline, and desipramine.[138] More recently, a useful correlation has been reported between nortriptyline clearance determined after a single dose and steady-state concentrations in depressed elderly patients, ranging in age from 69 to 100 yr.[150] The predicted dosage of nortriptyline required by individual patients to achieve steady-state plasma concentrations within the putative therapeutic range varied from 20 to 90 mg a day. Figure 15–7 compares predicted steady-state nortriptyline levels if all patients received a daily dose of 75 mg with levels actually achieved with individualized dosage.

Cooper and Simpson have proposed a much simpler method for predicting the dosage of tricyclics required to achieve a desired steady-state concentration.[151,152] This method is based on the relationship between clearance and the concentration of a drug in the plasma at a certain time after administration of a single test dose.[27,153] The 24-hr nortriptyline level after a 50-mg oral test dose accurately predicted steady-state plasma nortriptyline concentrations in human subjects ingesting 25 mg twice a day.[151] Similar success has been reported for imipramine, desipramine, and amitriptyline.[154–156] More recently, Sallee et al.[157] demonstrated that the combined plasma concentration of imipramine and desipramine 24 hr after a single 25-mg oral dose of imipramine correlates (r = 0.92) with steady-state imipramine + desipramine levels in children with depression receiving imipramine 3 mg/kg/day.

Methylxanthines

Caffeine, theophylline, and theobromine have been used as mild stimulants by societies through the ages. One or more of these alkaloids is found in tea, coffee, cola-flavored drinks, cocoa, and chocolate. Theobromine is rarely used as a drug today. Caffeine is widely available in the form of chewable tablets to overcome drowsiness. It is also used in the treatment of apnea in premature infants.

Theophylline and related compounds are the most important drugs in this category. Knowledge of its pharmacokinetic characteristics and the use of therapeutic drug concentration monitoring are critical factors in the resurgence of interest and use of theophylline in the U.S. for the treatment of bronchial asthma.

Theophylline. Theophylline-containing drugs include aminophylline, a 1:1 complex of theophylline and ethylenediamine containing about 80 to 85% anhydrous theophylline, oxtriphylline, a choline salt of theophylline containing 64% anhydrous theophylline, and anhydrous theophylline. Dyphylline is a different but closely related drug and is presumed to have the same mechanism of action as theophylline.

Aminophylline and oxtriphylline are more soluble than theophylline. Aminophylline is the form of theophylline used for intravenous administration. At one time it was thought that the solubility of theophylline was too low for effective oral administration. Today we recognize that theophylline is well absorbed after oral administration and the use of oral aminophylline has declined.

Theophylline competitively inhibits phosphodiesterase, the enzyme that degrades cyclic AMP. Presumably through this mechanism, theophylline relaxes smooth muscle of the bronchial airway and pulmonary blood vessels to relieve bronchospasm and increase flow rates and vital capacity.

The clinical pharmacokinetics of theophylline has been reviewed by Ogilvie.[158] Theophylline is rapidly and completely absorbed from oral solutions and conventional tablets or capsules; bioavailability problems may be encountered with prolonged-release dosage forms and rectal suppositories. Theophylline is eliminated by hepatic metabolism; less than 10% of a dose is excreted unchanged in the urine. In the neonate, theophylline is metabolized in part to caffeine; this may contribute to its efficacy in the treatment of apnea. There is evidence in children that the metabolism of theophylline is capacity-limited.

The half-life of theophylline is about 7 to 8 hr in nonsmoking, healthy adults but is considerably shorter (about 3 to 4 hr) in smokers and in children 1 to 9 years of age; these patients require higher mg/kg doses. Theophylline dosage may need to be reduced in patients with CHF or liver disease. The short half-life of theophylline in children has encouraged the widespread use of prolonged-release preparations that are given less frequently than conventional oral dosage forms.

The large variability in the dosage requirements of theophylline, its low therapeutic index and serious toxicity at excessive doses, and the good correlation between plasma theophylline levels and both efficacy and toxicity are the principal reasons that therapeutic drug concentration monitoring is recommended in certain patients.[159–161] Studies have shown that improvement of pulmonary function in asthmatic patients is related to the concentration of theophylline in the blood or plasma. For example, plasma theophylline levels of 5 μg/ml, 10 μg/ml, and 20 μg/ml were associated with average improvements in forced expiratory volume of 29%, 58%, and 85%, respectively.[162] These studies suggest that the optimal plasma theophylline concentration is about 10 to 15 μg/ml, on the average. Some patients, however, may benefit from plasma theophylline levels of 20 μg/ml or higher. Concentrations below 5 μg/ml are ordinarily considered subtherapeutic. Plasma theophylline levels of 20 to 35 μg/ml can cause adverse effects, which include anorexia, nausea, vomiting, agitation, tachycardia, and hypotension. It is generally believed that there is the potential for cardiac arrhythmias, seizures, and death with plasma theophylline concentrations exceeding 35 μg/ml. On the other hand, Aitken and Martin[163] have reported that serum levels were not useful in predicting life-threatening theophylline toxicity.

Children and perhaps other patients are at greater risk when theophylline is maintained in the high therapeutic plasma concentration range (i.e., 15 to 20 μg/ml). Relatively small changes in health status (e.g., fever or influenza) may decrease theophylline clearance, resulting in excessive blood levels and drug toxicity. Plasma concentrations of theophylline should be determined every 6 to 12 mo in children because clearance decreases with age between childhood and adulthood, and dosage may need to be reduced.

The value of monitoring theophylline concentration in saliva has also been investigated. The use of saliva as a substitute for serum or plasma theophylline determinations is usually not recommended, however, because a relatively high degree of intersubject variability in serum-to-saliva concentration ratio has been reported and, in some patients, the ratio does not remain constant. Contrary to this view, Vaughan et al.[164] have suggested that measuring theophylline concentration in passively absorbed saliva is useful for determining bioavailability of prolonged-release theophylline products in children.

Guidelines for dosing children and other patients with theophylline are available.[159,161] Koup and associates described a pharmacokinetic method for determining dosage requirements in individual patients to achieve a desired steady-state concentration of theophylline.[165] Asthmatic children were given 1 dose of theophylline (5 mg/kg); 6 hr later serum theophylline concentration was determined and used with a clearance nomogram to predict the dosage regimen needed to achieve a steady-state theophylline level of 10 μg/ml.[166] Individual daily dosage requirements ranged from 10 to 32 mg/kg. These individualized doses resulted in an average concentration of 12.0 μg/ml. Individual steady-state serum theophylline concentrations ranged from 6.2 to 16.0 μg/ml. This approach appears to be a safe and effective method for initiating theophylline dosage.

The widespread interest in monitoring theophylline therapy has prompted two manufacturers to market kits to measure serum levels in a physician's office in as little as 15 minutes. One kit, the Seralyzer-ARIS Theophylline Test, is available from Ames and the other, called Accu-Level, is available from Syntex. Unlike the Ames kit, the Accu-Level test does not require an analytical instrument and can use whole blood, eliminating the need for centrifugation and dilution. Both kits have been described in the Medical Letter.[167] The accuracy and precision of each kit has been evaluated by Vaughan et al.[168,169] Both methods are considered useful.

CONCLUSIONS

Therapeutic drug concentration monitoring as a guide to drug therapy is a small but definite part of clinical pharmacokinetics. Twenty years ago many of us hoped that it would grow in importance as our understanding of drug effects improved and better methods for drug and metabolite analysis were developed. This has not been the case.

In 1985, Sjoqvist[170] observed that "data supporting the clinical value of measuring plasma drug levels are still limited and it is not uncommon that therapeutic drug monitoring leads to 'treatment' of the plasma level rather than the patient."

In 1988, Spector et al.[171] announced that the time had come to validate the 'intuitive logic' that underlies therapeutic drug monitoring. They called for controlled, prospective clinical trials designed to test and prove the practical utility of therapeutic drug monitoring and thereby define the specific conditions and drugs for which it may prove beneficial. "The clinical utility of the target concentration strategy needs to be confirmed or the concept rejected if found useless."

In 1989, McInnes[172] observed that the value of therapeutic drug monitoring to the practicing physician is a hypothesis in need of testing. He asks that "in the light of all the uncertainties, why is therapeutic drug monitoring so widely advocated?" and concludes that "too much enthusiasm for therapeutic drug monitoring as an essential component of rational prescribing confront the practicing physician. Too little effort has gone into testing the hypothesis."

Even today, however, therapeutic drug monitoring still has its ardent defenders. Vozeh[173] evaluated the cost-effectiveness of therapeutic drug monitoring and concluded that although there is little direct evidence concerning the cost-benefit of therapeutic drug monitoring and prospective evaluation is needed, "there are sufficient data to conclude that the cost-benefit ratio can be improved by performing therapeutic drug monitoring with the appropriate expertise."

Setting this debate aside, it is undeniable that there is a need today for individualized approaches to drug therapy, be they based on serum levels, clinical response, or laboratory tests. There is considerable room for improvement in how we use the drugs available today and those that will be available in the years that lie ahead.

REFERENCES

1. Rowland, M., and Tozer, T.N.: Clinical Pharmacokinetics. Concepts and Applications. 2nd Ed., Philadelphia, Lea & Febiger, 1989.
2. Koch-Weser, J.: The serum level approach to individualization of drug dosage. Eur. J. Clin. Pharmacol., 9:1, 1975.
3. Koch-Weser, J.: Serum drug concentrations as therapeutic guides. N. Engl. J. Med., 287:227, 1972.
4. Evans, W.E., Schentag, J.J., and Jusko, W.J.L. (eds.): Applied Pharmacokinetics. Principles of Therapeutic Drug Monitoring. 2nd Ed., Spokane, Applied Therapeutics, 1986.
5. Pippenger, C.E.: Therapeutic drug monitoring: An overview. Ther. Drug Monit., 1:3, 1979.
6. Avery, G.S.: Editor's note. Clin. Pharmacokinet., 1:1, 1976.
7. Winter, M.E.: Basic Clinical Pharmacokinetics. 2nd Ed., Spokane, Applied Therapeutics, 1986.
8. Taylor, W.J., and Finn, A.L. (eds.): Individualizing Drug Therapy. Practical Applications of Drug Monitoring. Vols. 1–3. New York, Gross, Townsend, Frank, 1981.
9. Koch-Weser, J.: Serum drug concentrations in clinical perspective. Ther. Drug Monit., 3:3, 1981.
10. Richens, A., and Warrington, S.: When should plasma drug levels be monitored? Drugs, 17:488, 1979.
11. Duhme, D.W., Greenblatt, D.J., and Koch-Weser, J.: Reduction of digoxin toxicity associated with measurement of serum levels. Ann. Intern. Med., 80:516, 1974.
12. Sokolow, M., and Edgar, A.L.: Blood quinidine concentrations as a guide in the treatment of cardiac arrhythmias. Circulation, 1:576, 1950.
13. Brown, J.E., and Shand, D.G.: Therapeutic drug monitoring of antiarrhythmic agents. Clin. Pharmacokinet., 7:125, 1982.
14. Woosley, R.L.: Role of plasma concentration monitoring in the evaluation of response to antiarrhythmic drugs. Am. J. Cardiol., 62:9H, 1988.
15. Koch-Weser, J.: Serum procainamide levels as therapeutic guides. Clin. Pharmacokinet., 2:389, 1977.
16. Karlsson, E.: Clinical pharmacokinetics of procainamide. Clin. Pharmacokinet., 3:97, 1978.
17. Koch-Weser, J., and Klein, S.W.: Procainamide dosage schedules, plasma concentrations, and clinical effects. JAMA, 215:1454, 1971.
18. Ueda, C.T., and Dzindzio, B.S.: Bioavailability of quinidine in congestive heart failure. Br. J. Clin. Pharmacol., 11:571, 1981.
19. Ochs, H.R., Greenblatt, D.J., and Woo, E.: Clinical pharmacokinetics of quinidine. Clin. Pharmacokinet., 5:150, 1980.
20. Ueda, C.T.: Quinidine. In Applied Pharmacokinetics. Principles of Therapeutic Monitoring. 2nd Ed., Edited by W.E. Evans, J.J. Schentag, and W.J.L. Jusko. Spokane, Applied Therapeutics, 1986, pp. 712–734.
21. Garfinkel, D., Mamelok, R.D., and Blaschke, T.F.: Altered therapeutic range for quinidine after myocardial infarction and cardiac surgery. Ann. Intern. Med., 107:48, 1987.
22. Benowitz, N.L., and Meister, W.: Clinical pharmacokinetics of lignocaine. Clin. Pharmacokinet., 3:177, 1978.
23. Deglin, S.M., et al.: Rapid serum lidocaine determination in the coronary care unit. JAMA, 244:571, 1980.
24. Routledge, P.A., et al.: A free lignocaine index as a guide to unbound drug concentration. Br. J. Clin. Pharmacol., 20:695, 1985.
25. Zito, R.A., and Reid, P.R.: Lidocaine kinetics predicted by indocyanine green clearance. N. Engl. J. Med., 298:1160, 1978.
26. Bax, N.D.S., Tucker, G.T., and Woods, H.F.: Lidocaine and indocyanine green kinetics in patients following myocardial infarction. Br. J. Clin. Pharmacol., 10:353, 1980.
27. Slattery, J.T.: Single-point maintenance dose prediction: Role of interindividual differences in clearance and volume of distribution in choice of sampling time. J. Pharm. Sci., 70:1174, 1981.
28. Routledge, P.A., et al.: Control of lidocaine therapy. New perspectives. Ther. Drug. Monit., 4:265, 1982.
29. Stargel, W.W., et al.: Therapeutic monitoring of lidocaine concentrations. Clin. Pharmacol. Ther., 29:284, 1981.
30. Lopez, L.M., et al.: Optimal lidocaine dosing in patients with myocardial infarction. Ther. Drug Monit., 4:271, 1982.
31. Vozeh, S., et al.: Computer-assisted individualized lidocaine dosage: clinical evaluation and comparison with physician performance. Am. Heart J., 113:928, 1987.
32. Sheiner, L.B., et al.: Forecasting individual pharmacokinetics. Clin. Pharmacol. Ther., 26:294, 1979.
33. Salerno, D.M., et al.: Pharmacodynamics and side effects of flecainide acetate. Clin. Pharmacol. Ther., 40:101, 1986.
34. Wang, T., et al.: The development and testing of intravenous dosing regimens: application to flecainide for the suppression of ventricular arrhythmias. Clin. Pharmacol. Ther., 43:499, 1988.
35. Rylance, G.W., and Moreland, T.W.: Drug level monitoring in paediatric practice. Arch. Dis. Child., 55:89, 1980.
36. Neu, H.C.: Current practices in antimicrobial dosing. Rev. Infect. Dis., 3:12, 1981.
37. Henricks, J.N., and Schumacher, G.E.: Using pharmacokinetics in drug therapy. VIII. Pharmacokinetic evaluation of antibiotic dosage regimens. Am. J. Hosp. Pharm., 37:1356, 1980.
38. Nightingale, C., French, M.A., and Quintiliani, R.: Cephalosporins. In Applied Pharmacokinetics. Principles of Therapeutic Monitoring. Edited by W.E. Evans, J.J. Schentag, and W.J.L. Jusko. San Francisco, Applied Therapeutics, 1980, pp. 240–274.
39. Pechere, J.-C., and Dugal, R.: Clinical pharmacokinetics of aminoglycoside antibiotics. Clin. Pharmacokinet., 4:170, 1979.
40. Zaske, D.: Aminoglycosides. In Applied Pharmacokinetics. Principles of Therapeutic Drug Monitoring. Edited

by W.E. Evans, J.J. Schentag, and W.J.L. Jusko. Spokane, Applied Therapeutics, 1986, pp. 331–381.

41. Bowles, S.K., and Schentag, J.J.: Aminoglycosides commentary. *In* Applied Pharmacokinetics. Principles of Therapeutic Drug Monitoring. Edited by W.E. Evans, J.J. Schentag, and W.J.L. Jusko. Spokane, Applied Therapeutics, 1986, pp. 382–398.

42. Zaske, D.E., Russo, M.E., and Strate, R.G.: Amikacin/Kanamycin. Therapeutic use and serum concentration monitoring. *In* Individualizing Drug Therapy. Practical Applications of Drug Monitoring. Vol. 1. Edited by W.J. Taylor and A.L. Finn. New York, Gross, Townsend, Frank, 1980, pp. 67–111.

43. Cipolle, R.J., Zaske, D.E., and Crossley, K.: Gentamicin/Tobramycin. Therapeutic use and serum concentration monitoring. *In* Individualizing Drug Therapy. Practical Applications of Drug Monitoring. Vol. 1. Edited by W.J. Taylor and A.L. Finn. New York, Gross, Townsend, Frank, 1980, pp. 113–147.

44. Yee, G.C., and Evans, W.E.: Reappraisal of guidelines for pharmacokinetic monitoring of aminoglycosides. Pharmacotherapeutics, *1*:55, 1981.

45. Moore, R.D., Smith, C.R., and Lietman, P.S.: The association of aminoglycoside plasma levels with mortality in patients with gram-negative bacteremia. J. Inf. Dis., *149*:443, 1984.

46. Echeverria, P., et al.: Ototoxicity of gentamicin: Clinical experience in a children's hospital. Chemotherapy, *24*:267, 1978.

47. Smith, C.R., et al.: Nephrotoxicity induced by gentamicin and amikacin. Johns Hopkins Med. J., *142*:85, 1978.

48. Schentag, J.J., Cerra, F.B., and Plaut, M.E.: Clinical and pharmacokinetic characteristics of aminoglycoside nephrotoxicity in 201 critically ill patients. Antimicrob. Agents Chemother., *21*:721, 1982.

49. Hull, J.H., and Sarubbi, F.A.: Gentamicin serum concentrations: Pharmacokinetic predictions. Ann. Intern. Med., *85*:183, 1976.

50. Sarubbi, F.A., and Hull, J.H.: Amikacin serum concentrations: Prediction of levels and dosage guidelines. Ann. Intern. Med., *89*:612, 1978.

51. Begg, E.J., et al.: Individualised aminoglycoside dosage based on pharmacokinetic analysis is superior to dosage based on physician intuition at achieving target plasma drug concentrations. Br. J. Clin. Pharmacol., *28*:137, 1989.

52. Zokufa, H.Z., et al.: Simulation of vancomycin peak and trough concentrations using five dosing methods in 37 patients. Pharmacother., *9*:10, 1989.

53. Ackerman, B.H.: Evaluation of three methods for determining initial vancomycin doses. Drug Intell. Clin. Pharm., *23*:123, 1989.

54. Rodvold, K.A., Zokufa, H., and Rotschafer, J.C.: Routine monitoring of serum vancomycin concentrations: can waiting be justified? Clin. Pharm., *6*:655, 1987.

55. Edwards, D.J., and Pancorbo, S.: Routine monitoring of serum vancomycin concentrations: waiting for proof of its value. Clin. Pharm., *6*:652, 1987.

56. Reynolds, E.H.: Serum levels of anticonvulsant drugs. Interpretation and clinical value. Pharmacol. Ther., *8*:217, 1979.

57. Morselli, P.L., and Franco-Morselli, R.: Clinical pharmacokinetics of antiepileptic drugs in adults. Pharmacol. Ther., *10*:65, 1980.

58. Johannessen, S.I.: Antiepileptic drugs: Pharmacokinetic and clinical aspects. Ther. Drug Monit., *3*:17, 1981.

59. MacKichan, J.J., and Kutt, H.: Carbamazepine. Therapeutic use and serum concentration monitoring. *In* Individualizing Drug Therapy. Practical Applications of Drug

Monitoring. Vol. 2. Edited by W.J. Taylor and A.L. Finn. New York, Gross, Townsend, Frank, 1980, pp. 1–25.

60. Theodore, W.H., et al.: Carbamazepine and its epoxide: relation of plasma levels to toxicity and seizure control. Ann. Neurol., *25*:194, 1989.

61. Hoppener, R.J., et al.: Correlation between daily fluctuations of carbamazepine serum levels and intermittent side effects. Epilepsia, *21*:341, 1980.

62. Danhof, M., and Breimer, D.D.: Therapeutic drug monitoring in saliva. Clin. Pharmacokinet., *3*:39, 1978.

63. Mucklow, J.C.: The use of saliva in therapeutic drug monitoring. Ther. Drug Monit., *4*:229, 1982.

64. Froscher, W., et al.: Free level monitoring of carbamazepine and valproic acid: clinical significance. Clin. Neuropharmacol., *8*:362, 1985.

65. Stoehr, G.P., and Sherwin, A.L.: Ethosuximide. Therapeutic use and serum concentration monitoring. *In* Individualizing Drug Therapy. Practical Applications of Drug Monitoring. Vol. 2. Edited by W.J. Taylor and A.L. Finn. New York, Gross, Townsend, Frank, 1980, pp. 27–48.

66. Saunders, G.H., and Penry, J.K.: Phenobarbital/Primidone. Therapeutic use and serum concentration monitoring. *In* Individualizing Drug Therapy. Practical Applications of Drug Monitoring. Vol. 2. Edited by W.J. Taylor and A.L. Finn. New York, Gross, Townsend, Frank, 1980, pp. 49–62.

67. Winter, M.E., and Tozer, T.N.: Phenytoin. *In* Applied Pharmacokinetics. Principles of Therapeutic Drug Monitoring. Edited by W.E. Evans, J.J. Schentag, and W.J.L. Jusko. Spokane, Applied Therapeutics, 1986, pp. 493–539.

68. Finn, A.L., and Olanow, C.W.: Phenytoin. Therapeutic use and serum concentration monitoring. *In* Individualizing Drug Therapy. Practical Applications of Drug Monitoring. Vol. 2. Edited by W.J. Taylor and A.L. Finn. New York, Gross, Townsend, Frank, 1980, pp. 63–85.

69. Lund, L.: Effects of phenytoin in patients with epilepsy in relation to its concentration in plasma. *In* Biological Effects of Drugs in Relation to their Plasma Concentration. Edited by D.S. Davies and B.N.C. Prichard. London, Macmillan Press Ltd., 1973, p. 227.

70. Kutt, H., et al.: Diphenylhydantoin metabolism, blood levels and toxicity. Arch. Neurol., *11*:642, 1964.

71. Kapur, R.N., et al.: Diphenylhydantoin-induced gingival hyperplasia: Its relationship to dose and serum level. Dev. Med. Child Neurol., *15*:483, 1973.

72. Vozeh, S., et al.: Predictability of phenytoin serum levels by nomograms and clinicians. Eur. Neurol., *19*:345, 1980.

73. Murphy, J.E., Bruni, J., and Stewart, R.B.: Clinical utility of six methods of predicting phenytoin doses and plasma concentrations. Am. J. Hosp. Pharm., *38*:348, 1981.

74. Vozeh, S., et al.: Predicting individual phenytoin dosage. J. Pharmacokinet. Biopharm., *9*:131, 1981.

75. Rambeck, B., et al.: Predicting phenytoin dose. A revised nomogram. Ther. Drug Monit., *1*:325, 1979.

76. Richens, A.: Clinical pharmacokinetics of phenytoin. Clin. Pharmacokinet., *4*:153, 1979.

77. Peterson, G.M., et al.: Audit of a monitoring service for free phenytoin. Br. J. Clin. Pharmacol., *19*:693, 1985.

78. Rimmer, E.M., et al.: Should we routinely measure free plasma phenytoin concentration? Br. J. Clin. Pharmacol., *17*:99, 1984.

79. Theodore, W.H., et al.: The clinical value of free phenytoin levels. Ann. Neurol., *18*:90, 1985.

80. Schmidt, D., Einicke, I., and Haenel, F.: The influence of seizure type on the efficacy of plasma concentrations

of phenytoin, phenobarbital, and carbamazepine. Arch. Neurol., *43*:263, 1986.

81. Woo, E., et al.: If a well-stabilized epileptic patient has a subtherapeutic antiepileptic drug level, should the dose be increased? A randomized prospective study. Epilepsia, *29*:129, 1988.
82. Gugler, R., and von Unruh, G.E.: Clinical pharmacokinetics of valproic acid. Clin. Pharmacokinet., *5*:67, 1980.
83. Cloyd, J.C., and Leppik, I.E.: Valproic acid. Therapeutic use and serum concentration monitoring. *In* Individualizing Drug Therapy. Practical Applications of Drug Monitoring. Vol. 2. Edited by W.J. Taylor and A.L. Finn. New York, Gross, Townsend, Frank, 1980, pp. 87–108.
84. Levy, R.: Monitoring of free valproic acid levels. Ther. Drug Monit., *2*:199, 1980.
85. Dromgoole, S.H., and Furst, D.E.: Salicylates. *In* Applied Pharmacokinetics. Principles of Therapeutic Drug Monitoring. Edited by W.E. Evans, J.J. Schentag, and W.J.L. Jusko. Spokane, Applied Therapeutics, 1986, pp. 944–977.
86. Mandelli, M., and Tognoni, G.: Monitoring plasma concentrations of salicylate. Clin. Pharmacokinet., *5*:424, 1980.
87. Mongan, E., et al.: Tinnitus as an indication of therapeutic serum salicylate levels. JAMA, *226*:142, 1973.
88. Brash, A.R., et al.: Pharmacokinetics of indomethacin in the neonate. Relation of plasma indomethacin levels to response of the ductus arteriosus. N. Engl. J. Med., *305*:67, 1981.
89. Shapiro, S., et al.: The epidemiology of digoxin: A study in three Boston hospitals. J. Chronic Dis., *22*:361, 1969.
90. Beller, G.A., et al.: Digitalis intoxication. A prospective study with serum level correlations. N. Engl. J. Med., *284*:989, 1971.
91. Aronson, J.K.: Clinical pharmacokinetics of digoxin 1980. Clin. Pharmacokinet., *5*:137, 1980.
92. Wettrell, G., and Andersson, K.-E.: Clinical pharmacokinetics of digoxin in infants. Clin. Pharmacokinet., *2*:17, 1977.
93. Smith, T.W., and Haber, E.: Digoxin intoxication: The relationship of clinical presentation to serum digoxin concentration. J. Clin. Invest., *49*:2377, 1970.
94. Huffman, D.H., et al.: Association between clinical cardiac status, laboratory parameters and digoxin usage. Am. Heart J., *9*:28, 1976.
95. Ingelfinger, J.A., and Goldman, P.: The serum digitalis concentration: Does it diagnose digitalis toxicity? N. Engl. J. Med., *294*:867, 1976.
96. Weintraub, M.: Interpretation of the serum digoxin concentration. Clin. Pharmacokinet., *2*:205, 1977.
97. Holford, N., and Sheiner, L.B.: The digoxin concentration: before and after the fact. Am. Heart J., *94*:529, 1977.
98. Doherty, J.E.: How and when to use the digitalis serum levels. JAMA, *239*:2594, 1978.
99. Aronson, J.K.: Monitoring digoxin therapy: III. How useful are the nomograms? Br. J. Clin. Pharmacol., *5*:55, 1978.
100. Hyneck, M.L., et al.: Comparison of methods for estimating digoxin dosing regimens. Am. J. Hosp. Pharm., *38*:69, 1981.
101. Tsujimoto, G., et al.: Re-examination of digoxin dosage regimen: Comparison of the proposed nomograms or formulae in elderly patients. Br. J. Clin. Pharmacol., *13*:493, 1982.
102. Nicholson, P.W., et al.: A score for prescribing digoxin. Br. Heart J., *40*:177, 1978.
103. Sheiner, L.B., et al.: Forecasting individual pharmacokinetics. Clin. Pharmacol. Ther., *26*:294, 1979.
104. Snidero, M., Traina, G.L., and Bonati, M.: Is ambulatory

105. Hallworth, M.J., and Brodie, M.J.: Whithering look at serum digoxin requests. Lancet, *1*:95, 1986.
106. Perrier, D., Mayersohn, M., and Marcus, F.I.: Clinical pharmacokinetics of digitoxin. Clin. Pharmacokinet., *2*:292, 1977.
107. Yee, G.C., and Kennedy, M.S.: Cyclosporine. *In* Applied Pharmacokinetics. Principles of Therapeutic Drug Monitoring. Edited by W.E. Evans, J.J. Schentag, and W.J.L. Jusko. Spokane, Applied Therapeutics, 1986, pp. 826–851.
108. Ptachcinski, R.J., Burckart, G.J., and Venkataramanan, R.: Cyclosporine. Drug Intell. Clin. Pharm., *19*:90, 1985.
109. Burkle, W.S.: Cyclosporine pharmacokinetics and blood level monitoring. Drug Intell. Clin. Pharm., *19*:101, 1985.
110. Burckart, G.J., Canafax, D.M., and Yee, G.C.: Cyclosporine monitoring. Drug Intell. Clin. Pharm., *20*:649, 1986.
111. Ptachcinski, R.J., et al.: Cyclosporine concentration determinations for monitoring and pharmacokinetic studies. J. Clin. Pharmacol., *26*:358, 1986.
112. Rodighiero, V.: Therapeutic drug monitoring of cyclosporin. Practical applications and limitations. Clin. Pharmacokin., *16*:27, 1989.
113. Yee, G.C., et al.: Serum cyclosporine concentration and risk of acute graft-versus-host disease after allogeneic marrow transplantation. N. Engl. J. Med., *319*:65, 1988.
114. Evans, W.E., et al.: Methotrexate cerebrospinal fluid and serum concentrations after intermediate-dose methotrexate infusion. Clin. Pharmacol. Ther., *33*:310, 1983.
115. Evans, W.E., et al.: Methotrexate systemic clearance influences probability of relapse in children with standard risk acute lymphocytic leukaemia. Lancet, *1*:359, 1984.
116. Evans, W.E., et al.: Clinical pharmacodynamics of high-dose methotrexate in acute lymphocytic leukemia: identification of a relation between concentration and effect. N. Engl. J. Med., *314*:471, 1986.
117. Meyer, B.R., et al.: Optimizing metoclopramide control of cisplatin-induced emesis. Ann. Intern. Med., *100*:393, 1984.
118. Hirsch, J.: Therapeutic range for the control of oral anticoagulant therapy. Arch. Intern. Med., *145*:1187, 1985.
119. Breckenridge, A.M.: Interindividual differences in the response to oral anticoagulants. Drugs, *14*:367, 1977.
120. Holford, N.H.G.: Clinical pharmacokinetics and pharmacodynamics of warfarin. Understanding the dose-effect relationship. Clin. Pharmacokin., *11*:483, 1986.
121. Sheety, H.G.M., Fennerty, A.G., and Routledge, P.A.: Clinical pharmacokinetic considerations in the control of oral anticoagulant therapy. Clin. Pharmacokin., *16*:238, 1989.
122. Routledge, P.A., et al.: Predicting patients' warfarin requirements. Lancet, *2*:854, 1977.
123. Sawyer, W.T.: Predictability of warfarin dose requirements: Theoretical considerations. J. Pharm. Sci., *68*:432, 1979.
124. Cooper, T.B.: Plasma level monitoring of antipsychotic drugs. Clin. Pharmacokinet., *3*:14, 1978.
125. Dahl, S.G.: Plasma level monitoring of antipsychotic drugs. Clinical utility. Clin. Pharmacokin., *11*:36, 1986.
126. Sramek, J.J., Potkin, S.G., and Hahn, R.: Neuroleptic plasma concentrations and clinical response: in search of a therapeutic window. Drug Intell. Clin. Pharm., *22*:373, 1988.
127. Volavka, J., and Cooper, T.B.: Review of haloperidol blood level and clinical response: looking through the window. J. Clin. Psychopharmacol., *7*:25, 1987.

therapeutic digoxin monitoring useful? Drug Intell. Clin. Pharm., *19*:660, 1985.

128. Perry, P.J., Pfohl, B.M., and Kelly, M.W.: The relationship of haloperidol concentrations to therapeutic response. J. Clin. Psychopharmacol., 8:38, 1988.

129. Amdisen, A., and Carson, S.W.: Lithium. In Applied Pharmacokinetics. Principles of Therapeutic Drug Monitoring. Edited by W.E. Evans, J.J. Schentag, and W.J.L. Jusko. Spokane, Applied Therapeutics, 1986, pp. 978–1008.

130. Amdisen, A.: Serum level monitoring and clinical pharmacokinetics of lithium. Clin. Pharmacokinet., 2:73, 1977.

131. Cooper, T.B., Bergner, P.E., and Simpson, G.M.: The 24-hour serum lithium level as a prognosticator of dosage requirements. Am. J. Psychiatry, 130:601, 1973.

132. Cooper, T.B., and Simpson, G.M.: The 24-hour lithium level as a prognosticator of dosage requirements: A 2-year follow-up study. Am. J. Psychiatry, 133:440, 1976.

133. Schou, M.: Serum lithium monitoring of prophylactic treatment. Critical review and updated recommendations. Clin. Pharmacokin., 15:283, 1988.

134. Lobeck, F.: A review of lithium dosing methods. Pharmacother., 8:248, 1988.

135. DeVane, C.L.: Cyclic antidepressants. In Applied Pharmacokinetics. Principles of Therapeutic Drug Monitoring. Edited by W.E. Evans, J.J. Schentag, and W.J.L. Jusko. Spokane, Applied Therapeutics, 1986, pp. 852–907.

136. Risch, S.C., Huey, L.Y., and Janowsky, D.S.: Plasma levels of tricyclic antidepressants and clinical efficacy: Review of the literature. J. Clin. Psychiatry, 40:4, 58, 1979.

137. Montgomery, S.A.: Measurement of serum drug levels in the assessment of antidepressants. Br. J. Clin. Pharmacol., 10:411, 1980.

138. Amsterdam, J., Brunswick, D., and Mendels, J.: The clinical application of tricyclic antidepressant pharmacokinetics and plasma levels. Am. J. Psychiatry, 137:653, 1980.

139. Sjoqvist, F., Bertilsson, L., and Asberg, M.: Monitoring tricyclic antidepressants. Ther. Drug Monit., 2:85, 1980.

140. Gram, L.F., et al.: Drug level monitoring in psychopharmacology: Usefulness and clinical problems, with special reference to tricyclic antidepressants. Ther. Drug Monit., 4:17, 1982.

141. Gram, L.F., et al.: Methodology in studies on plasma level/effect relationship of tricyclic antidepressants. In Clinical Pharmacology in Psychiatry. Edited by E. Usdin et al. New York, Elsevier North-Holland, 1981, pp. 155–179.

142. Asberg, M., et al.: Relationship between plasma level and therapeutic effect of nortriptyline. Br. Med. J., 3:331, 1971.

143. Breyer-Pfaff, U., et al.: Validation of a therapeutic plasma level range in amitriptyline treatment of depression. J. Clin. Psychopharmacol., 9:116, 1989.

144. Rigal, J.G., et al.: Imipramine blood levels and clinical outcome. J. Clin. Psychopharmacol., 7:222, 1987.

145. Simpson, G.M., et al.: Relationship between plasma desipramine levels and clinical outcome for RDC major depressive inpatients. Psychopharmacol., 80:240, 1983.

146. Nelson, J.C., et al.: Desipramine plasma concentration and antidepressant response. Arch. Gen. Psychiatry, 39:1419, 1982.

147. Nelson, J.C., Jatlow, P.I., and Mazure, C.: Desipramine plasma levels and response in elderly melancholic patients. J. Clin. Psychopharmacol., 5:217, 1985.

148. Boehnert, M.T., and Lovejoy, F.H., Jr.: Value of the QRS duration versus the serum drug level in predicting seizures and ventricular arrhythmias after an acute overdose of tricyclic antidepressants. N. Engl. J. Med., 313:474, 1985.

149. Burrows, G.D., et al.: Should plasma level monitoring of tricyclic antidepressants be introduced in clinical practice? Commun. Psychopharmacol., 2:393, 1978.

150. Dawling, S., et al.: Nortriptyline therapy in elderly patients: Dosage prediction after single dose pharmacokinetic study. Eur. J. Clin. Pharmacol., 18:147, 1980.

151. Cooper, T.B., and Simpson, G.M.: Prediction of individual dosage of nortriptyline. Am. J. Psychiatry, 135:333, 1978.

152. Schneider, L.S., et al.: Prediction of individual dosage of nortriptyline in depressed elderly outpatients. J. Clin. Psychopharmacol., 7:311, 1987.

153. Slattery, J.T., Gibaldi, M., and Koup, J.R.: Prediction of maintenance dose required to attain a desired drug concentration at steady state from a single determination of concentration after an initial dose. Clin. Pharmacokinet., 5:377, 1980.

154. Brunswick, D.J., et al.: Prediction of steady-state imipramine and desmethylimipramine plasma concentrations from single-dose data. Clin. Pharmacol. Ther., 25:605, 1979.

155. Cooper, T.B., Bark, N., and Simpson, G.M.: Prediction of steady-state plasma and saliva levels of desmethylimipramine using a single dose, single time point procedure. Psychopharmacology, 74:115, 1981.

156. Madakasira, S., et al.: Single dose prediction of steady state plasma levels of amitriptyline. J. Clin. Psychopharmacol., 2:136, 1982.

157. Sallee, F., et al.: Targeting imipramine dose in children with depression. Clin. Pharmacol. Ther., 40:8, 1986.

158. Ogilvie, R.I.: Clinical pharmacokinetics of theophylline. Clin. Pharmacokinet., 3:267, 1978.

159. Hendeles, L., Massanari, M., and Weinberg, M.: Theophylline. In Applied Pharmacokinetics. Principles of Therapeutic Drug Monitoring. Edited by W.E. Evans, J.J. Schentag, and W.J.L. Jusko. Spokane, Applied Therapeutics. 1986, pp. 1105–1188.

160. Slaughter, R.L.: Theophylline commentary. In Applied Pharmacokinetics. Principles of Therapeutic Drug Monitoring. Edited by W.E. Evans, J.J. Schentag, and W.J.L. Jusko. Spokane, Applied Therapeutics, 1986, pp. 1189–1209.

161. Hendeles, L., and Weinberger, M.: Theophylline. Therapeutic use and serum concentration monitoring. In Individualizing Drug Therapy. Practical Applications of Drug Monitoring. Vol. 1. Edited by W.J. Taylor and A.L. Finn. New York, Gross, Townsend, Frank, 1980, pp. 31–65.

162. Mitenko, P.A., and Ogilvie, R.I.: Rational intravenous doses of theophylline. N. Engl. J. Med., 289:600, 1973.

163. Aitken, M.L., and Martin, T.R.: Life-threatening theophylline toxicity is not predictable by serum levels. Chest, 91:10, 1987.

164. Vaughan, L.M., et al.: Evaluation of passively absorbed saliva for determination of oral slow-release theophylline bioavailability in children. Drug Intell. Clin. Pharm., 22:684, 1988.

165. Koup, J.R., et al.: Hypothesis for the individualization of drug dosage. Clin. Pharmacokinet., 4:460, 1979.

166. Shapiro, G.G., et al.: Individualization of theophylline dosage using a single serum sample following a test dose. Pediatrics, 69:70, 1982.

167. Office tests for serum theophylline. Med. Lett. Drugs Ther., 27:102, 1985.

168. Vaughan, L.M., Weinberger, M.M., and Milavetz, G.: Evaluation of the Ames Seralyzer for therapeutic drug monitoring of theophylline. Drug Intell. Clin. Pharm., 20:118, 1986.

169. Vaughan, L.M., et al.: Multicentre evaluation of disposable visual measuring device to assay theophylline from capillary blood sample. Lancet, 1:184, 1986.

170. Sjoqvist, F.: Interindividual differences in drug response; an overview. In Variability in Drug Therapy, Edited by M. Rowland, L.B. Sheiner, and J.-L. Steimer. New York, Raven Press, 1985, pp. 1–10.

171. Spector, R., et al.: Therapeutic drug monitoring. Clin. Pharmacol. Ther., 43:345, 1988.

172. McInnes, G.T.: The value of therapeutic drug monitoring to the practising physician—an hypothesis in need of testing. Br. J. Clin. Pharmacol., 27:281, 1989.

173. Vozeh, S.: Cost-effectiveness of therapeutic drug monitoring. Clin. Pharmacokin., 13:131, 1987.

Estimation of Area Under the Curve

There are several methods for estimating the area under a drug concentration-time curve. An estimate of area is required to determine bioavailability, clearance, apparent volume of distribution, and other pharmacokinetic parameters. The most common method of estimating area is the use of the *trapezoidal rule*.

A blood level-time curve can be described by a series of trapezoids that are determined by each concentration-time point (Fig. I–1). The area bounded by the trapezoids approximates the area under the curve; the greater the number of data points, the closer is the approximation.

The area of a trapezoid is equal to one half the product of the sum of the heights times the width. The area under a drug concentration in plasma versus time curve is approximated by the following equation:

$$\text{Area} = (\tfrac{1}{2})(C_1 + C_2)(t_2 - t_1)$$
$$+ (\tfrac{1}{2})(C_2 + C_3)(t_3 - t_2). \ldots \quad \text{(I–1)}$$
$$+ (\tfrac{1}{2})(C_{n-1} + C_n)(t_n - t_{n-1})$$

where C denotes drug concentration, t denotes time, and the subscript refers to the sample number.

The use of the trapezoidal rule is illustrated in Table I–1. By way of example, the areas of the first, fifth, and seventh trapezoids are calculated as follows:

$$\text{Area (1)} = (\tfrac{1}{2})(0 + 6.6)(1 - 0)$$
$$= 3.3 \ \mu\text{g-hr/ml} \quad \text{(I–2)}$$

$$\text{Area (5)} = (\tfrac{1}{2})(9.4 + 8.7)(6 - 4)$$
$$= 18.1 \ \mu\text{g-hr/ml} \quad \text{(I–3)}$$

$$\text{Area (7)} = (\tfrac{1}{2})(6.6 + 3.7)(12 - 8)$$
$$= 20.6 \ \mu\text{g-hr/ml} \quad \text{(I–4)}$$

The area under the curve from $t = 0$ to $t = 12$ hr is the sum of the areas of all trapezoids or 83.3 μg-hr/ml.

Table I–1. Drug Concentration as a Function of Time after Oral Administration

Sample	Time (hr)	Concentration (μg/ml)	Area
1	0	0.0	3.30
2	1	6.6	7.55
3	2	8.5	9.00
4	3	9.5	9.45
5	4	9.4	18.10
6	6	8.7	15.30
7	8	6.6	20.60
8	12	3.7	—
		Total	83.3
			(μg/ml per hr)

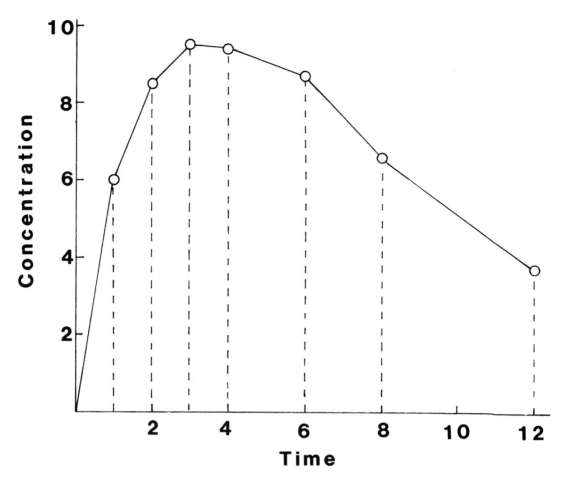

Fig. I–1. Drug concentration (μg/ml) as a function of time (hr) after oral administration. The data points are connected by straight line segments, rather than a smooth curve, to apply the trapezoidal rule. The area of each trapezoid is delineated.

Method of Superposition

The method of superposition is a useful non-compartmental approach for predicting drug accumulation and steady-state concentrations on repetitive dosing from data obtained after a single dose. The theoretical basis for superposition is merely that drug concentration is proportional to dose.

The application of superposition to predict the time course of drug concentration under different conditions requires several assumptions. The first is that, irrespective of time of administration, a given single dose administered by a given route will always give rise to the same drug concentration-time curve. A change in dose, but not in route of administration, is reflected by a proportional change in drug concentration at any time after administration. During repetitive administration, blood levels arising from a given dose are simply an additive function of the blood levels associated with that dose and the blood levels resulting from previous doses. This principle is illustrated in Table II–1.

Table II–1 shows how the method of superposition can be used to predict drug concentrations during multiple dosing. In this particular example, drug concentration-time data was obtained after a single dose (see column 2). We wish to predict drug concentrations on repetitive administration of the same dose given every 3 hr. Each subsequent dose, if given independently, would give rise to the same concentrations as the first dose; this is indicated by the values in parentheses. The net concentration after the second, third, or subsequent doses, however, must also reflect the contribution of previous doses.

If given independently, the second dose would provide a drug concentration of 7 μg/ml 1 hr after administration. When given after the first dose, however, the second dose gives rise to a drug concentration of 9.5 μg/ml 1 hr after dosing; 2.5 μg/ml of drug concentration is contributed by the first dose. One hr after giving the third dose, drug concentration equals 9.7 μg/ml (rather than 7 μg/ml) because of the contributions from the two previous doses.

The data in Table I–1 also indicate that steady state is achieved after the third dose, because drug concentrations following the third, fourth, and subsequent doses are identical.

Table II–1. Drug Concentrations (μg/ml) During 4 Consecutive Doses Given at 3-hr Intervals (See Text for Detailed Explanation)

Time	First dose	Second dose		Third dose		Fourth dose	
0	0						
1	7						
2	10						
3	5	(+0)	5				
4	2.5	(+7)	9.5				
5	1.25	(+10)	11.25				
6	0.6	(+5)	5.6	(+0)	5.6		
7	0.2	(+2.5)	2.7	(+7)	9.7		
8	0	(+1.25)	1.25	(+10)	11.25		
9	—	(+0.6)	0.6	(+5)	5.6	(+0)	5.6
10	—	(+0.2)	0.2	(+2.5)	2.7	(+7)	9.7
11	—	(+0)	0	(+1.25)	1.25	(+10)	11.25
12	—		—	(+0.6)	0.6	(+5)	5.6

Index

Page numbers in *italic* refer to illustrations; numbers followed by "t" refer to tables.